AF678969

Sickle Cell Anemia

Fernando Ferreira Costa • Nicola Conran
Editors

Sickle Cell Anemia

From Basic Science to Clinical Practice

Springer

Editors
Fernando Ferreira Costa
Centro de Hematologia e Hemoterapia
Unicamp
Campinas, São Paulo, Brazil

Nicola Conran
Centro de Hematologia e Hemoterapia
Unicamp
Campinas, São Paulo, Brazil

ISBN 978-3-319-06712-4 ISBN 978-3-319-06713-1 (eBook)
DOI 10.1007/978-3-319-06713-1

Library of Congress Control Number: 2016933678

Springer Cham Heidelberg New York Dordrecht London
© Springer International Publishing Switzerland 2016
This work is subject to copyright. All rights are reserved by the Publisher, whether the whole or part of the material is concerned, specifically the rights of translation, reprinting, reuse of illustrations, recitation, broadcasting, reproduction on microfilms or in any other physical way, and transmission or information storage and retrieval, electronic adaptation, computer software, or by similar or dissimilar methodology now known or hereafter developed.
The use of general descriptive names, registered names, trademarks, service marks, etc. in this publication does not imply, even in the absence of a specific statement, that such names are exempt from the relevant protective laws and regulations and therefore free for general use.
The publisher, the authors and the editors are safe to assume that the advice and information in this book are believed to be true and accurate at the date of publication. Neither the publisher nor the authors or the editors give a warranty, express or implied, with respect to the material contained herein or for any errors or omissions that may have been made.

Printed on acid-free paper

Springer International Publishing AG Switzerland is part of Springer Science+Business Media
(www.springer.com)

To all those with sickle cell disease, their families and their caregivers.

Preface

Although sickle cell anemia was the first molecular disease to be identified, its complex and fascinating pathophysiology is still not fully understood. A single mutation in the beta-globin gene incurs numerous molecular and cellular mechanisms that contribute to the plethora of manifestations and complications associated with the disease. Knowledge regarding sickle cell disease mechanisms, while still not complete, has broadened considerably over the last decades.

Sickle Cell Anemia: From Basic Science to Clinical Practice aims to provide an update on some aspects of our current understanding of the disease's pathophysiology and use this information as a basis to discuss its manifestations in childhood and adulthood, as well as therapeutic approaches to the disease. An introductory chapter (Chap. 1) describes the structure and function of hemoglobin, giving us a clue as to why a single gene mutation can wreak such havoc in the red blood cell. Chapter 2 describes the current theories regarding the emergence of the sickle mutation and the subsequent epidemiology of sickle cell anemia. Chapter 3 presents an overview of sickle cell disease pathophysiology, describing how the polymerization of the abnormal sickle hemoglobin injures the red cell, causing its membrane injury and ultimate failure, and producing a population of heterogeneous red blood cells, hemolysis, and reduced nitric oxide bioavailability. In a process that is driven by vascular inflammation and oxidative stress, interactions of the sickle red cells and leukocytes with the endothelium prolong the transit of the red cells through hypoxic vascular beds, resulting in red cell sickling and ultimately in the vaso-occlusive processes that are the hallmark of the disease. Some of these aspects are described in greater detail in Chaps. 4 (red cells), 5 (leukocytes), and 8 (inflammation), while Chap. 6 relates the evidence for a hypercoagulable state in sickle cell anemia and its role in disease pathophysiology and Chap. 7 looks at the endothelium and how the anemia that results from red cell destruction affects the cardiovascular system.

Recurrent vaso-occlusive processes, together with hemolytic anemia, result in end-organ damage and the diversity of complications of this disease, which can include stroke, pulmonary hypertension, osteonecrosis, leg ulcer, nephropathy, retinopathy, and priapism among numerous others. The complications of childhood sickle cell anemia, and their treatment, are considered in Chaps. 9 and 10, while priapism and the manifestations and current treatment and therapy of adult sickle cell anemia are presented in Chaps. 11 and 12, respectively. Some of the other more common sickle cell diseases (caused by the inheritance of the HbS gene along with another abnormal Hb variant) are explored in Chap. 13, while Chap. 14 looks at the management of sickle cell disease in Africa, the region with the highest burden of sickle cell disease, and in the Arabian Peninsula, which displays a great variety in terms of sickle cell disease genotype and phenotype; the challenges faced by clinicians in these regions are discussed. The clinical severity of sickle cell disease is extremely heterogeneous, and co-inheritance of numerous other genetic factors can significantly alter the course of the disease, for better or for worse; some of these genetic modifiers are discussed in Chap. 15. Finally, prospects for the development of new approaches for the management of the disease, many of which have been developed based on our progressive understanding of the pathophysiology of the disease, are explored in Chap. 16, in addition to discussion regarding the expansion of the use of hematopoietic stem cell transplantation as a curative option for sickle cell anemia and perspectives for the development of gene therapy/gene editing approaches for the disease.

Campinas, São Paulo, Brazil

Fernando Ferreira Costa
Nicola Conran

Acknowledgments

The editors greatly appreciate the time and expertise of all the authors who have contributed to this book. We would also like to thank Gabriel Natan Pires (Springer) for all his assistance and support during the compilation of this book.

Contents

Contributors

Miguel R. Abboud Department of Pediatrics and Adolescent Medicine, American University of Beirut Medical Center, Beirut, Lebanon

Rouba Abdennour Department of Pediatrics and Adolescent Medicine, American University of Beirut Medical Center, Beirut, Lebanon

Hans C. Ackerman Physiology Section, Sickle Cell Branch, National Heart, Lung, and Blood Institute, Bethesda, MD, USA

Adekunle Adekile Faculty of Medicine, Department of Pediatrics, Kuwait University, Safat, Kuwait

Camila Bononi de Almeida Instituto Israelita de Ensino e Pesquisa Albert Einstein, Hospital Israelita Albert Einstein, São Paulo, São Paulo, Brazil

Mário A. Claudino Laboratory of Multidisciplinary Research, São Francisco University – USF, Braganca Paulista, São Paulo, Brazil

Marina Pereira Colella Hematology Center, School of Medical Sciences, University of Campinas – UNICAMP, Campinas, São Paulo, Brazil

Nicola Conran Hematology Center, School of Medical Science, University of Campinas – UNICAMP, Campinas, São Paulo, Brazil

Fernando Ferreira Costa Hematology Center, School of Medical Sciences, University of Campinas – UNICAMP, Campinas, São Paulo, Brazil

Jeremie Estepp Department of Hematology, St. Jude Children's Research Hospital, Memphis, TN, USA

Kleber Yotsumoto Fertrin Hematology Center, School of Medical Sciences, University of Campinas – UNICAMP, Hemocentro, Rua Carlos Chagas, Campinas, São Paulo, Brazil

Paul S. Frenette Ruth L. and David S. Gottesman Institute for Stem Cell and Regenerative Medicine Research, Albert Einstein College of Medicine, Bronx, NY, USA

Department of Cell Biology, Albert Einstein College of Medicine, Bronx, NY, USA

Department of Medicine, Albert Einstein College of Medicine, Bronx, NY, USA

Kate Gardner Molecular Haematology, Division of Cancer Studies, Faculty of Life Sciences & Medicine, King's College London, London, UK

Department of Haematological Medicine, King's College Hospital NHS Foundation Trust, London, UK

Simone O. Gilli Hematology Center, School of Medical Sciences, University of Campinas – UNICAMP, Rua Carlos Chagas, Campinas, São Paulo, Brazil

Jane Hankins Department of Hematology, St. Jude Children's Research Hospital, Memphis, TN, USA

Cheryl A. Hillery Department of Pediatrics and Children's Research Institute, Medical College of Wisconsin, Milwaukee, WI, USA

Blood Research Institute, Medical Sciences Institute, BloodCenter of Wisconsin, Milwaukee, WI, USA

Department of Pediatrics, Division of Hematology/Oncology, Children's Hospital of Pittsburgh of UPMC, University of Pittsburgh School of Medicine, Pittsburgh, PA, USA

Lewis L. Hsu University of Illinois, Chicago, IL, USA

Susan E. Jorge Department of Clinical Pathology, School of Medical Sciences, University of Campinas-UNICAMP, Campinas, São Paulo, Brazil

Gregory J. Kato Sickle Cell Center of Excellence, University of Pittsburgh Medical Center, Pittsburgh, PA, USA

Julie Makani Department of Hematology and Blood Transfusion, Muhimbili University of Health and Allied Sciences, Dar-es-Salaam, Tanzania

University of Oxford, Oxford, UK

Robert Sheppard Nickel Children's National Health System, George Washington University School of Medicine and Health Sciences, Washington, DC, USA

Kerri Nottage Department of Hematology, St. Jude Children's Research Hospital, Memphis, TN, USA

Margareth Castro Ozelo Hematology Center, School of Medical Sciences, University of Campinas – UNICAMP, Campinas, São Paulo, Brazil

Erich Vinicius de Paula Hematology Center, School of Medical Sciences, University of Campinas – UNICAMP, Campinas, São Paulo, Brazil

Lydia H. Pecker Center for Cancer and Blood Disorders, Children's National Medical Center, Washington, DC, USA

Physiology Section, Sickle Cell Branch, National Heart, Lung, and Blood Institute, Center Drive, Bethesda, MD, USA

Carla F. Franco Penteado Hematology Center, School of Medical Sciences, University of Campinas – UNICAMP, Campinas, São Paulo, Brazil

Frédéric B. Piel Department of Zoology, University of Oxford, Oxford, UK

Daniela M. Ribeiro Department of Clinical Pathology, School of Medical Sciences, University of Campinas-UNICAMP, Campinas, São Paulo, Brazil

Sara T. Olalla Saad Hematology Center, School of Medical Sciences, University of Campinas – UNICAMP, Campinas, São Paulo, Brazil

Magnun N.N. Santos Department of Clinical Pathology, School of Medical Sciences, University of Campinas-UNICAMP, Campinas, São Paulo, Brazil

Maria de Fatima Sonati Department of Clinical Pathology, School of Medical Sciences, University of Campinas-UNICAMP, Campinas, São Paulo, Brazil

Martin H. Steinberg, MD Department of Medicine, Pediatrics, Pathology and Laboratory Medicine, Boston University School of Medicine, Boston, MA, USA

Swee Lay Thein Molecular Haematology, Division of Cancer Studies, Faculty of Life Sciences & Medicine, King's College London, London, UK

Department of Haematological Medicine, King's College Hospital NHS Foundation Trust, London, UK

Sickle Cell Branch, NIH/National Heart, Lung, and Blood Institute, Bethesda, MD, USA

Fabiola Traina Department of Internal Medicine, University of São Paulo at Ribeirão Preto Medical School, Ribeirão Preto, São Paulo, Brazil

Nancy J. Wandersee Department of Pediatrics and Children's Research Institute, Medical College of Wisconsin, Milwaukee, WI, USA

Blood Research Institute, Medical Sciences Institute, BloodCenter of Wisconsin, Milwaukee, WI, USA

Thomas N. Williams Kenya Medical Research Institute/Wellcome Trust Programme, Centre for Geographic Medicine Research-Coast, Kilifi District Hospital, Kilifi, Kenya

Department of Medicine, Imperial College, St Mary's Hospital, London, UK

Dachuan Zhang Ruth L. and David S. Gottesman Institute for Stem Cell and Regenerative Medicine Research, Albert Einstein College of Medicine, Bronx, NY, USA

Department of Cell Biology, Albert Einstein College of Medicine, Bronx, NY, USA

Chapter 1
Hemoglobin: Structure, Synthesis and Oxygen Transport

Susan E. Jorge, Daniela M. Ribeiro, Magnun N.N. Santos, and Maria de Fátima Sonati

Abstract Human hemoglobin (Hb) is the erythrocyte hemeprotein resulting from the combination of one pair of α-like (α or ζ) chains and another pair of β-like (β, δ, γ or ε) chains. Each of these chains is associated with a *heme* prosthetic group, a tetrapyrrole ring (protoporphyrin IX) containing a central ferrous atom (Fe^{2+}), which can reversibly bind to a molecule of O_2, being, therefore, responsible for its transport from the lungs to the tissues. This introductory chapter summarizes these important aspects, including findings of protein structure, synthesis and function, as well as its gene organization and regulation. We also describe the developmental switches in globin chain production (from the embryonic period until hematological adult life), *heme* synthesis and globin gene expression/regulation, besides functional aspects of the hemoglobin molecule. The chapter also includes models that predict the mechanisms of Hb-O_2 ligation, mediated by the presence of allosteric effectors, such as H^+/CO_2, Cl^- and organic phosphates, such as 2,3-biphosphoglycerate (2,3-BPG, from erythrocyte metabolism).

Keywords Hemeproteins • Human hemoglobin • Globin chains • Globin genes • Oxygen transport

1.1 Human Hemoglobins

Hemoglobins (Hb) are hemeproteins that transport oxygen (O_2). These proteins, or the genes expressing them, seem to be present in all living organisms. Like other vertebrate organisms, human hemoglobins are found in high concentrations in erythrocytes (around 640 million molecules/cell), and are their main component

S.E. Jorge • D.M. Ribeiro • M.N.N. Santos • M.d.F. Sonati (✉)
Department of Clinical Pathology, School of Medical Sciences, University of Campinas – UNICAMP, P.O. Box 6111, 13083-970 Campinas, São Paulo, Brazil
e-mail: susan@fcm.unicamp.br; ribeiro.danielamaria@gmail.com; magnun.nunes@gmail.com; sonati@fcm.unicamp.br; sonati_mf@yahoo.com.br

© Springer International Publishing Switzerland 2016

F.F. Costa, N. Conran (eds.), *Sickle Cell Anemia*,
DOI 10.1007/978-3-319-06713-1_1

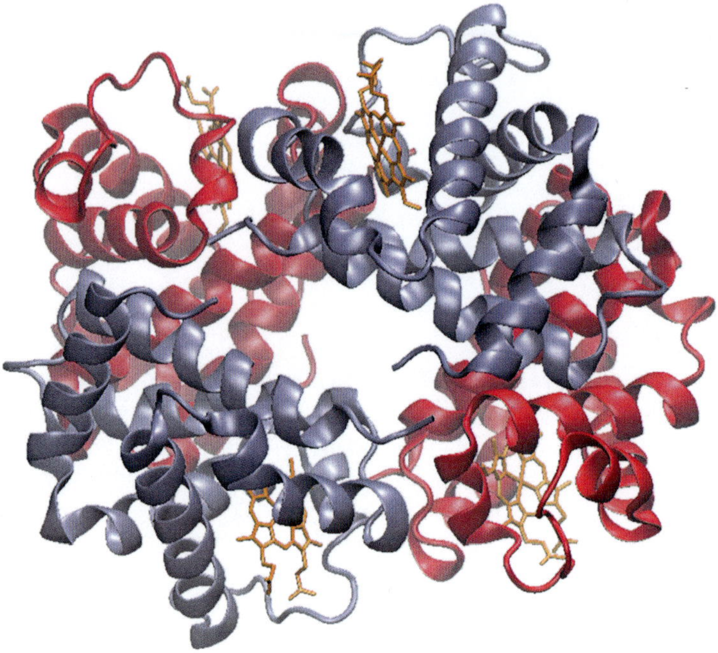

Fig. 1.1 Human Hb A, represented by two α-chains (in ice *blue*), two β-chains (in *red*) and four *heme* groups (in *orange*). Obtained from *Protein Data Bank* 1ZGX coordinates, using Visual Molecular Dynamics (VMD) software

(Shikama 2006). Despite hemoglobin diversity, the molecular structures of hemoglobins are very similar, showing a high degree of conservation during evolution. Hemoglobins are globular tetramers (molecular weight, 64,450 Daltons), comprised of two pairs of polypeptide chains (globins); one pair of α-like (α or ζ) chains and another pair of β-like (β, δ, γ or ε) chains. Each chain is associated with a *heme* prosthetic group, a tetrapyrrole ring (protoporphyrin IX) containing a central ferrous atom (Fe^{2+}), which can reversibly bind to a molecule of O_2 to transport oxygen from lungs to tissues (Fig. 1.1) (Antonini and Brunori 1971; Hoffbrand and Moss 2011).

The α and ζ globin chains have 141 residues, while the β, γ, δ and ε globins have 146 residues. Different combinations of these chains result in the formation of different types of hemoglobins, adapted for distinct periods of human development. During the embryonic period, hemoglobin synthesis starts at the end of the third week of pregnancy in primitive erythroblasts derived from the hematopoietic stem cells in the vitelline sac, with the production of the embryonic hemoglobins Gower 1 ($\zeta_2\varepsilon_2$), Hb Gower 2 ($\alpha_2\varepsilon_2$), Hb Portland I ($\zeta_2\gamma_2$) and Portland II ($\zeta_2\beta_2$). After the tenth week of pregnancy, hemopoiesis occurs in the liver and spleen (visceral phase) and the embryonic hemoglobins are replaced with fetal Hb, or Hb F ($\alpha_2\gamma_2$), which is predominant during the entire fetal period. During adult life the main site of erythropoiesis is the bone marrow and Hb F is replaced by hemoglobins A ($\alpha_2\beta_2$) and A_2 ($\alpha_2\delta_2$). Hb A predominates, comprising more than 95 % of the total hemoglobin,

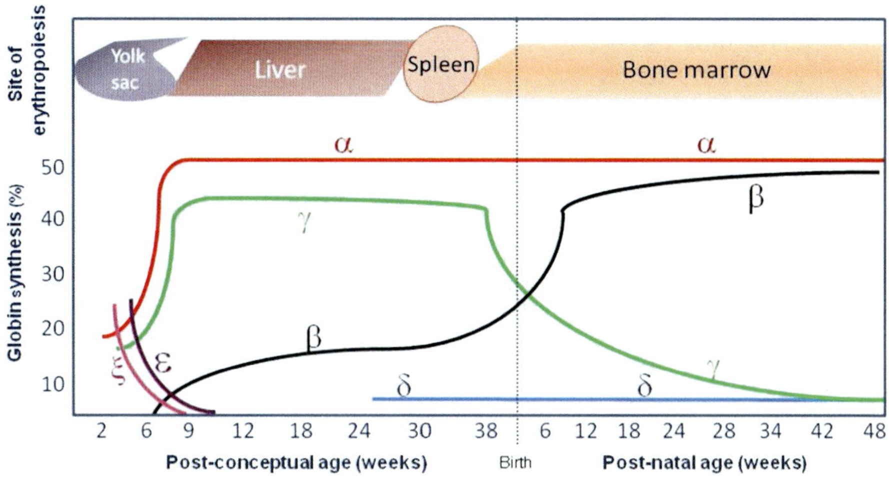

Fig. 1.2 Normal developmental switches in globin chain production. Adapted from Hoffbrand and Moss (2011)

Table 1.1 Normal hemoglobin profile in healthy adults

	Hb A	Hb F	Hb A_2
Globin chains	$\alpha_2\beta_2$	$\alpha_2\gamma_2$	$\alpha_2\delta_2$
Normal (%)	95–98	up to 2.0	2.0–3.0

while Hb A_2 corresponds to 2–3 % and Hb F to a maximum of 2 % of total hemoglobin. The 'adult' hemoglobin profile is generally established by the sixth post-birth month (Steinberg et al. 2001; Hoffbrand and Moss 2011) (Fig. 1.2) (Table 1.1).

1.1.1 Heme Synthesis

As previously mentioned, the tetrapyrrole ring (protoporphyrin IX) containing a bivalent iron atom (*heme*) constitutes the hemoglobin core, where the reversible binding of O_2 occurs. During the process of *heme* synthesis, the beginning and the end of the protoporphyrin production and the incorporation of iron take place in the mitochondria, which are arranged around the nuclei of erythroid precursors. The intermediate steps of protoporphyrin synthesis occur outside these organelles, in the soluble portion of the cytoplasm. Initially, the process involves condensation of succinyl-coenzyme A, formed in the mitochondria after the Krebs cycle (aerobic respiration), with amino acid glycine, to produce δ-Aminolevulinic acid (δ-ALA), a reaction stimulated by erythropoietin and catalyzed by ALA-synthetase, employing vitamin B6 as a coenzyme. Consequently, two molecules of δ-ALA produce porphobilinogen, a pyrrole, where four molecules of porphobilinogen, arranged in a ring structure (tetrapyrrole ring), yield uroporphyrinogen, which, after successive decarboxylation of side-chains, originates coproporphyrinogen, followed by

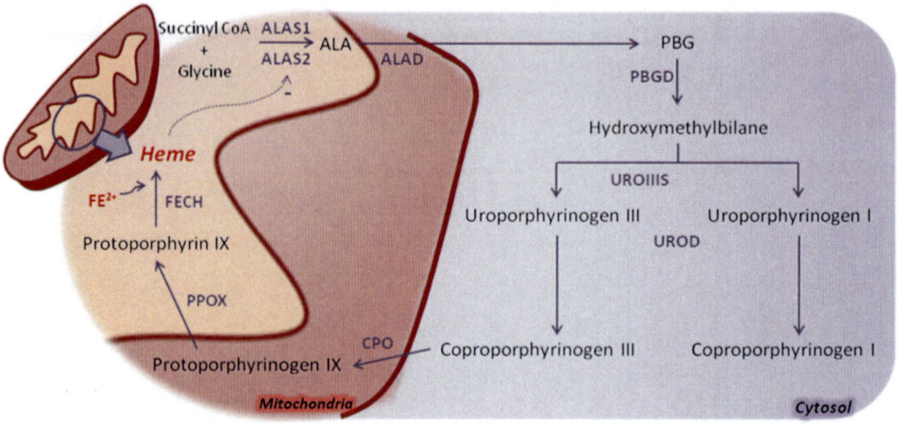

Fig. 1.3 *Heme* biosynthetic pathway. *ALA* 5-aminolaevulinic acid, *PBG* porphobilinogen, *ALAS1* ALA synthase 1, *ALAS2* ALA synthase 2, *ALAD* ALA dehydratase, *PBGD* porphobilinogen deaminase, *UROIIIS* uroporphyrinogen-III synthase, *UROD* uroporphyrinogen decarboxylase, *CPO* coproporphyrinogen oxidase, *PPOX* protoporphyrinogen oxidase, *FECH* ferrochelatase. Adapted from Puy et al. (2010)

protoporphyrin (protoporphyrin IX). In the final phase, protoporphyrin binds to an atom of iron in the ferrous state to produce *heme*. All these reactions are mediated by enzymes, including alanine synthetase, alanine dehydratase, porphobilinogen deaminase, uroporphyrinogen synthetase, uroporphyrinogen decarboxylase, coproporphyrinogen oxidase, ferrochelatase and *heme* synthetase (Fig. 1.3). In the human organism, biosynthesis of *heme* occurs predominantly in erythroid cells, where it is incorporated into recently synthesized hemoglobin, although *heme* can also be produced in hepatic cells, where it is used as part of cytochrome p-450 (Puy et al. 2010; Hoffbrand and Moss 2011).

Each gram of hemoglobin contains 3.4 mg iron which, before being incorporated into the molecule, is stored in macrophages located in the liver, spleen and bone marrow, and in cells of the liver parenchyma. Iron is transported in plasma by the transferrin protein and delivered to transferrin receptors present on the surface of the red blood cell membrane, before its incorporation into hemoglobin. Iron can be stored for prompt use in ferritin, a water-soluble protein, comprised of 22 subunits (apoferritin), arranged as a shell around a central storage cavity, where variable amounts of iron are found as ferric hydroxyphosphate microcrystals. Iron moves freely inside and outside this cavity, through channels in the protein shell and, therefore, is readily available for metabolic use. Iron can also be stored in the form of hemosiderin, an insoluble iron-protein complex, comprised of aggregates of partially denatured ferritin molecules. Iron release from hemosiderin is slower than from ferritin. In both ferritin and hemosiderin, iron is in the ferric state and, to be mobilized, it must be reduced to the ferrous state in a reaction that involves vitamin C (Puy et al. 2010; Hoffbrand and Moss 2011).

1.1.2 Globin Synthesis

Globin synthesis occurs in the polyribosomes, in the cytoplasm of erythroblasts and reticulocytes, where specific messenger RNAs (mRNAs) are translated into different globin chains. The globin mRNA is relatively stable and, therefore, reticulocytes are able to synthesize hemoglobin for at least 2 days after loss of the nucleus. A balanced globin synthesis is critical to the development and function of erythroid cells; every α chain should have a non-α chain, so that neither is in excess or deficient. Although the quantity of mRNA encoding α globins in normal reticulocytes exceed the quantity of mRNA encoding β globins, the efficiency of the translation of β globin mRNA seems to be higher to compensate and maintain the important balance between both chains (Stamatoyannopoulos et al. 2001; Weatherall et al. 2001). Moreover, during the synthesis process, free alpha globin chains are stabilized by the alpha-hemoglobin stabilizing protein (ASHP), an erythroid molecular chaperone that binds to α-hemoglobin (α-Hb) or α-globin until its association with beta globin to form the Hb tetramer (Khandros et al. 2012; Domingues-Hamdi et al. 2014).

The polypeptide chains (primary structure), released by ribosomes, assume their tridimensional configuration spontaneously due to the interactions of their residues (Fig. 1.4). The protein folding of the alpha helix structure of hemoglobin (secondary structure) involves a very stable ligation to the *heme* group, in the globin chain core, favored by the creation of a hydrophobic environment that protects the *heme* group from oxidation (tertiary structure) (Figs. 1.4 and 1.5). Subsequently, a tetramer of globin chains is created by the association of the tertiary conformations (quaternary structure) (Figs. 1.4 and 1.5). Each chain is constituted by seven or eight α-helical segments (named A through H, from the amino-terminal) followed by non-helical segments (Fig. 1.5a). The flexibility of the chain permits oxygen to access the *heme* pocket (Antonini and Brunori 1971; Mairbäurl and Weber 2012) (Fig .1.5b).

1.1.3 Globin Chain Genes

Globin genes are arranged in groups, or gene clusters, that organize the balanced production of globins during the different pre- and post-birth stages. Cluster α, located in a 30-kb DNA segment on the short arm of chromosome 16 (16p13.3), contains embryonic gene ζ, pseudogenes $\psi\zeta$ and $\psi\alpha_1$, double α globin genes (α_2 and α_1) and genes θ and α^D, of undetermined functions. The arrangement in the chromosome is the same as that expressed during human development, i.e., $5'$ - ζ - $\psi\zeta$ - α^D - $\psi\alpha_1$ - α_2 - α_1 - θ - $3'$ (Weatherall et al. 2001; Harteveld and Higgs 2010) (Fig. 1.6). Cluster β, located in an approximately 50-kb DNA segment on the short arm of chromosome 11 (11p15.5), includes genes ε, $^G\gamma$, $^A\gamma$, δ, β and pseudogene $\psi\beta$, in the following order: $5'$ - ε - $^G\gamma$ - $^A\gamma$ - $\psi\beta$ - δ - β - $3'$ (Fig. 1.7).

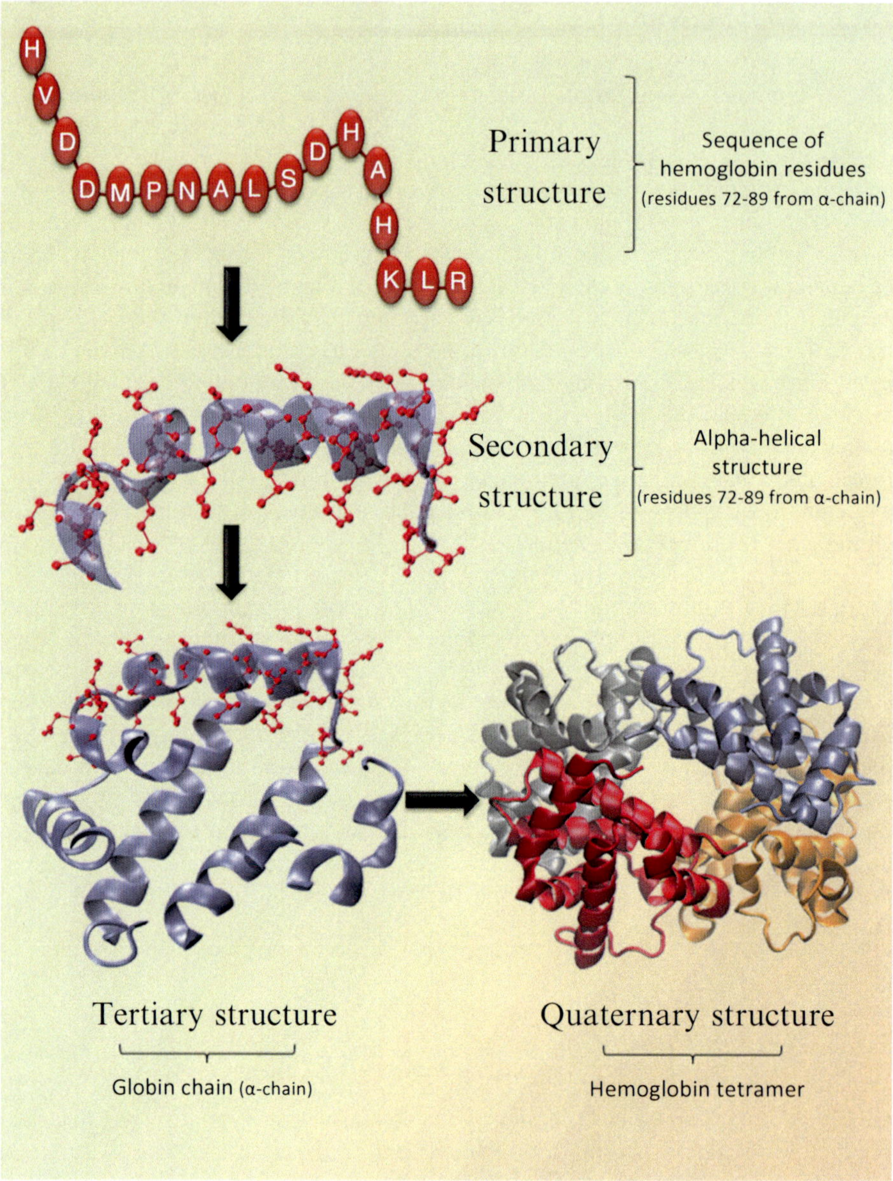

Fig. 1.4 Hemoglobin formation. A fragment of the alpha globin chain (residues from the position 72 to 89, in *red*), was used to represent primary, secondary and tertiary conformation. Structure obtained from *Protein Data Bank* 1GZX coordinates, using Visual Molecular Dynamics (VMD) software

Pseudogenes (ψ) are not functional genes, i.e. they are unable to encode proteins, although it has been demonstrated that they may have an important role in the regulation of transcription and translation in human cells. The globin pseudogenes have

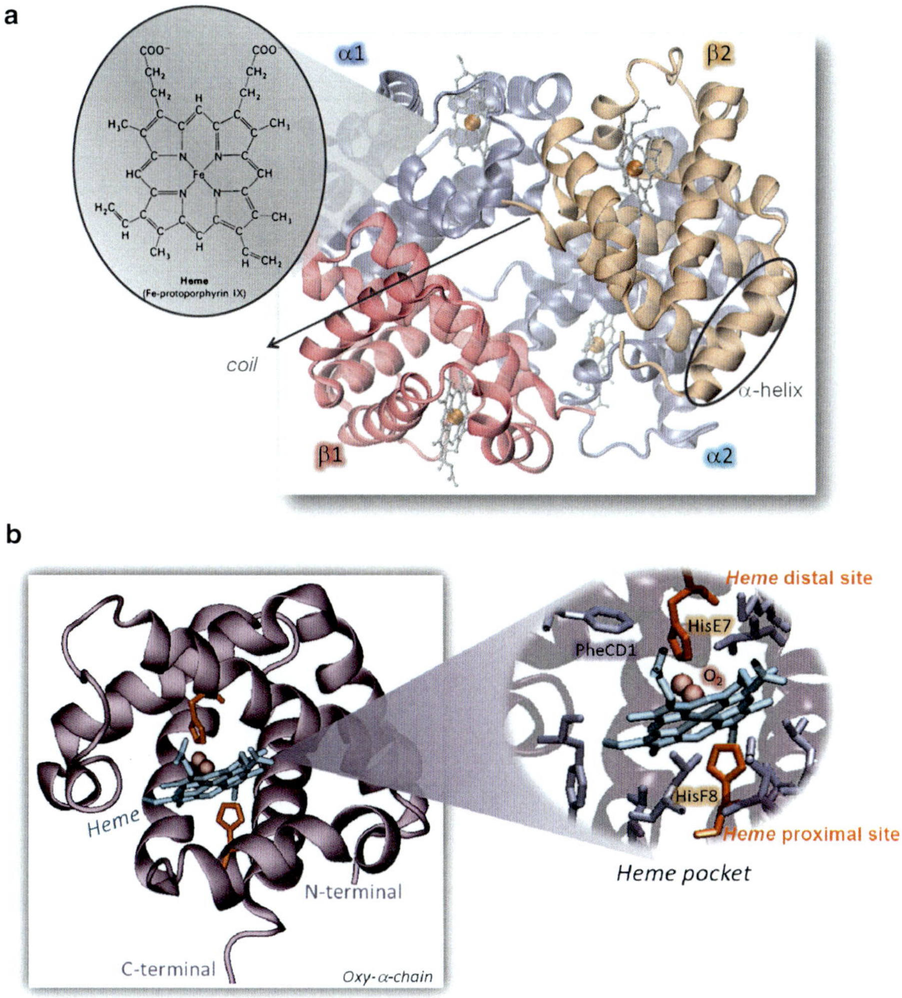

Fig. 1.5 Hemoglobin structure. (**a**) Tetramer of Hb A with *heme* featured and globin chains highlighted; coil and α-helical regions are indicated. Structure obtained from *Protein Data Bank* 1GZX coordinates, using Visual Molecular Dynamics (VMD) software. (**b**) Structure of the Oxy-alpha chain in globin (*purple*); C- and N-terminals are indicated. *Heme* in *cyan blue*, distal and proximal histidines in *orange*, oxygen in *red* and other residues from the *heme* pocket (active site) in *purple*. Structure obtained from *Protein Data Bank* 1GZX coordinates, using Visual Molecular Dynamics (VMD) software

developed from protogenes α and β through replicating events and have been disabled by mutations (substitution of bases, deletions and/or insertions) that have determined their loss of expression. Genes θ and α^D do not have a specific function; they are expressed at very low levels in vivo and their protein products have not been identified (Johnsson et al. 2013).

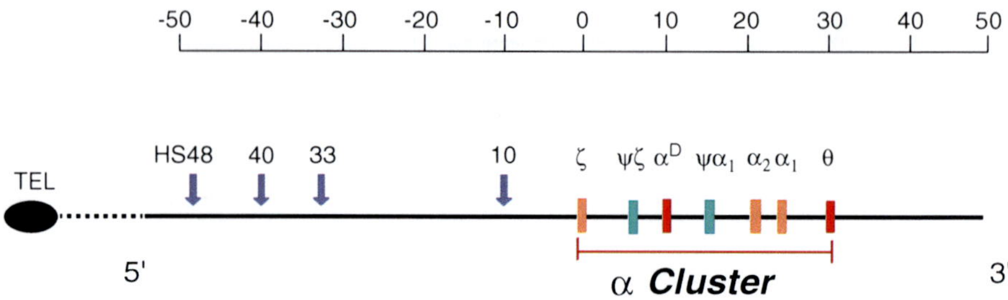

Fig. 1.6 Structure of the α cluster on chromosome 16. The telomere is shown as an oval, the *orange boxes* represent functional genes, while *blue boxes* are pseudogenes and the *red boxes* represent genes of undetermined function. *Arrows* represent the α-globin regulatory region. The scale is in kilobases as indicated above, counting from the ζ-globin gene. Adapted from Harteveld and Higgs (2010)

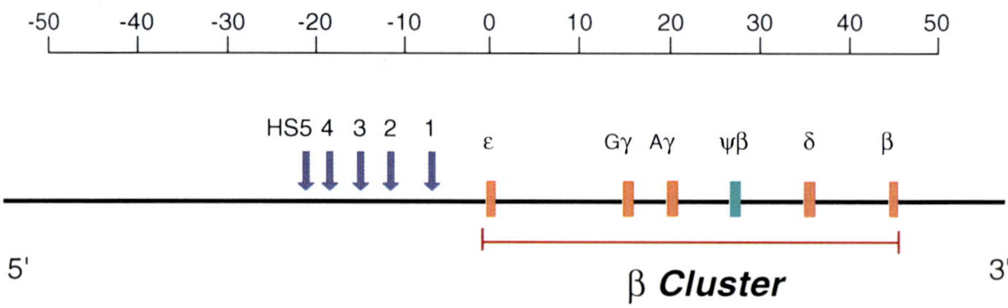

Fig. 1.7 Structure of the β cluster on chromosome 11. The *orange boxes* represent the functional genes and the *blue box* depicts a pseudogene. The *arrows* represent the β-globin regulatory region. Distances are in kilobases, counting from the ε-globin gene, as indicated above. Adapted from Patrinos et al. (2004)

Globin genes are compact, measuring 1–2 kb in length, and they have three exons and two introns. Amino acids involved in binding to the *heme* group (*heme* pocket), essential for the ability of hemoglobin to bind O_2 and total stability of the molecule, and involved in $\alpha_1\beta_2$ contacts, are mainly coded by exon 2, while those that intermediate $\alpha_1\beta_1$ contacts (increasing molecule stability and involving numerous amino acids in the chain interaction) are mostly coded by exon 3; the residues related to the binding affinity of hemoglobin for O_2 (Bohr effect and binding to 2,3- BPG) are randomly distributed among exons (Steinberg et al. 2001; Hoffbrand and Moss 2011). Genes γ and α are duplicated in chromosomes 11 and 16, respectively. Gene γ encodes different polypeptide chains ($^{G}\gamma$ and $^{A}\gamma$), which contain alanine or glycine, respectively, at position 136 of the chain. Genes α_2 and α_1 encode identical proteins and are very similar, presenting only 17 % structural divergence, limited to intron 2 (IVS-II) and exon 3, in the 3′ non-coding region (Weatherall et al. 2001; Higgs et al. 2012; Richard et al. 2012). Although it produces identical α chains, the expression level of gene α_2 is around 2.5 times greater than the expression level of gene α_1, as evaluated by the proportion of synthesized messenger RNA (mRNA) and experiments with mutants (Liebhaber and Kan 1982). Another particularity of the α genes is that they are inserted, as every group, in a GC-rich DNA segment, characteristic of genes expressed in all tissues (housekeeping genes); however, although it has been demonstrated that endothelial cells can also produce alpha-hemoglobin, the expression of these genes is highly erythroid specific (Straub et al. 2012).

A balanced globin synthesis is critical for the development and function of erythroid cells. As mentioned above, the quantity of mRNA encoding α globin in normal reticulocytes exceeds the quantity of mRNA encoding β globin, but the efficiency of the translation of this second mRNA seems to be higher to compensate and maintain the balance between both chains. Although a balanced expression of globin chains occurs during development, no feedback mechanism has been identified through which the expression of a globin may affect the expression of another globin; both seem to function coordinately, but with independent regulation (Liebhaber and Kan 1982; Weatherall et al. 2001; Higgs et al. 2012; Richard et al. 2012).

1.1.4 Regulation of Globin Gene Expression

Globin gene expression in both clusters is controlled according to the human developmental stage and in a tissue-specific manner. This complex control is dependent on *cis-acting* regulatory sequences (such as promoters and 3′ non-coding regions) that are close to and far from the globin genes (enhancers and negative regulatory elements), and the interaction of trans-acting factors with proteins, i.e. transcription factors. The interaction of transcription factors and regulatory elements close to the globin genes is similar to the regulatory mechanisms used by other human genes; however, the remote *cis-acting* control involves some particularities (Weatherall et al. 2001).

The expression of genes in the β cluster is controlled by regulatory sequences located upstream of the ε gene, which are five erythroid-specific DNase I hypersensitive sites (HS 1-5) (Fig. 1.7). The DNA segment that contains these sites is called the β Locus Control Region (β-LCR). The β-LCR, besides acting as an enhancer that activates the expression of β genes, has the additional function of changing the chromatin structure where these genes are inserted, allowing their transcription (Patrinos et al. 2004).

The β cluster is located in an AT-rich genome region of highly condensed chromatin. A few cell types have active genes in these regions. In non-erythroid cells, the chromatin domain in which this group is located is not sensitive to DNase I, demonstrating delayed replication (in the second half of the S phase of the cell cycle) and transcriptional inaction. In contrast, in erythroid cells, this domain is sensitive to DNase I, replicates at the beginning of the S phase and is transcriptionally active. Tissue-specific changes in chromatin structure are attributed to the β-LCR, which interacts via a loop with promoters of the active genes, creating a single chromatic structure, known as the active chromatin hub (ACH), causing chromatin decondensation and promoting the interaction of regulatory proteins with

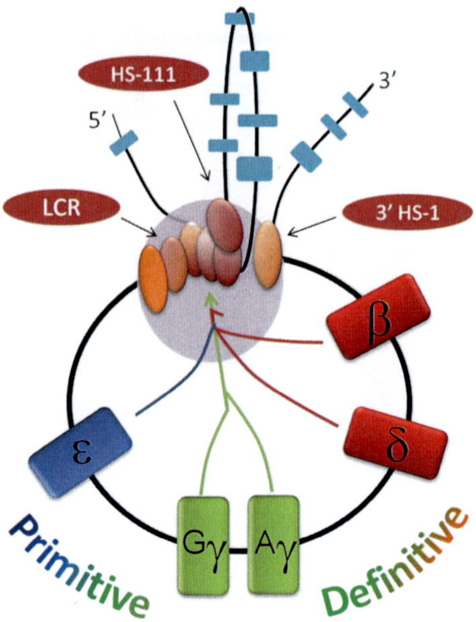

Fig. 1.8 Representation of the interactions between the β-Locus Control Region (LCR and the β cluster genes in erythroid cells. The Active Chromatin Hub (ACH), indicated as a lilac sphere, is formed by LCR and Hypersensitive Sites (HSs). The genes are depicted in different colors, indicative of their interaction with the β-LCR within the ACH during development. The embryonic ε- and fetal γ-globin genes are expressed during primitive hematopoiesis and the switch to the fetal γ- and adult δ- and β-globin genes occurs during early definitive hematopoiesis. Adapted from Patrinos et al. (2004)

DNA and the activation of the expression of genes from the respective group. This erythroid-specific chromatic structure is also regulated according to different stages of human development as, during each developmental stage, only one gene interacts with the β-LCR to yield a single ACH (Patrinos et al. 2004) (Fig. 1.8).

Due to the common ancestry of the α and β clusters (they diverged around 500 million years ago) and their similar arrangements, it was assumed for some time that the expression of these genes was controlled similarly. However, in vitro and in vivo studies employing transgenic mice suggest that these clusters are controlled in different manners. The regulation of the expression of the α cluster in humans is dependent upon a regulatory element located 40 kb upstream of the ζ gene, close to the telomere, denominated HS-40, which is an erythroid-specific DNase I hypersensitive site (Fig. 1.6). Its existence was perceived at first, due to deletions in this region that resulted in an α-thalassemia phenotype, although the α genes in these individuals presented a normal structure (Weatherall et al. 2001; Higgs et al. 2012).

HS-40 (today referred to as α-Major Regulatory Element, or α-MRE) does not change the chromatic structure in which the α cluster is inserted; its function is to act as an enhancer, activating the expression of genes in this cluster, located in a GC-rich genome region, of decondensed chromatin in both erythroid and

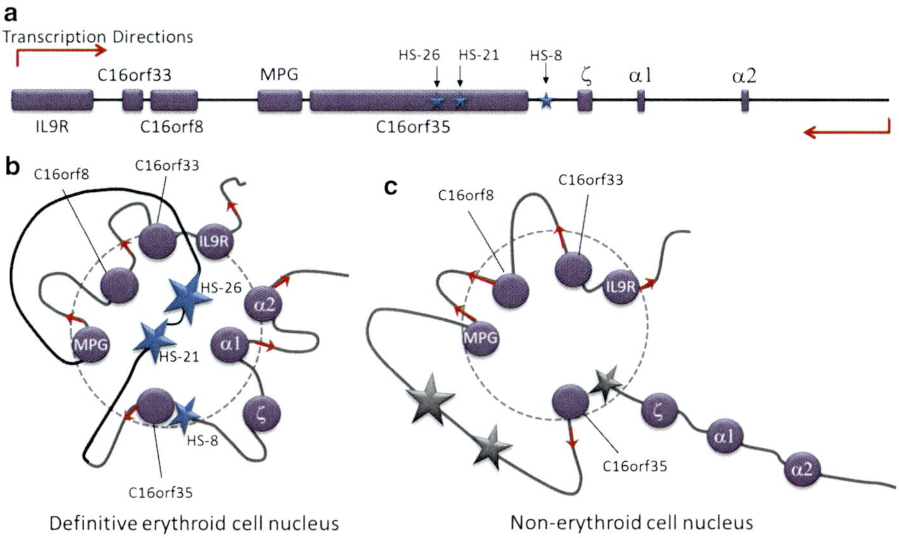

Fig. 1.9 The linear structure of the mouse α cluster (**a**) and putative chromatin structure in murine definitive erythroid cells (**b**) and murine nonerythroid cells (**c**). In panel **a**, the *blue stars* indicate hypersensitive sites (HSs) and the *purple boxes* indicate genes. In panels **b** and **c**, the *blue* and *gray stars* show the positions of HSs, the *purple spheres* represent protein complexes on gene promoters, the *gray* and *black strings* represent chromatin and the *red arrows* indicate transcription direction. Adapted from Zhou et al. (2006)

non-erythroid cells. Thus, the main question is to understand how HS-40 controls the expression of the α genes without interfering in adjacent gene expression. In fact, a permanent chromatin structure is created and maintained (Vernimmen et al. 2009). In murine erythroid cells, the recruitment of promoters of active genes from the α cluster and the regulatory element for this ACH results in the gene expression of globins. Furthermore, the exclusion of α globin genes and their regulatory element from this chromatin structure in non-erythroid cells disables gene expression (Zhou et al. 2006) (Fig. 1.9).

1.2 Oxygen Transport

Hb A results from the combination of two α and two β chains. These segments consist, respectively, of seven and eight α-helical structures, named from A to H, which are intermediated by non-helical sequences (AB, BC, and so on). The terminal portions of each globin, NA and HC, are short non-helical extensions from helix A to the C-terminal. Thus, all residues are numbered according to the coordinates presented in the structure, from the N-terminal and/or according to its position on the segment (Antonini and Brunori 1971; Mairbäurl and Weber 2012) (helix, coil, etc.—Fig. 1.5a).

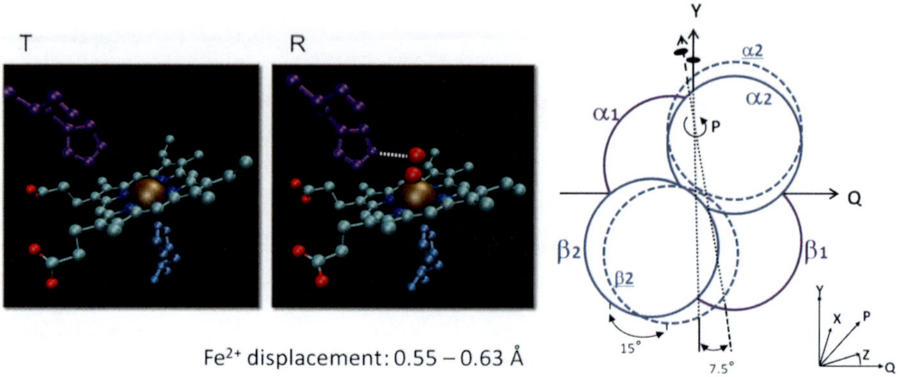

Fig. 1.10 Proximal (*blue*) and distal histidines (*purple*) in the *heme* pocket, in the T (deoxy) and R (oxy) hemoglobin states. Oxygen (*red*) is bound to Fe^{2+} (*brown*) in the R conformation of hemoglobin—figure produced from *Protein Data Bank* 1GZX and 2DN1 coordinates, using Visual Molecular Dynamics (VMD) software. The chain movements are represented in the *right panel*

The *heme* group is located under the E, F and G helixes and CD contacts. The stability of the binding of O_2 to *heme* is, therefore, affected by a number of residue interactions located at these contact regions. Of these, the most important are formed by proximal histidines [α87 (F8) or β92 (F8)], which bind directly to the iron of protoporphyrin IX, and distal histidines [α58 (E7) or β63 (E7)], which then interact with iron-bound O_2 (Antonini and Brunori 1971; Shikama 2006; Mairbäurl and Weber 2012) (Fig. 1.5b). During oxygen binding, the iron atom moves 0.55–0.63 Å, which results in conformational changes on the residues surrounding the active *heme* pocket site. This event also causes significant changes in the remaining globin chains, in both the tertiary and quaternary structures (Antonini and Brunori 1971; Mairbäurl and Weber 2012). These structural alterations confer two stable states to the hemoglobin molecule; the tense form (T or "*deoxy*-Hb", with a lower affinity for O_2) and the relaxed form (R or "*oxy*-Hb", with increased affinity for O_2), as described by Perutz, in 1970, using crystallography (Perutz 1970) (Fig. 1.10).

The protein stability of the tetramer is controlled by the interface contacts $\alpha_1\beta_1$ and $\alpha_2\beta_2$, also called packing contacts, where the α- and β- chains are connected by 34 residues located in the C, G and H helices and the BC corner. The $\alpha_1\beta_2/\alpha_2\beta_1$ interdimer interface is less extensive and contains 19 residues in total. This characteristic ensures the stability of the T-R transition during oxygen binding. Besides being shorter, the $\alpha_1\beta_2/\alpha_2\beta_1$ interface is located close to the *heme* group, promoting conformational changes in the active *heme* site. Simultaneously, structural changes in the *heme* pocket also mediate allosteric interactions in the $\alpha_1\beta_2$ area. Therefore, any substitution of residues at the $\alpha_1\beta_2/\alpha_2\beta_1$ interface may result in reduced *heme-heme* cooperativity and changes in the affinity of hemoglobin for O_2, demonstrating the extreme importance that $\alpha_1\beta_1$ and $\alpha_2\beta_2$ dimer interactions have in balancing T-R conformational changes when binding to O_2 (Antonini and Brunori 1971; Eaton et al. 2007).

1.2.1 Functional Aspects of Hemoglobin

The main function of hemoglobin is to transport O_2 from the lungs to peripheral tissues, and to take carbon dioxide from tissues back to the lungs. Usually, 95 % of O_2 molecules transported from the lungs to tissues are maintained in chemical combination with hemoglobin in the red blood cells, while the remaining 5 % are transported dissolved in plasma and cell water (Hoffbrand and Moss 2011).

The mechanism of the Hb-O_2 ligation is mediated by homotropic (*heme-heme* cooperativity) and heterotropic events, such as differences in O_2 pressures. Under high pressures of O_2 (PO_2), as in pulmonary capillaries, O_2 binds to hemoglobin; when PO_2 is decreased, as in tissue capillaries, O_2 is released from the hemoglobin, in an event that is modulated by allosteric effectors, such as H^+/CO_2, Cl^- and organic phosphates, such as 2,3-biphosphoglycerate (2,3-BPG). O_2 binding can be mathematically represented by the oxygen-dissociation curve (ODC), which is obtained from the PO_2 *versus* saturated *heme* site under standard conditions of temperature, pH, atmospheric pressure, PCO_2 and concentration of organic phosphates, such as 2,3-BPG. Due to *heme-heme* cooperativity, the ODC results in a sigmoidal shape, and any change in the concentrations of gases, ions or 2,3-BPG concentration, among other factors, may affect the affinity of hemoglobin for O_2 (Antonini and Brunori 1971; Shikama 2006; Mairbäurl and Weber 2012) (Fig. 1.11).

The affinity of hemoglobin for O_2 is expressed by the P_{50}: the partial pressure of O_2 required for 50 % hemoglobin saturation (Fig. 1.11). The standard P_{50} value for

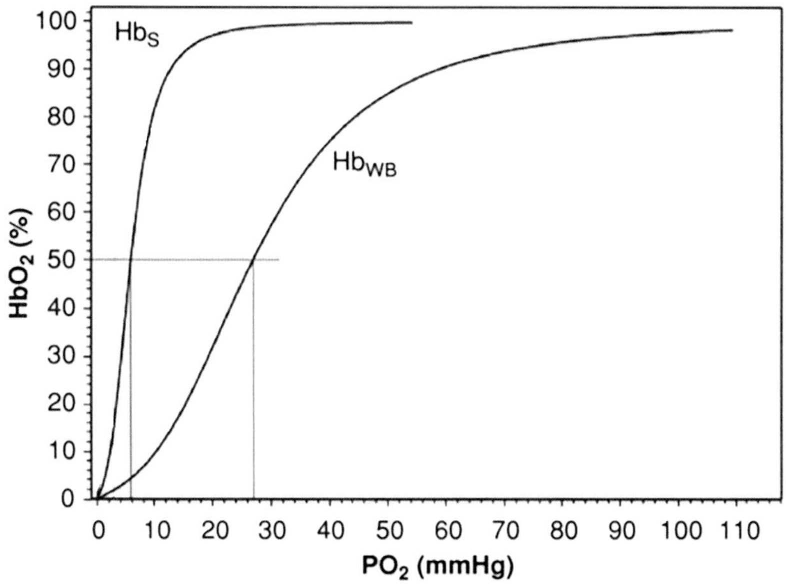

Fig. 1.11 Oxygen dissociation curves (ODCs) for stripped Hb in buffered solution (Hb_S), and human RBCs in whole blood (Hb_{WB}). Adapted from Mairbäurl and Weber (2012)

Hb A is 26.6 mmHg; thus, higher P_{50} values signify a decreased affinity for O_2, and vice versa. Several genetic and environmental factors may affect O_2 affinity and the great variation observed in hemoglobin P_{50} values occurs, partially, due to structural differences among the hemoglobins and, partially, due to differences in the intracellular environment. Native human hemoglobin affinity may vary by as much as 100-fold, as a result of changes in pH and/or PCO_2 (Bohr effect), salt ion concentrations (such as Cl^-) and, in particular, due to the concentration of organic phosphates (e.g. 2,3-BPG), which can shift the dissociation curve to the right (favoring the T conformation and a decreased oxygen affinity) (Antonini and Brunori 1971; Shikama 2006; Mairbäurl and Weber 2012) (Fig. 1.11).

During the last two decades, a number of different quaternary states of hemoglobin, such as R_2, RR_2, RR_3, T_{high}, have been reported. These states represent different conformations and comprise from canonical T-(deoxy) to R-(ligated) quaternary structures, depending on the experimental conditions, although the T and R states are the most stable. It is assumed that hemoglobin exists in allosteric equilibrium between two functional states, the **T** (lower-affinity) and **R** (higher-affinity) states, and that successive O_2-binding shifts the allosteric equilibrium towards the higher-affinity R states, therefore, explaining the sigmoidal Hb-O_2 binding curve (Fig. 1.11). The allosterism of the T-R transition is modulated by homotropic and heterotropic mechanisms, which comprehend the *heme-heme* cooperativity and the allosteric modifications promoted by non-specific ligands that interfere in the affinity for O_2 at the active *heme* site, respectively (Bruno et al. 2001; Eaton et al. 2007; Yonetani and Laberge 2008).

1.2.2 Homotropic Interactions: Heme-Heme Cooperativity

Heme-heme cooperativity can numerically be represented by the Hill coefficient ('*n*') as a global event, or calculated by the Adair equation, which considers four O_2-binding *hemes*, with, therefore, four equilibrium constants ($K_1<K_2<K_3<K_4$). Several models predict the T-R transition due to *heme-heme* cooperativity and heterotropic interactions (Antonini and Brunori 1971; Eaton et al. 2007).

Allosteric Regulation: Symmetry Model—MWC

The first T-R transition model was proposed by Monod, Wyman and Changeux (MWC, symmetry model) in 1965. The model describes two stable states for hemoglobin: the T and R states, which are independent of the presence of O_2, where hemoglobin has a higher affinity for O_2 in its R state, and a lower affinity for O_2 in the T conformation. This model predicts the T-R transition as a global allosteric event, not based on chain-by-chain conformational changes; as such, in this model, hemoglobin has only two constants of O_2 ligation-dissociation K_{high} or K_R for the R state and K_{low} or K_T for the T state. The Hb-O_2 ligation occurs, therefore, as the result of the balanced presence of hemoglobin in its more reactive R form (with a higher affinity for O_2) and less reactive T form (with a lower affinity for O_2) (Fig. 1.12a). This model, however, does not take into consideration environmental factors and conditions, such as buffers, pH, and the types and the nature of heterotropic effectors (Monod et al. 1965).

Based on the MWC model, Brunoni and coworkers proposed the 'Cooperon' model, which considers the cooperative free energy in the microstates from R to T (Brunori et al. 1986) (Fig. 1.12b).

Allosteric Regulation: Sequential Model—The Adair and KNF Model

The second model of allosteric regulation, denominated the sequential or KNF model, was proposed by Koshland, Nemethy and Filmer in 1966, and is based on calculations established by Adair in 1925. The model predicts a T-R dynamic transition, considering conformational changes that occur chain by chain, and assuming the existence of 4 O_2-ligation/dissociation constants (K_1, K_2, K_3, K_4). This model, therefore, proposes a "globin centric" mechanism of regulation of the T-R equilibrium (Koshland et al. 1966) (Fig. 1.12c).

Stereochemical Model of Perutz, SK, SKL and TTS

Based on the MWC and KNF models of allosteric regulation, other T-R mechanisms have been proposed to explain intermediary states in the T-R equilibrium. Perutz, in 1970, for example, proposed the stereochemical model, which integrated the previous MWC and KNF models. This model considers the structural changes in the globin subunits during the T-R transition, as well as the T and R stable protein conformations (Perutz 1970) (Fig. 1.12d).

Szabo and Karplus (SK), in 1972, developed a mathematical model for hemoglobin based on Perutz's stereochemical mechanism. The SK model represents the statistical thermodynamical formulation of the Perutz mechanism (Szabo and Karplus 1972). This model was revised by Karplus and Lee (SKL), who developed the concept of the 'allosteric core' upon oxygen binding, particularly proposing the steric repulsion between the proximal histidine and the pyrrole nitrogens of the porphyrin ring, associated with the motion of the iron into the *heme* plane (Lee and Karplus 1983) (Fig. 1.12e).

The 'Tertiary Two-State' (TTS) allosteric model was predicted by Henry et al. (2002), and was also based on Perutz model, as well as on experiments performed by Herzfeld and Stanley (1974) and Mozzarelli et al. (1997). The model is essentially similar to the MWC model, but differs in that an equilibrium of tertiary conformations is proposed, involving high and low affinity conformations of individual subunits, called **r** and **t**, which exist in equilibrium within each quaternary structure. The quaternary structures influence the affinity of hemoglobin by biasing the **t**-**r** conformation equilibrium, where the **T** conformation favors **t** and the **R** conformation

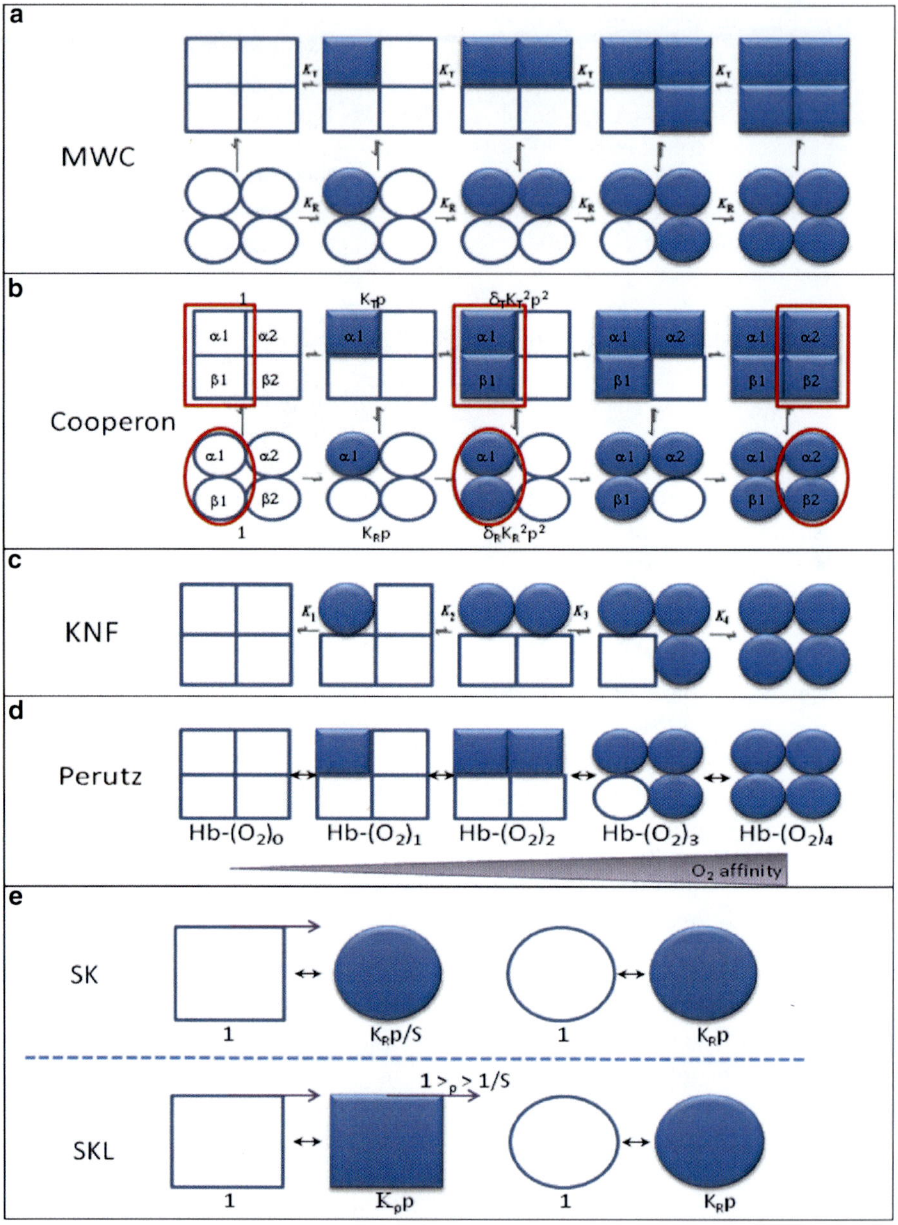

Fig. 1.12 Predictions of allosterism for Human Hemoglobin. *Empty symbols* correspond to unligated subunits and filled subunits correspond to ligated subunits. (**a**) The MWC (Monod, Wyman and Changeux) model of allosteric regulation. Adapted from Eaton et al. (2007); (**b**) Cooperon binding model. Adapted from Eaton et al. (2007); (**c**) The KNF (Koshland, Némethy and Filmer) allosteric binding model. Adapted from Yonetani and Laberge (2008); (**d**) Perutz model of hemoglobin cooperativity. Adapted from Eaton et al. (2007); (**e**) SK (Szabo and Karplus) and SKL (Szabo, Karplus and Lee) simplified binding systems. Adapted from Eaton et al. (2007)

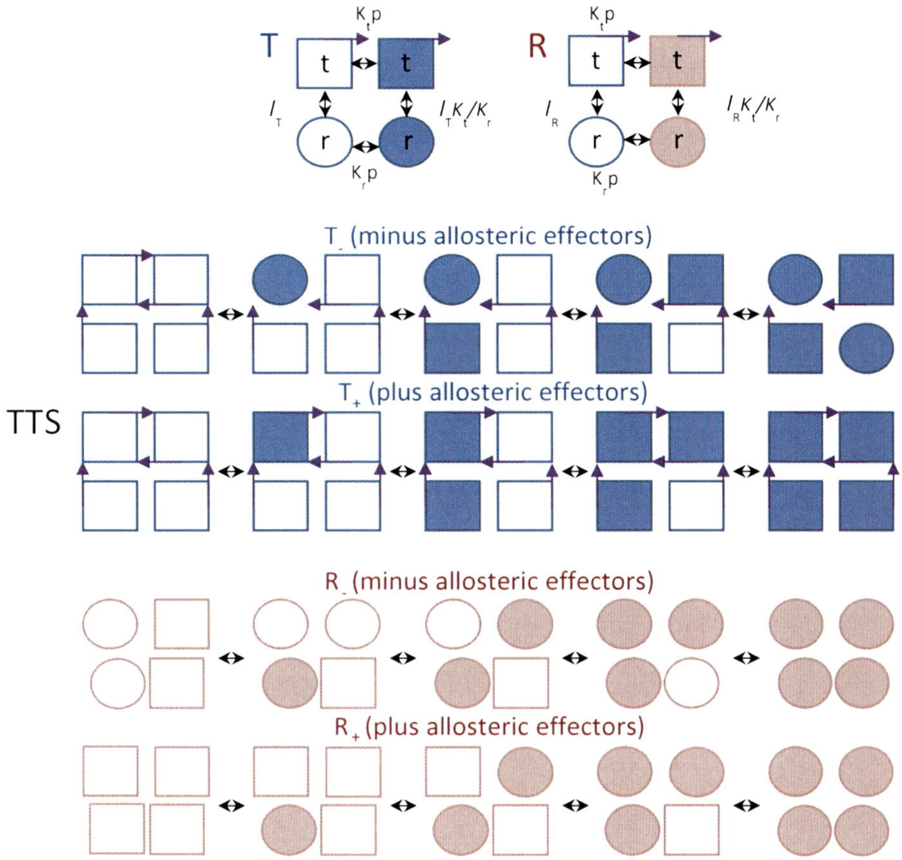

Fig. 1.13 Tertiary Two-State (TTS) allosteric model predicted by Henry et al. (2002). *Empty symbols* correspond to unligated subunits and *filled symbols* correspond to ligated subunits. Adapted from Eaton et al. (2007)

favors **r**. Ligand binding to both **R** and to **T** favors **r** (Herzfeld and Stanley 1974; Mozzarelli et al. 1997; Henry et al. 2002; Eaton et al. 2007) (Fig. 1.13).

1.2.3 Heterotropic Interactions: Allosteric Effectors

The affinity of hemoglobin for O_2 is also modulated by heterotropic interactions (outside the *heme* pocket); examples of these effectors are H^+, Cl^- and CO_2, which shift the T-R balance of hemoglobin to the T state (with lower affinity for O_2). Physiological organic phosphates, such as 2,3-Bisphosphoglycerate (2,3-BPG), ATP and ADP, also act at heterotropic sites, shifting the equilibrium towards to T. Other allosteric effectors, such as inositol hexaphosphate (IHP), and other

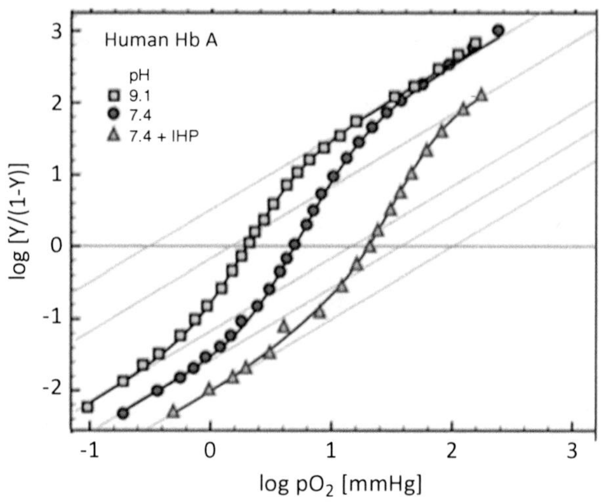

Fig. 1.14 Oxygen equilibrium curves for human hemoglobin at different pH values and in the presence of inositol hexaphosphate (IHP). Adapted from Brunori (2014)

hydrophobic compounds, including bezafibrate (BZF) and L35, which lead to reduced states of K_T and K_R, have been used for the study of the T-R equilibrium (Baldwin and Chothia 1979; Yonetani and Kanaori 2013) (Fig. 1.14).

2,3-Bisphosphoglycerate (2,3-BPG)

The presence of organic phosphates reduces the affinity of hemoglobin for O_2. The principal organic phosphate allosteric effector is 2,3-BPG. Physiologically, 2,3-BPG binds to hemoglobin at a heterotropic site, located at the $\beta_1\beta_2$ interface, in the central axis of the symmetry plane of the protein, which lies in the central cavity of the protein. At low O_2 tension in peripheral tissues, hemoglobin tends towards the T form, exposing the positively-charged portions of the side chains of histidine 2 and 143, lysine 82 residues and the amino-terminal groups of Val1 of the β chains. As such, the negatively-charged 2,3-BPG stabilizes the spatial conformation of the protein in its T form, allowing the release of O_2 (Antonini and Brunori 1971; Baldwin and Chothia 1979; Mairbäurl and Weber 2012; Yonetani and Kanaori 2013) (Fig. 1.15).

The Bohr Effect

In the deoxyhemoglobin form, H^+ ions establish salt bridges between individual globin chains, consequently the β chains separate and allow the entry of CO_2 and 2,3-BPG, which binds to the N-terminal group and amino groups of lysines at positions 143 and 82 of the same β chains, hindering the interaction of hemoglobin with O_2. In the oxyhemoglobin form, a sudden change in the tertiary structure of the molecule occurs, with the rupture of salt bridges and repositioning of the β

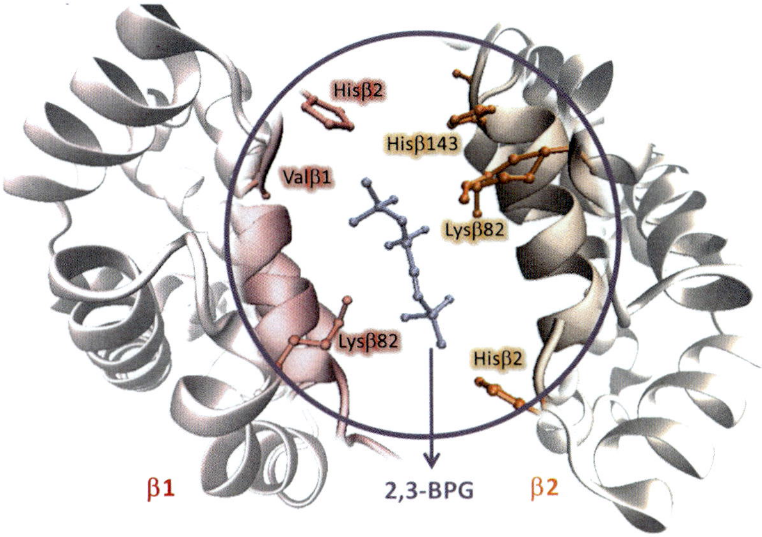

Fig. 1.15 The 2,3-biphosphoglycerate (2,3-BPG) binding pocket—from *Protein Data Bank* 1B86 coordinates, using Visual Molecular Dynamics (VMD) software. 2,3-BPG (*purple*) in the β_1 (*red*)/ β_2 (*orange*) interface. Some of the important residues involved in this allosteric pocket are represented in *red* (Hisβ2, Valβ1 and Lysβ82, from the β_1 chain) and *orange* (Hisβ2, Lysβ82 and Hisβ143, from the β_2 chain)

chains, leading to the removal of CO_2 and 2,3-BPG. Thus, although the H^+ ion concentration (pH) and partial pressure of CO_2 (PCO_2) have an important influence on the affinity of hemoglobin for O_2, its major physiological mediator is 2,3-BPG, an intermediary molecule of glucose metabolism, which is the most abundant phosphate in red blood cells, and present in very low concentrations in tissues (Antonini and Brunori 1971; Mairbäurl and Weber 2012; Yonetani and Kanaori 2013; Brunori 2014).

The ability of H^+ ions to change hemoglobin's affinity for O_2 is known as the Bohr effect; this mechanism can be subdivided into alkaline and acid effects. According to the basic Bohr effect, the presence of H^+ ions reduces the affinity of hemoglobin for O_2, while the absence of H^+ ions, and therefore a more alkaline pH, leads to increased affinity for O_2 (Antonini and Brunori 1971; Shikama 2006) (Fig. 1.14).

Chloride Anions – Cl^-

Chloride anions reduce the affinity of hemoglobin for O_2 by stabilizing the protein structure in the T form (deoxyhemoglobin). This stabilization occurs as the result of the interaction of the chloride anions with positively-charged residues (such as Arginine 141 in the α chain) in the central cavity of hemoglobin, which are exposed when the protein is in the T state (Perutz et al. 1994).

Transport of CO_2

Hemoglobin also transports carbon dioxide (CO_2) from the peripheral tissues to the lungs via two mechanisms:

- The Bohr effect: When oxyhemoglobin loses O_2 and binds to H^+ ions present in the medium, this causes a change in the balanced ionization of carbon dioxide, increasing the transport of CO_2, in the form of bicarbonate ions.
- The production of carbaminohemoglobin, derived from the reaction of CO_2 with groups of non-proton coupled amino acids (α– or ε–) in the hemoglobin. The constants of CO_2 binding to oxyhemoglobin and deoxyhemoglobin are distinct for this mechanism.

The transport of CO_2 via hemoglobin is not exclusively performed by either of the mechanisms above, but probably by both of them, in a higher or lower proportion. In addition, hemoglobin performs only 5 % of CO_2 transport from the tissues to the lungs (Antonini and Brunori 1971; Shikama 2006; Mairbäurl and Weber 2012).

Effect of Temperature

Hb-O_2 binding is exothermal. As such, the affinity of hemoglobin for O_2 is reduced as temperature increases. An increase of 10 °C reduces the affinity of hemoglobin for O_2 by 1.5–2.5-fold, depending on the experimental conditions (Antonini and Brunori 1971).

1.3 Hemoglobin Variants

Differences in the structure of hemoglobin can determine its ability to transport O_2. Hb F is not able to bind 2,3-BPG with the same affinity as Hb A. This results in a displacement of the oxygen-dissociation curve to the left, with decreased P_{50}. The reduced affinity for 2,3-BPG confers high stability of the Hb F-O_2 complex and better access to oxygen from maternal umbilical cord blood (Antonini and Brunori 1971).

Differences in Hb function can also be observed in some rare hemoglobin variants, due to the substitution of residues at important sites, such as in the *heme* pocket and at the $\alpha_1\beta_2/\alpha_2\beta_1$ dimer interface. For example, Hb Coimbra [HBB:c.300 T>A or 300 T>G p.99Asp>Glu] has increased O_2 affinity and confers polycythemia to its carriers (Tamagnini et al. 1991), while the double mutant HbS-São Paulo [HBB:c.20A>T p.Glu6Val; c.196A>G p.Lys65Glu] has decreased O_2 affinity and stable polymers, resulting in moderate anemia in its carriers (Jorge et al. 2012).

1.3.1 Methemoglobin

Methemoglobin is the non-functional molecule of hemoglobin, where the ferrous iron (Fe^{2+}) in the active *heme pocket* is inappropriately oxidized to ferric Fe^{3+}. The clinical condition, methemoglobinemia, results from the formation of oxidized hemoglobin (methemoglobin, Fe^{3+}), which is unable to bind oxygen. Among different reasons, this methemoglobinemia may be genetically caused by hemoglobins with structural anomalies (Hb M-), in which the residue substitutions affect principally the *heme* pocket, leading to iron oxidation, deficiency of the methemoglobin reductase enzyme, or due to the reactivity of some drugs, such as the highly oxidant effects conferred by sulfa drugs, which may lead to toxic methemoglobinemia. Cyanosis is, therefore, the main clinical sign of this condition (Percy et al. 2005; Hoffbrand and Moss 2011).

References

Antonini E, Brunori M (1971) Hemoglobin and myoglobin in their reaction with ligands. North-Holland, Amsterdam

Baldwin J, Chothia C (1979) Haemoglobin: the structural changes related to ligand binding and its allosteric mechanism. J Mol Biol 129(2):175–220

Bruno S, Bonaccio M, Bettati S et al (2001) High and low oxygen affinity conformations of T state hemoglobin. Protein Sci 10(11):2401–2407

Brunori M (2014) Variations on the theme: allosteric control in hemoglobin. FEBS J 281(2): 633–643

Brunori M, Coletta M, Di Cera E (1986) A cooperative model for ligand binding to biological macromolecules as applied to oxygen carriers. Biophys Chem 23(3–4):215–222

Domingues-Hamdi E, Vasseur C, Fournier JB, Marden MC, Wajcman H, Baudin-Creuza V (2014) Role of α-globin H helix in the building of tetrameric human hemoglobin: interaction with α-hemoglobin stabilizing protein (AHSP) and heme molecule. PLoS One 9(11), e111395

Eaton WA, Henry ER, Hofrichter J, Bettati S, Viappiani C, Mozzarelli A (2007) Evolution of allosteric models for hemoglobin. IUBMB Life 59(8–9):586–599

Harteveld CL, Higgs DR (2010) Alpha-thalassaemia. Orphanet J Rare Dis 5:13

Henry ER, Bettati S, Hofrichter J, Eaton WA (2002) A tertiary two-state allosteric model for hemoglobin. Biophys Chem 98(1–2):149–164

Herzfeld J, Stanley HE (1974) A general approach to co-operativity and its application to the oxygen equilibrium of hemoglobin and its effectors. J Mol Biol 82(2):231–265

Higgs DR, Engel JD, Stamatoyannopoulos G (2012) Thalassaemia. Lancet 379(9813):373–383

Hoffbrand AV, Moss PAH (2011) Essential Haematology, 6th edn. Blackwell Science, Malden

Johnsson P, Ackley A, Vidarsdottir L et al (2013) A pseudogene long-noncoding-RNA network regulates PTEN transcription and translation in human cells. Nat Struct Mol Biol 20(4):440–446

Jorge SE, Petruk AA, Kimura EM et al (2012) Hb S-São Paulo: a new sickling hemoglobin with stable polymers and decreased oxygen affinity. Arch Biochem Biophys 519(1):23–31

Khandros E, Mollan TL, Yu X et al (2012) Insights into hemoglobin assembly through in vivo mutagenesis of α-hemoglobin stabilizing protein. J Biol Chem 287(14):11325–11337

Koshland DE Jr, Némethy G, Filmer D (1966) Comparison of experimental binding data and theoretical models in proteins containing subunits. Biochemistry 5(1):365–385

Lee AW, Karplus M (1983) Structure-specific model of hemoglobin cooperativity. Proc Natl Acad Sci U S A 80(23):7055–7059

Liebhaber SA, Kan YW (1982) Different rates of mRNA translation balance the expression of the two human α-globin loci. J Biol Chem 257(20):11852–11855

Mairbäurl H, Weber RE (2012) Oxygen transport by hemoglobin. Comp Physiol 2(2):1463–1489

Monod J, Wyman J, Changeux JP (1965) On the nature of allosteric transitions: a plausible model. J Mol Biol 12:88–118

Mozzarelli A, Rivetti C, Rossi GL, Eaton WA, Henry ER (1997) Allosteric effectors do not alter the oxygen affinity of hemoglobin crystals. Protein Sci 6(2):484–489

Patrinos GP, de Krom M, de Boer E et al (2004) Multiple interactions between regulatory regions are required to stabilize an active chromatin hub. Genes Dev 18(12):1495–1509

Percy MJ, McFerran NV, Lappin TR (2005) Disorders of oxidised haemoglobin. Blood Rev 19(2):61–68

Perutz MF (1970) Stereochemistry of cooperative effects in haemoglobin. Nature 228(5273): 726–739

Perutz MF, Shih DT, Williamson D (1994) The chloride effect in human haemoglobin. A new kind of allosteric mechanism. J Mol Biol 239(4):555–560

Puy H, Gouya L, Deybach JC (2010) Porphyrias. Lancet 375(9718):924–937

Richard NP, Haley KM, Recht M (2012) Thalassemia. In: Elzouki AY (ed) Textbook of clinical pediatrics, 2nd edn. Springer, Berlin, pp 3029–3036

Shikama K (2006) Nature of the FeO_2 bonding in myoglobin and hemoglobin: a new molecular paradigm. Prog Biophys Mol Biol 91(1–2):83–162

Stamatoyannopoulos G, Majerus PW, Perlmutter RM, Varmus H (2001) The molecular bases of blood diseases, 3rd edn. WB Sounders, Philadelphia

Steinberg MH, Forget BG, Higgs DR, Nagel RL (2001) Disorders of hemoglobin: genetics, pathophysiology and clinical management, 1st edn. Cambridge University Press, Cambridge

Straub AC, Lohman AW, Billaud M et al (2012) Endothelial cell expression of haemoglobin α regulates nitric oxide signalling. Nature 491(7424):473–477

Szabo A, Karplus M (1972) A mathematical model for structure-function relations in hemoglobin. J Mol Biol 72(1):163–197

Tamagnini GP, Ribeiro ML, Valente V et al (1991) Hb Coimbra or alpha 2 beta (2)99(G1)Asp>Glu, a newly discovered high oxygen affinity variant. Hemoglobin 15(6):487–496

Vernimmen D, Marques-Kranc F, Sharpe JA et al (2009) Chromosome looping at the human alpha-globin locus is mediated via the major upstream regulatory element (HS–40). Blood 114(19): 4253–4260

Weatherall DJ, Clegg JB, Gibbons R et al (2001) The thalassaemia syndromes, 4th edn. Blackwell Science, Oxford

Yonetani T, Kanaori K (2013) How does hemoglobin generate such diverse functionality of physiological relevance? Biochim Biophys Acta 1834(9):1873–1884

Yonetani T, Laberge M (2008) Protein dynamics explain the allosteric behaviour of hemoglobin. Biochem Biophys Acta 1784(9):1146–1158

Zhou GL, Xin L, Song W et al (2006) Active chromatin hub of the mouse α globin locus forms in a transcription factory of clustered housekeeping genes. Mol Cell Biol 26(13):5096–5105

Chapter 2
Sickle Cell Anemia: History and Epidemiology

Frédéric B. Piel and Thomas N. Williams

Abstract This chapter summarizes how a simple point mutation in the human genome has evolved to become a global public health problem, as well as a remarkable example of evolutionary biology, population genetics and clinical epidemiology. Through malaria selection and interactions with other genes, the sickle mutation of the *HBB* gene reached high population frequencies throughout much of sub-Saharan Africa and in parts of the Mediterranean, the Middle East and India before spreading globally through subsequent population migration. Sickle cell anemia is a severe disease that is still associated with a high mortality in low- and middle-income countries, where simple public health interventions could help significantly in reducing its long-term health burden, and with high health-care costs in high-income countries, where life expectancy and quality of life remain suboptimal. Alongside huge progress in the understanding of the natural history and epidemiology of sickle cell anemia during the last century, significant gaps, discussed in this chapter, still remain, highlighting the need for further research to better prevent the adverse consequences of this disease.

Keywords Evolution • Malaria selection • Geographic distribution • Population estimates • Health burden

F.B. Piel (✉)
Department of Zoology, University of Oxford, Oxford OX1 3PS, UK
e-mail: fred.piel@zoo.ox.ac.uk

T.N. Williams (✉)
Kenya Medical Research Institute/Wellcome Trust Programme, Centre for Geographic Medicine Research-Coast, Kilifi District Hospital, PO Box 230, Kilifi, Kenya

Department of Medicine, Imperial College, St Mary's Hospital,
Praed Street, London W21NY, UK
e-mail: tom.williams@imperial.ac.uk

© Springer International Publishing Switzerland 2016

F.F. Costa, N. Conran (eds.), *Sickle Cell Anemia*,
DOI 10.1007/978-3-319-06713-1_2

2.1 Natural History

2.1.1 Introduction

It is still unclear when the sickle mutation appeared in the human genome, but it is well established that sickle cell anemia has had a profound impact on human populations for centuries. In various African populations, such as the Igbo of Nigeria, the term "ogbanjes" has long been used to describe babies born with weak, disease-ridden bodies, who are chronically ill and die early in life and recent social studies have found a strong association between the use of this term and the diagnosis of sickle cell anemia (Nzewi 2001). In 1910, James Herrick and his intern Ernest Lyons described peculiar elongated red blood cells in a 20-year old patient presenting with severe anemia (Herrick 1910). The follow up of this patient of West Indian origins allowed the identification of some of the clinical complications (including "muscular rheumatism" and "bilious attacks") that are now recognized as common complications of sickle cell anemia, as well as the early mortality associated with it. The term "sickle cell anemia" was first used in a case report by Vernon Mason in 1922 (Mason 1922) since when the disease has been at the center of numerous discoveries in Medicine and Genetics. Sickle cell anemia has indeed become a textbook example of balanced polymorphism and was the first genetic condition to be characterized at the molecular level.

2.1.2 The Malaria Hypothesis

Early studies of patients with sickle cell anemia rapidly suggested an association with African descent, although patients with the disease were also observed in parts of the Mediterranean, the Middle East and India. In the middle of the twentieth century, both Anthony C. Allison and John B.S. Haldane hypothesized that the geographical correspondence between the distribution of disorders affecting hemoglobin—sickle cell anemia and the thalassemias respectively—might reflect a selective advantage conferred by such disorders in protecting against *Plasmodium falciparum* malaria in heterozygous individuals (Allison 1954b; Haldane 1949). Allison proposed that improved survival among carriers of the mutation (HbAS) in the face of *P. falciparum* exposure might confer an evolutionary advantage that could compensate for the early death of individuals affected by sickle cell anemia (HbSS). This hypothesis, now commonly referred to as the "malaria hypothesis", has since been confirmed by a range of clinical studies showing a remarkably high level of protection (>90 %) against severe and lethal malaria (Taylor et al. 2012). Although a wide range of other polymorphisms, including HbC, HbE, glucose-6-phosphate dehydrogenase (G6PD) deficiency and α-thalassemia and β-thalassemia, have also been shown to protect against malaria (Kwiatkowski 2005), a multicenter study based on nearly 12,000 cases of severe malaria and more than 17,000 controls, has recently confirmed the unique level of protection that is afforded by the HbS mutation (Rockett et al. 2014). Some of the proposed mechanisms for this

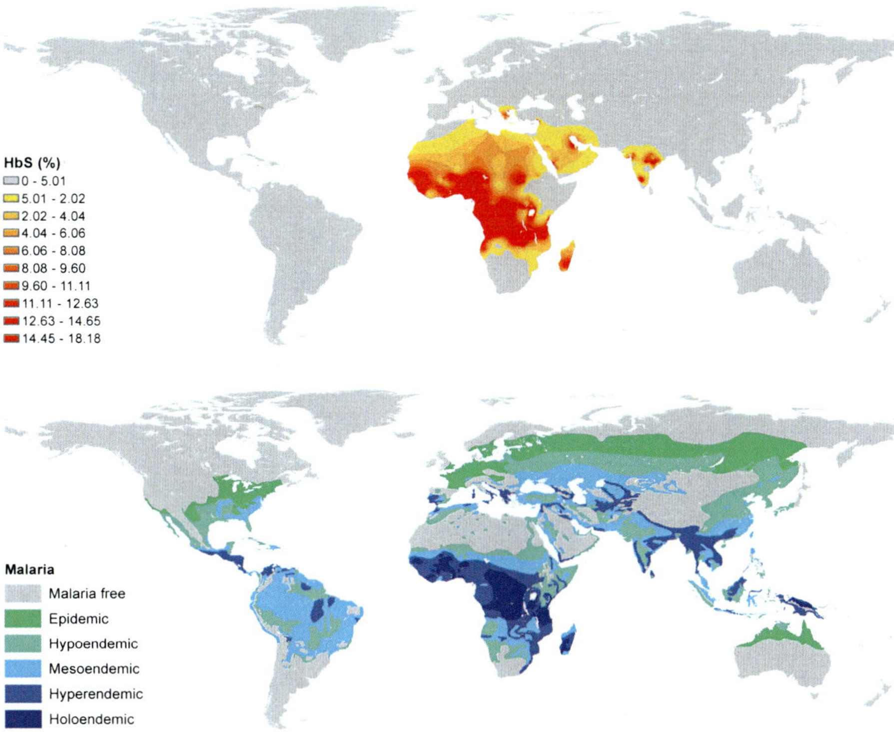

Fig. 2.1 (*Top*) Map of HbS allele frequency generated by a Bayesian model-based geostatistical framework; (*Bottom*) Historical map of malaria endemicity digitized from Lysenko and Semashko (1968). The classes are defined by parasite rates (PR_{2-10}, the proportion of 2- up to 10-year olds with the parasite in their peripheral blood): malaria free, $PR_{2-10} \approx 0$; epidemic, $PR_{2-10} \approx 0$; hypoendemic, $PR_{2-10} < 0.10$; mesoendemic, $PR_{2-10} \geq 0.10$ and <0.50; hyperendemic, $PR_{2-10} \geq 0.50$ and <0.75; holoendemic, $PR_{0-1} \geq 0.75$ (this class was measured in 0- up to 1-year olds). Adapted from Piel et al. (2010)

protection, which remain to be fully elucidated, are discussed below (see Sect. 2.1.3). In 2010, the geographical relationship between the frequency of the sickle cell allele and the level of transmission intensity of malaria was formally investigated and confirmed a strong relationship in Africa (Fig. 2.1) (Piel et al. 2010). The weak relationship found in India would benefit from further investigations, for example, on the role of social structure and *P. vivax* malaria.

2.1.3 Mechanisms of Malaria Protection

The full details of the cellular mechanisms by which HbAS protects against malaria are still unclear. Various hypotheses have been formulated, with more or less evidence supporting each of them, and it now seems increasingly likely that, rather than being explained by a single mechanism, a combination of mechanisms might well be at play (Lopez et al. 2010; Gong et al. 2013; Bunn 2013). Most proposals have so far involved innate immunity, i.e. the ability of host cells to resist infection by the parasite, irrespective of previous exposure. Although earlier studies suggested that HbAS might protect against parasitemia, more recent studies have shown that, rather than an absence of parasitemia, asymptomatic parasitemia was more common in HbAS children than in HbAA. The main mechanisms identified in vitro so far are:

Enhanced Removal (or "Suicide") of Parasitized Red Blood Cells Parasitized red blood cells have an increased (up to eight times) chance of sickling in HbAS than in HbAA individuals, which may enhance phagocytosis of infected red blood cells and, therefore, result in reduced parasitemia (Luzzatto et al. 1970; Roth et al. 1978; Ayi et al. 2004). This process might particularly affect red blood cells containing small parasite forms compared to larger trophozoite and schizont forms.

Impaired Growth of *P. falciparum* Parasites Under Low Oxygen Tension The rates of invasion and growth of *P. falciparum* parasites in individuals with the sickling disorders are markedly reduced under hypoxemic conditions (Pasvol et al. 1978). This reduction occurs even in the absence of morphologic sickling of the red blood cells. Impaired growth could be due to polymer-induced red blood cell dehydration (Griffiths et al. 2001) or to enhanced oxidant damage (Friedman 1979).

Decreased Rosette Formation Uninfected red blood cells can bind to *P. falciparum*-infected red blood cells, a process called rosette formation, which contributes to microcirculatory obstruction in cerebral malaria. Studies have found that modifications of the mechanical properties of red blood cells containing HbS under deoxygenated conditions result in a decreased ability to form rosettes. This mechanism would therefore be particularly protective against cerebral malaria (Carlson et al. 1994).

Reduced Cytoadherence Infected red blood cells express specific molecules on their surface. One such molecule, *P. falciparum* erythrocyte membrane protein 1 (*Pf*EMP-1), has been extensively studied (Cholera et al. 2008). This protein allows *P. falciparum*-infected red blood cells to adhere to the microvasculature endothelium, a process known as sequestration, and therefore to avoid clearance from the circulation by the spleen (Fairhurst et al. 2012). Sequestration can lead to endothelial activation and associated inflammation in the brain and other organs, and therefore contribute to the progression to severe malaria. *Pf*EMP-1 has been found to be reduced in HbAS red blood cells in comparison to HbAA red blood cells, and to be associated with reduced binding properties (Cholera et al. 2008; Opi et al. 2014). Reduced cytoadherence of HbAS and HbSS erythrocytes is likely to lead to increased splenic clearance, and may in part explain lower parasite densities and a lower incidence of severe malaria in HbAS individuals.

Accelerated Immunity Finally, Williams and colleagues recently hypothesized that an acquired immune response might also be part of the protective mechanisms. They found epidemiologic evidence of an increase in protection against malaria with age in HbAS Kenyan children. The protective effect of HbAS was increased by more than twofold between the ages of 2 and 10 years (Williams et al. 2005a).

2.1.4 Historical Distribution of the Sickle Mutation

Anthony C. Allison and Frank B. Livingstone were among the first to study the detailed distribution of the sickle mutation between the 1950s and the 1980s. Allison's work focused on sub-Saharan Africa for which he reported detailed surveys of tribes from Tanganyika (Tanzania), The Gambia, Sierra Leone, Nigeria and the Gold Coast (Ghana) (Allison 1956). He also reviewed and discussed the frequency of HbAS in different age groups based on published studies. This allowed him to estimate for the first time the fitness of each of the three genotypes (HbAA = 0.9511, HbAS = 1.1974, HbSS = 0.2029), estimates that supported the "malaria hypothesis" (see Sect. 2.1.2). Livingstone assembled the first global database of frequency data on hemoglobinopathies, G6PD deficiency and the Duffy blood group, compiling approximately 8000 frequencies from more than 2000 bibliographical references in the latest version of his work published in the mid-1980s (Livingstone 1985). He believed that his compilation would be useful in solving some of challenges in explaining the distributions of red blood cell disorders and in relating human genetic variation to human demographic, cultural, and epidemiological history. This unique resource was instrumental in the work later conducted by both Modell & Darlison and by Piel et al., in estimating the numbers of individuals born with HbS at national, regional and global scales (see Sect. 2.2.3) (Modell and Darlison 2008; Piel et al. 2013c).

Africa Through malaria selection, the sickle allele frequency reached 10 % in large parts of sub-Saharan Africa. A maximum allele frequency of about 18 % has been observed in pregnant women in Kaduna (Sadek 1974) and Abeokuta (Idowu et al. 2005), northern Angola (Fig. 2.1). Allele frequencies ranged between 1.5 and 12.1 % in southern Senegal, Guinea-Bissau, Guinea and Sierra Leone (Mauran-Sendrail et al. 1975; Trincao et al. 1950; Spivak et al. 1992). Frequencies were somewhat lower in Liberia, Burkina Faso and Côte d'Ivoire (Sansarricq et al. 1959; Bienzle et al. 1983; Devoucoux et al. 1991), where HbC frequencies are the highest (Livingstone 1976; Piel et al. 2013b), but increased again in Southern Ghana, Benin and Togo (Kreuels et al. 2008; Acquaye and Oldham 1973; Biondi et al. 1980; Bienzle et al. 1972). In Nigeria, frequencies of >10 % were seen in the southwest and northern central parts of the country (Sadek 1974; Odunvbun et al. 2008). Although limited surveys are available for the Democratic Republic of the Congo, data suggest that frequencies decrease from East (where they reach around 16 % near Kinshasa), to West (van den Berghe and Janssen 1950; Vandepitte and Motulsky

1956; Tshilolo et al. 2008). In Eastern Africa, the allele frequency for HbS is highest in historically malarious areas around Lake Victoria and along the coast (Foy et al. 1954; Allison 1954a; Enevold et al. 2007). In Madagascar, the overall frequency is approximately 1.5 % in the highland populations and 7.5 % in the lowland populations (Saugrain 1957; Hewitt et al. 1996). Frequencies of up to 2 % have been observed in North African populations including in Tunisia and Egypt (Selim et al. 1974; Fattoum 2006). HbS was historically absent from the Horn of Africa and from areas south of the Zambezi (Fig. 2.1).

The Mediterranean The sickle mutation is also present in parts of Greece, particularly in Khalkidhiki, and in southern Turkey, Lebanon and Israel (Aksoy 1961; Barnicot et al. 1963; Deliyannis and Tavlarakis 1955; Yuregir et al. 2001; Rachmilewitz et al. 1985).

The Middle East Frequencies up to 10 % are found in pockets within both the eastern and western coastal populations of Saudi Arabia, although frequencies are much lower in the rest of the country (Lehmann et al. 1963; Elhazmi and Warsy 1993; Elhazmi and Warsy 1987). Few data are available regarding the sickle prevalence in autochthonous populations from Iran and Pakistan (Farzana et al. 1975; Rahgozar et al. 2000).

India The sickle mutation has historically been confined to isolated tribal populations in which the sickle cell trait frequency ranges between 5 and 34 % (Shukla and Solanki 1958; Balgir 2006; Rao 1988; ICMR 2002; Colah et al. 2014). The mutation is thought to have been introduced into Southern India through migration of Dravidians from Nubia (Winters 2008).

HbS is not found in populations living further East than India (i.e. Southeast Asia and Australasia), or in indigenous populations in the Americas (Fig. 2.1).

2.1.5 Origin and Genetic Diversity

Anthropologists have long been interested in the origin of the HbS mutation. Two main hypotheses have been formulated since the 1980s. The first suggested that HbS arose just once in an isolated population and increased in frequency on a single haplotype. Through migration, the mutation was then exposed to populations with different haplotypic backgrounds and subsequently spread onto new haplotypes by gene conversion (Livingstone 1989a; Flint et al. 1993). The second hypothesis postulates that the current distribution of HbS has arisen from multiple independent mutations (Wainscoat 1987). The incredible developments of molecular biology in the late 1970s and 1980s, including the use of restriction fragment length polymorphism (RFLP) technology, favored the latter hypothesis (Kan and Dozy 1978). This method allowed for the definition of a range of haplotypes through the identification of different polymorphic sites in multiple African populations. Based on analysis of the β-globin gene cluster, Pagnier et al. suggested that three independent mutations had arisen in Senegal, the Central African Republic (CAR) and Benin (Pagnier et al. 1984), noting a remarkable homogeneity of the haplotypic background found in each of these populations. Subsequently, a survey of individuals from the eastern oases of Saudi Arabia and from the coast of India identified another haplotype, not found in African populations, consistent with a further independent occurrence, which was named the Arab-India haplotype (Kulozik et al. 1986). To date, it remains unclear whether the widespread distribution of this haplotype is related to historical population movements from the Middle East to India or vice versa. Finally, in the early 1990s, a French team identified yet another haplotype in members of the Eton ethnic group of Cameroon and argued that this supported a fourth independent African origin of the HbS mutation (Lapoumeroulie et al. 1992). Although many more haplotypes have been identified since then, all appear to be explained by genetic recombination. The five main haplotypes—Benin, Cameroon, CAR, Senegal and Arab-India—are often called "classical haplotypes", while less common haplotypes are usually termed "atypical haplotypes". Our knowledge of the distribution of both classical and atypical haplotypes remains relatively limited (Fig. 2.2).

To date, it has not been possible to firmly distinguish between the single and multi-centric origin hypotheses on the basis of genetic analyses (Antonarakis et al. 1984). Evidence cited in favor of multiple mutations includes the fact that the 5′ flanking region of the β-globin gene in African patients with sickle cell anemia displays a high level of population homogeneity, and that differences between any pair of the Benin, CAR and Senegal haplotypes occur both upstream and downstream to a putative recombination hotspot. Both of these observations remain consistent with new sickle cell haplotypes having arisen through gene conversion and then having rapidly increased in frequency through malaria-selection. Furthermore, the implicit assumption that the four independent mutations in Africa must have either appeared *de novo* within a short period of time, or have been part of the standing genetic variation when malaria selection began, is difficult to uphold—both scenarios are improbable given, respectively, the low mutation rate of a point mutation such as HbS and the deleterious nature of the HbS mutation in the absence of malaria selection.

Despite limitations to the multi-centric origin theory, efforts to explore the single-origin hypothesis have also been limited. Livingstone used a stochastic model of the diffusion of different HbA- and HbS-associated chromosomes to demonstrate that recombination and gene conversion readily give rise to multiple HbS haplotypes, with no need for recurrent mutation (Livingstone 1989b). He considered a linear meta-population in which the sickle mutation was introduced at a fixed point at the beginning of the simulation and explicitly modelled recombination between different haplotypic markers. He concluded that the single origin hypothesis was "*at least as plausible an explanation of the world distribution of this remarkable gene as is the assumption of several separate mutations, especially in Africa where the limited amount of S haplotype variation is more likely indicative of the recent diffusion of the S gene to these populations.*"

Various attempts have been made to date the HbS mutation, with published estimates ranging from 700 to 21,000 years ago based on Monte Carlo maximum

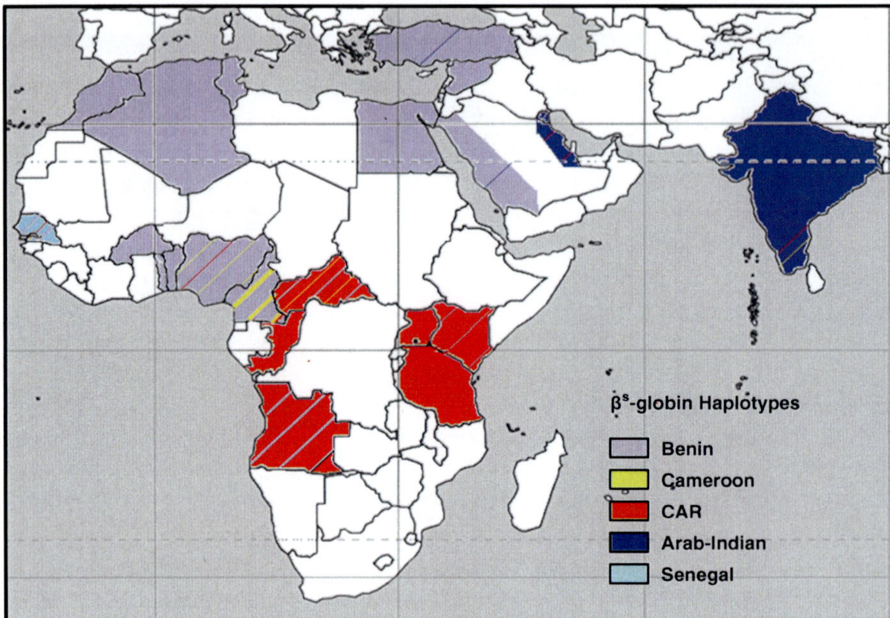

	β^S-associated haplotypes							β^S-associated haplotypes					
Country	Arab-Indian	Benin	Cameroon	CAR	Senegal	Other	Country	Arab-Indian	Benin	Cameroon	CAR	Senegal	Other
Angola	-	12.0	-	88.0	-	-	Eygypt	-	100.0	-	-	-	-
Benin	-	100.0	-	-	-	-	Morocco	-	100.0	-	-	-	-
Burkina Faso	-	100.0	-	-	-	-	Saudi Arabia	1.5	98.5	-	-	-	-
Cameroon	0.3	74.0	19.0	0.5	0.2	6.0	Saudi Arabia	94.0	-	-	4.0	-	2.0
CAR	-	6.9	3.4	82.8	3.4	3.5	Kuwait	77.8	16.7	-	-	-	-
Congo	-	-	-	91.0	-	9.0	Syria	-	100.0		-	-	-
Kenya	-	1.3	-	98.2	-	0.5	Tunisia	-	94.8	-	-	-	-
Nigeria	-	92.9	3.4	0.7	0.9	2.1	Turkey	0.4	96.3	-	-	-	3.3
Senegal	-	14.0	-	1.8	80.7	3.5	Turkey	-	100.0	-	-	-	-
Tanzania	-	-	-	100.0	-	-	India	100.0	-	-	-	-	-
Togo	-	100.0	-	-	-	-	India	90.7	-	-	-	-	9.3
Algeria	-	100.0	-	-	-	-	India	98.45	-	1.55	-	-	-
Uganda	-	-	-	99.5	0.5	-	India	91.67	-	2.78	1.39	-	4.17

Fig. 2.2 Distribution of the five major β-globin haplotypes (indicated by different *colors*) in individuals with sickle cell anemia in Sub-Saharan Africa, North Africa, Middle East and India. Haplotype data presented are summarized from genetic epidemiological studies of sickle-cell populations across different regions represented in the Table. For some countries, the Table presents data from different studies, of which some refer to different regions and study populations. CAR Central African Republic. Figure prepared from data obtained from Hockham et al. (2015), Gabriel and Przybylski (2010), Bitoungui et al. (2015) and from Nagel and Steinberg (2001) and references within each. Table adapted from Hockham et al. (2015) (with permission), references for each study are presented in the original table, with the exception of data for Cameroon, Uganda and Congo which were obtained from Bitoungui et al. (2015)

likelihood simulations for the Niokholo Mandenka populations of Senegal (Currat et al. 2002) and 70,000–150,000 years ago based on the association between the sickle variant of β-globin and a characteristic pattern of human platelet antigen (Hpa 1) recognition site (Kurnit 1979; Solomon and Bodmer 1979). It is usually considered that the frequency of the sickle mutation began to rise approximately 10,000 years ago following the developments of agriculture and human settlements which provided favorable conditions for malaria transmission (Wiesenfeld 1967) (see Sect. 2.1.2).

Using population dynamic modelling, Livingstone suggested that the rate of gene flow and population size were key parameters for dating the mutation and explaining its widespread distribution across sub-Saharan Africa, the Mediterranean, the Middle East and India (Livingstone 1969). Nevertheless, to our knowledge, phylogenetic studies and analyses of old DNA samples have so far provided limited support in dating the origin of the HbS mutation.

The severity of clinical complications in patients with sickle cell anemia varies widely. Soon after the various sickle cell haplotypes were identified, geneticists and clinicians attempted to explore relationships between haplotype and phenotype in patients with sickle cell anemia. Early on, it was suggested that the Arab-India haplotype was milder than the African haplotypes (Kulozik et al. 1986). This was later ascribed to the higher levels of HbF seen in patients with the Arab-India haplotype (Miller et al. 1987). Anecdotal observations later suggested that the Bantu haplotype was associated with a more severe clinical course, while patients with the Benin haplotype appeared to follow a milder clinical course (Steinberg 2005). Nevertheless, more recent studies conducted in Saudi Arabia and India have suggested that severe disease was more common than previously thought in patients with the Arab-India haplotype (Alsultan et al. 2014; Italia et al. 2015). Although, the frequency of some clinical complications associated with sickle cell anemia have also been reported to vary by haplotype (Adorno et al. 2008), a lack of systematic studies makes it difficult to confirm such relationships.

2.1.6 Epistatic Interactions

In recent years, interactions between different genes, termed epistatic interactions, have become increasingly relevant to a better understanding of the pathophysiology and geographic distribution of various genetic disorders, including hemoglobinopathies (Miko 2008). When gene interactions result in a milder phenotype, it is called "positive epistasis", while when they result in a more severe phenotype, they are termed "negative epistasis". In 2005, studying two cohorts of children in Kilifi District on the coast of Kenya, Williams and colleagues identified a remarkable example of negative epistasis by showing that the resistance conferred against malaria by HbAS was almost totally lost when co-inherited with α^+-thalassemia (Williams et al. 2005b) (Fig. 2.3). Further investigation into the underlying mechanisms of these interactions showed that, in individuals co-inheriting both HbAS and α^+-thalassemia, cytoadherence was not reduced, possibly due to a higher expression of PfEMP1, and the frequency of rosette formation was closer to that in normal HbAA individuals (Opi et al. 2014) (see Sect. 2.1.3). Interestingly, a recent study conducted among Cameroonians suggested that the phenotype and survival of patients with sickle cell anemia might be milder and improved, respectively, on co-inheritance with α-thalassemia (Rumaney et al. 2014).

Based on this clinical evidence, Penman et al. have used evolutionary mathematical models to support the idea that the complex distribution of hemoglobinopathies across Africa, the Mediterranean and South Asia can be explained by their specific

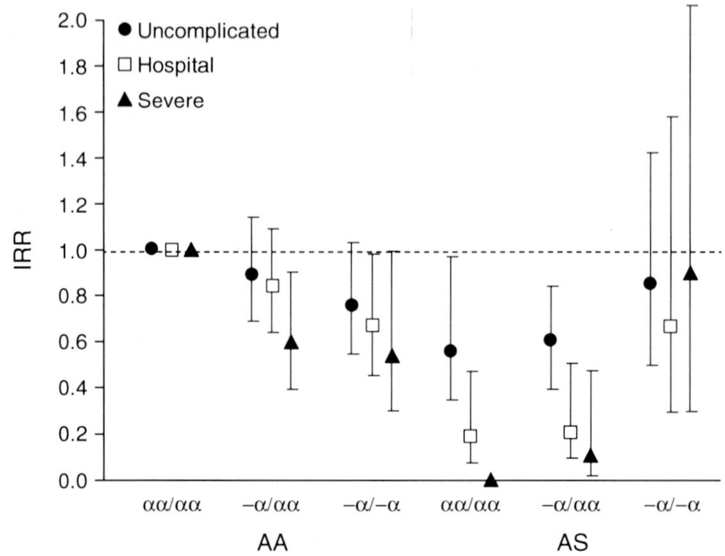

Fig. 2.3 Incidence rate ratio (IRR) of uncomplicated malaria, malaria requiring hospital admission and severe malaria for individuals with normal hemoglobin (AA) and the sickle cell trait (AS), with (one or two deletions: −α/αα and −α/−α, respectively) and without α^+-thalassemia (αα/αα). Reproduced with permission from (Williams et al. 2005b)

intracellular interactions. They suggest that the relative patchiness of the sickle mutation in the Mediterranean can be explained by interactions with α- and β-thalassemia, rather than a later introduction (Penman et al. 2009). In addition, by contrasting Southeast Asian and African populations, they hypothesized that the relatively low prevalence of α-thalassemia in Africa could be due to the presence of HbS (Penman et al. 2011).

2.2 Epidemiology

2.2.1 Contemporary Geographic Distribution

While natural selection shaped the historical distribution of the sickle mutation (see Sect. 2.1.4), its contemporary distribution has largely been driven by human diaspora (Cavalli-Sforza et al. 1994). Between the beginning of the sixteenth century and the end of the twentieth century, millions of Africans, mostly from West and Central Africa, were forced to move to the Caribbean and the Eastern coast of the Americas through the slave trade. This human traffic from areas of high prevalence of the sickle mutation to regions in which hemoglobinopathies were absent left a profound impact on populations of the Americas. The frequency of the HbS mutation in African Americans is often similar to those observed in the African subcontinent, resulting in sickle cell disease being the most common inherited blood disorder in the United States (Brousseau et al. 2010).

In recent decades, further expansion of the distribution of the sickle cell allele resulted from the globalization process (Roberts and de Montalembert 2007; Angastiniotis et al. 2013). This process has been the focus of a global retrospective quantitative study analyzing the number of migrants in 1960, 1970, 1980, 1990 and 2000 for all pairs of countries in relation to the prevalence of the sickle cell allele in the country of origin of the migrants (Piel et al. 2014b). It showed that, while the number of international migrants increased from 92.6 million in 1960 to 165.2 million in 2000, the estimated global number of migrants with HbS increased from about 1.6 million in 1960, to 3.6 million in 2000. This change was largely due to an increase in the number of migrants from countries with HbS allele frequencies of higher than 10 %, from 3.1 million in 1960, to 14.2 million in 2000. Additionally, the mean number of countries of origin for each destination country increased from 70 ± 46 in 1960, to 98 ± 48 in 2000, showing an increasing diversity in the network of international migrations between countries. This trend is well-illustrated, for example, by the case of Ireland where patients with sickle cell crises were very rarely seen by clinicians or registered with the Paediatric Haematology Service in the late 1990s but are relatively common nowadays, prompting the debate to implement a national newborn screening program for this disorder (McMahon et al. 2001).

As a result of these two processes, today, sickle cell disease is very much a global health problem and it seems likely that most countries now number carriers amongst their populations. Major changes in the global distribution of the HbS mutation are summarized by region below, and can be visualized by comparing Figs. 2.1 and 2.4. It is worth noting that due to both the presence of the HbS mutation in the Mediterranean region and to population admixture, sickle cell disorders occur in

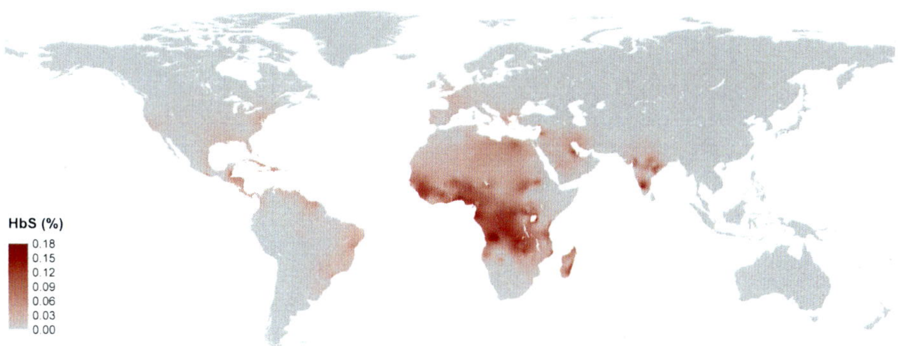

Fig. 2.4 Contemporary distribution and prevalence of the sickle cell allele. Adapted from (Piel et al. 2013c)

Caucasian individuals who have no known African ancestry. The assumption that sickle cell disorders only occur in Black populations, often leading to stigmatization, is therefore outdated.

The Americas In the United States, the vast majority of individuals carrying the sickle mutation are found in the eastern half of the country, which reflects the distribution of African Americans. Based on data from the National Newborn Screening Information System combined with population census data and corrected for early mortality, Hassell's population study suggested that the highest numbers of individuals with sickle cell disease were found in Florida, New York and Texas (Hassell 2010). The prevalence of HbS is substantially higher in California than in most states, falling in the Western half of the US. Overall, it is estimated that approximately one out of every 500 Black or African-American births are affected by sickle cell disease as are one out of every 36,000 Hispanic-American births. Approximately one in 12 Black or African Americans are carriers of the HbS allele. In Canada, HbS is mostly found in British Columbia, Ontario, Quebec and Nova Scotia. The birth prevalence of sickle cell anemia was found to be 1 in 2500 in the greater Montreal region and 1 in 134 in a targeted population in Quebec (Robitaille et al. 2006). In Brazil, the sickle mutation is common in the north-eastern region and the States of São Paulo, Rio de Janeiro and Minas Gerais. The prevalence of HbAS has been estimated to vary between 1.1 % in Rio Grande do Sul and 9.8 % in Bahia, while between 0.8 and 60 per 100,000 births are affected by sickle cell anemia (Lervolino et al. 2011).

The Caribbean Screening of 100,000 consecutive non-operative deliveries in the Jamaica Cohort Study conducted in the early 1980s found HbAS in 10.0 % (Serjeant et al. 1986). A follow up study conducted between 1995 and 2003 found similar frequencies, suggesting that the absence of malaria selection has not led to a decline in the frequency of the HbS allele in Jamaica (Hanchard et al. 2005). In Martinique, about 8 % of babies are born with HbAS while in Guadeloupe, the prevalence is one in 575 births, based on 27 years of universal newborn screening (Saint-Martin et al. 2013). Data from Aruba, St Maarten and Curacao found that 0.3, 0.7 and 2.2 newborns per year, respectively, were suffering from sickle cell anemia (van Heyningen et al. 2009).

Europe The prevalence of the sickle allele varies substantially within Europe, as well as within each European country, with a majority of cases being seen in capital cities in France (Paris) and the United Kingdom (London). In an epidemiological overview of hemoglobin disorders across Europe, Modell et al. estimated that sickle cell disorders occurred in 0 per 1000 newborns in eastern (Bulgaria and Romania) and parts of southern Europe (Malta and Former Yugoslavia), but in more than 0.3 per 1000 newborns in Albania (0.99), England and Wales (0.63), the Netherlands (0.32), Portugal (0.31) and France (0.30) (Modell et al. 2007). In Scandinavian countries and Germany, the estimated prevalence of sickle cell disorders ranged between 0.03 per 1000 births in Finland and 0.10 in Norway and Sweden.

Australasia Epidemiological data on sickle cell disease from Australia and New Zealand are relatively limited. Cases are rare, concentrated in large cities (particularly Sydney) (Harley and Concannon 1978) and are most commonly individuals of Greek or Italian ancestry (Wilkinson 1981).

2.2.2 *Mortality*

Data on mortality rates of sickle cell anemia patients are relatively limited, particularly in low- and middle-income countries. Based on a review of prospective cohort studies, age-stratified cross-sectional surveys and other cross-sectional surveys conducted in sub-Saharan Africa, Grosse et al. concluded that, although existing data were inadequate to support definitive statements, they were consistent with an early-life mortality of 50–90 % among children born in Africa with sickle cell anemia. Due to differences in access to health care and infectious disease control, it is likely that the mortality rate varies considerably between rural and urban areas. With substantial progress made towards the Millennium Development Goals (MDG), particularly in reducing childhood mortality (Rajaratnam et al. 2010), the situation of newborns with sickle cell anemia in low- and middle-income countries should progressively improve. Further studies are nevertheless necessary to quantify this impact. Appropriate measures are essential to provide adequate health care and to prevent clinical complications in sickle cell anemia patients surviving through childhood and adulthood (Piel et al. 2014a).

By contrast to the developing world, data on life expectancy of patients with sickle cell anemia for the United States are detailed and have allowed the tracking of substantial improvements in recent decades following the implementation of a range of interventions (see Sect. 2.2.6). Median age at death attributed to sickle cell anemia in 1967 was around 20 years old, primarily due to infections (Scott 1970). In the mid-1990s, the median age at death was 42 years for males and 48 years for females (Platt et al. 1994). Between the early 1980s and the late 1990s, it is estimated that mortality at age 0–3 years, 4–9 years and 10–14 years decreased by 68 %, 39 % and 24 %, respectively (Yanni et al. 2009). Similar trends have been observed in Jamaica (King et al. 2007). Despite these improvements, the life expectancy of patients with sickle cell anemia is still typically reduced by 20–30 years while, additionally, quality of life is substantially altered (Barakat et al. 2008; McClish et al. 2005). Furthermore, the financial costs of routine treatment and emergency care for these patients is huge (Kauf et al. 2009), to which social and psychological effects on both the patients and their families need to be added (Jenerette and Brewer 2010). Finally, recent data from the New York newborn screening program highlighted the fact that mortality rates were significantly lower among children of foreign-born mothers compared to US-born mothers, and significantly higher among preterm infants with low birth weight, which warrants further investigations on the impact of genetic and environmental factors (Wang et al. 2014).

2.2.3 Newborn and Population Estimates

Only a limited number of studies have so far attempted to estimate the number of newborns affected by sickle cell anemia and the number of carriers of the HbS allele on national, regional and global scales. With support from the World Health Organization (WHO), Modell and Darlison assembled a global epidemiological database for hemoglobin disorders by country and derived several service indicators to reflect the needs for care and prevention (Modell and Darlison 2008). Using demographic data from the 2003 United Nations Demographic Yearbook and correcting for consanguinity based on limited data from the Bittles's database (Bittles and Black 2014) and Murdock's ethnographic atlas (Murdock 1967), they estimated the number of annual births with sickle cell anemia at 222,785 worldwide, 83 % of which were occurring in the AFRO region. More recently, Piel et al. developed a novel Bayesian geo-statistical method to account for sub-national heterogeneities and to assess the uncertainty associated with the estimates (Patil et al. 2011). Using an updated database of epidemiological surveys, their global annual estimates for 2010 were 312,000 (inter-quartile range (IQR): 294,000–330,000) newborns with sickle cell anemia and 5,476,000 (IQR: 5,291,000–5,679,000) newborns with the sickle cell trait (Piel et al. 2013c). Regional estimates are presented in Table 2.1. Due to ongoing changes in the distribution of the HbS allele it is important to calculate new estimates at regular intervals in order to assess the current and future burdens of this disorder (see Sects. 2.2.1 and 2.2.5).

Population estimates for individuals affected by and carrying the sickle mutation are much harder to calculate, particularly on national, regional and global scales. This is well illustrated by the fact that despite having a universal newborn screening program in place and relatively good data on mortality, the number of individuals with sickle cell disease in the U.S. is unknown. Recent estimates based on birth-cohort disease prevalence ranged from 104,000 to 138,900, and between 72,000 and 98,000 when corrected for early mortality (Hassell 2010; Brousseau et al. 2010). Due mostly to limited availability of mortality data, similar estimates for other countries, particularly those with a high-prevalence or a high-burden for sickle cell disease, are currently missing.

Finally, hemoglobinopathies were recently included in the Global Burden of Diseases, Injuries, and Risk Factors Study (GBD). This project is the largest systematic effort yet to describe the global distribution and causes of a wide array of major diseases, injuries, and health risk factors. It estimated that, in 2010, sickle cell disorders accounted for 0.42 deaths per 100,000; 28.69 years of life lost (YLLs) per 100,000 and 53.21 years lived with disability (YLDs) per 100,000, adding up to 81.9 disability-adjusted life years (DALYs) per 100,000 (Murray et al. 2012b). Although these estimates have large uncertainties associated with them and need to be interpreted with caution, they allow the comparison of the burden of sickle cell disorders with those of other communicable and non-communicable diseases (Murray et al. 2012a).

Table 2.1 Regional estimates of newborns affected by sickle cell anemia (HbSS) and carrying sickle cell trait (HbAS)

	Population[a]	CBR[b]	HbAS newborns/year					HbSS newborns/year					
			Mean	Median	*IQR*[c]		%	Mean	Median	*IQR*[c]		%	M&D[d]
WHO regions[e]													
AFRO	888,817	0.0357	3,607,022	3,610,851	*3,498,595*	*3,704,303*	64.2	239,547	238,083	*224,003*	*253,047*	75.4	184,812**
AMRO	939,833	0.0162	398,279	391,257	*358,199*	*435,894*	7.6	13,708	13,104	*11,126*	*15,606*	4.6	4432**
EMRO	560,803	0.0249	275,365	256,643	*199,839*	*327,983*	5.7	10,007	8239	*6012*	*11,951*	3.6	7389
EURO	893,002	0.0123	127,494	121,601	*99,414*	*147,505*	2.6	3653	3271	*2408*	*4366*	1.3	376**
SEARO	1,789,082	0.0200	1,040,033	1,020,489	*900,452*	*1,154,480*	20.0	44,132	42,597	*35,022*	*50,750*	15.1	25,768**
WPRO	1,840,667	0.0128	2292	1150	*477*	*2374*	0.0	4	9	*2*	*33*	0.0	9
HbS regions													
Americas	939,724	0.0162	389,892	386,430	*349,253*	*425,791*	7.4	13,309	12,802	*10,869*	*15,210*	4.6	/
Arab-India	1,771,305	0.0219	1,168,805	1,147,477	*1,010,443*	*1,299,147*	22.7	48,951	46,826	*39,147*	*56,000*	16.9	/
Eurasia	1,098,104	0.0139	271,474	256,163	*216,499*	*310,758*	5.4	8784	7493	*5919*	*10,090*	3.0	/
Southeast Asia	2,215,004	0.0133	4854	2535	*1324*	*5171*	0.1	80	21	*7*	*63*	0.0	/
Sub-Saharan Africa	888,065	0.0365	3,579,982	3,580,207	*3,473,117*	*3,684,718*	64.4	237,253	235,681	*220,993*	*250,568*	75.5	/

Adapted from Piel et al. (2013c)

[a]In thousands

[b]Crude birth rate

[c]Interquartile range

[d]SS newborn estimates from Modell and Darlison (2008). A double asterisk (**) indicates M&D estimates falling outside our 90 % credible interval

[e]*AFRO* Regional Office for Africa, *AMRO* Regional Office for the Americas, *EMRO* Regional Office for the Eastern Mediterranean Countries, *EURO* Regional Office for Europe, *SEARO* Regional Office for South-East Asia, *WPRO* Regional Office for the Western Pacific

2.2.4 Screening Programs

Newborn screening programs allow for early diagnosis, parental education and comprehensive care, which results in a marked impact on mortality and morbidity throughout infancy, childhood and adulthood (see Sect. 2.2.2).

The United States was the first country to implement large scale universal newborn screening programs, starting as early as 1975 across New York State, following the enactment of the Sickle Cell Anemia Control Act in 1972, and resulting in required newborn screening programs in all 50 states and the District of Columbia by 2006 (Benson and Therrell 2010). Data management by each state makes it challenging to get an accurate picture at the national level, although various initiatives have recently aimed at bridging this gap (e.g. RuSH's CDC project[1]).

In the United Kingdom, the National Health Service (NHS) implemented a linked antenatal and universal newborn screening program for sickle cell disease in 2004 with the aim of achieving the lowest possible childhood death rate and to minimize childhood morbidity from sickle cell disease (Streetly et al. 2009). This program has resulted in substantial improvements in the detection rate of sickle cell disorders in the UK. Nevertheless, the impact of this program on the prevalence of these disorders remains unclear (Streetly and Rees 2013). France has chosen to implement a targeted screening program based on populations at risks, while universal screening is performed in its overseas territories (Bardakdjian-Michau et al. 2009). Although it could be argued that this option is more cost-effective than universal screening, it raises complex ethical issues including the objectivity of selection criteria potentially resulting in discrimination and stigmatization of populations affected (Panepinto et al. 2000). Other European countries, including Belgium and Italy, have effective local screening programs but lack national policies (Gulbis et al. 2009; Ballardini et al. 2013).

Both newborn screening and premarital screening have been implemented in the Middle East, often resulting in substantial decreases in the prevalence of sickle cell anemia at birth. In Saudi Arabia, policies including compulsory screening, genetic counselling and optional marriage cancellations for couples at risk have contributed to lowering the birth rate of children with sickle cell disease, although such policies seemed to have had a more pronounced impact on the prevention of β-thalassemia than on sickle cell disease between 2004 and 2009 (Memish and Saeedi 2011). In Bahrain, the birth prevalence of sickle cell disease declined from 2.1 % in 1985 to 0.4 % in 2010 (Al Arrayed and Al Hajeri 2012).

No African country has so far implemented a large-scale universal screening program for sickle cell disorders. Various local programs have been launched, including in Benin, Ghana, Kenya, Tanzania and The Democratic Republic of the Congo (DRC) (Makani et al. 2015; Ohene-Frempong et al. 2008; Tshilolo et al. 2009; Rahimy et al. 2009; William et al. 2009). Considering the large burden associated with this disease, particularly in Nigeria and the DRC, appropriate policies are urgently needed in sub-Saharan Africa.

[1] http://www.cdc.gov/ncbddd/hemoglobinopathies/rush.html.

Finally, awareness about sickling disorders has substantially increased in India in recent years and this has led to the launch of various screening initiatives, for example in Chhattisgarh (Patra et al. 2011; Panigrahi et al. 2012), Gujarat (Patel et al. 2013) and Maharashtra (Jain et al. 2012). While these initiatives are still very recent, they will hopefully result in the release of a large amount of epidemiological data in the near future, allowing further studies of the natural history of this disease and the development of effective and appropriate models of care (Patel and Serjeant 2014).

2.2.5 *Future Burden*

Various publications have suggested that the global burden of hemoglobinopathies has been increasing and that appropriate public health policies need to be developed accordingly (Weatherall and Clegg 2001; Weatherall 2010, 2011a, b). In low- and middle-income countries, in which the prevalence of sickle cell disorders is high, this increase is due to the epidemiologic transition, which involves a shift from high infant and child mortality caused by infectious diseases to lower mortality caused by non-communicable diseases. Practically, this means that newborns affected by sickle cell anemia were previously dying undiagnosed in early life. Due to better health care and access to health facilities, a substantial proportion of these newborns are now surviving to adulthood. Early diagnosis is essential for preventing severe complications and adequate counselling is needed to inform patients' parents about the risks for the offspring once they reach reproductive age. This alarming situation has been described in detail for Nigeria (Akinyanju 2010). In high-income countries, the increasing health burden caused by hemoglobinopathies is due to large population movements from areas of high prevalence to low-prevalence areas, as described in detail in Sect. 2.2.1 of this chapter. The recent impact of sickle cell disorders in high-income countries is best illustrated by the implementation of universal newborn screening programs for sickle cell disorders in various countries including the USA and the UK (see Sect. 2.2.4).

In order to define appropriate public health policies in relation to hemoglobinopathies, it is nevertheless essential to quantify the magnitude of this increase. In order to do this, Piel et al. combined national allele frequency estimates for sickle cell anemia with demographic projections for 2010–2050. The study concluded that it was likely that Nigeria (2010: 91,000 newborns with SCA [confidence interval (CI): 77,900–106,100]; 2050: 140,800 [CI: 95,500–200,600]) and the Democratic Republic of the Congo (2010: 39,700 [CI: 32,600–48,800]; 2050: 44,700 [CI: 27,100–70,500]) would remain the countries most in need of policies for the prevention and management of SCA, and predicted a decrease in the annual number of newborns with SCA in India (2010: 44,400 [CI: 33,700–59,100]; 2050: 33,900 [CI: 15,900–64,700]) (Piel et al. 2013a). Furthermore, it suggested that the implementation of basic health interventions for SCA in 2015, including prenatal diagnosis, penicillin prophylaxis, and vaccination, could lead to significant reductions in excess mortality among children under-five with SCA. By 2050, this would result in prolonging the lives of 5,302,900 [CI: 3,174,800–6,699,100] newborns with SCA. Similarly, the implementation of large-scale universal screening programs could save the lives of up to 9,806,000 (CI: 6,745,800–14,232,700) newborns with SCA globally, 85 % (CI: 81–88 %) of whom will be born in sub-Saharan Africa (Piel et al. 2013a). Rigorous epidemiological evaluation of the impact of implementing such interventions through time is necessary to confirm the accuracy of such projections based on demographic data.

2.2.6 Public Health Interventions

There is currently no cure for sickle cell anemia. Existing treatments and future options, including stem cell transplant and gene therapy, are described in detail in Chaps. 15 and 16, respectively.

Systematic use of penicillin prophylaxis and pneumococcal conjugate vaccines has resulted in remarkable improvement in the survival of children with sickle cell anemia in high-income countries (Gaston et al. 1986; Telfer et al. 2007). Similar impact has been found in more resource-limited settings, particularly in Jamaica (King et al. 2007). Although education is usually considered to have a limited impact, parental education on the detection of enlarged spleens and need for medical attention was found to have an important effect in Jamaica.

More recently, hydroxyurea, a drug boosting the level of HbF in patients with sickle cell anemia (Platt et al. 1984), appeared as a safe and effective drug for preventive therapy in adult patients (Charache et al. 1995). Safety trials were later conducted in adolescents and children with positive results (Scott et al. 1996; Kinney et al. 1999). Despite some studies suggesting that the use of hydroxyurea can lead to fertility problems or increased frequency of malignancies, current evidence suggests that the benefits of this drug far outweigh these potential risks (Ware 2010).

Awareness about the disease is a key element to preventing and managing it. Although positive advances have been made towards this goal, including the recognition by the WHO in 2006 of sickle cell disease as a worldwide public health issue and the adoption of a resolution on the prevention and management of birth defects, including those resulting from sickle cell disease, at the 63rd World Health Assembly, the real impact of these events is hard to assess, particularly from the perspective of patients living in resource-poor regions.

References

Acquaye CT, Oldham JH (1973) Variants of haemoglobin and glucose-6-phosphate dehydrogenase-I. distribution in Southern Ghana. Ghana Med J 12(4):412–418

Adorno EV, Zanette A, Lyra I, Seixas MO, Reis MG, Goncalves MS (2008) Clinical and molecular characteristics of sickle cell anemia in the northeast of Brazil. Genet Mol Biol 31(3):621–625

Akinyanju O (2010) The national burden of sickle cell disorder and the way forward http://www.sicklecellfoundation.com/wp-content/uploads/2015/05/Nat-Burden-SCD.pdf
Aksoy M (1961) Hemoglobin S in Eti-Turks and the Allewits in Lebanon. Blood 17:657–659
Al Arrayed S, Al Hajeri A (2012) Newborn screening services in Bahrain between 1985 and 2010. Adv Hematol 2012:903219
Allison AC (1954a) The distribution of the sickle-cell trait in East Africa and elsewhere, and its apparent relationship to the incidence of subtertian malaria. Trans R Soc Trop Med Hyg 48(4):312–318
Allison AC (1954b) Notes on sickle-cell polymorphism. Ann Hum Genet 19(1):39–51
Allison AC (1956) The sickle-cell and haemoglobin C genes in some African populations. Ann Hum Genet 21(1):67–89
Alsultan A, Alabdulaali MK, Griffin PJ et al (2014) Sickle cell disease in Saudi Arabia: the phenotype in adults with the Arab-Indian haplotype is not benign. Br J Haematol 164(4): 597–604
Angastiniotis M, Vives Corrons J-L, Soteriades ES, Eleftheriou A (2013) The impact of migrations on the health services for rare diseases in Europe: the Example of haemoglobin disorders. Sci World J 2013:727905
Antonarakis SE, Boehm CD, Serjeant GR, Theisen CE, Dover GJ, Kazazian HH Jr (1984) Origin of the beta S-globin gene in blacks: the contribution of recurrent mutation or gene conversion or both. Proc Natl Acad Sci U S A 81(3):853–856
Ayi K, Turrini F, Piga A, Arese P (2004) Enhanced phagocytosis of ring-parasitized mutant erythrocytes: a common mechanism that may explain protection against falciparum malaria in sickle trait and beta-thalassemia trait. Blood 104(10):3364–3371
Balgir R (2006) Genetic heterogeneity of population structure in 15 major scheduled tribes in central-eastern India: a study of immuno-hematological disorders. Indian J Hum Genet 12(2):86–92
Ballardini E, Tarocco A, Marsella M et al (2013) Universal neonatal screening for sickle cell disease and other haemoglobinopathies in Ferrara, Italy. Blood Transfus 11(2):245–249
Barakat L, Patterson C, Daniel L, Dampier C (2008) Quality of life among adolescents with sickle cell disease: mediation of pain by internalizing symptoms and parenting stress. Health Qual Life Outcomes 6(1):60
Bardakdjian-Michau J, Bahuau M, Hurtrel D et al (2009) Neonatal screening for sickle cell disease in France. J Clin Pathol 62(1):31–33
Barnicot NA, Allison AC, Blumberg BS, Deliyannis G, Krimbas C, Ballas A (1963) Haemoglobin types in Greek populations. Ann Hum Genet 26:229–236
Benson JM, Therrell BL Jr (2010) History and current status of newborn screening for hemoglobinopathies. Semin Perinatol 34(2):134–144
Bienzle U, Okoye VC, Gogler H (1972) Haemoglobin and glucose-6-phosphate dehydrogenase variants: distribution in relation to malaria endemicity in a Togolese population. Z Tropenmed Parasitol 23(1):56–62
Bienzle U, Komp H, Feldheim M, Reimer A, Steffen E, Guggenmoos-Holzmann I (1983) The distribution and interaction of haemoglobin variants and the beta thalassaemia gene in Liberia. Hum Genet 63(4):400–403
Biondi G, Calandra PL, Coppa A, Falcone G, Rickards O, Vecchi F (1980) Distribution of the S and C hemoglobins in Atakora District (Benin). Hum Biol 52(2):205–213
Bitoungui, V. J., Pule, G. D., Hanchard, N., Ngogang, J., & Wonkam, A. (2015). Beta-globin gene haplotypes among cameroonians and review of the global distribution: Is there a case for a single sickle mutation origin in Africa? *OMICS, 19*(3), 171–179.
Bittles AH, Black ML (2014) Global patterns and tables of consanguinity. http://consang.net
Brousseau DC, Panepinto JA, Nimmer M, Hoffmann RG (2010) The number of people with sickle-cell disease in the United States: national and state estimates. Am J Hematol 85(1): 77–78
Bunn HF (2013) The triumph of good over evil: protection by the sickle gene against malaria. Blood 121(1):20–25

Carlson J, Nash GB, Gabutti V, al-Yaman F, Wahlgren M (1994) Natural protection against severe Plasmodium falciparum malaria due to impaired rosette formation. Blood 84(11):3909–3914

Cavalli-Sforza LL, Menozzi P, Piazza A (1994) The history and geography of human genes. Princeton University Press, Princeton

Charache S, Terrin ML, Moore RD et al (1995) Effect of hydroxyurea on the frequency of painful crises in sickle cell anemia. Investigators of the Multicenter Study of Hydroxyurea in Sickle Cell Anemia. N Engl J Med 332(20):1317–1322

Cholera R, Brittain NJ, Gillrie MR et al (2008) Impaired cytoadherence of Plasmodium falciparum-infected erythrocytes containing sickle hemoglobin. Proc Natl Acad Sci U S A 105(3): 991–996

Colah R, Mukherjee M, Ghosh K (2014) Sickle cell disease in India. Curr Opin Hematol 21(3): 215–223

Currat M, Trabuchet G, Rees D et al (2002) Molecular analysis of the beta-globin gene cluster in the Niokholo Mandenka population reveals a recent origin of the beta(S) Senegal mutation. Am J Hum Genet 70(1):207–223

Deliyannis GA, Tavlarakis N (1955) Sickling phenomenon in Northern Greece. Br Med J 2(4934):299–301

Devoucoux R, Hurpin C, Baudon D et al (1991) Population genetics of abnormal haemoglobins in Burkina Faso, west Africa. Ann Hum Biol 18(4):295–302

Elhazmi MAF, Warsy AS (1987) Interaction between glucose-6-phosphate-dehydrogenase deficiency and sickle-cell gene in Saudi-Arabia. Trop Geogr Med 39(1):32–35

Elhazmi MAF, Warsy AS (1993) The frequency of Hbs and glucose-6-phosphate-dehydrogenase phenotypes in relation to malaria in Western Saudi-Arabia. Saudi Med J 14(2):121–125

Enevold A, Alifrangis M, Sanchez JJ et al (2007) Associations between alpha(+)-thalassemia and Plasmodium falciparum malarial infection in northeastern Tanzania. J Infect Dis 196(3): 451–459

Fairhurst RM, Bess CD, Krause MA (2012) Abnormal PfEMP1/knob display on Plasmodium falciparum-infected erythrocytes containing hemoglobin variants: fresh insights into malaria pathogenesis and protection. Microbes Infect 14(10):851–862

Farzana F, Zuberi SJ, Hashmi JA (1975) Prevalence of abnormal hemoglobin and thalassemia trait in a group of professional blood donors and hospital staff in Karachi. J Pak Med Assoc 25(9):237–239

Fattoum S (2006) Hemoglobinopathies in Tunisia. An updated review of the epidemiologic and molecular data. Tunis Med 84(11):687–696

Flint J, Harding RM, Boyce AJ, Clegg JB (1993) The population genetics of the haemoglobinopathies. Baillieres Clin Haematol 6(1):215–262

Foy H, Kondi A, Timms GL, Brass W, Bushra F (1954) The variability of sickle-cell rates in the tribes of Kenya and the Southern Sudan. Br Med J 1(4857):294–297

Friedman MJ (1979) Oxidant damage mediates variant red cell resistance to malaria. Nature 280(5719):245–247

Gabriel A, Przybylski J (2010) Sickle-cell anemia: A Look at Global Haplotype Distribution. Nat Educ 3(3):2

Gaston MH, Verter JI, Woods G et al (1986) Prophylaxis with oral penicillin in children with sickle cell anemia. N Engl J Med 314(25):1593–1599

Gong L, Parikh S, Rosenthal PJ, Greenhouse B (2013) Biochemical and immunological mechanisms by which sickle cell trait protects against malaria. Malar J 12:317

Griffiths MJ, Ndungu F, Baird KL et al (2001) Oxidative stress and erythrocyte damage in Kenyan children with severe Plasmodium falciparum malaria. Br J Haematol 113(2):486–491

Gulbis B, Cotton F, Ferster A et al (2009) Neonatal haemoglobinopathy screening in Belgium. J Clin Pathol 62(1):49–52

Haldane JBS (1949) The rate of mutation of human genes. Hereditas 35(S1):267–273

Hanchard NA, Hambleton I, Harding RM, McKenzie CA (2005) The frequency of the sickle allele in Jamaica has not declined over the last 22 years. Br J Haematol 130(6):939–942

Harley JD, Concannon AJ (1978) Eleven cases of sickle cell disease in Sydney. Med J Aust 2(9):401–404

Hassell KL (2010) Population estimates of sickle cell disease in the U.S. Am J Prev Med 38 (4 Suppl):S512–S521

Herrick JB (1910) Peculiar elongated and sickle-shaped red blood corpuscles in a case of severe anemia. Arch Intern Med 6(5):517–521

Hewitt R, Krause A, Goldman A, Campbell G, Jenkins T (1996) Beta-globin haplotype analysis suggests that a major source of Malagasy ancestry is derived from Bantu-speaking Negroids. Am J Hum Genet 58(6):1303–1308

Hockham, C., Piel, F. B., Gupta, S., & Penman, B. S. (2015). Understanding the contrasting spatial haplotype patterns of malaria-protective β-globin polymorphisms. *Infection, Genetics and Evolution, 36*, 174–183. doi:10.1016/j.meegid.2015.09.018.

ICMR (2002) Sickle cell anemia control project, Government of Gujarat. Sickle cell anaemia control project. Ahmedabad: Govt. of Gujarat; 2012. Available at: http://www.academia.edu/4913389/Sickle_Cell_Anemia_Control_Project

Idowu OA, Mafiana CF, Dapo S (2005) Anaemia in pregnancy: a survey of pregnant women in Abeokuta, Nigeria. Afr Health Sci 5(4):295–299

Italia K, Kangne H, Shanmukaiah C, Nadkarni AH, Ghosh K, Colah RB (2015) Variable phenotypes of sickle cell disease in India with the Arab-Indian haplotype. Br J Haematol 168(1): 156–159

Jain DL, Sarathi V, Upadhye D et al (2012) Newborn screening shows a high incidence of sickle cell anemia in Central India. Hemoglobin 36(4):316–322

Jenerette CM, Brewer C (2010) Health-related stigma in young adults with sickle cell disease. J Natl Med Assoc 102(11):1050–1055

Kan YW, Dozy AM (1978) Polymorphism of DNA sequence adjacent to human beta-globin structural gene: relationship to sickle mutation. Proc Natl Acad Sci U S A 75(11):5631–5635

Kauf TL, Coates TD, Huazhi L, Mody-Patel N, Hartzema AG (2009) The cost of health care for children and adults with sickle cell disease. Am J Hematol 84(6):323–327

King L, Fraser R, Forbes M, Grindley M, Ali S, Reid M (2007) Newborn sickle cell disease screening: the Jamaican experience (1995–2006). J Med Screen 14(3):117–122

Kinney TR, Helms RW, O'Branski EE et al (1999) Safety of hydroxyurea in children with sickle cell anemia: results of the HUG-KIDS study, a phase I/II Trial. Blood 94(5):1550–1554

Kreuels B, Kobbe R, Adjei S et al (2008) Spatial variation of malaria incidence in young children from a geographically homogeneous area with high endemicity. J Infect Dis 197(1):85–93

Kulozik AE, Wainscoat JS, Serjeant GR et al (1986) Geographical survey of beta S-globin gene haplotypes: evidence for an independent Asian origin of the sickle-cell mutation. Am J Hum Genet 39(2):239–244

Kurnit D (1979) Evolution of sickle variant gene. Lancet 1(8107):104

Kwiatkowski DP (2005) How malaria has affected the human genome and what human genetics can teach us about malaria. Am J Hum Genet 77(2):171–192

Lapoumeroulie C, Dunda O, Ducrocq R et al (1992) A novel sickle-cell mutation of yet another origin in Africa - the Cameroon type. Hum Genet 89(3):333–337

Lehmann H, Maranjian G, Mourant AE (1963) Distribution of sickle-cell hemoglobin in Saudi Arabia. Nature 198:492–493

Lervolino LG, Baldin PEA, Picado SM, Calil KB, Viel AA, Campos LAF (2011) Prevalence of sickle cell disease and sickle cell trait in national neonatal screening studies. Rev Bras Hematol Hemoter 33(1):49–54

Livingstone FB (1969) Gene frequency clines of the beta-hemoglobin locus in various human populations and their simulation by models involving differential selection. Hum Biol 41(2):223–236

Livingstone FB (1976) Hemoglobin history in West Africa. Hum Biol 48(3):487–500

Livingstone FB (1985) Frequencies of hemoglobin variants. Thalassemia, the glucose-6-phosphate dehydrogenase deficiency, G6PD variants, and ovalocytosis in human populations. Oxford University Press, New York

Livingstone FB (1989a) Simulation of the diffusion of the beta-globin variants in the Old World. Hum Biol 61(3):297–309

Livingstone FB (1989b) Who gave whom hemoglobin S: the use of restriction site haplotype variation for the interpretation of the evolution of the βS-globin gene. Am J Hum Biol 1(3):289–302

Lopez C, Saravia C, Gomez A, Hoebeke J, Patarroyo MA (2010) Mechanisms of genetically-based resistance to malaria. Gene 467(1–2):1–12

Luzzatto L, Nwachuku-Jarrett ES, Reddy S (1970) Increased sickling of parasitised erythrocytes as mechanism of resistance against malaria in the sickle-cell trait. Lancet 1(7642):319–321.

Lysenko AJ, Semashko IN (1968) In: Lebedew AW (ed) Itogi Nauki: Medicinskaja Geografija. Academy of Sciences, USSR, pp 25–146

Makani J, Soka D, Rwezaula S, Krag M, Mghamba J, Ramaiya K, Cox SE, Grosse SD (2015) Health policy for sickle cell disease in Africa: experience from Tanzania on interventions to reduce under-five mortality. Trop Med Int Health 20(2):184–187

Mason VR (1922) Sickle cell anemia. J Am Med Assoc 79(16):1318–1320

Mauran-Sendrail A, Bouloux C, Gomila J, Langaney A (1975) Comparative study of haemoglobin types of two populations of eastern Senegal--Bedik and Niokholonko. Ann Hum Biol 2(2):129–136

McClish D, Penberthy L, Bovbjerg V et al (2005) Health related quality of life in sickle cell patients: the PiSCES project. Health Qual Life Outcomes 3(1):50

McMahon C, Callaghan CO, O'Brien D, Smith OP (2001) The increasing prevalence of childhood sickle-cell disease in Ireland. Ir J Med Sci 170(3):183–185

Memish ZA, Saeedi MY (2011) Six-year outcome of the national premarital screening and genetic counseling program for sickle cell disease and beta-thalassemia in Saudi Arabia. Ann Saudi Med 31(3):229–235

Miko I (2008) Epistasis: gene interaction and phenotype effects. Nat Educ 1(1):197

Miller BA, Olivieri N, Salameh M et al (1987) Molecular analysis of the high-hemoglobin-F phenotype in Saudi Arabian sickle cell anemia. N Engl J Med 316(5):244–250

Modell B, Darlison M (2008) Global epidemiology of haemoglobin disorders and derived service indicators. Bull World Health Organ 86(6):480–487

Modell B, Darlison M, Birgens H et al (2007) Epidemiology of haemoglobin disorders in Europe: an overview. Scand J Clin Lab Invest 67(1):39–70

Murdock GP (1967) Ethnographic atlas. University of Pittsburgh Press, Pittsburgh

Murray CJ, Ezzati M, Flaxman AD et al (2012a) GBD 2010: a multi-investigator collaboration for global comparative descriptive epidemiology. Lancet 380(9859):2055–2058

Murray CJ, Vos T, Lozano R et al (2012b) Disability-adjusted life years (DALYs) for 291 diseases and injuries in 21 regions, 1990–2010: a systematic analysis for the Global Burden of Disease Study 2010. Lancet 380(9859):2197–2223

Nagel, R. L., & Steinberg, M. H. (2001). Genetics of the βs gene: Origins, epidemiology and epistasis. In M. H. Steinberg, B. G. Forget, D. R. Higgs, & D. J. Weatherall (Eds.), *Disorders of Hemoglobin: Genetics, Pathophysiology and Clinical Management* (pp. 711–755). Cambridge, MA: Cambridge University Press.

Nzewi E (2001) Malevolent ogbanje: recurrent reincarnation or sickle cell disease? Soc Sci Med 52(9):1403–1416

Odunvbun ME, Okolo AA, Rahimy CM (2008) Newborn screening for sickle cell disease in a Nigerian hospital. Public health 122(10):111–116

Ohene-Frempong K, Oduro J, Tetteh H, Nkrumah F (2008) Screening newborns for sickle cell disease in Ghana. Paediatrics 121(2 Suppl):S120–S121

Opi DH, Ochola LB, Tendwa M et al (2014) Mechanistic studies of the negative epistatic malaria-protective Interaction between sickle cell trait and α+thalassemia. EBioMedicine 1:29–36

Pagnier J, Mears JG, Dunda-Belkhodja O et al (1984) Evidence for the multicentric origin of the sickle cell hemoglobin gene in Africa. Proc Natl Acad Sci U S A 81(6):1771–1773

Panepinto JA, Magid D, Rewers MJ, Lane PA (2000) Universal versus targeted screening of infants for sickle cell disease: a cost-effectiveness analysis. J Pediatr 136(2):201–208

Panigrahi S, Patra PK, Khodiar PK (2012) Neonatal screening of sickle cell anemia: a preliminary report. Indian J Pediatr 79(6):747–750

Pasvol G, Weatherall DJ, Wilson RJ (1978) Cellular mechanism for the protective effect of haemoglobin S against P. falciparum malaria. Nature 274(5672):701–703

Patel J, Serjeant G (2014) Newborn screening for sickle cell disease in India: the need for defining optimal clinical care. Indian J Pediatr 81(3):229–230

Patel J, Patel B, Gamit N, Serjeant GR (2013) Screening for the sickle cell gene in Gujarat, India: a village-based model. J Community Genet 4(1):43–47

Patil AP, Gething PW, Piel FB, Hay SI (2011) Bayesian geostatistics in health cartography: the perspective of malaria. Trends Parasitol 27(6):246–253

Patra PK, Chauhan VS, Khodiar PK, Dalla AR, Serjeant GR (2011) Screening for the sickle cell gene in Chhattisgarh state, India: an approach to a major public health problem. J Community Genet 2(3):147–151

Penman BS, Pybus OG, Weatherall DJ, Gupta S (2009) Epistatic interactions between genetic disorders of hemoglobin can explain why the sickle-cell gene is uncommon in the Mediterranean. Proc Natl Acad Sci U S A 106(50):21242–21246

Penman BS, Habib S, Kanchan K, Gupta S (2011) Negative epistasis between alpha + thalassaemia and sickle cell trait can explain interpopulation variation in South Asia. Evolution 65(12): 3625–3632

Piel FB, Patil AP, Howes RE, Nyangiri OA et al (2010) Global distribution of the sickle cell gene and geographical confirmation of the malaria hypothesis. Nat Commun 1:104

Piel FB, Hay SI, Gupta S, Weatherall DJ, Williams TN (2013a) Global burden of sickle cell anaemia in children under five, 2010–2050: modelling based on demographics, excess mortality, and interventions. PLoS Med 10(7):e1001484

Piel FB, Howes RE, Patil AP et al (2013b) The distribution of haemoglobin C and its prevalence in newborns in Africa. Sci Rep 3:1671

Piel FB, Patil AP, Howes RE et al (2013c) Global epidemiology of sickle haemoglobin in neonates: a contemporary geostatistical model-based map and population estimates. Lancet 381(9861): 142–151

Piel FB, Rees DC, Williams TN (2014a) Managing the burden of sickle-cell disease in Africa. Lancet Haematol 1(1):e11–e12

Piel FB, Tatem AJ, Huang Z, Gupta S, Williams TN, Weatherall DJ (2014b) Global migration and the changing distribution of sickle haemoglobin: a quantitative study of temporal trends between 1960 and 2000. Lancet Glob Health 2(2):e80–e89

Platt OS, Orkin SH, Dover G et al (1984) Hydroxyurea enhances fetal hemoglobin production in sickle cell anemia. J Clin Invest 74(2):652–656

Platt OS, Brambilla DJ, Rosse WF et al (1994) Mortality in sickle cell disease. Life expectancy and risk factors for early death. N Engl J Med 330(23):1639–1644

Rachmilewitz EA, Tamari H, Liff F, Ueda Y, Nagel RL (1985) The Interaction of Hemoglobin-O Arab with Hb-S and Beta+–thalassemia among Israeli Arabs. Hum Genet 70(2):119–125

Rahgozar S, Poorfathollah AA, Moafi AR, Old JM (2000) Beta(S) gene in Central Iran is in linkage disequilibrium with the Indian-Arab haplotype. Am J Hematol 65(3):192–195

Rahimy MC, Gangbo A, Ahouignan G, Alihonou E (2009) Newborn screening for sickle cell disease in the Republic of Benin. J Clin Pathol 62(1):46–48

Rajaratnam JK, Marcus JR, Flaxman AD et al (2010) Neonatal, postneonatal, childhood, and under-5 mortality for 187 countries, 1970–2010: a systematic analysis of progress towards Millennium Development Goal 4. Lancet 375(9730):1988–2008

Rao VR (1988) Genetics and epidemiology of sickle cell anemia in India. ICMR Bull 9:87–90

Roberts I, de Montalembert M (2007) Sickle cell disease as a paradigm of immigration hematology: new challenges for hematologists in Europe. Haematologica 92(7):865–871

Robitaille N, Delvin EE, Hume HA (2006) Newborn screening for sickle cell disease: a 1988–2003 Quebec experience. Paediatr Child Health 11(4):223–227

Rockett KA, Clarke GM, Hubbart C et al (2014) Reappraisal of known malaria resistance loci in a large multicenter study. Nat Genet 46(11):1197–1204

Roth E, Friedman M, Ueda Y, Tellez I, Trager W, Nagel R (1978) Sickling rates of human AS red cells infected in vitro with Plasmodium falciparum malaria. Science 202(4368):650–652

Rumaney MB, Ngo Bitoungui VJ, Vorster AA et al (2014) The co-inheritance of alpha-thalassemia and sickle cell anemia is associated with better hematological indices and lower consultations rate in Cameroonian patients and could improve their survival. PLoS One 9(6):e100516

Sadek SH (1974) Sickle cell trait in North Nigeria. J Trop Med Hyg 77(3):61–64

Saint-Martin C, Romana M, Bibrac A et al (2013) Universal newborn screening for haemoglobinopathies in Guadeloupe (French West Indies): a 27-year experience. J Med Screen 20(4): 177–182

Sansarricq H, Marill G, Portier A, Cabannes R (1959) Les hémoglobinopathies en Haute-Volta. Sangre 30:503–511

Saugrain J (1957) New research on drepanocytosis in Madagascar. Bull Soc Pathol Exot Filiales 50(3):480–486

Scott RB (1970) Health care priority and sickle cell anemia. JAMA 214(4):731–734

Scott JP, Hillery CA, Brown ER, Misiewicz V, Labotka RJ (1996) Hydroxyurea therapy in children severely affected with sickle cell disease. J Pediatr 128(6):820–828

Selim O, Kamel K, Azim AA et al (1974) Genetic markers and anthropometry in the populations of the Egyptian oases of El-Kharga and El-Dakhla. Hum Hered 24(3):259–272

Serjeant GR, Serjeant BE, Forbes M, Hayes RJ, Higgs DR, Lehmann H (1986) Haemoglobin gene frequencies in the Jamaican population: a study in 100,000 newborns. Br J Haematol 64(2):253–262

Shukla RN, Solanki BR (1958) Sickle-cell trait in Central India. Lancet 1(7015):297–298

Solomon E, Bodmer WF (1979) Evolution of sickle variant gene. Lancet 1(8122):923

Spivak VA, Sou A, Lutsenko IN (1992) Distribution of abnormal hemoglobins S and C in the Republic of Guinea. Genetika 28(8):159–165

Steinberg MH (2005) Predicting clinical severity in sickle cell anaemia. Br J Haematol 129(4): 465–481

Streetly A, Rees DC (2013) Newborn screening for haematological disorders. Paediatr Child Health 23(11):472–479

Streetly A, Latinovic R, Hall K, Henthorn J (2009) Implementation of universal newborn bloodspot screening for sickle cell disease and other clinically significant haemoglobinopathies in England: screening results for 2005–7. J Clin Pathol 62(1):26–30

Taylor SM, Parobek CM, Fairhurst RM (2012) Haemoglobinopathies and the clinical epidemiology of malaria: a systematic review and meta-analysis. Lancet Infect Dis 12(6):457–468

Telfer P, Coen P, Chakravorty S et al (2007) Clinical outcomes in children with sickle cell disease living in England: a neonatal cohort in East London. Haematologica 92(7):905–912

Trincao C, Pinto AR, de Almeida CL, Gouveia E (1950) Drepanocythemia in the papel tribe of Portuguese Guinea. An Inst Med Trop 7:125–129

Tshilolo L, Kafando E, Sawadogo M et al (2008) Neonatal screening and clinical care programmes for sickle cell disorders in sub-Saharan Africa: lessons from pilot studies. Public Health 122(9):933–941

Tshilolo L, Aissi LM, Lukusa D et al (2009) Neonatal screening for sickle cell anaemia in the Democratic Republic of the Congo: experience from a pioneer project on 31 204 newborns. J Clin Pathol 62(1):35–38

van den Berghe LJ, Janssen P (1950) Maladie a sickle cells en Afrique noire. Ann Soc Belg Med Trop 30:1553–1566

van Heyningen A, Levenston M, Tamminga N et al (2009) Estimated incidence of sickle-cell disease in Aruba and St Maarten suggests cost-effectiveness of a universal screening programme for St Maarten. West Indian Med J 58(4):301–304

Vandepitte J, Motulsky AG (1956) Abnormal haemoglobins in the Kasai province of the Belgian Congo. Nature 177(4512):757

Wainscoat JS (1987) The origin of mutant beta-globin genes in human populations. Acta Haematol 78(2–3):154–158

Wang Y, Liu G, Caggana M et al (2014) Mortality of New York children with sickle cell disease identified through newborn screening. Genet Med. doi:10.1038/gim.2014.123

Ware RE (2010) How I use hydroxyurea to treat young patients with sickle cell anemia. Blood 115(26):5300–5311

Weatherall DJ (2010) The inherited diseases of hemoglobin are an emerging global health burden. Blood 115(22):4331–4336

Weatherall DJ (2011a) The inherited disorders of haemoglobin: an increasingly neglected global health burden. Indian J Med Res 134:493–497

Weatherall DJ (2011b) The challenge of haemoglobinopathies in resource-poor countries. Br J Haematol 154(6):736–744

Weatherall DJ, Clegg JB (2001) Inherited haemoglobin disorders: an increasing global health problem. Bull World Health Organ 79(8):704–712

Wiesenfeld SL (1967) Sickle-cell trait in human biological and cultural evolution. Development of agriculture causing increased malaria is bound to gene-pool changes causing malaria reduction. Science 157(3793):1134–1140

Wilkinson T (1981) Haemoglobinopathies in Australia and New Zealand. Hemoglobin 5(5): 525–530

Williams TN, Mwangi TW, Roberts DJ et al (2005a) An immune basis for malaria protection by the sickle cell trait. PLoS Med 2(5):e128

Williams TN, Mwangi TW, Wambua S et al (2005b) Negative epistasis between the malaria-protective effects of alpha+–thalassemia and the sickle cell trait. Nat Genet 37(11): 1253–1257

Williams TN, Uyoga S, Macharia A, Ndila C, McAuley CF, Opi H, Mwarumba S, Makani J, Komba A, Ndiritu MN, Sharif SK, Marsh K, Berkley JA, Scott JAG (2009) Bacteraemia in Kenyan children with sickle cell anaemia: a retrospective cohort and case-control study. Lancet 374:1364–1370, PMID: 19747721. PMCID: PMC2768782

Winters C (2008) Origin and spread of Dravidian speakers. Int J Hum Genet 8(4):325–329

Yanni E, Grosse SD, Yang Q, Olney RS (2009) Trends in pediatric sickle cell disease-related mortality in the United States, 1983–2002. J Pediatr 154(4):541–545

Yuregir GT, Kilinc M, Ekerbicer H, Bilaloglu N, Tekin N (2001) Screening of hemoglobinopathies in Kahramanmaras Province (Turkey) situated in a high prevalence area. J Trop Pediatr 47(2):124–125

Chapter 3
Overview of Sickle Cell Anemia Pathophysiology

Martin H. Steinberg

Abstract Sickle cell disease, caused by a mutation in the β-hemoglobin gene, is a Mendelian disorder with a very diverse phenotype. The primary cause of disease pathophysiology is the deoxygenation-induced polymerization of the mutant sickle hemoglobin. This ultimately leads to vasoocclusion by damaged sickle erythrocytes that interact with the endothelium and other blood cells, and the hemolysis of sickle cells within and outside of the vasculature. Treatment can target these separate but interconnected pathophysiologic pathways of sickle vasoocclusion and hemolytic anemia but targeting effectively a single limb or aspect of pathophysiology might have unintended consequences and increase the chance of complications closely associated with the other pathophysiologic pathway. The prime approach to treatment would be to effectively increase the level of the antisickling fetal hemoglobin in most sickle erythrocytes thereby thwarting all downstream effects of this primary pathophysiologic event.

Keywords Fetal hemoglobin • Polymerization • Hemolytic anemia • Vasoocclusion • Cell adhesion

3.1 Introduction

A point mutation in the β-hemoglobin gene (*HBB*; 11p15.4, β6 GAG-GTG; glutamic acid-valine) encodes the sickle β-globin chain (β^S) (Ingram 1956; Marotta et al. 1976; Pauling et al. 1949). Dimers of α-globin and β^S globin combine to form the sickle hemoglobin (HbS) tetramer ($\alpha_2\beta_2{}^S$) (Bunn 1987). Homozygosity for this sickle cell mutation is called sickle cell anemia. Compound heterozygosity for HbS and another hemoglobin gene mutation that changes the structure of the β-globin chain, like HbC ($\alpha_2\beta_2{}^C$) or reduces the expression of *HBB* like β thalassemia, or affects the structure or expression of the α-globin genes (*HBA2, HBA1*) make up other genotypes that cause the phenotype of sickle cell disease (Steinberg 2009). Some of the common genotypes of sickle hemoglobinopathies are shown in Table 3.1. Many

M.H. Steinberg, M.D. (✉)
Department of Medicine, Pediatrics, Pathology and Laboratory Medicine,
Boston University School of Medicine, 72 E. Concord St., Boston, MA 02118, USA
e-mail: mhsteinb@bu.edu; http://www.bu.edu/sicklecell

© Springer International Publishing Switzerland 2016

F.F. Costa, N. Conran (eds.), *Sickle Cell Anemia*,
DOI 10.1007/978-3-319-06713-1_3

Table 3.1 Common genotypes of sickle hemoglobinopathies

	Percent HbS[b]	Percent HbF[b]	Other variant[b]/ thalassemia type	Ethnicity[c]	Comments
HbS/HbS	Usually >90	5–20	No HbA	African, Arab, Indian, Greek	Most common genotype
HbS/HbC	50	~2	50 % HbC	West African	Less hemolysis
HbS/β^0 thal[d]	Usually >90	5–20	No HbA		Many different β^0 and β^+ thalassemia mutations exist
HbS/β^+ thal[d]	70–90	2–10	10–30 % HbA	African, Greek	
HbS/$\delta\beta^0$ thal	~75	10–25	Low HbA_2	Varied	Different $\delta\beta^0$ thalassemia mutations exist
HbS/HbO Arabia	~50	~5	~45 % HbO Arab	Mixed black/caucasian	Can be mistaken for severe HbSC disease
HbS/HbD Los Angeles	~60	~2	HbD Punjab ~40 %	HbD found in the Punjab	Severe disease like HbS/HbS
HbS/HbE	~70	~2	~30 % HbE	African/SE Asian	"Mild" disease like some HbS-β^+ thal
HbS/HbS/HbG Philadelphia	~60	~3	HbS/G hybrid ~30 %	African	HbG Philadelphia is an α-globin variant (*HBA* asn68lys)
HbA/HbS	30–40	Normal	60–70 % HbA	African, Arab, Indian, Greek	No hemolysis or vasoocclusion
HbS/HPFH	~70	~30	~30	African	Pancellular distribution of HbF

Provided are average percent hemoglobin fractions in untransfused young adults with each genotype, in the absence hydroxyurea treatment. Findings in young children will differ. Within a genotype, results in an individual patient can vary widely. Many other compound heterozygotes with HbS have been reported, with and without a clinical phenotype. These have been summarized (Steinberg & Embury 1986)

[a] All β-globin genotypes can be accompanied by heterozygosity or homozygosity for mutations causing α thalassemia

[b] Approximate percent of HbS or other hemoglobin present in the hemolysate

[c] Ethnicity where the variant arose or is most common

[d] β^+ or β^0 thalassemia

other less common and some rare genotypes are also found. Depending on the population studied, the incidence of the various common genotypes of sickle cell disease can vary greatly. The pathophysiology of these disorders has many commonalities but differences are present that can be ascribed to the pathological effects of the other globin gene or genes. For example, in HbSC disease, the most common compound heterozygous form of sickle cell disease, HbC affects cation transport leading to cellular dehydration and increased mean corpuscular HbS concentration (MC[HbS]C). In HbS-β thalassemia or sickle cell anemia with concurrent α thalassemia, cell density is decreased compared with sickle cell anemia. The pathophysiology of the sickle hemoglobinopathies has been reviewed extensively (Steinberg et al. 2009; Dean and Schechter 1978a, b, c; Embury et al. 1994; Frenette and Atweh 2007; Bunn and Forget 1986; Bunn 1997; Hebbel 1991; Hebbel et al. 2004).

3.2 The Phenotype of Sickle Hemoglobinopathies

The phenotype of sickle hemoglobinopathies results from injury to the sickle erythrocyte caused by HbS and deoxyHbS polymerization. This injury leads to extra and intravascular hemolysis, sickle vasculopathy and vasoocclusive disease. All sickle erythrocytes do not share a similar degree of cellular damage. This is due to both intrinsic properties of the erythrocyte that include fetal hemoglobin (HbF, $\alpha_2\gamma_2$) concentration and cell density and its state of hydration, and the environment the circulating erythrocyte encounters. The erythrocyte population in sickle cell disease is noted for its heterogeneity: some cells are young and short-lived; others are young and long-lived; some are extraordinarily dense; others unusually light. Anisocytosis is a result of many reticulocytes and dense cells and poikilocytosis is caused by the mixture of normal biconcave discoid cells, target cells, dense pointed, elongated contracted cells, sickle-like shapes and holly leaf-like forms. In HbSC disease target cells predominate and oxygenated cells can have crystals of HbC. In the sickle thalassemias, microcytosis and hypochromia are prevalent.

Sickle cells are in dynamic flux as their environment constantly cycles from laminar to microcirculatory flow, macro to microcirculation, high to low oxygen content, normal to low pH and normal to high solute concentration. The cycle of HbS polymerization and depolymerization can continue infinitely but the process of deoxyHbS polymerization and oxidant-induced damage to the cell membrane and contents ultimately injures the sickle erythrocyte membrane irreversibly fixing the cell in a variety of abnormal, or "sickle" shapes regardless of whether or not its HbS is polymerized. Prominent among these damaged cells is the irreversibly sickled cell or ISC. It was these cells that were first glimpsed by Herrick (1910) and that gave the disease its present name (Mason 1922). Examining the interactions among the primary and secondary pathophysiologic components of sickling hemoglobinopathies, the former due to HbS polymerization, the latter a downstream effect of polymer—whose complexity is compounded by genetic and environmental modulatory factors—provides some basis for appreciating the well-known heterogeneity of the clinical features associated with sickle cell disease.

3.3 HbS and the HbS Polymer

Polymerization of deoxyHbS is dependent on HbS concentration, pH, oxygen saturation and temperature (Eaton and Hofrichter 1987). In experiments designed to study polymerization, a delay occurs between the induction of the gelation and the detection of HbS polymer (Mozzarelli et al. 1987). It has been estimated that the delay time varies inversely with the 30th–50th power of HbS concentration (Hofrichter et al. 1974). This means that small decreases in MC[HbS]C can have substantial effects on polymerization and some of the pathophysiologic features of disease and has spurred efforts to develop agents that can reduce cell density, improving cell hydration and thereby decreasing MC[HbS]C) and the polymerization tendency of HbS.

The deoxyHbS polymer forms by homogeneous and heterogeneous processes of nucleation (Ferrone et al. 1985; Eaton and Hofrichter 1987). In the former, the structure of deoxyHbS tetramers allows them to adhere to each other forming a polymer composed of elementary fibers whose helix comprises 14 strands and is 210 Å thick (Fig. 3.1a). The hydrophobic site of the HbS mutation finds a properly registered hydrophobic receptor in another molecule forming a double strand. The lateral contacts of the fiber are the most crucial for polymerization where the β6 valine is within a hydrophobic pocket formed by β88 leucine, β85 phenylalanine and several heme atoms. Some mutant sites are on the polymer surface and uninvolved in homogeneous nucleation. These surface valine residues provide the stability for the nucleation of new fibers at the polymer surface, a process called heterogeneous nucleation, which explains the exponential growth of the polymer phase once the process begins after the delay time (Fig. 3.1b). Critical for understanding the pathophysiology of sickle cell anemia, neither HbA_2 nor HbF can co-polymerize with HbS because of the presence of a glutamine residue at δ87 in the former and an aspartic acid residue at γ80 and glutamine residue at γ87 in the latter (Nagel et al. 1979). HbA and HbC are able to co-polymerize extensively with HbS as neither hemoglobin has these amino acid residues at the corresponding position. Hence, neither hemoglobin has the polymerization-sparing effects of HbF or HbA_2 and their sole effect when present with HbS in the cell is to reduce its concentration.

Oxygen binding by HbS is normal in dilute solutions but in concentrated solutions, like those in the sickle erythrocyte, the hemoglobin-oxygen dissociation curve is right-shifted. This is an effect of the deoxyHbS polymer with some contribution from the high levels of 2, 3 BPG in the sickle erythrocyte.

3.3.1 HbF, HbS Polymer, and the Phenotype of Sickle Cell Anemia

Infants have few signs or symptoms of sickle cell anemia (Watson et al. 1948). Their high HbF retards the polymerization of deoxyHbS as neither HbF nor its mixed hybrid tetramer ($\alpha_2\beta^S\gamma$) enters the deoxyHbS polymer phase (Noguchi et al. 1993; Eaton and

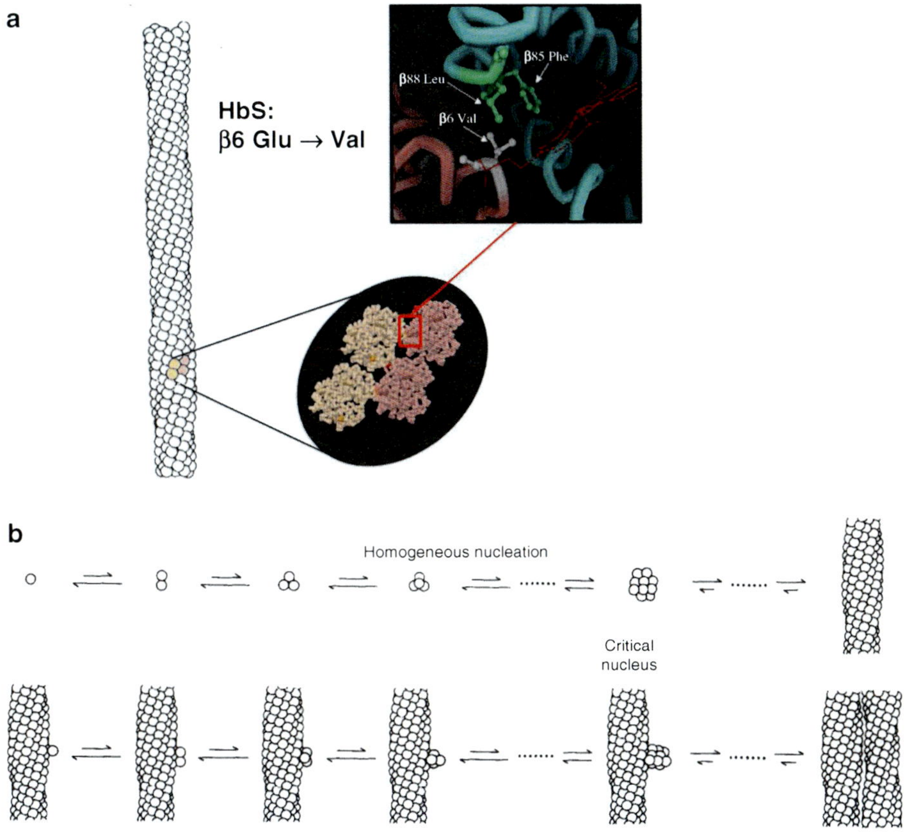

Fig. 3.1 HbS polymer (**a**) The 14-strand HbS fiber is the basic unit of the HbS polymer. Adapted with permission from a figure kindly provided by Prof. Stuart J. Edelstein (http://www.unige.ch/sciences/biochimie/Edelstein/sldHbS.htm) (HbS-HbS image from the Protein Data Bank). (**b**) The homogeneous and heterogeneous 2-phase model for sickle polymer growth structure, reproduced with permission from (Ferrone et al. 1985)

Hofrichter 1987). The phenotype of sickle cell disease becomes manifest within 6 months to 2 years of age as HbF levels decline. Because of these effects on HbS polymerization, HbF is the predominant genetic modulator of the phenotype of sickle cell anemia (Akinsheye et al. 2011; Steinberg and Sebastiani 2012). Sufficient HbF in each sickle cell can prevent deoxyHbS polymerization at physiologic oxygen saturations and abrogate the tissue injury and hemolytic anemia exemplifying this disease (Maier-Redelsperger et al. 1994; Brittenham et al. 1985). The best evidence supporting the relevance of high concentrations of HbF within the sickle erythrocyte is the naturally occurring example of individuals who are compound heterozygotes for HbS and gene deletion hereditary persistence of HbF. In this genotype, about one third of the total hemoglobin in each sickle erythrocyte (~10 pg) is HbF. This is the concentration of HbF needed to protect the cell from deoxyHbS polymer induced damage. In HbS homozygotes HbF is distributed heterogeneously among erythrocytes.

Individuals with HbS-gene deletion hereditary persistence of HbF are asymptomatic and have nearly normal total hemoglobin levels (Conley et al. 1963; Ngo et al. 2012). To "cure" sickle cell disease pharmacologically similar HbF concentrations in most sickle erythrocytes would need to be achieved (Steinberg et al. 2014).

The average HbF level in cases of sickle cell anemia where the HbS gene had its origin in Africa is between 5 and 8 % (Solovieff et al. 2010). HbF levels are associated with haplotypes of the β-globin gene complex (Labie et al. 1985, 1989; Nagel et al. 1984; Nagel and Labie 1989; Kan and Dozy 1980; Costa et al. 1994; Lapoumeroulie et al. 1989; Kulozik et al. 1986, 1987). Four common haplotypes had an African origin and 1 haplotype originated in India and/or the Middle East. In the Middle East and in India the HbS gene is often on the Arab-Indian (AI) *HBB* haplotype that is associated with HbF levels 3–5 times as high as those found with African haplotypes (Miller et al. 1986; Ngo et al. 2013). The youngest individuals with the AI haplotype have the mildest phenotype of all sickle cell anemia patients, although when HbF levels fall from about 30 % in children to 15–20 % in adults, the disease becomes more severe (Perrine et al. 1972, 1978; Padmos et al. 1991; Adekile 2011; Marouf et al. 2003a, b; Alsultan et al. 2014). A hierarchy of HbF levels is present among the HbS haplotypes after HbF levels have stabilized at age 5–10 years, with a mean of about 5 % in the Bantu haplotype to about 20 % in the AI haplotype (Akinsheye et al. 2011). However, within each haplotype group there is considerable heterogeneity of HbF levels suggesting that the cis-acting regulatory elements have key roles to play in HbF gene expression. In population-based studies, any increment in HbF had a beneficial effect on mortality in sickle cell anemia (Platt et al. 1994). F cells are erythrocytes that have sufficient HbF to be enumerated by flow cytometry. It takes only 5–6 pg HbF/F cell for the cell to be visualized. Modeling the distribution of HbF/F cell suggests that very few F cells are protected from deoxyHbS polymer induced damage when HbF levels are approximately 5 %, larger numbers of protected cells are possible when HbF reaches levels of 10 %; HbF concentrations of about 30 % can provide protection to more than 70 % of cells (Steinberg et al. 2014). Figure 3.2 shows the sub-phenotypes found in sickle cell anemia in patients with African-origin *HBB* haplotypes and HbF levels of 5–8 % (L panel) compared with that seen in patients with the AI haplotype and HbF of 20 % (R panel). Because of less hemolysis, the hemoglobin level of AI haplotype patients is higher than that of African-origin haplotype carriers. They have a nearly similar incidence of complications most often associated with sickle vasoocclusion. Less hemolysis might account for a reduced incidence of leg ulcers and stroke.

3.4 The Sickle Erythrocyte Membrane

The erythrocyte membrane is a lipid bilayer linked to an underlying protein membrane skeleton that is penetrated by integral proteins that interact with the lipid core and skeletal proteins. Integral membrane proteins include but are not limited to; glycophorins, the Rh proteins, transport proteins like band 3, the sodium pump, Ca2+ ATPase and Mg2+ ATPase. Skeletal proteins include the structural proteins of the spectrin-actin based membrane cytoskeleton. The lipid bilayer is made of

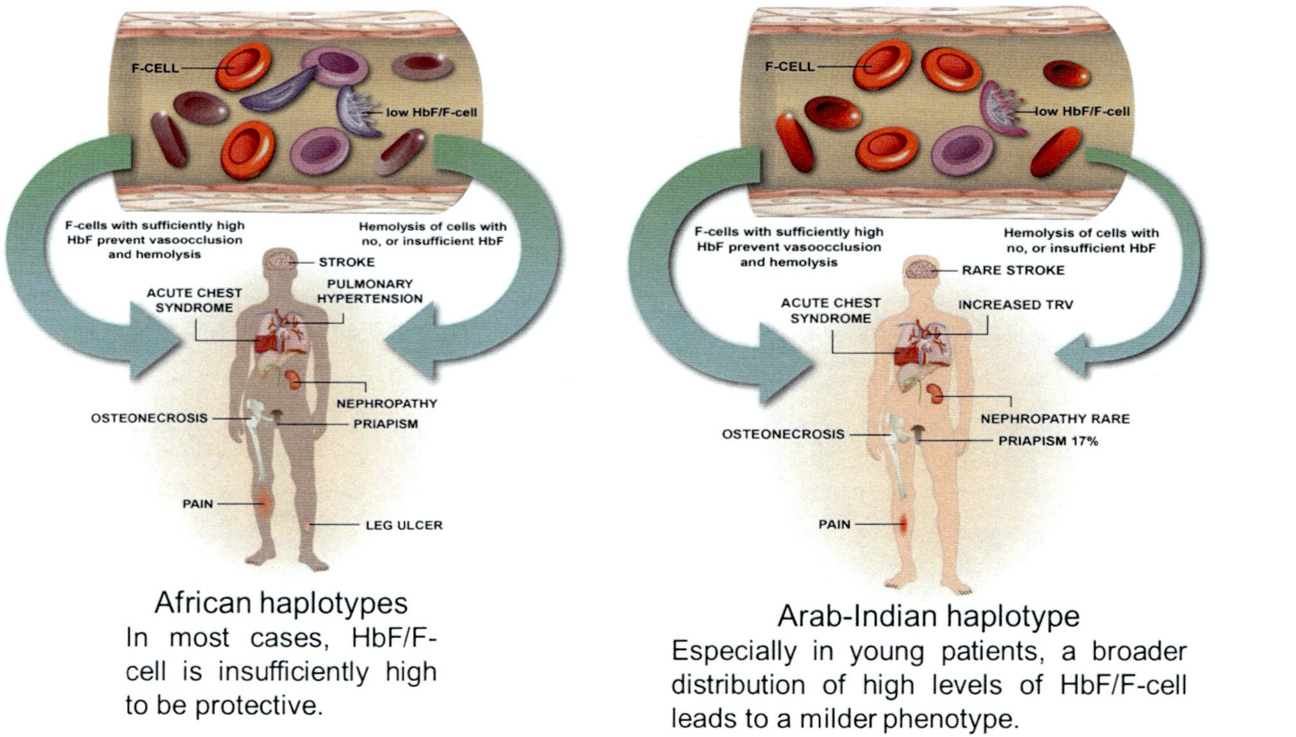

Fig. 3.2 HbF and the phenotype of sickle cell anemia. The *left panel* shows a typical adult patient with an African HbS haplotype and HbF level. Rare F-cells have sufficient HbF to protect them from polymer-induced damage; other cells are unprotected and can hemolyze intravascularly promoting the subphenotypes closely associated with hyperhemolysis, like stroke, pulmonary hypertension, priapism in males, leg ulcers and nephropathy. The *right panel* depicts an adult with the Arab-Indian haplotype of the HbS gene and ~20% HbF. With a high total HbF it is now possible to have greater numbers of F cells where deoxyHbS polymerization does not occur at physiologic oxygen saturations. This reduces the rate of hemolysis and the incidence of hemolysis-associated complications. A version of this research was originally published in Blood (Akinsheye et al. Fetal hemoglobin in sickle cell anemia. Blood. 2011; 118(1):19–27. © The American Society of Hematology)

phospholipids intercalated with unesterified cholesterol and some glycolipids. The major lipids are phosphatidyl choline (PC), phosphatidyl ethanolamine (PE), sphingomyelin (SM) and phosphatidyl serine (PS) that are asymmetrically distributed, with PC and SM primarily in the outer monolayer, and most of PE, all of PS—the amino phospholipids—and the phosphoinositides in the inner monolayer. This distribution is actively maintained by several enzymes. With erythrocyte sickling, the normal lipid asymmetry is lost as PS translocates to the outer membrane leaflet. PS-exposing surfaces propagate proteolytic reactions that result in thrombin formation and activation of fibrinolysis. Some studies suggest that PS exposure is related to stroke, activation of coagulation and extravascular hemolysis (Brugnara 2001; de Jong et al. 2001; Joiner and Gallagher 2009; Franck et al. 1985; Kuypers et al. 1996; Westerman et al. 1984; Tait and Gibson 1994; Lane et al. 1994; Setty et al. 2002; Kuypers 2008).

The membrane contacts HbS and its polymer leading to distortion by physical effects (Wagner et al. 1986; Liu et al. 1991; Allan et al. 1981, 1982). DeoxyHbS polymer forms spicules that can physically dissociate fragments of the lipid bilayer from the membrane skeleton. The membrane spicule is composed of spectrin-poor lipid vesicles with some integral membrane proteins. Perhaps the loss of complement regulatory proteins in these vesicles leaves the erythrocyte susceptible to complement-mediated intravascular hemolysis and facilitates erythrocyte recognition and removal by macrophages (Wang et al. 1993; Test and Woolworth 1994). Membrane proteins are also subjected to oxidative stress induced by hemoglobin oxygenation and deoxygenation that generates reactive oxygen species.(Hebbel 1984, 1985; Hebbel et al. 1982, 1988). Decompartmentalization of erythrocyte iron also contributes to oxidant radical generation via Fenton chemistry. Unstable HbS can precipitate on the membrane in the form of hemichromes (Browne et al. 1998; Repka and Hebbel 1991; Schwartz et al. 1987; Sugihara et al. 1992) (Fig. 3.3). The ISC is a result of permanent deformation of the spectrin-actin membrane skeleton and perhaps a defect in β-actin caused by oxidative changes (Lux et al. 1976; Horiuchi et al. 1988; Goodman 2004; Bertles and Milner 1968; Bencsath et al. 1996; Shartava et al. 1995).

Red cell volume and density must be closely controlled to maintain cell flexibility and permit flow through the microcirculation. Maintenance of normal density is especially critical in the sickle erythrocyte because the MC[HbS]C is a dominant factor for deoxyHbS polymerization. Erythrocyte cation content is the major determinant of cell volume and is regulated by several transport channels whose activity can be altered in the sickle erythrocyte (Brugnara 1993, 1997). Erythrocyte heterogeneity in sickle cell disease is contributed to by variation in cell volume and water content. Increased numbers of reticulocytes and young red cells have low density and increased volume; dense, rigid, dehydrated cells, some with extraordinarily high hemoglobin concentrations can be both young and old cells, especially ISCs (Franco et al. 1996, 2006; Joiner and Gallagher 2009; Fabry et al. 1984, 1991; Fabry and Nagel 1982; Evans et al. 1984). Dense, dehydrated cells are due in part to damage of cation transport systems that have different activities in different segments of the erythrocyte population. Two have been studied most intensively. The Gardos pathway, a Na/K exchange channel activated by calcium is a 428 amino acid, 6 transmembrane domain protein with about 150 copies per red cell. Inhibitors of this pathway can reduce cell

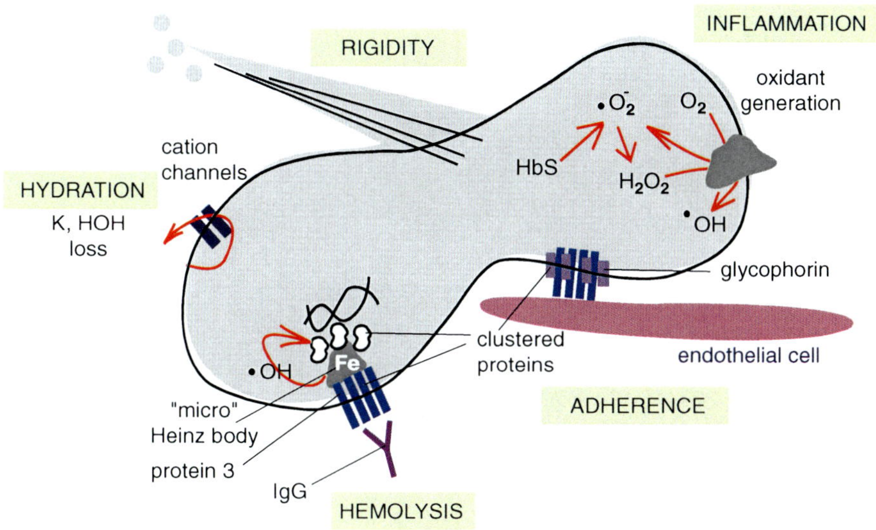

Fig. 3.3 Loci of damage of the sickle erythrocyte membrane. HbS polymer can directly injure the membrane causing release of lipid rich microparticles that lead to the evolution of dense cells with a reduced membrane:cytoplasmic ratio. This increases MC(HbS)C and because of the extreme dependence of HbS polymerization on HbS concentration favors polymerization. Unstable and oxidizing sickle hemoglobin can also damage the membrane leading to altered cation transport, exposure of epitopes favoring cell adhesion and premature cell destruction in the reticuloendothelial system and intravascularly. The life expectancy of red cells in sickle cell anemia is about 20 days compared with 120 days in normal individuals. Hemolytic anemia is always present, regardless of whether acute vasoocclusive event are taking place. Illustration kindly provided by Prof. O.Platt and adapted from (Platt 1994)

density and hemolysis but have not yet been shown to decrease sickle vasoocclusive events. A K/Cl cotransport pathway, the products of the *KCC4*, *KCC1* and *KCC3* genes, is most active in reticulocytes and young cells and has little activity in older and dense sickle erythrocytes (Joiner and Gallagher 2009). K/Cl cotransport is stimulated by the reduced levels of cellular magnesium found in sickle erythrocytes and by acid pH. Magnesium supplementation can improve cell hydration but therapeutic trials of this agent to date have not been encouraging (Hankins et al. 2008; De Franceschi et al. 1997, 2000). Pathways characterized by deoxygenation-induced cation permeability and sensitive to physical perturbation of the membrane are also present (Gallagher 2013). All pathways are activated in sickle erythrocytes leading to cation and water loss and cell dehydration. Some of these pathways are amenable to targeted inhibition providing a means to prevent erythrocyte cell dehydration and the tendency for HbS polymerization thereby reducing hemolysis.

Disappointingly, clinical trials aimed at rehydrating dehydrated sickle cells by inhibiting the Gardos channel did not achieve their primary endpoint of reducing sickle vasoocclusion (Ataga et al. 2008, 2011). The Gardos channel inhibitor worked as anticipated; cell density fell and hemolysis was reduced. As a result the hemoglobin level rose. Unfortunately, more cells with primarily HbS likely increased blood viscosity and failed to reduce, or even increased the likelihood of vasoocclusive complications. These results might have been predicted based on the naturally occurring example of sickle cell anemia-α-thalassemia (Steinberg and Embury 1986; Steinberg and Sebastiani 2012). In compound heterozygotes with this genotype—about 30 % of all patients homozygous for the HbS gene—the presence of α thalassemia reduces the density of the sickle erythrocyte and improves its lifespan. Higher total hemoglobin levels associated with this genotype of disease are associated with an increased prevalence of some vasoocclusive complications of the disease. Other complications more closely linked to hemolytic anemia are reduced. These examples highlight the difficulties of treating directly one downstream consequence of deoxyHbS polymerization without considering the critical primary process of polymer formation.

A failed erythrocyte membrane, damaged by the pathophysiologic effects of HbS and HbS polymer, is responsible for the hemolysis and vasoocclusion that are the hallmarks of sickle cell disease. An injured and abnormal red cell membrane is likely to initiate intercellular interactions with the endothelium and leukocytes that trigger sickle vasoocclusion (Hebbel et al. 2004; Kaul et al. 1996; Kaul 2009; Frenette and Atweh 2007).

3.5 Cellular Interactions

Sickle erythrocyte and leukocyte interaction with the endothelium prolongs erythrocyte transit through hypoxic vascular beds, providing the time needed for deoxyHbS to polymerize (Fig. 3.4). Adhesive interactions require the expression of certain epitopes on erythrocytes, leukocytes and the endothelium along with soluble plasma factors. Two non-mutually exclusive constructs of the adhesion process have been proposed. An “erythrocentric” theory posits that sickle erythrocytes interact directly with endothelium (Fig. 3.4a) (Hebbel 1984, 1997). A “leukocentric” theory proposes that sickle erythrocytes interact with leukocytes that then contact and damage the endothelium (Turhan et al. 2002) (Fig. 3.4b). There is ample evidence from human in vitro studies and murine in vivo and ex vivo studies that both means of adherence can occur, but limited data that the acute vasoocclusive events, hallmarks of sickle cell disease, are a direct result of adhesive interactions. In vitro studies of human sickle erythrocytes first showed in a static adherence assay that these cells could adhere to endothelium with physiologically relevant forces and that more tenacious adherence was correlated with an estimate of disease severity. In more physiologically relevant conditions of flow, sickle cells also show increased ability to adhere (Hoover et al. 1979; Hebbel 1997; Hebbel et al. 1980; Zennadi et al. 2004; Mohandas and Evans 1984; Burns et al. 1985; Kaul et al. 1989). Ex vivo murine studies confirmed adherence in the microvasculature to the precapillary venules with similar observations in some strains of sickle transgenic mice (Kaul et al. 1981, 1983, 1995; Lipowsky et al. 1982; Smith and La Celle 1986).

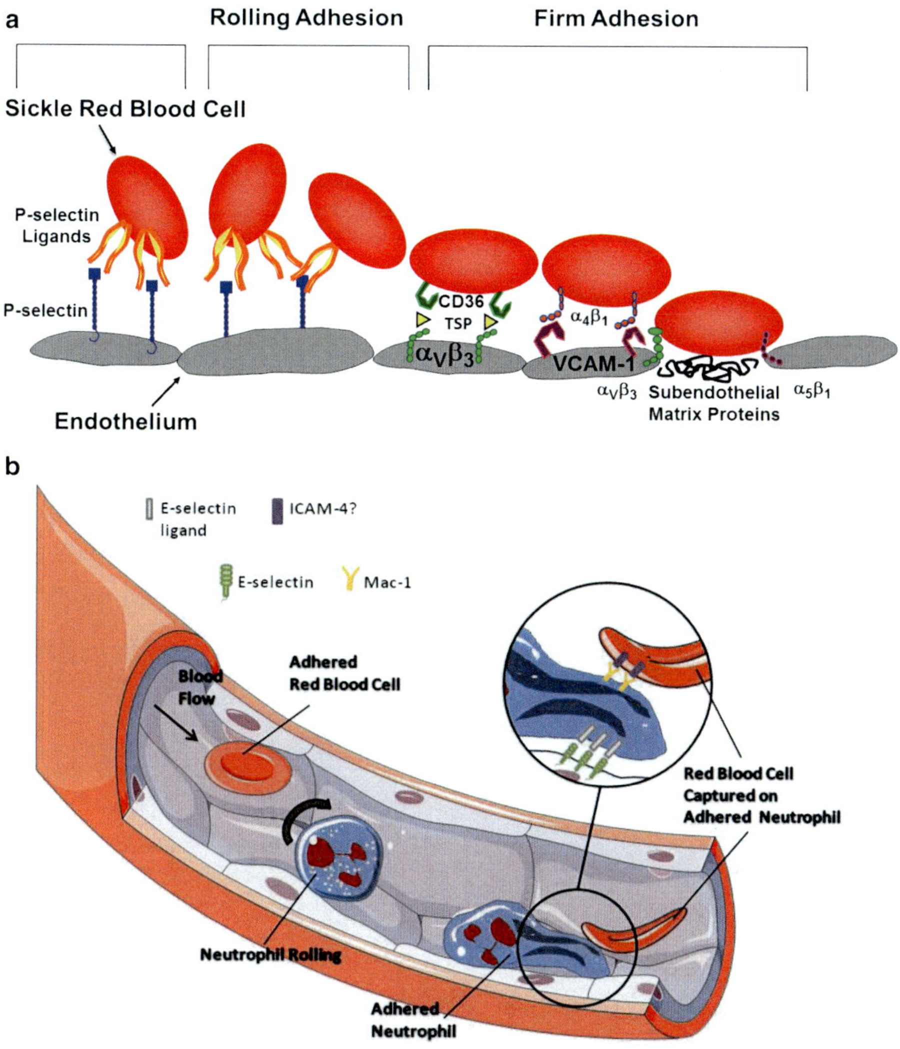

Fig. 3.4 Mechanisms of cellular interactions. (**a**) In an "erythrocentric" view of sickle vasoocclusion, initial contact with endothelium is caused by the adherence of sickle erythrocyte to endothelium via P-selectin. The subsequent strengthening of this interaction and firm adherence is mediated by other adhesion molecules (Illustration kindly provided by S.H. Embury). (**b**) In a "leukocentric" view of sickle vasoocclusion, sickle erythrocytes and inflammatory mediators activate endothelium that then recruits leukocytes and generates additional signals that produce polarized expression of activated αMβ2 integrin (Mac-1) at the leading edge of the crawling neutrophil. This permits the capture of sickle erythrocytes. These events culminate in vasoocclusion in the postcapillary venules. Figure drawn from information from (Manwani and Frenette 2013)

Many different molecules have been implicated in the process of sickle erythrocyte adhesion to endothelium (Fig. 3.5) (Hebbel et al. 2004). Characteristically, the least dense cells and reticulocytes are the most adherent. Some adhesion molecules can interact directly with the endothelial cell membrane without bridging plasma proteins. Others need a soluble bridge molecule; some epitopes interact with subendothelial matrix proteins. All these interactions have the potential of further injuring the endothelium and can lead to reperfusion injury provoking inflammation and oxidant radical generation. Neutrophils can bind sickle erythrocytes but in this case, the most dense cells and ISCs are most adherent (Frenette and Atweh 2007). In sickle mice, leukocyte-erythrocyte interactions were most prominent and were potentiated following an inflammatory stimulus that provoked vasoocclusion (Turhan et al. 2002). One reflection of endothelial damage in sickle cell disease is increased numbers of circulating activated endothelial cells. Compared with circulating endothelial cells from control subjects, sickle cell disease-derived endothelial cells produced more IL-8 and were more adherent to normal erythrocytes than cultured endothelium from normal subjects (Solovey et al. 1997; Sakamoto et al. 2013).

Selectins mediate intercellular interactions that include the adhesion of sickle cells to endothelium. P-selectin has been proposed as the initiating step in sickle-endothelial adhesion process. E-selectin mediates leukocyte-endothelial interactions and the capture of sickle cells by neutrophils. Early phase clinical trials of an oral P-selectin blocking agent and an intravenous pan-selectin inhibitor, mainly active against E-selectin, have shown some clinical activity and further trials of these agents and an anti-P-selectin antibody are in process (Kutlar and Embury 2014; Chang et al. 2010).

Sickle vasoocclusion, hemolysis and nitric oxide (NO) depletion causes inflammation. Another source of inflammation in sickle cell disease is mediated by invariant natural killer T-lymphocytes (iNKT cells). Ischemia-reperfusion can be initiated by the activation of iNKT cells and sickle mice have increased numbers of these cells compared with control animals (Field et al. 2013; Nathan et al. 2012; Lin et al. 2013). Antibodies targeting iNKT cells reversed pulmonary dysfunction in sickle mice. Patients also have increased numbers of activated circulating iNKT cells. Activation of the adenosine A_2 receptor on iNKT cells reduces pulmonary injury in sickle mice (Wallace et al. 2009). A clinically approved adenosine A_2 receptor agonist, regadenoson, is in early-phase trials in sickle cell disease. Preliminary studies suggest that iNKT cells can be safely depleted by an antibody suggesting a possible approach to inflammation-induced tissue damage.

There has been little evidence to support the role of coagulation in sickle vasoocclusion despite studies showing activation of both the intrinsic and extrinsic coagulation systems. Nevertheless, activated endothelial cells with exposure of membrane PS and generation of tissue factor might activate the coagulation system and contribute to vasoocclusion (Stuart and Setty 2001; Sparkenbaugh and Pawlinski 2013; Lim et al. 2013).

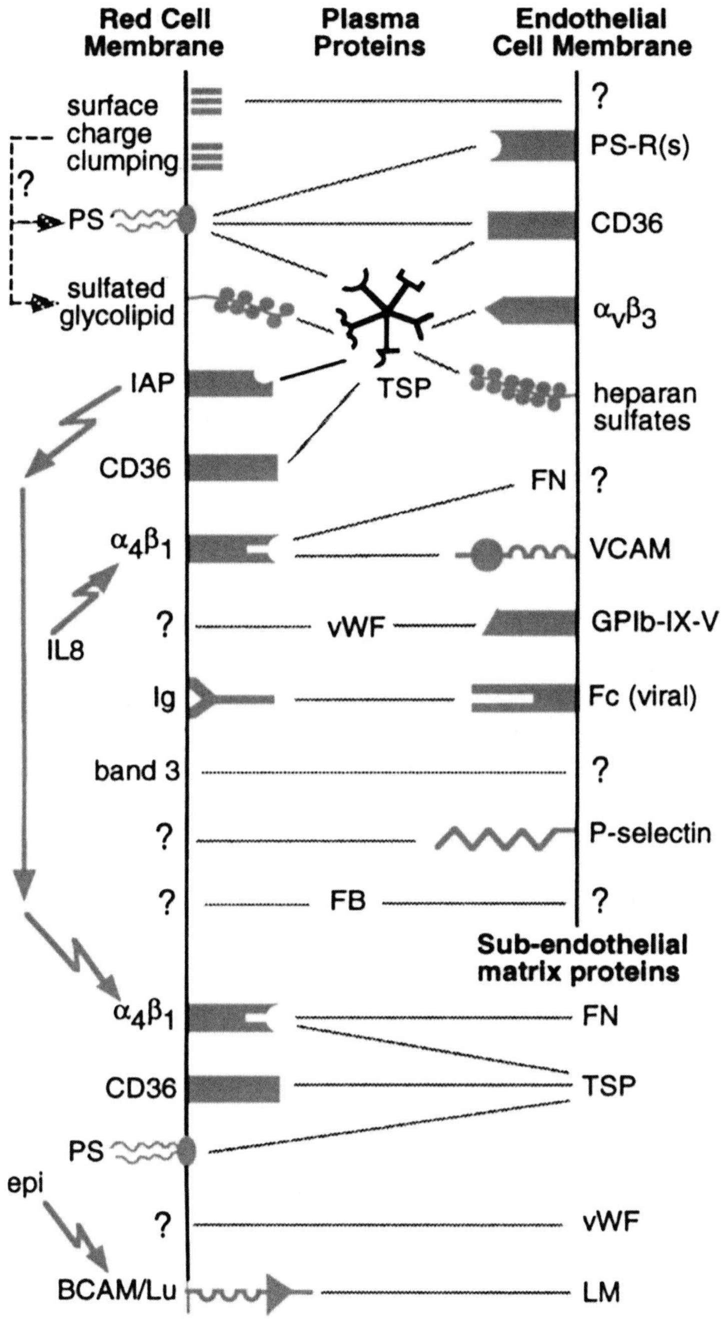

Fig. 3.5 Multiple molecules can account for the adhesion of sickle cells to the endothelium. Figure reproduced with permission from Hebbel et al. (2004)

3.6 Hemolytic Anemia and the Nitric Oxide Paradigm

Injury to the sickle erythrocyte membrane results in their premature removal from the circulation. The lifespan of sickle erythrocytes is 7–14 days compared with 120 days for normal erythrocytes. To compensate, the hematopoietic bone marrow increases erythropoiesis and hypertrophies while spreading into long bones. But, compensation is incomplete and less than expected. This is likely to be a result of the decreased oxygen affinity of sickle cell blood and damage to the marrow with regions of necrosis. Compared with other types of anemia, erythropoietin levels are inappropriately low in sickle cell anemia and decrease further as renal function deteriorates (Sherwood et al. 1986). In distinction to severe β thalassemia, there is little intramedullary destruction of erythroid precursors and ineffective erythropoiesis in sickle cell disease is minimal. Stress reticulocytes, the product of expanded erythropoiesis are the first cells to adhere in the microcirculation facilitating the further entrapment of other erythrocytes and leukocytes. This is likely to provide the nexus between complications of the disease that are believed to be a result of hemolytic anemia and disease complications that are closely associated with sickle vasoocclusion and blood viscosity. Reticulocytes are not always long-lived. Their complement of HbF is uneven and those with higher levels of HbF survive longer while those with little or no HbF die more rapidly (Franco et al. 2006).

Damaged erythrocytes are removed from circulation by two pathophysiologic routes: extravascular catabolism within the reticuloendothelial system; intravascular lysis. Extravascular hemolysis is prompted by membrane PS exposure, exposure of epitopes that are recognized by macrophages and perhaps by the physical properties of rigid and deformed sickle cells. Intravascular hemolysis is related to oxidant radical generation within the sickle erythrocyte (Fig. 3.3) and exposure to external oxidants generated by xanthine oxidase, NADPH oxidase and uncoupled NO synthase causing reduced abundance of reduced sulfhydryl groups and increased lipid peroxidation. Also contributing to intravascular hemolysis is increasing cell density resulting from hyperactive cation transport channels and loss of membrane lipid-rich microparticles (Fig. 3.3). Sickle cells have a defect in activity of the membrane attack complex, C5b-9, as C5b-7 and C9 binds to the most dense cells. Exposure of PS and PE might facilitate this binding (Liu et al. 1999). This leads to C5b-9-mediated lysis initiated by C5b-6.

Based on measurement of plasma hemoglobin, an accurate biomarker of intravascular hemolysis, the fraction of cells lysing within the circulation varies from less than 10 % to more than 30 % and plasma heme can vary from 0.25 to more than 20 μM (Reiter et al. 2002). Other more easily obtainable surrogate biomarkers of hemolysis are reticulocyte count, bilirubin level, AST, LDH, haptoglobin and urine hemosiderin. Combinations of some of these biomarkers have been used in a principle component analysis as a measure of the degree of intravascular hemolysis (Nouraie et al. 2013; Milton et al. 2013; Gordeuk et al. 2009).

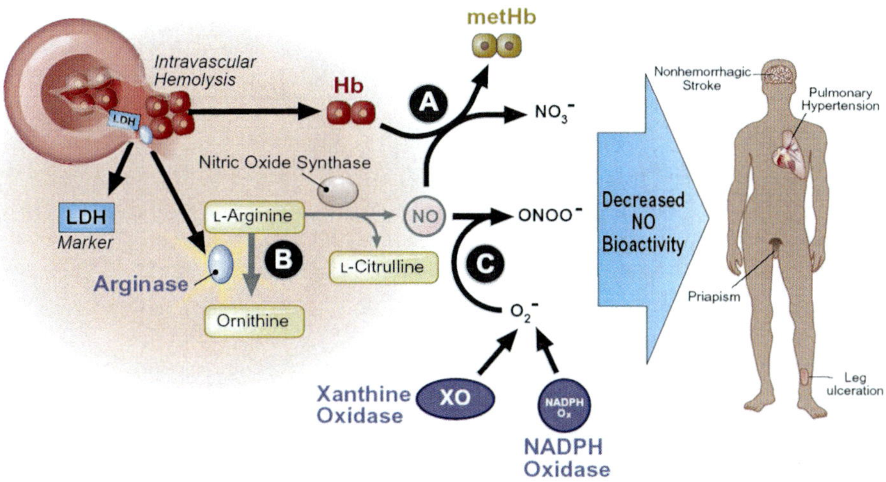

Fig. 3.6 The NO biology of sickle cell disease. Intravascular hemolysis liberates heme and hemoglobin that scavenges NO producing nitrate and methemoglobin. Arginase is also released into the plasma and can catabolize L-arginine, the substrate for the NO synthases. NO is also oxidized by xanthine oxidase and NAPPH oxidase to peroxynitrite and superoxide. Together these scavenge bioavailable NO. LDH isozymes released during intravascular hemolysis are a marker of the extent of intravascular hemolysis. Figure reproduced with permission from (Kato et al. 2007)

3.6.1 Subphenotypes of Disease

Dozens of studies of hundreds of patients have firmly established the association of markers of hemolysis with certain complications of disease (Fig. 3.6) (Gladwin et al. 2004; Nolan et al. 2005, 2006; Taylor et al. 2008; Bernaudin et al. 2008; Guasch et al. 1999; Kato et al. 2006a, b; Liem et al. 2007; Nouraie et al. 2013; Saraf et al. 2014; Minniti et al. 2011; Hamideh et al. 2014; van der Land et al. 2013). These observations have established the generally accepted hypothesis of a hemolysis-driven phenotype of sickle cell anemia characterized by a higher incidence of pulmonary hypertension, stroke, leg ulcers, priapism and renal failure in patients with hyperhemolysis compared with patients with less intense hemolysis (Kato et al. 2007). Tricuspid regurgitant velocity (TRV) and serum nt-proBNP are markers of general vascular stress. Pulmonary arterial hypertension, ascertained by right heart catheterization, and TRV are both closely associated with the intensity of hemolysis and mortality in sickle cell anemia. Some aspects of the hemolytic phenotype are prevalent in other types of hemolytic anemia where intravascular hemolysis is common, like paroxysmal nocturnal hemolytic anemia, thalassemia and hereditary spherocytosis. Observational and epidemiological studies of widely varied patient cohorts that have shown associations of hemolysis with certain disease subphenotypes have been amply supported by mechanistic studies in animal models (Hu et al. 2010; Hsu et al. 2007).

The hyperhemolytic phenotype of sickle cell disease is driven by the liberation of hemoglobin into the plasma where it overwhelms the available detoxification mechanisms of haptoglobin and hemopexin binding and leads to vascular injury (Deonikar and Kavdia 2012; Jeffers et al. 2006). This is in distinction to red cell destruction within the macrophage where only small amounts of hemoglobin escape its intracellular catabolism. The presence of free plasma hemoglobin and heme promotes the scavenging of NO and its downstream effects of endothelial damage, vasoconstriction, increased inflammation, hypercoagulability, increased expression of adhesion molecules like VCAM-1, P-selectin, E-selectin, altered platelet function, increased expression of the vasoconstrictor endothelin-1 and alteration of vascular redox balance. Acute sickle vasoocclusive events are the most dramatic manifestation of disease and are the greatest acute concern for the patient and treating physicians. However, hemolytic anemia never stops, even when patients are successfully treated with hydroxyurea. Perhaps by depleting bioavailable NO, the vasculopathy associated with chronic intravascular hemolysis, while clinically unapparent for long periods, might have a greater effect on mortality than acute vasoocclusive events.

NO is a free radical produced enzymatically by a family of NO synthases in endothelium, macrophages and neurons during the conversion of arginine to citrulline (Fig. 3.6) (Stamler et al. 1992, 1997). After its production, endothelial NO, a product of the endothelial NO synthase *NOS3*, diffuses to adjacent smooth muscle where it binds the heme of soluble guanylate cyclase that is activated and converts GTP to cGMP. This produces vasodilation by activating cGMP dependent protein kinases that causes calcium sequestration and relaxation of the perivascular smooth muscle (Cannon et al. 2001; Dejam et al. 2004; Kim-Shapiro et al. 2006). NO is also depleted by the liberation from the erythrocyte of arginase that can decrease the availability of arginine, the substrate for the NO synthases and by the conversion of NO to superoxide and peroxynitrite.

Based on this pathophysiology, restoration of vascular NO has been tested as potential treatment for the complications of sickle cell disease that are postulated to result from decreased NO bioavailability (Gladwin and Schechter 2001; Reiter and Gladwin 2003). Inhibiting the degradation of cyclic GMP, which is partly responsible for maintaining vascular dilation, using phosphodiesterase 5 inhibitors like sildenafil or tadalafil, has been studied as treatment for pulmonary hypertension (Machado et al. 2005, 2011). Arginine, the substrate of the nitric oxide synthases has had limited study for pulmonary hypertension (Morris et al. 2003). None of these treatments have reached the clinic. The trial of sildenafil was stopped prematurely because the treatment group had more sickle cell pain. Inhibiting phosphodiesterase 5, the predominant enzyme catabolizing cGMP in the corpora cavernosum was used to treat priapism in sickle cell anemia where it might restore toward normal dysregulated NO metabolism (Burnett 2003; Burnett et al. 2006; Champion et al. 2005). Inhaled NO reduced opioid use in a small study in children with acute vasoocclusive pain episodes (Weiner et al. 2003), but in a controlled randomized trial in adults it was no better than a placebo (Gladwin et al. 2011). A short-term phase 1 study of topical sodium nitrite cream, a NO donor, in sickle cell leg ulcers showed an increase in cutaneous blood flow and a dose dependent decrease in ulcer size with some ulcers healing completely.

3.7 Summary

One view of the pathophysiology of sickle cell disease is shown in Fig. 3.7. The HbS mutation allows deoxyHbS to polymerize at oxygen saturations that are present in some vascular beds. Sickle polymer injures the erythrocyte and is responsible for its membrane injury and ultimate failure that produces a population of heterogeneous red blood cells, many of which are very short-lived and adherent to other circulating cells and to the endothelium. Intravascular destruction of some sickle erythrocytes

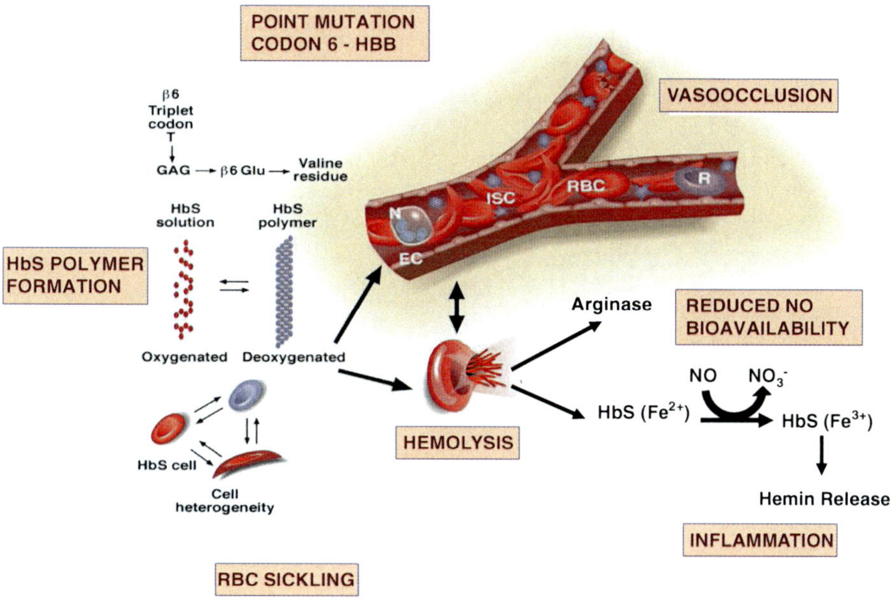

Fig. 3.7 The pathophysiology of sickle cell disease. The adenine (A) to thymidine (T) point mutation at codon 6 in the *HBB* substitutes a valine for the normal glutamic acid. This single and "simple" change leads to the synthesis of HbS that has the nearly unique property of polymerizing when it is deoxygenated. DeoxyHbS polymer injures the erythrocyte and leads to a heterogeneous population of sickle cells with a damaged membrane. In the vasculature, sickle cells interact with endothelium and other blood cells leading to vasoocclusion. Damaged erythrocytes are short-lived and while most hemolysis is extravascular 10–30% of hemolysis occurs intravascularly releasing hemoglobin into the plasma. Hemoglobin scavenges NO that binds soluble guanylate cyclase, converts cyclic guanosine triphosphate to guanosine monophosphate, and relaxes vascular smooth muscle vasodilation. Reduced endothelial NO bioavailability impairs the homeostatic vascular functions like inhibition of platelet activation and aggregation and transcriptional repression of genes transcribing cell adhesion molecules. Hemoglobin, hemin (or heme), and heme iron catalyze the production of oxygen radicals and protein nitration, potentially further limiting NO bioavailability and activating endothelium. Lysed erythrocytes also liberate arginase, which destroys L-arginine, the substrate for NO production, providing another mechanism for endothelial NO deficiency. Hemin is released from ferric hemoglobin (Fe^{3+}) and promotes inflammatory and oxidative effects; Adapted from (Steinberg 2006). *EC* = endothelial cell; *N* = neutrophil; *R* = reticulocyte; *RBC* = red blood cell

causes a state of NO deficiency with reduced bioavailability. Hemolytic anemia and sickle vasoocclusion are intimately linked. It should not be supposed that the subphenotypes of this very complex disease are driven exclusively by either hemolysis or vasoocclusion. Both processes influence each other at various points in their convergence, for example, reticulocytes reflect the intensity of hemolysis and are also the most adherent erythrocytes. Nevertheless, understanding the importance and contribution of each major pathophysiologic limb shown in Fig. 3.7 to the overall pathophysiology of disease can focus our approach to treatment modalities that are targeted to one or the other of these branches. Treatments directed at inhibiting endothelial adherence would mainly target the complications of presumed sickle vasoocclusion, like acute painful episodes; those reducing the density of the sickle erythrocyte would reduce presumed complications of hemolysis, like stroke. The naturally occurring example of sickle cell anemia-α thalassemia and the aforementioned results of a clinical trial of an agent that improved cell density and reduced hemolysis have shown that targeting effectively a single limb or aspect of pathophysiology might have unintended consequences and increase the chance of complications closely associated with the other pathophysiologic feature. Perhaps the best pharmacologic treatment approach is to focus on the most proximal driver of the disease, deoxyHbS polymerization, and inhibit this by increasing the intracellular concentration of HbF. To be most effective, the HbF level in each cell would have to approximate the level present in HbS-gene deletion hereditary persistence of HbF. Although this is not possible with the HbF-inducing drug, hydroxyurea, gene therapeutic approaches where this might be achievable, perhaps incorporating editing of the elements that modulate HbF gene expression, can be anticipated in the near future.

References

Adekile AD (2011) Limitations of Hb F as a phenotypic modifier in sickle cell disease: study of Kuwaiti Arab patients. Hemoglobin 35(5–6):607–617

Akinsheye I, Alsultan A, Solovieff N et al (2011) Fetal hemoglobin in sickle cell anemia. Blood 118(1):19–27

Allan D, Limbrick AR, Thomas P, Westerman MP (1981) Microvesicles from sickle erythrocytes and their relation to irreversible sickling. Br J Haematol 47(3):383–390

Allan D, Limbrick AR, Thomas P, Westerman MP (1982) Release of spectrin-free spicules on reoxygenation of sickled erythrocytes. Nature 295(5850):612–613

Alsultan A, Alabdulaali MK, Griffin PJ et al (2014) Sickle cell disease in Saudi Arabia: the phenotype in adults with the Arab-Indian haplotype is not benign. Br J Haematol 164(4):597–604

Ataga KI, Smith WR, De Castro LM et al (2008) Efficacy and safety of the Gardos channel blocker, senicapoc (ICA-17043), in patients with sickle cell anemia. Blood 111(8):3991–3997

Ataga KI, Reid M, Ballas SK et al (2011) Improvements in haemolysis and indicators of erythrocyte survival do not correlate with acute vaso-occlusive crises in patients with sickle cell disease: a phase III randomized, placebo-controlled, double-blind study of the Gardos channel blocker senicapoc (ICA-17043). Br J Haematol 153(1):92–104

Bencsath FA, Shartava A, Monteiro CA, Goodman SR (1996) Identification of the disulfide-linked peptide in irreversibly sickled cell á-actin. Biochemistry 35:4403–4408

Bernaudin F, Verlhac S, Chevret S et al (2008) G6PD deficiency, absence of alpha-thalassemia and hemolytic rate at baseline are significant independent risk factors for abnormally high cerebral velocities in patients with sickle cell anemia. Blood 112:4314–4317

Bertles JF, Milner PFA (1968) Irreversibly sickled erythrocytes: a consequence of heterogeneous distribution of hemoglobin types in sickle cell anemia. J Clin Invest 47:1731–1741

Brittenham GM, Schechter AN, Noguchi CT (1985) Hemoglobin S polymerization: primary determinant of the hemolytic and clinical severity of the sickling syndromes. Blood 65:183–189

Browne P, Shalev O, Hebbel RP (1998) The molecular pathobiology of cell membrane iron: the sickle red cell as a model. Free Radic Biol Med 24(6):1040–1048

Brugnara C (1993) Membrane transport of Na and K and cell dehydration in sickle erythrocytes. Experientia 49:100–109

Brugnara C (1997) Erythrocyte membrane transport physiology. Curr Opin Hematol 4(2):122–127

Brugnara C (2001) Red cell membrane in sickle cell disease. In: Steinberg MH, Forget BG, Higgs DR, Nagel RL (eds) Disorders of hemoglobin: genetics, pathophysiology, and clinical management, vol 1. Cambridge University Press, Cambridge, pp 550–576

Bunn HF (1987) Subunit assembly of hemoglobin: an important determinant of hematologic phenotype. [Review]. Blood 69:1–6

Bunn HF (1997) Pathogenesis and treatment of sickle cell disease. N Engl J Med 337(11): 762–769

Bunn HF, Forget BG (1986) Hemoglobin: molecular, genetic and clinical aspects. W.B. Saunders Company, Philadelphia

Burnett AL (2003) Pathophysiology of priapism: dysregulatory erection physiology thesis. J Urol 170(1):26–34

Burnett AL, Bivalacqua TJ, Champion HC, Musicki B (2006) Long-term oral phosphodiesterase 5 inhibitor therapy alleviates recurrent priapism. Urology 67(5):1043–1048

Burns ER, Wilkinson WH, Nagel RL (1985) Adherence properties of sickle erythrocytes in dynamic flow systems. J Lab Clin Med 105(6):673–678

Cannon RO III, Schechter AN, Panza JA et al (2001) Effects of inhaled nitric oxide on regional blood flow are consistent with intravascular nitric oxide delivery. J Clin Invest 108(2):279–287

Champion HC, Bivalacqua TJ, Takimoto E, Kass DA, Burnett AL (2005) Phosphodiesterase-5A dysregulation in penile erectile tissue is a mechanism of priapism. Proc Natl Acad Sci U S A 102(5):1661–1666

Chang J, Patton JT, Sarkar A et al (2010) GMI-1070, a novel pan-selectin antagonist, reverses acute vascular occlusions in sickle cell mice. Blood 116(10):1779–1786

Conley CL, Weatherall DJ, Richardson SN, Shepard MK, Charache S (1963) Hereditary persistence of fetal hemoglobin: a study of 79 affected persons in 15 Negro families in Baltimore. Blood 21:261–281

Costa FF, Arruda VR, Gon‡alves MG et al (1994) á S -gene-cluster haplotypes in sickle cell anemia patients from two regions of Brazil. Am J Hematol 45:96–97

Cretegny I, Edelstein SJ (1993) Double strand packing in hemoglobin S fibers. J Mol Biol 230(3):733–738

De Franceschi L, Bachir D, Galacteros F et al (1997) Oral magnesium supplements reduce erythrocyte dehydration in patients with sickle cell disease. J Clin Invest 100(7):1847–1852

De Franceschi L, Bachir D, Galacteros F et al (2000) Oral magnesium pidolate: effects of long-term administration in patients with sickle cell disease. Br J Haematol 108(2):284–289

de Jong K, Larkin SK, Styles LA, Bookchin RM, Kuypers FA (2001) Characterization of the phosphatidylserine-exposing subpopulation of sickle cells. Blood 98(3):860–867

Dean J, Schechter AN (1978a) Sickle-cell anemia: molecular and cellular bases of therapeutic approaches (third of three parts). N Engl J Med 299:863–870

Dean J, Schechter AN (1978b) Sickle-cell anemia: molecular and cellular bases of therapeutic approaches (first of three parts). N Engl J Med 299:752–763

Dean J, Schechter AN (1978c) Sickle-cell anemia: molecular and cellular bases of therapeutic approaches (second of three parts). N Engl J Med 299:804–811

Dejam A, Hunter CJ, Schechter AN, Gladwin MT (2004) Emerging role of nitrite in human biology. Blood Cells Mol Dis 32(3):423–429
Deonikar P, Kavdia M (2012) Low micromolar intravascular cell-free hemoglobin concentration affects vascular NO bioavailability in sickle cell disease: a computational analysis. J Appl Physiol 112(8):1383–1392
Dykes G, Crepeau RH, Edelstein SJ (1978) Three-dimensional reconstruction of the fibres of sickle cell haemoglobin. Nature 272(5653):506–510
Eaton WA, Hofrichter J (1987) Hemoglobin S gelation and sickle cell disease. Blood 70(5): 1245–1266
Embury SH, Hebbel RP, Mohandas N, Steinberg MH (1994) Sickle cell disease: basic principles and clinical practice, vol 1. Raven Press, New York
Evans E, Mohandas N, Leung A (1984) Static and dynamic rigidities of normal and sickle erythrocytes. Major influence of cell hemoglobin concentration. J Clin Invest 73(2):477–488
Fabry ME, Nagel RL (1982) The effect of deoxygenation on red cell density: significance for the pathophysiology of sickle cell anemia. Blood 60(6):1370–1377
Fabry ME, Mears JG, Patel P et al (1984) Dense cells in sickle cell anemia: the effects of gene interaction. Blood 64:1042–1046
Fabry ME, Romero JR, Buchanan ID et al (1991) Rapid increase in red blood cell density driven by K: Cl cotransport in a subset of sickle cell anemia reticulocytes and discocytes. Blood 78: 217–225
Ferrone FA, Hofrichter J, Eaton WA (1985) Kinetics of sickle hemoglobin polymerization. II. A double nucleation mechanism. J Mol Biol 183:611–631
Field JJ, Lin G, Okam MM et al (2013) Sickle cell vaso-occlusion causes activation of iNKT cells that is decreased by the adenosine A2A receptor agonist regadenoson. Blood 121(17): 3329–3334
Franck PF, Bevers EM, Lubin BH et al (1985) Uncoupling of the membrane skeleton from the lipid bilayer. The cause of accelerated phospholipid flip-flop leading to an enhanced procoagulant activity of sickled cells. J Clin Invest 75(1):183–190
Franco RS, Palascak M, Thompson H, Rucknagel DL, Joiner CH (1996) Dehydration of transferrin receptor-positive sickle reticulocytes during continuous or cyclic deoxygenation: role of KCl cotransport and extracellular calcium. Blood 88:4359–4365
Franco RS, Yasin Z, Palascak MB et al (2006) The effect of fetal hemoglobin on the survival characteristics of sickle cells. Blood 108(3):1073–1076
Frenette PS, Atweh GF (2007) Sickle cell disease: old discoveries, new concepts, and future promise. J Clin Invest 117(4):850–858
Gallagher PG (2013) Disorders of red cell volume regulation. Curr Opin Hematol 20(3):201–207
Gladwin MT, Schechter AN (2001) Nitric oxide therapy in sickle cell disease. Semin Hematol 38(4):333–342
Gladwin MT, Sachdev V, Jison ML et al (2004) Pulmonary hypertension as a risk factor for death in patients with sickle cell disease. N Engl J Med 350(9):886–895
Gladwin MT, Kato GJ, Weiner D et al (2011) Nitric oxide for inhalation in the acute treatment of sickle cell pain crisis: a randomized controlled trial. JAMA 305(9):893–902
Goodman SR (2004) The irreversibly sickled cell: a perspective. Cell Mol Biol 50(1):53–58
Gordeuk VR, Campbell A, Rana S et al (2009) Relationship of erythropoietin, fetal hemoglobin, and hydroxyurea treatment to tricuspid regurgitation velocity in children with sickle cell disease. Blood 114(21):4639–4644
Guasch A, Zayas CF, Eckman JR et al (1999) Evidence that microdeletions in the alpha globin gene protect against the development of sickle cell glomerulopathy in humans [In Process Citation]. J Am Soc Nephrol 10(5):1014–1019
Hamideh D, Raj V, Harrington T et al (2014) Albuminuria correlates with hemolysis and NAG and KIM-1 in patients with sickle cell anemia. Pediatr Nephrol 29(10):1997–2003
Hankins JS, Wynn LW, Brugnara C et al (2008) Phase I study of magnesium pidolate in combination with hydroxycarbamide for children with sickle cell anaemia. Br J Haematol 140(1):80–85

Hebbel RP (1984) Erythrocyte autoxidation and the membrane abnormalities of sickle red cells. Prog Clin Biol Res 159:219–225

Hebbel RP (1985) Auto-oxidation and a membrane-associated 'Fenton reagent': a possible explanation for development of membrane lesions in sickle erythrocytes. Clin Haematol 14:129–140

Hebbel RP (1991) Beyond hemoglobin polymerization: the red blood cell membrane and sickle disease pathophysiology. Blood 77:214–237

Hebbel RP (1997) Adhesive interactions of sickle erythrocytes with endothelium. J Clin Invest 99:2561–2564

Hebbel RP, Boogaerts MA, Koresawa S et al (1980) Erytrocyte adherence to endothelium as a determinant of vasocclusive severity in sickle cell disease. Trans Assoc Am Physicians 93:94–99

Hebbel RP, Eaton JW, Balasingam M, Steinberg MH (1982) Spontaneous oxygen radical generation by sickle erythrocytes. J Clin Invest 70:1253–1259

Hebbel RP, Morgan WT, Eaton JW, Hedlund BE (1988) Accelerated autoxidation and heme loss due to instability of sickle hemoglobin. Proc Natl Acad Sci U S A 85(1):237–241

Hebbel RP, Osarogiagbon UR, Kaul D (2004) The endothelial biology of sickle cell disease: inflammation and a chronic vasculopathy. Microcirculation 11:129–152

Herrick JB (1910) Peculiar elongated and sickle-shaped red blood corpuscles in a case of severe anemia. Arch Intern Med 6:517–521

Hofrichter J, Ross PD, Eaton WA (1974) Kinetics and mechanism of deoxyhemoglobin S gelation: a new approach to understanding sickle cell disease. Proc Natl Acad Sci U S A 71(12): 4864–4868

Hoover R, Rubin R, Wise G, Warren R (1979) Adhesion of normal and sickle erythrocytes to endothelial monolayer cultures. Blood 54(4):872–876

Horiuchi K, Ballas SK, Asakura T (1988) The effect of deoxygenation rate on the formation of irreversibly sickled cells. Blood 71(1):46–51

Hsu LL, Champion HC, Campbell-Lee SA et al (2007) Hemolysis in sickle cell mice causes pulmonary hypertension due to global impairment in nitric oxide bioavailability. Blood 109(7):3088–3098

Hu W, Jin R, Zhang J et al (2010) The critical roles of platelet activation and reduced NO bioavailability in fatal pulmonary arterial hypertension in a murine hemolysis model. Blood 116(9):1613–1622

Ingram VM (1956) A specific chemical difference between the globins of normal human and sickle-cell anaemia haemoglobin. Nature 178:792–794

Jeffers A, Gladwin MT, Kim-Shapiro DB (2006) Computation of plasma hemoglobin nitric oxide scavenging in hemolytic anemias. Free Radic Biol Med 41(10):1557–1565

Joiner CH, Gallagher PG (2009) The erythrocyte membrane. In: Steinberg MH, Forget BG, Higgs DR, Nagel RL (eds) Disorders of hemoglobin: genetics, pathophysiology, and clinical management, vol 2. Cambridge University Press, Cambridge

Kan YW, Dozy AM (1980) Evolution of the hemoglobin S and C genes in world populations. Science 209:388–391

Kato GJ, Hsieh M, Machado R et al (2006a) Cerebrovascular disease associated with sickle cell pulmonary hypertension. Am J Hematol 81(7):503–510

Kato GJ, McGowan V, Machado RF et al (2006b) Lactate dehydrogenase as a biomarker of hemolysis-associated nitric oxide resistance, priapism, leg ulceration, pulmonary hypertension, and death in patients with sickle cell disease. Blood 107(6):2279–2285

Kato GJ, Gladwin MT, Steinberg MH (2007) Deconstructing sickle cell disease: reappraisal of the role of hemolysis in the development of clinical subphenotypes. Blood Rev 21:37–47

Kaul DK (2009) Rheology and vascular pathobiology in sickle cell disease and thalassemia. In: Steinberg MH, Forget BG, Higgs D, Weatherall DJ (eds) Disorders of hemoglobin: genetics, pathophysiology and clinical management, 2nd edn. Cambridge University Press, Cambridge

Kaul DK, Baez S, Nagel RL (1981) Flow properties of oxygenated Hb S and Hb C erythrocytes in the isolated microvasculature of the rat: a contribution to the hemorheology of hemoglobinopathies. Clin Hemorheol 1:73–86

Kaul DK, Fabry ME, Windisch P, Baez S, Nagel RL (1983) Erythrocytes in sickle cell anemia are heterogeneous in their rheological and hemodynamic characteristics. J Clin Invest 72:22–29
Kaul DK, Fabry ME, Nagel RL (1989) Microvascular sites and characteristics of sickle cell adhesion to vascular endothelium in shear flow conditions: pathophysiological implications. Proc Natl Acad Sci U S A 86(9):3356–3360
Kaul DK, Fabry ME, Costantini F, Rubin EM, Nagel RL (1995) In vivo demonstration of red cell-endothelial interaction, sickling and altered microvascular response to oxygen in the sickle transgenic mouse. J Clin Invest 96:2845–2853
Kaul DK, Fabry ME, Nagel RL (1996) The pathophysiology of vascular obstruction in the sickle syndromes. Blood Rev 10:29–44
Kim-Shapiro DB, Schechter AN, Gladwin MT (2006) Unraveling the reactions of nitric oxide, nitrite, and hemoglobin in physiology and therapeutics. Arterioscler Thromb Vasc Biol 26(4):697–705
Kulozik AE, Wainscoat JS, Serjeant GR et al (1986) Geographical survey of the ás-globin gene haplotypes: evidence for an independent Asian origin of the sickle-cell mutation. Am J Hum Genet 39:239–244
Kulozik AE, Kar BC, Satapathy RK et al (1987) Fetal hemoglobin levels and áS globin haplotypes in an Indian population with sickle cell disease. Blood 69:1742–1746
Kutlar A, Embury SH (2014) Cellular adhesion and the endothelium: p-selectin. Hematol Oncol Clin North Am 28(2):323–339
Kuypers FA (2008) Red cell membrane lipids in hemoglobinopathies. Curr Mol Med 8(7):633–638
Kuypers FA, Lewis RA, Hua M et al (1996) Detection of altered membrane phospholipid asymmetry in subpopulations of human red blood cells using fluorescently labeled annexin V. Blood 87(3):1179–1187
Labie D, Pagnier J, Lapoumeroulie C et al (1985) Common haplotype dependency of high Gg-globin gene expression and high HbF levels in á_thalassemia and sickle cell anemia patients. Proc Natl Acad Sci U S A 82:2111–2114
Labie D, Srinivas R, Dunda O et al (1989) Haplotypes in tribal Indians bearing the sickle gene: evidence for the unicentric origin of the beta S mutation and the unicentric origin of the tribal populations of India. Hum Biol 61(4):479–491
Lane PA, O'Connell JL, Marlar RA (1994) Erythrocyte membrane vesicles and irreversibly sickled cells bind protein S. Am J Hematol 47:295–300
Lapoumeroulie C, Dunda O, Ducrocq R et al (1989) A novel sickle gene of yet another origin in Africa: the Cameroon type. Hum Genet 89:333–337
Liem RI, Young LT, Thompson AA (2007) Tricuspid regurgitant jet velocity is associated with hemolysis in children and young adults with sickle cell disease evaluated for pulmonary hypertension. Haematologica 92:1549–1552
Lim MY, Ataga KI, Key NS (2013) Hemostatic abnormalities in sickle cell disease. Curr Opin Hematol 20:472–477
Lin G, Field JJ, Yu JC et al (2013) NF-kappaB is activated in CD4+ iNKT cells by sickle cell disease and mediates rapid induction of adenosine A2A receptors. PLoS One 8(10), e74664
Lipowsky HH, Usami S, Chien S (1982) Human SS red cell rheological behavior in the microcirculation of cremaster muscle. Blood Cells 8(1):113–126
Liu SC, Derick LH, Zhai S, Palek J (1991) Uncoupling of the spectrin-based skeleton from the lipid bilayer in sickled red cells. Science 252(5005):574–576
Liu C, Marshall P, Schreibman I et al (1999) Interaction between terminal complement proteins C5b-7 and anionic phospholipids. Blood 93(7):2297–2301
Lux SE, John KM, Karnovsky MJ (1976) Irreversible deformation of the spectrin-actin lattice in irreversibly sickled cells. J Clin Invest 58:955–963
Machado RF, Martyr S, Kato GJ et al (2005) Sildenafil therapy in patients with sickle cell disease and pulmonary hypertension. Br J Haematol 130(3):445–453
Machado RF, Barst RJ, Yovetich NA et al (2011) Hospitalization for pain in patients with sickle cell disease treated with sildenafil for elevated TRV and low exercise capacity. Blood 118(4):855–864

Maier-Redelsperger M, Noguchi CT, De Montalembert M et al (1994) Variation in fetal hemoglobin parameters and predicted hemoglobin S polymerization in sickle cell children in the first two years of life: Parisian prospective study on sickle cell disease. Blood 84:3182–3188
Manwani D, Frenette PS (2013) Vaso-occlusion in sickle cell disease: pathophysiology and novel targeted therapies. Blood 122(24):3892–3898
Marotta CA, Forget BG, Cohen-Solal M, Weissman SM (1976) Nucleotide sequence analysis of coding and noncoding regions of human beta-globin mRNA. Prog Nucleic Acid Res Mol Biol 19:165–175
Marouf R, Gupta R, Haider MZ, Adekile AD (2003a) Silent brain infarcts in adult Kuwaiti sickle cell disease patients. Am J Hematol 73(4):240–243
Marouf R, Gupta R, Haider MZ, Al-Wazzan H, Adekile AD (2003b) Avascular necrosis of the femoral head in adult Kuwaiti sickle cell disease patients. Acta Haematol 110(1):11–15
Mason VR (1922) Sickle cell anemia. JAMA 79:1318–1320
Miller BA, Salameh M, Ahmed M et al (1986) High fetal hemoglobin production in sickle cell anemia in the eastern province of Saudi Arabia is genetically determined. Blood 67(5):1404–1410
Milton JN, Rooks H, Drasar E et al (2013) Genetic determinants of haemolysis in sickle cell anaemia. Br J Haematol 161(2):270–278
Minniti CP, Taylor JG, Hildesheim M et al (2011) Laboratory and echocardiography markers in sickle cell patients with leg ulcers. Am J Hematol 86(8):705–708
Mohandas N, Evans E (1984) Adherence of sickle erythrocytes to vascular endothelial cells: requirement for both cell membrane changes and plasma factors. Blood 64(1):282–287
Morris CR, Morris SM Jr, Hagar W et al (2003) Arginine therapy: a new treatment for pulmonary hypertension in sickle cell disease? Am J Respir Crit Care Med 168(1):63–69
Mozzarelli A, Hofrichter J, Eaton WA (1987) Delay time of Hb S gelation prevents most cells from sickling in vivo. Science 237:500–506
Nagel RL, Labie D (1989) DNA haplotypes and the beta s globin gene. [Review]. Prog Clin Biol Res 316B:371–393
Nagel RL, Bookchin RM, Labie D et al (1979) Structural basis for the inhibitory effects of hemoglobin F and hemoglobin A2 on the polymerization of hemoglobin S. Proc Natl Acad Sci U S A 76:670–672
Nagel RL, Fabry ME, Pagnier J et al (1984) Hematologically and genetically distinct forms of sickle cell anemia in Africa. The Senegal type and the Benin type. N Engl J Med 312:880–884
Nathan DG, Field J, Lin G et al (2012) Sickle cell disease (SCD), iNKT cells, and regadenoson infusion. Trans Am Clin Climatol Assoc 123:312–317, discussion 317–318
Ngo DA, Aygun B, Akinsheye I et al (2012) Fetal haemoglobin levels and haematological characteristics of compound heterozygotes for haemoglobin S and deletional hereditary persistence of fetal haemoglobin. Br J Haematol 156(2):259–264
Ngo D, Bae H, Steinberg MH et al (2013) Fetal hemoglobin in sickle cell anemia: genetic studies of the Arab-Indian haplotype. Blood Cells Mol Dis 51(1):22–26
Noguchi CT, Schechter AN, Rodgers GP (1993) Sickle cell disease pathophysiology. Baillieres Clin Haematol 6(1):57–91
Nolan VG, Wyszynski DF, Farrer LA, Steinberg MH (2005) Hemolysis-associated priapism in sickle cell disease. Blood 106(9):3264–3267
Nolan VG, Adewoye A, Baldwin C et al (2006) Sickle cell leg ulcers: associations with haemolysis and SNPs in Klotho, TEK and genes of the TGF-beta/BMP pathway. Br J Haematol 133(5):570–578
Nouraie M, Lee JS, Zhang Y et al (2013) The relationship between the severity of hemolysis, clinical manifestations and risk of death in 415 patients with sickle cell anemia in the US and Europe. Haematologica 98:464–472
Padmos MA, Roberts GT, Sackey K et al (1991) Two different forms of homozygous sickle cell disease occur in Saudi Arabia. Br J Haematol 79:93–98

Pauling L, Itano H, Singer SJ, Wells IC (1949) Sickle cell anemia: a molecular disease. Science 110:543–548

Perrine RP, Brown MJ, Clegg JB, Weatherall DJ, May A (1972) Benign sickle-cell anaemia. Lancet 2:1163–1167

Perrine RP, Pembrey ME, John P, Perrine S, Shoup F (1978) Natural history of sickle cell anemia in Saudi Arabs. A study of 270 subjects. Ann Intern Med 88(1):1–6

Platt OS (1994) Membrane proteins. In: Embury S, Hebbel RP, Mohandas N, Steinberg MH (eds) Sickle cell disease: basic principles and clinical practice. Raven Press, New York, pp 125–137

Platt OS, Brambilla DJ, Rosse WF et al (1994) Mortality in sickle cell disease. Life expectancy and risk factors for early death. N Engl J Med 330(23):1639–1644

Reiter CD, Gladwin MT (2003) An emerging role for nitric oxide in sickle cell disease vascular homeostasis and therapy. Curr Opin Hematol 10(2):99–107

Reiter CD, Wang X, Tanus-Santos JE et al (2002) Cell-free hemoglobin limits nitric oxide bioavailability in sickle-cell disease. Nat Med 8(12):1383–1389

Repka T, Hebbel RP (1991) Hydroxyl radical formation by sickle erythrocyte membranes: role of pathologic iron deposits and cytoplasmic reducing agents. Blood 78(10):2753–2758

Sakamoto TM, Lanaro C, Ozelo MC et al (2013) Increased adhesive and inflammatory properties in blood outgrowth endothelial cells from sickle cell anemia patients. Microvasc Res 90:173–179

Saraf SL, Zhang X, Kanias T et al (2014) Haemoglobinuria is associated with chronic kidney disease and its progression in patients with sickle cell anaemia. Br J Haematol 164(5): 729–739

Schwartz RS, Rybicki AC, Heath RH, Lubin BH (1987) Protein 4.1 in sickle erythrocytes. Evidence for oxidative damage. J Biol Chem 262(32):15666–15672

Setty BN, Kulkarni S, Stuart MJ (2002) Role of erythrocyte phosphatidylserine in sickle red cell-endothelial adhesion. Blood 99(5):1564–1571

Shartava A, Monteiro CA, Bencsath FA et al (1995) A posttranslational modification of á-actin contributes to the slow dissociation of the spectrin-protein 4.1-actin complex of irreversibly sickled cells. J Cell Biol 128:805–818

Sherwood JB, Goldwasser E, Chilcote R, Carmichael LD, Nagel RL (1986) Sickle cell anemia patients have low erythropoietin levels for their degree of anemia. Blood 67(1):46–49

Smith BD, La Celle PL (1986) Erythrocyte-endothelial cell adherence in sickle cell disorders. Blood 68(5):1050–1054

Solovey A, Lin Y, Browne P et al (1997) Circulating activated endothelial cells in sickle cell anemia. N Engl J Med 337(22):1584–1590

Solovieff N, Milton JN, Hartley SW et al (2010) Fetal hemoglobin in sickle cell anemia: genome-wide association studies suggest a regulatory region in the 5' olfactory receptor gene cluster. Blood 115(9):1815–1822

Sparkenbaugh E, Pawlinski R (2013) Interplay between coagulation and vascular inflammation in sickle cell disease. Br J Haematol 162(1):3–14

Stamler JS, Singel DJ, Loscalzo J (1992) Biochemistry of nitric oxide and its redox-activated forms. Science 258(5090):1898–1902

Stamler JS, Jia L, Eu JP et al (1997) Blood flow regulation by S-nitrosohemoglobin in the physiological oxygen gradient. Science 276:2034–2037

Steinberg MH (2006) Pathophysiologically based drug treatment of sickle cell disease. Trends Pharmacol Sci 27(4):204–210

Steinberg MH (2009) Other sickle hemoglobinopathies. In: Steinberg MH, Forget BG, Higgs DR, Weatherall DJ (eds) Disorders of hemoglobin, 2nd edn. Cambridge University Press, Cambridge, pp 564–586

Steinberg MH, Embury SH (1986) Alpha-thalassemia in blacks: genetic and clinical aspects and interactions with the sickle hemoglobin gene. [Review]. Blood 68:985–990

Steinberg MH, Sebastiani P (2012) Genetic modifiers of sickle cell disease. Am J Hematol 87:824–826

Steinberg MH, Forget BG, Higgs DR, Weatherall DJ (2009) Disorders of hemoglobin: genetics, pathophysiology, clinical management, 2 edn, vol 2. Cambridge University Press, Cambridge

Steinberg MH, Chui DH, Dover GJ, Sebastiani P, Alsultan A (2014) Fetal hemoglobin in sickle cell anemia: a glass half full? Blood 123(4):481–485

Stuart MJ, Setty BN (2001) Hemostatic alterations in sickle cell disease: relationships to disease pathophysiology. Pediatr Pathol Mol Med 20(1):27–46

Sugihara T, Repka T, Hebbel RP (1992) Detection, characterization, and bioavailability of membrane- associated iron in the intact sickle red cell. J Clin Invest 90:2327–2332

Tait JF, Gibson D (1994) Measurement of membrane phospholipid asymmetry in normal and sickle-cell erythrocytes by means of annexin V binding. J Lab Clin Med 123:741–748

Taylor JG, Nolan VG, Mendelsohn L et al (2008) Chronic hyper-hemolysis in sickle cell anemia: association of vascular complications and mortality with less frequent vasoocclusive pain. PLoS One 3(5), e2095

Test ST, Woolworth VS (1994) Defective regulation of complement by the sickle erythrocyte: evidence for a defect in control of membrane attack complex formation. Blood 83:842–852

Turhan A, Weiss LA, Mohandas N, Coller BS, Frenette PS (2002) Primary role for adherent leukocytes in sickle cell vascular occlusion: a new paradigm. Proc Natl Acad Sci U S A 99(5):3047–3051

van der Land V, Peters M, Biemond BJ et al (2013) Markers of endothelial dysfunction differ between subphenotypes in children with sickle cell disease. Thromb Res 132(6):712–717

Wagner GM, Chiu DT, Yee MC, Lubin BH (1986) Red cell vesiculation--a common membrane physiologic event. J Lab Clin Med 108(4):315–324

Wallace KL, Marshall MA, Ramos SI et al (2009) NKT cells mediate pulmonary inflammation and dysfunction in murine sickle cell disease through production of IFN-gamma and CXCR3 chemokines. Blood 114(3):667–676

Wang RH, Phillips G Jr, Medof ME, Mold C (1993) Activation of the alternative complement pathway by exposure of phosphatidylethanolamine and phosphatidylserine on erythrocytes from sickle cell disease patients. J Clin Invest 92:1326–1335

Watson J, Stahman AW, Bilello FP (1948) Significance of paucity of sickle cells in newborn negro infants. Am J Med Sci 215:419–423

Weiner DL, Hibberd PL, Betit P et al (2003) Preliminary assessment of inhaled nitric oxide for acute vaso-occlusive crisis in pediatric patients with sickle cell disease. JAMA 289(9):1136–1142

Westerman MP, Cole ER, Wu K (1984) The effect of spicules obtained from sickle red cells on clotting activity. Br J Haematol 56(4):557–562

Zennadi R, Hines PC, De Castro LM et al (2004) Epinephrine acts through erythroid signaling pathways to activate sickle cell adhesion to endothelium via LW-alphavbeta3 interactions. Blood 104(12):3774–3781

Chapter 4
Red Blood Cells and the Vaso-Occlusive Process

Nancy J. Wandersee and Cheryl A. Hillery

Abstract While the definitive genetic defect in sickle cell disease (SCD) is sickle hemoglobin (HbS), the relationship between the HbS mutation and the pathogenesis of vaso-occlusion in SCD remains incompletely understood and likely involves multiple complex and heterogeneous steps. Since chronic transfusion can prevent stroke and reduce the frequency of acute vaso-occlusive events, it is clear that the sickle red blood cell (RBC) plays a critical role in this process. Numerous sickle RBC factors contribute to the vaso-occlusive process, including: HbS polymerization; RBC cation loss and resultant cellular dehydration; oxidative injury of RBC membrane proteins and lipids; band 3 clustering; loss of phospholipid asymmetry and phosphatidylserine exposure; reduced RBC deformability; irreversibly sickled RBCs; increased adhesion of sickle RBCs to the endothelium and other circulating blood cells; intravascular hemolysis with the release of cell-free hemoglobin, arginase, and adenosine deaminase; and RBC microvesiculation. These sickle RBC properties initiate and propagate endothelial injury, vascular stasis, and activation of the coagulation and inflammatory pathways, precipitating acute vaso-occlusion.

Keywords Sickle red blood cell • Adhesion • Oxidative injury • Vaso-occlusion • Hemolysis

---

N.J. Wandersee
Department of Pediatrics and Children's Research Institute, Medical College of Wisconsin, Milwaukee, WI, USA

Blood Research Institute, Medical Sciences Institute, BloodCenter of Wisconsin, 8727 Watertown Plank Rd., Milwaukee, WI 53226, USA
e-mail: nancy.wandersee@bcw.edu

C.A. Hillery (✉)
Department of Pediatrics and Children's Research Institute, Medical College of Wisconsin, Milwaukee, WI, USA

Blood Research Institute, Medical Sciences Institute, BloodCenter of Wisconsin, 8727 Watertown Plank Rd., Milwaukee, WI 53226, USA

Department of Pediatrics, Division of Hematology/Oncology, Children's Hospital of Pittsburgh of UPMC, University of Pittsburgh School of Medicine, 5119 Rangos Research Building, 4401 Penn Avenue, Pittsburgh, PA 15224, USA
e-mail: cheryl.hillery@chp.edu

© Springer International Publishing Switzerland 2016

F.F. Costa, N. Conran (eds.), *Sickle Cell Anemia*,
DOI 10.1007/978-3-319-06713-1_4

4.1 The Sickle Red Blood Cell (RBC)

Sickle cell disease (SCD) is caused by a single amino acid substitution in the beta chain of hemoglobin (hemoglobin β Glu6Val) that predisposes deoxyhemoglobin S to polymerize and form long crystals that distort and damage the red cell membrane (Hillery and Panepinto 2004; Hebbel 1991; Bunn 1997). In addition, sickle hemoglobin (HbS) is moderately unstable, with oxidized hemoglobin binding avidly to the lipid bilayer and contributing to multiple membrane defects. The link between HbS polymerization, its many effects on the sickle red blood cell (RBC), and the pathobiology of vaso-occlusion remains incompletely understood and likely involves many complex and heterogeneous steps. The evidence that chronic RBC transfusion effectively prevents most primary or recurrent stroke events (Adams et al. 1998; Russell et al. 1984) and reduces the incidence of pain and acute chest syndrome (Miller et al. 2001) indicates a critical role for the sickle RBC in the pathophysiology of vaso-occlusion. Sickle RBC characteristics that appear to contribute to acute vaso-occlusion include the extent of HbS polymerization, oxidant injury of membrane proteins and lipids, cation loss resulting in cellular dehydration, reduced deformability with a propensity for vesiculation, cellular lysis and enhanced adhesive properties. These sickle RBC characteristics also contribute to chronic endothelial injury, vascular stasis and increased activation of the inflammatory and coagulation pathways. This chapter will focus on the role of the sickle red blood cell (RBC) in the vaso-occlusive process.

4.2 Hemoglobin S Polymerization

The substitution of valine for glutamic acid at the sixth position of the beta chain of sickle hemoglobin creates a hydrophobic pocket in the hemoglobin tetramer that polymerizes upon deoxygenation. This polymerization process is reversed with reoxygenation. The polymerization of deoxy-HbS involves a two-step, double-nucleation process, followed by a rapid increase in polymer/fiber formation that results in RBC "sickling" (Eaton and Hofrichter 1987). There is a delay time between HbS deoxygenation and the onset of exponential polymerization, which is markedly influenced by the intracellular hemoglobin concentration (MCHC), temperature, pH, and the presence of non-S hemoglobins, such as HbF or HbA. For example, the delay time of polymer formation is dependent on the 15th to 30th power of hemoglobin concentration (Eaton and Hofrichter 1987). Thus, the dehydration found in subpopulations of sickle RBCs (described in Sect. 4.3) can greatly promote HbS polymerization.

The estimated delay time of greater than 15 s predicts that an unimpeded sickle RBC should return to the lung for reoxygenation before HbS is fully polymerized (Mozzarelli et al. 1987; Du et al. 2015). In agreement, the majority of sickle RBCs in the returning venous circulation are not polymerized. However, any event that delays the return of the sickle RBC to the pulmonary circulation will permit progression to full polymerization. RBC adhesion to the vascular endothelium, either directly to endothelial cells or via bridging adhesive ligands or bound leukocytes will also promote HbS polymerization due to delay in return to the pulmonary circulation for reoxygenation. Reduced sickle RBC deformability will also slow trafficking through the microcirculation and prolong the time in the hypoxic environment. Finally, any pre-existing polymer that does not completely solubilize in the lung circulation may have a markedly shortened or absent delay time such that polymerization can more rapidly proceed in the microcirculation following delivery of oxygen to tissue beds (Huang et al. 2003).

While the definitive genetic defect in SCD is HbS, the direct link between HbS polymerization and the pathobiology of vaso-occlusion is more complex. Since HbS will only polymerize after delivery of oxygen, uninterrupted blood return to the lungs for reoxygenation is essential to prevent RBC sickling. Risk factors that promote sickling include RBC dehydration, lung or vascular disease that prevents optimal oxygenation, any right shift in oxygen binding curve (acidosis and fever), low HbF levels and delayed microvascular transit time due to leukocyte and sickle RBC adhesion to injured or inflamed endothelium. Because of this, clinical care for sickle cell disease is often targeted to limit HbS polymerization, such as with generous hydration, optimizing oxygenation and raising HbF levels with hydroxyurea therapy.

4.3 Cation Loss and Dehydration

Since the polymerization rate of deoxyHbS is critically dependent on the intracellular concentration of hemoglobin, sickle RBC dehydration will promote sickling and may contribute to the development of vaso-occlusion in SCD cell disease; this may be best exemplified by the papillary necrosis that occurs in the hyperosmolar kidney medulla. Additionally, RBC dehydration status can directly affect the adhesive phenotype, possibly by exposing or altering adhesive components of the membrane (Stone et al. 1996; Hebbel et al. 1989; Wandersee et al. 2005).

A significant proportion of sickle RBCs are inherently dehydrated, primarily due to intracellular K^+ and water losses via the erythrocyte Ca^{2+}-dependent K^+ (Gardos) channel (Brugnara et al. 1986) and the K/Cl cotransport system (Franco et al. 1996). In sickle RBCs, the pathologic activation of the Gardos channel that results in water loss is aggravated by transient increases in Ca^{2+} permeability induced in sickle RBCs with every deoxygenation-reoxygenation cycle (Lew et al. 1997). In SCD, RBC K-Cl cotransport is activated by low pH (Brugnara et al. 1986), low magnesium content, oxidative damage, positively charged hemoglobin (HbS, HbC) and cell swelling. Clotrimazole specifically inhibits the Gardos channel (Brugnara et al. 1993). Magnesium decreases the K^+ and water losses via the K/Cl cotransport system. Both dietary magnesium supplementation (De Franceschi et al. 1996) and oral clotrimazole therapy (De Franceschi et al. 1994) improved the hydration status and hemoglobin levels of a transgenic sickle cell mouse model.

Despite the likely important link between polymerization of HbS with cellular dehydration, and the potential contribution of RBC dehydration to RBC adhesive properties (Wandersee et al. 2005), clinical trials to date using agents to improve sickle RBC hydration have shown minimal effects on clinically significant vaso-occlusive events. A short term study of five patients with SCD treated with oral clotrimazole also reduced RBC dehydration and resulted in a striking reduction of the number of dense red cells (Brugnara et al. 1996). While the Phase II study using the novel inhibitor of the Gardos channel, ICA-17043, showed improvement of anemia and reduction in reticulocytosis in patients with SCD (Ataga et al. 2006), the subsequent Phase III study was prematurely terminated due to lack of clinical efficacy in reducing acute painful events in patients with sickle cell syndromes (Ataga et al. 2011). In addition, while preliminary studies using Mg pidolate to block the K/CL cotransport system confirmed the beneficial effects on red cell dehydration (De Franceschi et al. 2000; Hankins et al. 2008), the Phase III trial was terminated due to a slow rate of enrollment.

4.4 Oxidant Injury of the Sickle RBC Membrane

Hemoglobin S has a higher auto-oxidation rate compared to hemoglobin A; oxidized hemoglobin has an affinity for the lipid bilayer and can expel its heme group with subsequent liberation of free iron (Hebbel et al. 1988; Sheng et al. 1998). Membrane associated iron is catalytically active and likely contributes to the increased susceptibility of sickle RBC membranes to lipid peroxidation (Chiu et al. 1979). This also promotes further hemoglobin denaturation, including the formation of irreversibly oxidized hemichromes located near the membrane inner surface. As a consequence, the sickle RBC membrane is uniquely targeted for oxidant stress, effectively bypassing or depleting the RBC of natural antioxidants, such as vitamin E (α- and γ-tocopherol) glutathione or ascorbic acid (Darghouth et al. 2011). The increased oxidative damage to membrane proteins and lipids contributes to sickle RBC membrane abnormalities, including aberrant clustering of surface proteins, disruption of phospholipid asymmetry, dysregulated cation homeostasis, reduced deformability, formation of irreversibly sickled cells (ISC), increased fragility and release of microvesicles.

4.5 Clusters of Band 3

Clustered Band 3 can also participate in sickle RBC adhesion and promote vaso-occlusion. Band 3 is an abundant RBC anion exchanger that spans the plasma membrane multiple times and is linked to the RBC cytoskeleton. Band 3 is abnormally clustered on the sickle RBC surface due to binding of its cytosolic sections to denatured HbS hemichromes found at the inner sickle membrane (Waugh et al. 1986). Denatured hemoglobin also colocalizes glycophorin and ankyrin on sickle RBC membranes, although to a lesser extent than band 3. Clustering of band 3 binds naturally occurring anti-band 3 autoantibodies (Kannan et al. 1988). Opsonized band 3 promotes sickle RBC phagocytosis by the reticuloendothelial system that will shorten the sickle RBC lifespan. Band 3 mediates the adhesion of malaria-infected RBCs to the vascular endothelium via exposure of previously cryptic adhesive sites (Crandall et al. 1993). Peptides from sites of clustered Band 3 that are aberrantly exposed on sickle RBCs will also inhibit sickle RBC adhesion to cultured endothelial cells in vitro (Thevenin et al. 1997).

4.6 Increased Phosphatidylserine (PS) Exposure

The normal lipid bilayer maintains phosphatidylserine (PS) and phosphatidylethanolamine sequestered on the inner leaflet. In SCD, PS is abnormally exposed on the outer surface of the sickle RBC membrane (Choe et al. 1986). This impairment of the normal phospholipid asymmetry on the sickle RBC membrane may be due to thiol oxidation of the translocase that moves PS to the inner layer and increased calcium activation of the scramblase that permits PS to move outward (Zachowski et al. 1985).

When PS translocates to the cell surface under normal physiologic circumstances, such as during platelet activation, externalized PS serves as an anchor for factors in the hemostatic system, promoting the activation of the coagulation cascade (Zwaal and Schroit 1997). In agreement, there is a correlation between the level of sickle RBC PS exposure and the activity of the coagulation cascade in human and murine SCD (Setty et al. 2000, 2001). This suggests that this loss of sickle RBC membrane asymmetry, which results in increased PS exposure, contributes to the well described prothrombotic state found in individuals with SCD (Singer and Ataga 2008). Sickle membrane PS exposure also promotes RBC adhesion to endothelial cells (Setty et al. 2002; Schlegel et al. 1985; Manodori et al. 2000). In addition, PS exposure on sickle RBCs shortens RBC survival in sickle mice effectively increasing hemolytic rate (de Jong et al. 2001). Thus, increased PS exposure on sickle RBCs may participate in the vaso-occlusive process by increased adhesion to the microvasculature, activation of the coagulation cascade, and decreased RBC lifespan.

4.7 Membrane Deformability and Irreversibly Sickled Cells (ISC)

There is reduced deformability of sickle RBCs even when oxygenated and when HbS is fully solubilized (Chien et al. 1970). Both cellular dehydration and irreversible membrane changes contribute to this effect. This includes abnormal associations and crosslinking of cytoskeletal proteins and membrane components that result from both repeated HbS polymerization and oxidative injury of the membrane lipids and proteins.

Irreversibly sickled RBCs (ISCs) are the predominant form of "sickled" RBCs seen on typical blood smears. ISCs are due to a permanent shape change as a product of damage to membrane and cytoskeletal proteins enabling the retention of the elongated RBC shape regardless of hemoglobin polymerization status (Lux et al. 1976).

Consequently, even when the HbS is oxygenated and fully soluble, the ISC retains its abnormal elongated shape. ISCs tend to be very dense (MCHC greater than 44 g/dL), externalize PS, have low HbF levels and very short survival (Bertles and Milner 1968). Clinically, ISCs are important in diagnosis of a sickling disorder from a blood smear, vary greatly in number between individual patients and contribute to the hemolytic rate from the shortened life span. While ISCs likely participate in RBC blockage associated with vaso-occlusion (Kaul et al. 1986), it is less clear whether the ISC count correlates with vaso-occlusive severity (Barabino et al. 1987b).

4.8 Adhesive Properties of Sickle RBCs

The increased adhesion of sickle RBCs to vascular endothelium in vitro has been described using both static adhesion assays (Hebbel et al. 1980b; Mohandas and Evans 1984) and endothelialized flow chambers (Barabino et al. 1987a). These observations have been confirmed using live animal models by either infusing human sickle RBCs into rats (Fabry et al. 1989; Kaul et al. 1989; French et al. 1997) or by studying transgenic sickle cell mouse models (Kaul et al. 1995; Wood et al. 2004). In addition, leukocyte and platelet interactions with sickle RBC and vascular endothelium are important components of the vaso-occlusive process (Turhan et al. 2002; Dominical et al. 2015; Conran and Costa 2009). The enhanced interactions between sickle RBCs, leukocytes, platelets and the vessel wall play important roles in the pathogenesis of vascular occlusion in sickle cell disease.

The early findings that sickle RBCs adhere to the endothelium to a variable degree and that the level of adhesion may correlate with disease severity (Hebbel et al. 1980a) prompted further investigation into potential receptors and signaling pathways involved in the adhesive processes. Reticulocytes from both normal and sickle individuals express the adhesion molecules integrin $\alpha4\beta1$ (Swerlick et al. 1993; Joneckis et al. 1993) and CD36 (GP IV) (Joneckis et al. 1993; Sugihara et al. 1992; Browne and Hebbel 1996). Immature reticulocytes have greater levels of adhesion to endothelial cells compared to mature RBCs, pointing to a potential unique role for reticulocyte adhesion under select experimental and physiologic conditions (Mohandas and Evans 1984; Brittain et al. 1993; Fabry et al. 1992; Joneckis et al. 1993; Sugihara et al. 1992). Potential RBC adhesion molecules that remain present on mature RBCs include basal cell adhesion molecule-1/Lutheran (BCAM/LU), intercellular adhesion molecule-4 (ICAM-4) (Zennadi et al. 2004), integrin associated protein (CD47), phosphatidylserine (PS) (Setty et al. 2002) and sulfated glycolipids (Hillery et al. 1996; Joneckis et al. 1996).

Integrin $\alpha4\beta1$ is a receptor for both fibronectin and vascular cell adhesion molecule-1 (VCAM-1) (Humphries et al. 1995). Sickle RBCs bind to VCAM-1 on cytokine-stimulated endothelial cells (Swerlick et al. 1993) or transfected COS cells (Gee and Platt 1995), as well as immobilized fibronectin (Kasschau et al. 1996) via $\alpha4\beta1$. The activation state of $\alpha4\beta1$ is regulated by several factors, including divalent cation concentration and agonist-induced cell signaling (Han et al. 2003). The $\alpha4$

cytoplasmic domain is directly phosphorylated in vitro by cAMP-dependent protein kinase A (PKA) (Goldfinger et al. 2003), suggesting a role for PKA in activation of α4β1. In agreement, ligation of CD47 on sickle reticulocytes activates α4β1 via a PKA-dependent phosphorylation of the α4 cytoplasmic tail (Brittain et al. 2004). Sickle RBC α4β1 binding to endothelial VCAM-1 likely contributes to the adherence of sickle reticulocytes to cytokine-stimulated retinal microvascular endothelial cells in vitro (Setty and Stuart 1996).

CD36 is a non-integrin adhesive receptor that binds thrombospondin (TSP) and collagen and is present on the surface of endothelial cells, platelets, and a reticulocyte-rich subpopulation of normal and sickle RBCs (Joneckis et al. 1993; Sugihara et al. 1992). Sickle RBCs bind to endothelial cells in the presence of soluble TSP and this adhesion is blocked by anti-CD36 monoclonal antibodies in both static adhesion assays (Sugihara et al. 1992) and under flow conditions (Brittain et al. 1993).

The Lutheran blood group proteins, basal cell adhesion molecule-1 and Lutheran (BCAM/Lu) are derived by alternative splicing from the same gene and differ only in the length of their cytoplasmic tails. Sickle RBCs over express BCAM/Lu, which specifically binds to the alpha 5 subunit of the extracellular matrix protein laminin (Udani et al. 1998; Parsons et al. 2001). RBC intercellular adhesion molecule-4 (ICAM-4), otherwise known as blood group Landsteiner-Weiner (LW), binds β3 integrins, including αvβ3 expressed on vascular endothelial cells (Parsons et al. 1999). In a rat ex vivo microvascular flow model, ICAM-4-specific peptides inhibited human sickle RBC adhesion to the activated ex vivo microvascular endothelium (Kaul et al. 2006). Interestingly, both BCAM/Lu and ICAM-1 can be activated by epinephrine in a subset of sickle RBCs via a cAMP-dependent pathway that likely involves PKA (Zennadi et al. 2004; Hines et al. 2003).

Integrin-associated protein (CD47) is a 50 kDa integral membrane protein found on RBCs and many other cells that associates with integrins and binds to the C-terminal cell binding domain of thrombospondin-1 (TSP) (Gao et al. 1996). CD47 is expressed in RBCs and protects normal RBCs from immune clearance (Oldenborg et al. 2000). CD47 on sickle RBCs binds immobilized TSP under both static and flow conditions (Brittain et al. 2001). Furthermore, soluble TSP binds CD47 and induces an increase in sickle RBC adhesion via shear stress-dependent and G protein-mediated signal transduction pathways (Brittain et al. 2001).

Lipids naturally present in the red cell membrane that have been abnormally exposed or modified on the sickle RBC also contribute to their adhesive properties. For example, increased exposure of phosphatidylserine (PS) on the sickle RBC likely contributes to its proadhesive phenotype (Setty et al. 2002; Schlegel et al. 1985; Manodori et al. 2000). Sulfated glycolipids avidly bind TSP, von Willebrand factor, and laminin and may also play a role in sickle red cell adhesion (Hillery et al. 1996; Joneckis et al. 1996; Barabino et al. 1999; Zhou et al. 2011).

A disturbed endothelium contributes to sickle RBC, leukocyte and platelet adhesion. Endothelial adhesive molecules that bind sickle RBCs include VCAM-1, integrin αVβ3, E-selectin and P-selectin (Swerlick et al. 1993; Gee and Platt 1995;

Brittain et al. 1993; Natarajan et al. 1996; Matsui et al. 2001). For example, monoclonal antibodies directed against αVβ3 inhibited human sickle RBC adhesion to platelet-activating factor (PAF)-treated rat mesocecum vasculature ex vivo (Kaul et al. 2000b). In agreement, αVβ3 antagonists also reduced sickle RBC adhesion to human endothelial cell monolayers under venular shear flow conditions (Finnegan et al. 2007). P-selectin is rapidly expressed on the surface of activated endothelial cells and promotes sickle RBC rolling and adhesion (Embury et al. 2004). Optimal surface expression of these endothelial adhesion molecules requires induction by cytokines, shear stress or other perturbations of the endothelium. In fact, exposure of endothelium to inflammatory agonists is associated with increased RBC adhesion (Wick and Eckman 1996; Manodori 2001).

Adhesive plasma and extracellular matrix proteins may also contribute to sickle RBC adhesion. Thrombospondin (TSP) is a 450 kDa, homotrimeric glycoprotein present in the subendothelial matrix, plasma and platelet alpha storage granules; it can be released in high local concentrations by activated platelets (Santoro and Frazier 1987). In SCD, both soluble and immobilized TSP can bind sickle RBCs. In its soluble form, TSP may serve as a linker molecule between sickle RBCs and endothelial cells (Brittain et al. 1993; Gupta et al. 1999). TSP also interacts with sickle RBC CD47 (Brittain et al. 2001), sulfated glycolipids (Barabino et al. 1999), and a normally cryptic domain of the dominant membrane protein, band 3, which is subject to rearrangement in hematologic disorders (Thevenin et al. 1997; Sherman et al. 1992). Laminin, a major constituent of the extracellular matrix, is composed of a family of large heterotrimeric glycoproteins that support cell adhesion and migration (Tryggvason 1993). Sickle RBCs avidly bind both immobilized and soluble laminin (Udani et al. 1998; Hillery et al. 1996). Vitronectin, fibrinogen, and von Willebrand factor also support sickle RBC adherence (Wick and Eckman 1996).

Sickle RBCs also bind leukocytes and platelets (Sakamoto et al. 2013; Frenette 2004). In fact, the leukocyte-endothelial cell adhesive event may initiate and precede sickle RBC adhesion in the microvascular bed (Turhan et al. 2002; Dominical et al. 2015; Conran and Costa 2009). The sickle RBC likely utilizes multiple adhesive pathways, potentially first binding to the endothelium and inducing localized pathologic changes, followed by a second adhesive event with the sickle RBC binding to leukocytes, platelets, or the newly exposed endothelial or subendothelial adhesive ligands.

4.9 Increased Fragility and Microvesiculation

Sickle RBCs have increased fragility with a propensity for vesiculation and cellular lysis. The shortened lifespan of sickle RBCs includes both extravascular mechanisms of removal, primarily through the reticuloendothelial system, and intravascular hemolysis. Intravascular RBC lysis releases intracellular components and generates RBC microvesicles and likely contributes most directly to the vaso-occlusive process.

4.9.1 Intravascular Hemolysis

Intravascular hemolysis contributes to the vascular pathologies associated with SCD. RBC lysis releases Hb into the plasma compartment; consequently plasma levels of cell-free Hb (CF-Hb) from individuals with SCD are elevated. CF-Hb is present mainly in the ferrous oxygenated form (oxyHb) with a smaller contribution of the ferric form (metHb) (Reiter et al. 2002). Normal individuals have plasma CF-Hb levels of less than 1 μM, whereas individuals with SCD have variable levels up to ~20 μM (Reiter et al. 2002). CF-Hb is an efficient scavenger of nitric oxide (NO), a critical regulator of vascular homeostasis (Datta et al. 2004; Gladwin et al. 2004; Jison and Gladwin 2003; Liao 2002; Pawloski 2003; Jeffers et al. 2006; Kim-Shapiro et al. 2006; Lancaster Jr 1994). OxyHb reacts with NO with a rate constant in excess of 10^7 $M^{-1}s^{-1}$ to form metHb and inert nitrate. In individuals with SCD, oxidation of CF-Hb by NO inhalation therapy improves forearm blood flow in response to nitrovasodilators, suggesting that CF-Hb has an acute effect on the bioavailability of NO (Reiter et al. 2002). However, chronic vascular dysfunction in isolated vessels has been observed in animal models of SCD and other intravascular hemolytic models (Kaul et al. 2000a; Frei et al. 2008; Ou et al. 2003). The role played by CF-Hb in chronic vascular dysfunction is less clear, but it is conceivable that long-term loss of NO bioavailability, due to the presence of CF-Hb, could lead to significant changes in endothelial function, including a switch to alternate mechanisms of vascular control (Godecke and Schrader 2000; Zatz and Baylis 1998). The chronic presence of CF-Hb is also associated with other pathological presentations of SCD, including hemoglobinuria, increased blood pressure and vasoconstriction, decreased inhibition of platelet activation, a prothrombotic tendency, and increased expression of endothelial cell adhesion molecules such as ICAM-1, VCAM-1 and E-selectin (Rother et al. 2005; Villagra et al. 2007; Silva et al. 2009).

Other cytoplasmic components of lysed RBCs also accumulate in the plasma during chronic intravascular hemolysis, and may be important contributors to overall vascular dysfunction. RBC arginase has been specifically highlighted as arginase will deplete the substrate for nitric oxide formation with a negative impact on vasoreactivity. In this regard it is worth highlighting that there is significant evidence that RBC arginase, in humans, may contribute to loss of NO function through its ability to deplete arginine, the substrate for nitric oxide synthase (Rother et al. 2005; Gladwin 2006; Morris et al. 2008).

In addition, hemolysis releases adenosine deaminase (ADA) from the RBC into plasma, reducing extracellular adenosine stores via the conversion of adenosine to inosine (Tofovic et al. 2009). Since adenosine is involved in protective responses against vasculopathy, the reduction of adenosine by ADA released from RBCs may exacerbate vascular pathology initiated by cell-free hemoglobin and heme (Tofovic et al. 2009).

4.9.2 *Microvesiculation*

Patients with SCD have elevated RBC, platelet, monocyte, and endothelial microvesicles that increase further during crisis (Shet et al. 2003). RBC sickling, induced by hypoxia and subsequent reoxygenation, causes the loss of 2–3 % of sickled RBC lipids in the form of microvesicles (Allan et al. 1982). RBC-derived microvesicles house hemoglobin, which scavenges NO with comparable kinetics to soluble hemoglobin (Donadee et al. 2011). Circulating RBC fragments and microparticles may directly injure the endothelium and promote coagulation and inflammation (Setty et al. 2001). Interestingly, when children with SCD were treated with hydroxyurea therapy, which should improve sickling and provide a new source of nitric oxide, there were reduced levels of RBC and platelet-derived microvesicles compared to untreated counterparts (Nebor et al. 2013).

Incubation of sickle RBC microvesicles with cultured endothelial cells induced reactive oxygen species (ROS) formation to a much greater extent than control RBC microvesicles (Camus et al. 2012). The ROS formation was also inhibited by pretreating the microvesicles with annexin V to "cover" microvesicle anionic phospholipids. When RBC microvesicles were injected into a mouse model of sickle cell disease, acute "vaso-occlusion" of the kidneys was observed, suggesting a potential role for microvesicles in the evolution of vaso-occlusion (Camus et al. 2012, 2015).

In summary, the sickle RBC is a critical participant in the vaso-occlusive process, which is the major clinical manifestation of sickle cell disease. HbS directly injures the sickle RBC through polymerization of deoxyHbS that distorts and perturbs the red blood cell membrane and through oxidized HbS that binds to the lipid bilayer, causing further membrane damage. This results in a wide array of sickle RBC abnormalities, including cellular dehydration, clustering of band, increased PS exposure, reduced RBC deformability, increased hemolysis with release of intracellular contents and microvesicles, and increased adhesion to the vascular endothelium and non-erythroid blood cells. These aberrant sickle RBC properties initiate and propagate endothelial injury, vascular stasis, and activation of the coagulation and inflammatory pathways, ultimately precipitating acute vascular occlusion.

References

Adams RJ, McKie VC, Hsu L, Files B, Vichinsky E, Pegelow C, Abboud M, Gallagher D, Kutlar A, Nichols FT, Bonds DR, Brambilla D, Woods G, Olivieri N, Driscoll C, Miller S, Wang W, Hurlett A, Scher C, Berman B, Carl E, Jones AM, Roach ES, Wright E (1998) Prevention of a first stroke by transfusions in children with sickle, cell anemia and abnormal results on transcranial Doppler ultrasonography. N Engl J Med 339:5–11

Allan D, Limbrick AR, Thomas P, Westerman MP (1982) Release of spectrin-free spicules on reoxygenation of sickled erythrocytes. Nature 295:612–613

Ataga KI, Orringer EP, Styles L, Vichinsky EP, Swerdlow P, Davis GA, Desimone PA, Stocker JW (2006) Dose-escalation study of ICA-17043 in patients with sickle cell disease. Pharmacotherapy 26:1557–1564

Ataga KI, Reid M, Ballas SK, Yasin Z, Bigelow C, James LS, Smith WR, Galacteros F, Kutlar A, Hull JH, Stocker JW (2011) Improvements in haemolysis and indicators of erythrocyte survival do not correlate with acute vaso-occlusive crises in patients with sickle cell disease: a phase III randomized, placebo-controlled, double-blind study of the Gardos channel blocker senicapoc (ICA-17043). Br J Haematol 153:92–104

Barabino GA, McIntire LV, Eskin SG, Sears DA, Udden M (1987a) Endothelial cell interactions with sickle cell, sickle trait, mechanically injured, and normal erythrocytes under controlled flow. Blood 70:152–157

Barabino GA, McIntire LV, Eskin SG, Sears DA, Udden M (1987b) Rheological studies of erythrocyte-endothelial cell interactions in sickle cell disease. Prog Clin Biol Res 240:113–127

Barabino GA, Liu XD, Ewenstein BM, Kaul DK (1999) Anionic polysaccharides inhibit adhesion of sickle erythrocytes to the vascular endothelium and result in improved hemodynamic behavior. Blood 93:1422–1429

Bertles JF, Milner PF (1968) Irreversibly sickled erythrocytes: a consequence of the heterogeneous distribution of hemoglobin types in sickle-cell anemia. J Clin Invest 47:1731–1741

Brittain HA, Eckman JR, Swerlick RA, Howard RJ, Wick TM (1993) Thrombospondin from activated platelets promotes sickle erythrocyte adherence to human microvascular endothelium under physiologic flow: a potential role for platelet activation in sickle cell vaso-occlusion. Blood 81:2137–2143

Brittain JE, Mlinar KJ, Anderson CS, Orringer EP, Parise LV (2001) Integrin-associated protein is an adhesion receptor on sickle red blood cells for immobilized thrombospondin. Blood 97:2159–2164

Brittain JE, Han J, Ataga KI, Orringer EP, Parise LV (2004) Mechanism of CD47-induced alpha-4beta1 integrin activation and adhesion in sickle reticulocytes. J Biol Chem 279: 42393–42402

Browne PV, Hebbel RP (1996) CD36-positive stress reticulocytosis in sickle cell anemia. J Lab Clin Med 127:340–347

Brugnara C, Bunn HF, Tosteson DC (1986) Regulation of erythrocyte cation and water content in sickle cell anemia. Science 232:388–390

Brugnara C, de Franceschi L, Alper SL (1993) Inhibition of Ca(2+)-dependent K+ transport and cell dehydration in sickle erythrocytes by clotrimazole and other imidazole derivatives. J Clin Invest 92:520–526

Brugnara C, Gee BE, Armsby CC, Kurth S, Sakamoto M, Rifai N, Alper SL, Platt OS (1996) Therapy with oral clotrimazole induces inhibition of the Gardos channel and reduction of erythrocyte dehydration in patients with sickle cell disease. J Clin Invest 97:1227–1234

Bunn HF (1997) Pathogenesis and treatment of sickle cell disease. N Engl J Med 337:762–769

Camus SM, Gausseres B, Bonnin P, Loufrani L, Grimaud L, Charue D, De Moraes JA, Renard JM, Tedgui A, Boulanger CM, Tharaux PL, Blanc-Brude OP (2012) Erythrocyte microparticles can induce kidney vaso-occlusions in a murine model of sickle cell disease. Blood 120:5050–5058

Camus SM, De Moraes JA, Bonnin P, Abbyad P, Le JS, Lionnet F, Loufrani L, Grimaud L, Lambry JC, Charue D, Kiger L, Renard JM, Larroque C, Le CH, Tedgui A, Bruneval P, Barja-Fidalgo C, Alexandrou A, Tharaux PL, Boulanger CM, Blanc-Brude OP (2015) Circulating cell membrane microparticles transfer heme to endothelial cells and trigger vasoocclusions in sickle cell disease. Blood 125:3805–3814

Chien S, Usami S, Bertles JF (1970) Abnormal rheology of oxygenated blood in sickle cell anemia. J Clin Invest 49:623–634

Chiu D, Lubin B, Shohet SB (1979) Erythrocyte membrane lipid reorganization during the sickling process. Br J Haematol 41:223–234

Choe HR, Schlegel RA, Rubin EM, Williamson P, Westerman MP (1986) Alteration of red cell membrane organization in sickle cell anaemia. Br J Haematol 63:761–773

Conran N, Costa FF (2009) Hemoglobin disorders and endothelial cell interactions. Clin Biochem 42:1824–1838

Crandall I, Collins WE, Gysin J, Sherman IW (1993) Synthetic peptides based on motifs present in a human band 3 protein inhibit cytoadherence/sequestration of the malaria parasite *Plasmodium falciparum*. Proc Natl Acad Sci U S A 90:4703–4707

Darghouth D, Koehl B, Madalinski G, Heilier JF, Bovee P, Xu Y, Olivier MF, Bartolucci P, Benkerrou M, Pissard S, Colin Y, Galacteros F, Bosman G, Junot C, Romeo PH (2011) Pathophysiology of sickle cell disease is mirrored by the red blood cell metabolome. Blood 117:e57–e66

Datta B, Tufnell-Barrett T, Bleasdale RA, Jones CJ, Beeton I, Paul V, Frenneaux M, James P (2004) Red blood cell nitric oxide as an endocrine vasoregulator: a potential role in congestive heart failure. Circulation 109:1339–1342

De Franceschi L, Saadane N, Trudel M, Alper SL, Brugnara C, Beuzard Y (1994) Treatment with oral clotrimazole blocks Ca(2+)-activated K+ transport and reverses erythrocyte dehydration in transgenic SAD mice. A model for therapy of sickle cell disease. J Clin Invest 93:1670–1676

De Franceschi L, Beuzard Y, Jouault H, Brugnara C (1996) Modulation of erythrocyte potassium chloride cotransport, potassium content, and density by dietary magnesium intake in transgenic SAD mouse. Blood 88:2738–2744

De Franceschi L, Bachir D, Galacteros F, Tchernia G, Cynober T, Neuberg D, Beuzard Y, Brugnara C (2000) Oral magnesium pidolate: effects of long-term administration in patients with sickle cell disease. Br J Haematol 108:284–289

de Jong K, Emerson RK, Butler J, Bastacky J, Mohandas N, Kuypers FA (2001) Short survival of phosphatidylserine-exposing red blood cells in murine sickle cell anemia. Blood 98: 1577–1584

Dominical VM, Vital DM, O'Dowd F, Saad ST, Costa FF, Conran N (2015) In vitro microfluidic model for the study of vaso-occlusive processes. Exp Hematol 43:223–228

Donadee C, Raat NJ, Kanias T, Tejero J, Lee JS, Kelley EE, Zhao X, Liu C, Reynolds H, Azarov I, Frizzell S, Meyer EM, Donnenberg AD, Qu L, Triulzi D, Kim-Shapiro DB, Gladwin MT (2011) Nitric oxide scavenging by red blood cell microparticles and cell-free hemoglobin as a mechanism for the red cell storage lesion. Circulation 124:465–476

Du E, Diez-Silva M, Kato GJ, Dao M, Suresh S. (2015) Kinetics of sickle cell biorheology and implications for painful vasoocclusive crisis. Proc Natl Acad Sci USA. 112(5):1422–1427

Eaton WA, Hofrichter J (1987) Hemoglobin S gelation and sickle cell disease. Blood 70: 1245–1266

Embury SH, Matsui NM, Ramanujam S, Mayadas TN, Noguchi CT, Diwan BA, Mohandas N, Cheung AT (2004) The contribution of endothelial cell P-selectin to the microvascular flow of mouse sickle erythrocytes in vivo. Blood 104:3378–3385

Fabry ME, Rajanayagam V, Fine E, Holland S, Gore JC, Nagel RL, Kaul DK (1989) Modeling sickle cell vasoocclusion in the rat leg: quantification of trapped sickle cells and correlation with 31P metabolic and 1H magnetic resonance imaging changes. Proc Natl Acad Sci U S A 86:3808–3812

Fabry ME, Fine E, Rajanayagam V, Factor SM, Gore J, Sylla M, Nagel RL (1992) Demonstration of endothelial adhesion of sickle cells in vivo: a distinct role for deformable sickle cell discocytes. Blood 79:1602–1611

Finnegan EM, Barabino GA, Liu XD, Chang HY, Jonczyk A, Kaul DK (2007) Small-molecule cyclic alpha V beta 3 antagonists inhibit sickle red cell adhesion to vascular endothelium and vasoocclusion. Am J Physiol Heart Circ Physiol 293:H1038–H1045

Franco RS, Palascak M, Thompson H, Rucknagel DL, Joiner CH (1996) Dehydration of transferrin receptor-positive sickle reticulocytes during continuous or cyclic deoxygenation: role of KCl cotransport and extracellular calcium. Blood 88:4359–4365

Frei AC, Guo Y, Jones DW, Pritchard KA Jr, Fagan KA, Hogg N, Wandersee NJ (2008) Vascular dysfunction in a murine model of severe hemolysis. Blood 112:398–405

French JA, Kenny D, Scott JP, Hoffmann RG, Wood JD, Hudetz AG, Hillery CA (1997) Mechanisms of stroke in sickle cell disease: sickle erythrocytes decrease cerebral blood flow in rats after nitric oxide synthase inhibition. Blood 89:4591–4599

Frenette PS (2004) Sickle cell vasoocclusion: heterotypic, multicellular aggregations driven by leukocyte adhesion. Microcirculation 11:167–177
Gao AG, Lindberg FP, Finn MB, Blystone SD, Brown EJ, Frazier WA (1996) Integrin-associated protein is a receptor for the C-terminal domain of thrombospondin. J Biol Chem 271:21–24
Gee BE, Platt OS (1995) Sickle reticulocytes adhere to VCAM-1. Blood 85:268–274
Gladwin MT (2006) Role of the red blood cell in nitric oxide homeostasis and hypoxic vasodilation. Adv Exp Med Biol 588:189–205
Gladwin MT, Crawford JH, Patel RP (2004) The biochemistry of nitric oxide, nitrite, and hemoglobin: role in blood flow regulation. Free Radic Biol Med 36:707–717
Godecke A, Schrader J (2000) Adaptive mechanisms of the cardiovascular system in transgenic mice--lessons from eNOS and myoglobin knockout mice. Basic Res Cardiol 95:492–498
Goldfinger LE, Han J, Kiosses WB, Howe AK, Ginsberg MH (2003) Spatial restriction of alpha4 integrin phosphorylation regulates lamellipodial stability and alpha4beta1-dependent cell migration. J Cell Biol 162:731–741
Gupta K, Gupta P, Solovey A, Hebbel RP (1999) Mechanism of interaction of thrombospondin with human endothelium and inhibition of sickle erythrocyte adhesion to human endothelial cells by heparin. Biochim Biophys Acta 1453:63–73
Han J, Rose DM, Woodside DG, Goldfinger LE, Ginsberg MH (2003) Integrin alpha 4 beta 1-dependent T cell migration requires both phosphorylation and dephosphorylation of the alpha 4 cytoplasmic domain to regulate the reversible binding of paxillin. J Biol Chem 278:34845–34853
Hankins JS, Wynn LW, Brugnara C, Hillery CA, Li CS, Wang WC (2008) Phase I study of magnesium pidolate in combination with hydroxycarbamide for children with sickle cell anaemia. Br J Haematol 140:80–85
Hebbel RP (1991) Beyond hemoglobin polymerization: the red blood cell membrane and sickle disease pathophysiology. Blood 77:214–237
Hebbel RP, Boogaerts MA, Eaton JW, Steinberg MH (1980a) Erythrocyte adherence to endothelium in sickle-cell anemia. A possible determinant of disease severity. N Engl J Med 302:992–995
Hebbel RP, Yamada O, Moldow CF, Jacob HS, White JG, Eaton JW (1980b) Abnormal adherence of sickle erythrocytes to cultured vascular endothelium: possible mechanism for microvascular occlusion in sickle cell disease. J Clin Invest 65:154–160
Hebbel RP, Morgan WT, Eaton JW, Hedlund BE (1988) Accelerated autoxidation and heme loss due to instability of sickle hemoglobin. Proc Natl Acad Sci U S A 85:237–241
Hebbel RP, Ney PA, Foker W (1989) Autoxidation, dehydration, and adhesivity may be related abnormalities of sickle erythrocytes. Am J Physiol 256:C579–C583
Hillery CA, Panepinto JA (2004) Pathophysiology of stroke in sickle cell disease. Microcirculation 11:195–208
Hillery CA, Du MC, Montgomery RR, Scott JP (1996) Increased adhesion of erythrocytes to components of the extracellular matrix: isolation and characterization of a red blood cell lipid that binds thrombospondin and laminin. Blood 87:4879–4886
Hines PC, Zen Q, Burney SN, Shea DA, Ataga KI, Orringer EP, Telen MJ, Parise LV (2003) Novel epinephrine and cyclic AMP-mediated activation of BCAM/Lu-dependent sickle (SS) RBC adhesion. Blood 101:3281–3287
Huang Z, Hearne L, Irby CE, King SB, Ballas SK, Kim-Shapiro DB (2003) Kinetics of increased deformability of deoxygenated sickle cells upon oxygenation. Biophys J 85:2374–2383
Humphries MJ, Sheridan J, Mould AP, Newham P (1995) Mechanisms of VCAM-1 and fibronectin binding to integrin alpha 4 beta 1: implications for integrin function and rational drug design. Ciba Found Symp 189:177–191
Jeffers A, Gladwin MT, Kim-Shapiro DB (2006) Computation of plasma hemoglobin nitric oxide scavenging in hemolytic anemias. Free Radic Biol Med 41:1557–1565
Jison ML, Gladwin MT (2003) Hemolytic anemia-associated pulmonary hypertension of sickle cell disease and the nitric oxide/arginine pathway. Am J Respir Crit Care Med 168:3–4

Joneckis CC, Ackley RL, Orringer EP, Wayner EA, Parise LV (1993) Integrin alpha 4 beta 1 and glycoprotein IV (CD36) are expressed on circulating reticulocytes in sickle cell anemia. Blood 82:3548–3555

Joneckis CC, Shock DD, Cunningham ML, Orringer EP, Parise LV (1996) Glycoprotein IV-independent adhesion of sickle red blood cells to immobilized thrombospondin under flow conditions. Blood 87:4862–4870

Kannan R, Labotka R, Low PS (1988) Isolation and characterization of the hemichrome-stabilized membrane protein aggregates from sickle erythrocytes. Major site of autologous antibody binding. J Biol Chem 263:13766–13773

Kasschau MR, Barabino GA, Bridges KR, Golan DE (1996) Adhesion of sickle neutrophils and erythrocytes to fibronectin. Blood 87:771–780

Kaul DK, Fabry ME, Nagel RL (1986) Vaso-occlusion by sickle cells: evidence for selective trapping of dense red cells. Blood 68:1162–1166

Kaul DK, Fabry ME, Nagel RL (1989) Microvascular sites and characteristics of sickle cell adhesion to vascular endothelium in shear flow conditions: pathophysiological implications. Proc Natl Acad Sci U S A 86:3356–3360

Kaul DK, Fabry ME, Costantini F, Rubin EM, Nagel RL (1995) In vivo demonstration of red cell-endothelial interaction, sickling and altered microvascular response to oxygen in the sickle transgenic mouse. J Clin Invest 96:2845–2853

Kaul DK, Liu XD, Fabry ME, Nagel RL (2000a) Impaired nitric oxide-mediated vasodilation in transgenic sickle mouse. Am J Physiol Heart Circ Physiol 278:H1799–H1806

Kaul DK, Tsai HM, Liu XW, Nakada MT, Nagel RL, Coller BS (2000b) Monoclonal antibodies to alphaVbeta3 (7E3 and LM609) inhibit sickle red blood cell-endothelium interactions induced by platelet-activating factor. Blood 95:368–374

Kaul DK, Liu XD, Zhang X, Mankelow T, Parsons S, Spring F, An X, Mohandas N, Anstee D, Chasis JA (2006) Peptides based on alphaV-binding domains of erythrocyte ICAM-4 inhibit sickle red cell-endothelial interactions and vaso-occlusion in the microcirculation. Am J Physiol Cell Physiol 291:C922–C930

Kim-Shapiro DB, Schechter AN, Gladwin MT (2006) Unraveling the reactions of nitric oxide, nitrite, and hemoglobin in physiology and therapeutics. Arterioscler Thromb Vasc Biol 26:697–705

Lancaster JR Jr (1994) Simulation of the diffusion and reaction of endogenously produced nitric oxide. Proc Natl Acad Sci USA 91:8137–8141

Lew VL, Ortiz OE, Bookchin RM (1997) Stochastic nature and red cell population distribution of the sickling-induced Ca^{2+} permeability. J Clin Invest 99:2727–2735

Liao JC (2002) Blood feud: keeping hemoglobin from nixing NO. Nat Med 8:1350–1351

Lux SE, John KM, Karnovsky MJ (1976) Irreversible deformation of the spectrin-actin lattice in irreversibly sickled cells. J Clin Invest 58:955–963

Manodori AB (2001) Sickle erythrocytes adhere to fibronectin-thrombospondin-integrin complexes exposed by thrombin-induced endothelial cell contraction. Microvasc Res 61:263–274

Manodori AB, Barabino GA, Lubin BH, Kuypers FA (2000) Adherence of phosphatidylserine-exposing erythrocytes to endothelial matrix thrombospondin. Blood 95:1293–1300

Matsui NM, Borsig L, Rosen SD, Yaghmai M, Varki A, Embury SH (2001) P-selectin mediates the adhesion of sickle erythrocytes to the endothelium. Blood 98:1955–1962

Miller ST, Wright E, Abboud M, Berman B, Files B, Scher CD, Styles L, Adams RJ (2001) Impact of chronic transfusion on incidence of pain and acute chest syndrome during the Stroke Prevention Trial (STOP) in sickle-cell anemia. J Pediatr 139:785–789

Mohandas N, Evans E (1984) Adherence of sickle erythrocytes to vascular endothelial cells: requirement for both cell membrane changes and plasma factors. Blood 64:282–287

Morris CR, Gladwin MT, Kato GJ (2008) Nitric oxide and arginine dysregulation: a novel pathway to pulmonary hypertension in hemolytic disorders. Curr Mol Med 8:620–632

Mozzarelli A, Hofrichter J, Eaton WA (1987) Delay time of hemoglobin S polymerization prevents most cells from sickling in vivo. Science 237:500–506

Natarajan M, Udden MM, McIntire LV (1996) Adhesion of sickle red blood cells and damage to interleukin-1 beta stimulated endothelial cells under flow in vitro. Blood 87:4845–4852

Nebor D, Romana M, Santiago R, Vachiery N, Picot J, Broquere C, Chaar V, Doumdo L, Odievre MH, Benkerrou M, Elion J (2013) Fetal hemoglobin and hydroxycarbamide moduate both plasma concentration and cellular origin of circulating microparticles in sickle cell anemia children. Haematologica 98:862–867

Oldenborg PA, Zheleznyak A, Fang YF, Lagenaur CF, Gresham HD, Lindberg FP (2000) Role of CD47 as a marker of self on red blood cells. Science 288:2051–2054

Ou J, Ou Z, Jones DW, Holzhauer S, Hatoum OA, Ackerman AW, Weihrauch DW, Gutterman DD, Guice K, Oldham KT, Hillery CA, Pritchard KA Jr (2003) L-4F, an apolipoprotein A-1 mimetic, dramatically improves vasodilation in hypercholesterolemia and sickle cell disease. Circulation 107:2337–2341

Parsons SF, Spring FA, Chasis JA, Anstee DJ (1999) Erythroid cell adhesion molecules Lutheran and LW in health and disease. Baillieres Best Pract Res Clin Haematol 12:729–745

Parsons SF, Lee G, Spring FA, Willig TN, Peters LL, Gimm JA, Tanner MJ, Mohandas N, Anstee DJ, Chasis JA (2001) Lutheran blood group glycoprotein and its newly characterized mouse homologue specifically bind alpha5 chain-containing human laminin with high affinity. Blood 97:312–320

Pawloski JR (2003) Hemoglobin and nitric oxide. N Engl J Med 349:402–405

Reiter CD, Wang X, Tanos-Santos JE, Hogg N, Cannon RO III, Schechter A, Gladwin MT (2002) Cell-free hemoglobin limits nitric oxide bioavailability in sickle-cell disease. Nat Med 8:1383–1389

Rother RP, Bell L, Hillmen P, Gladwin MT (2005) The clinical sequelae of intravascular hemolysis and extracellular plasma hemoglobin: a novel mechanism of human disease. JAMA 293:1653–1662

Russell MO, Goldberg HI, Hodson A, Kim HC, Halus J, Reivich M, Schwartz E (1984) Effect of transfusion therapy on arteriographic abnormalities and on recurrence of stroke in sickle cell disease. Blood 63:162–169

Sakamoto TM, Canalli AA, Traina F, Franco-Penteado CF, Gambero S, Saad ST, Conran N, Costa FF (2013) Altered red cell and platelet adhesion in hemolytic diseases: hereditary spherocytosis, paroxysmal nocturnal hemoglobinuria and sickle cell disease. Clin Biochem 46:1798–1803

Santoro SA, Frazier WA (1987) Isolation and characterization of thrombospondin. Methods Enzymol 144:438–446

Schlegel RA, Prendergast TW, Williamson P (1985) Membrane phospholipid asymmetry as a factor in erythrocyte-endothelial cell interactions. J Cell Physiol 123:215–218

Setty BN, Stuart MJ (1996) Vascular cell adhesion molecule-1 is involved in mediating hypoxia-induced sickle red blood cell adherence to endothelium: potential role in sickle cell disease. Blood 88:2311–2320

Setty BN, Kulkarni S, Rao AK, Stuart MJ (2000) Fetal hemoglobin in sickle cell disease: relationship to erythrocyte phosphatidylserine exposure and coagulation activation. Blood 96:1119–1124

Setty BN, Rao AK, Stuart MJ (2001) Thrombophilia in sickle cell disease: the red cell connection. Blood 98:3228–3233

Setty BN, Kulkarni S, Stuart MJ (2002) Role of erythrocyte phosphatidylserine in sickle red cell-endothelial adhesion. Blood 99:1564–1571

Sheng K, Shariff M, Hebbel RP (1998) Comparative oxidation of hemoglobins A and S. Blood 91:3467–3470

Sherman IW, Crandall I, Smith H (1992) Membrane proteins involved in the adherence of Plasmodium falciparum-infected erythrocytes to the endothelium. Biol Cell 74:161–178

Shet AS, Aras O, Gupta K, Hass MJ, Rausch DJ, Saba N, Koopmeiners L, Key NS, Hebbel RP (2003) Sickle blood contains tissue factor-positive microparticles derived from endothelial cells and monocytes. Blood 102:2678–2683

Silva G, Jeney V, Chora A, Larsen R, Balla J, Soares MP (2009) Oxidized hemoglobin is an endogenous proinflammatory agonist that targets vascular endothelial cells. J Biol Chem 284:29582–29595

Singer ST, Ataga KI (2008) Hypercoagulability in sickle cell disease and beta-thalassemia. Curr Mol Med 8:639–645

Stone PC, Stuart J, Nash GB (1996) Effects of density and of dehydration of sickle cells on their adhesion to cultured endothelial cells. Am J Hematol 52:135–143

Sugihara K, Sugihara T, Mohandas N, Hebbel RP (1992) Thrombospondin mediates adherence of CD36+ sickle reticulocytes to endothelial cells. Blood 80:2634–2642

Swerlick RA, Eckman JR, Kumar A, Jeitler M, Wick TM (1993) Alpha 4 beta 1-integrin expression on sickle reticulocytes: vascular cell adhesion molecule-1-dependent binding to endothelium. Blood 82:1891–1899

Thevenin BM, Crandall I, Ballas SK, Sherman IW, Shohet SB (1997) Band 3 peptides block the adherence of sickle cells to endothelial cells in vitro. Blood 90:4172–4179

Tofovic SP, Jackson EK, Rafikova O (2009) Adenosine deaminase-adenosine pathway in hemolysis-associated pulmonary hypertension. Med Hypotheses 72:713–719

Tryggvason K (1993) The laminin family. Cell Biol 5:877–882

Turhan A, Weiss LA, Mohandas N, Coller BS, Frenette PS (2002) Primary role for adherent leukocytes in sickle cell vascular occlusion: a new paradigm. Proc Natl Acad Sci U S A 99:3047–3051

Udani M, Zen Q, Cottman M, Leonard N, Jefferson S, Daymont C, Truskey G, Telen MJ (1998) Basal cell adhesion molecule/lutheran protein. The receptor critical for sickle cell adhesion to laminin. J Clin Invest 101:2550–2558

Villagra J, Shiva S, Hunter LA, Machado RF, Gladwin MT, Kato GJ (2007) Platelet activation in patients with sickle disease, hemolysis-associated pulmonary hypertension and nitric oxide scavenging by cell-free hemoglobin. Blood 110(6):2166–2172

Wandersee NJ, Punzalan RC, Rettig MP, Kennedy MD, Pajewski NM, Sabina RL, Paul SJ, Low PS, Hillery CA (2005) Erythrocyte adhesion is modified by alterations in cellular tonicity and volume. Br J Haematol 131:366–377

Waugh SM, Willardson BM, Kannan R, Labotka RJ, Low PS (1986) Heinz bodies induce clustering of band 3, glycophorin, and ankyrin in sickle cell erythrocytes. J Clin Invest 78:1155–1160

Wick TM, Eckman JR (1996) Molecular basis of sickle cell-endothelial cell interactions. Curr Opin Hematol 3:118–124

Wood KC, Hebbel RP, Granger DN (2004) Endothelial cell P-selectin mediates a proinflammatory and prothrombogenic phenotype in cerebral venules of sickle cell transgenic mice. Am J Physiol Heart Circ Physiol 286:H1608–H1614

Zachowski A, Craescu CT, Galacteros F, Devaux PF (1985) Abnormality of phospholipid transverse diffusion in sickle erythrocytes. J Clin Invest 75:1713–1717

Zatz R, Baylis C (1998) Chronic nitric oxide inhibition model six years on. Hypertension 32:958–964

Zennadi R, Hines PC, De Castro LM, Cartron JP, Parise LV, Telen MJ (2004) Epinephrine acts through erythroid signaling pathways to activate sickle cell adhesion to endothelium via LW-alphavbeta3 interactions. Blood 104:3774–3781

Zhou Z, Thiagarajan P, Udden M, Lopez JA, Guchhait P (2011) Erythrocyte membrane sulfatide plays a crucial role in the adhesion of sickle erythrocytes to endothelium. Thromb Haemost 105:1046–1052

Zwaal RF, Schroit AJ (1997) Pathophysiologic implications of membrane phospholipid asymmetry in blood cells. Blood 89:1121–1132

Chapter 5
Leukocytes in the Vaso-Occlusive Process

Dachuan Zhang and Paul S. Frenette

Abstract Sickle cell disease (SCD) results from a single mutation in the *β-globin* gene, leading to clinical manifestations that extend far beyond the mutated hemoglobin in red blood cells (RBCs). SCD is associated with a chronic inflammatory condition that, in the presence of a "second hit", can produce vaso-occlusive crises (VOC), the major cause of morbidity and mortality of the disease. Leukocytes play an important role in the vaso-occlusive phenomenon, as suggested initially by the findings of clinical studies that high leukocyte count strongly correlates with clinical severity of the disease. Further, intravital microscopy studies in SCD mice have revealed that sickle RBCs directly interact with adherent neutrophils in post-capillary and collecting venules. These heterotypic interactions are mediated by activated $\alpha_M\beta_2$ (Mac-1) integrin polarized on the leading edge of adherent neutrophils, resulting in severe VOC. A multistep and multicellular model for the vaso-occlusive process is proposed in which endothelial cells are activated by sickle RBCs and multiple inflammatory mediators, leading to the recruitment of adherent leukocytes. The recruited adherent neutrophils capture circulating sickle RBCs, resulting in reduced blood flow and vascular occlusion in the microcirculation. This model has triggered several clinical trials targeting drivers of vaso-occlusion, and suggests a major contribution of leukocytes to sickle cell VOC.

Keywords Adherent leukocyte • Heterotypic interaction • Vaso-occlusion

---

D. Zhang
Ruth L. and David S. Gottesman Institute for Stem Cell and Regenerative Medicine Research, Albert Einstein College of Medicine, Bronx, NY 10461, USA

Department of Cell Biology, Albert Einstein College of Medicine, Bronx, NY 10461, USA
e-mail: dachuan.zhang@phd.einstein.yu.edu

P.S. Frenette (✉)
Ruth L. and David S. Gottesman Institute for Stem Cell and Regenerative Medicine Research, Albert Einstein College of Medicine, Bronx, NY 10461, USA

Department of Cell Biology, Albert Einstein College of Medicine, Bronx, NY 10461, USA

Department of Medicine, Albert Einstein College of Medicine, Bronx, NY 10461, USA
e-mail: paul.frenette@einstein.yu.edu

© Springer International Publishing Switzerland 2016
F.F. Costa, N. Conran (eds.), *Sickle Cell Anemia*,
DOI 10.1007/978-3-319-06713-1_5

5.1 Inflammation in Sickle Cell Disease

5.1.1 Sickle RBCs Promote Inflammation

Repeated cycles of RBC sickling and the generation of oxygen radicals in sickle RBCs lead to profound changes in the surface membrane that promote their adhesion to the endothelium (Kaul et al. 2009). The interactions between sickle RBCs and the endothelium lead to the activation of endothelial cells. For example, co-culture of human umbilical vein endothelial cells (HUVECs) with sickle RBCs in presence of von Willebrand factor (vWf) derived from endothelial cell-conditioned medium results in a dramatic increase of lipid peroxide formation and activation of the transcription factor NFκB in endothelial cells (Sultana et al. 1998). Activation of NFκB signaling leads to up-regulation of several adhesion molecules on endothelial cells, including E-selectin, vascular cell adhesion molecule 1 (VCAM-1) and intercellular adhesion molecule 1 (ICAM-1) (Sultana et al. 1998), which mediate leukocyte recruitment and adhesion (Ley et al. 2007). The interactions of sickle RBCs with leukocytes also lead to the activation of leukocytes. For example, sickle RBCs have been shown to adhere to neutrophils in vitro, resulting in respiratory burst in neutrophils (Hofstra et al. 1996). In addition, sickle RBCs also produces higher amount of oxygen radicals compared to normal RBCs, thus promoting inflammation and tissue damage (Hebbel et al. 1982).

Damaged surface membranes also enhance hemolysis, resulting in anemia and the release of hemoglobin into the circulation. Extracellular hemoglobin promotes inflammation in sickle cell disease (SCD) by depleting nitric oxide (NO), triggering oxidative stress and releasing heme, the prosthetic moiety of hemoglobin (Schaer et al. 2013). Extracellular heme could increase the expression of adhesion molecules on endothelial cells, thus enhancing leukocyte recruitment and adhesion (Wagener et al. 2001). In both SCD patients and mice, plasma heme levels are elevated during vaso-occlusive crisis (VOC), leading to activation of circulating neutrophils and the formation of neutrophil extracellular traps (NETs) in the pulmonary vasculature and causing acute lung injury (Chen et al. 2014). In addition, administration of exogenous heme or hemin, the oxidized form of heme, can trigger VOC or acute chest syndrome (ACS) in SCD mice, respectively. Heme/hemin-induced VOC and ACS could be largely prevented by toll-like receptor 4 (TLR4) inhibition, suggesting that extracellular heme/hemin signals through TLR4 to trigger an inflammatory response (Ghosh et al. 2013; Belcher et al. 2014).

5.1.2 Hypoxia-Reoxygenation Promotes Inflammation

Recurrent vaso-occlusive events in individuals with SCD evoke repeated transient cycles of hypoxia-reoxygenation in the microcirculation. Using a transgenic sickle cell mouse model, Kaul and Hebbel showed that the induction of hypoxia followed by reoxygenation enhances peroxide production by endothelial cells and increases leukocyte recruitment in the venules of sickle cell mice but not of normal mice (Kaul and Hebbel 2000). Hypoxia-reoxygenation promotes leukocyte recruitment by activating NFκB signaling in endothelial cells, leading to increased expressions of endothelial adhesion molecules, including ICAM-1 and VCAM-1 (Kaul et al. 2004; Belcher et al. 2005). Administration of corticosteroid drug dexamethasone or NFκB inhibitor sulfasalazine prevents the activation of endothelial cells induced by hypoxia-reoxygenation, leading to marked decreases in leukocyte adhesion and increased blood flow (Kaul et al. 2004; Belcher et al. 2005).

5.1.3 Monocytes and iNKT Cells Promote Inflammation

Several leukocyte populations exhibit an activated phenotype and promote inflammation even under steady state conditions in SCD. For example, monocytes from SCD patients express higher levels of the activation marker CD11b, and can activate endothelial cells by secreting higher levels of tumor necrosis factor-alpha (TNF-α) and interleukin-1-beta (IL-1β) compared to normal monocytes (Belcher et al. 2000). Co-culture of monocytes from SCD patients with pulmonary microvascular and arterial endothelial cells results in activation of NFκB signaling and up-regulation of multiple adhesion molecules and cytokines in endothelial cells (Safaya et al. 2012; Belcher et al. 2000). One possible mechanism for monocyte activation in SCD individuals is the increased production of placental growth factor (PlGF), an angiogenic growth factor produced by erythroblasts. Levels of PlGF are elevated in the plasma of individuals with SCD and correlate with disease severity. Treating monocytes with PlGF stimulates monocyte chemotaxis and increases the expressions of IL-1β, IL-8, monocyte chemoattractant protein-1 (MIP-1), and vascular endothelial growth factor (VEGF) in monocytes, thus activating endothelial cells and promoting inflammation (Perelman et al. 2003).

The inflammatory condition is also amplified by CD1d-restricted invariant natural killer T (iNKT) cells. Compared to normal mice, SCD mice have more numerous and activated iNKT cells (CD69$^+$ IFN-γ^+) in lung, liver and spleen that are hypersensitive to hypoxia-reoxygenation (Wallace et al. 2009). SCD mice have increased pulmonary levels of IFN-γ and IFN-γ-inducible CXCR3 chemokine CXCL9 and CXCL10, and increased numbers of CXCR3$^+$ lymphocytes in the lung. Baseline pulmonary dysfunction in SCD mice can be reversed by inhibiting iNKT cell activation using a CD1d antibody, by neutralizing CXCR3 on lymphocytes, or by completely depleting lymphocytes using genetic models (Wallace et al. 2009). Activated iNKT cells also exhibit a dramatic increase in the expression of an anti-inflammatory receptor, adenosine A_{2A} receptor ($A_{2A}R$). Treating SCD mice with $A_{2A}R$ agonists decreases the activation of iNKT cells, producing an effective reversal of the baseline pulmonary dysfunction (Wallace and Linden 2010). Patients with SCD also show increased activation of iNKT cells in the circulation during painful VOC, leading to NFκB activation and increased expression of $A_{2A}R$ (Lin et al.

2013). An $A_{2A}R$ agonist, regadenoson, has been shown to reverse iNKT cell activation during VOC in SCD patients. Currently a phase 2 trial is ongoing to determine the therapeutic efficacy of regadenoson infusion (Field et al. 2013; Nathan et al. 2012).

5.1.4 Cytokine Profile in SCD

Elevation of multiple cytokines in the circulation, including TNF-α (Francis and Haywood 1992; Malave et al. 1993), IL-1β (Francis and Haywood 1992; Croizat 1994), granulocyte macrophage colony-stimulating factor (GM-CSF), IL-3 (Croizat 1994), endothelin-1 and prostaglandin E2 (Graido-Gonzalez et al. 1998), have been reported in SCD. However, contradictory observations were also noted for TNF-α and IL-1β (Graido-Gonzalez et al. 1998), suggesting that the cytokine profile in SCD patients might be affected by disease manifestations.

These pro-inflammatory cytokines can activate NFκB signaling in leukocytes and endothelial cells, resulting in a feed-forward pro-inflammatory response to produce more cytokines and chemokines. The importance of these inflammatory mediators is highlighted by observations that anti-inflammatory drugs can alleviate SCD symptoms in patients and mouse models (Kaul et al. 2004; Solovey et al. 2001; Griffin et al. 1994; Belcher et al. 2005). Although the strong adverse effects of corticosteroid therapy precludes a prolonged use, high-dose intravenous methylprednisolone therapy was shown to significantly shorten the duration of the pain crisis in patients (Griffin et al. 1994). Similarly, treatment with dexamethasone or NFκB inhibitor sulfasalazine prevents endothelial cell activation and improves the disease outcome (Belcher et al. 2005; Kaul et al. 2004; Solovey et al. 2001).

5.1.5 A "Second Hit" for Vaso-Occlusive Crisis

Interplay of these above-described factors perpetuates a continuous inflammatory condition that predisposes SCD patients and mice to VOC. However, the initiation of VOC often requires a "second hit" or triggering event, such as infection, ischemia-reperfusion or hemolysis, which could induce an acute inflammatory response that precipitates the crisis. For example, infection can induce a cytokine storm in which the levels of many cytokines, including TNF-α and IL-1β, are elevated (Ahmed 2011). In fact, TNF-α alone plus surgical injury can induce lethal VOC in SCD mice (Turhan et al. 2002). Delayed hemolytic transfusion reaction can also trigger VOC by elevating plasma CXCL1 levels. Exogenous administration of CXCL1 alone is sufficient to induce VOC and inhibition of CXCR2, the receptor for CXCL1, prevents the hemolytic transfusion reaction-induced VOC (Jang et al. 2011). In addition, infusion of heme can also trigger VOC by activating endothelial cells through TLR4 (Belcher et al. 2014).

5.2 Leukocytes in Sickle Cell Disease

5.2.1 *Leukocyte Count Is a Major Risk Factor for VOC*

A role for leukocytes in the pathophysiology of SCD is suggested by clinical epidemiological studies. For many years, it has been noted that marked variation in disease severity exists between patients with SCD. For example, in a longitudinal cohort study of 280 subjects with homozygous SCD, benign disease occurred in 15 % patients (Thomas et al. 1997). In patients with painful crisis, the most common disease manifestation, the severity varies between individuals, with rates of crisis episodes ranging from 0 per year to 10+ per year. Patients with high rates of painful crisis tend to die earlier than those with low rates of crisis (Platt et al. 1991). Such striking variation between patients with an identical genetic mutation raised the challenge to identify the risk factors for clinical severity of the disease so that proactive treatment can be applied before irreversible damage to vital organs occurs. Among the factors that showed statistically significant correlation with disease severity in SCD, steady-state neutrophil count was identified to be a major risk factor (Anyaegbu et al. 1998). The patients with severe clinical manifestations have significantly more circulating neutrophils compared to racially matched controls (Anyaegbu et al. 1998). High leukocyte counts in SCD patients also positively correlate with early SCD-related death (Platt et al. 1994), silent brain infarcts (Kinney et al. 1999), and acute chest syndrome (Castro et al. 1994). High leukocyte counts in SCD infants also appear to be one of the three manifestations that can predict disease severity later in life (Miller et al. 2000).

5.2.2 *Myeloid Growth Factors Are Contraindications in SCD*

An important role of leukocytes in SCD is further demonstrated by clinical studies that administration of myeloid growth factors, including granulocyte macrophage colony-stimulating factor (GM-CSF) and granulocyte colony-stimulating factor (G-CSF), can cause severe disease outcome. In the first report, local injection of GM-CSF to treat leg ulcers in a sickle cell patient triggered a crisis (Pieters et al. 1995). In two reports attempting to mobilize hematopoietic stem and progenitor cells for gene therapy, administration of G-CSF resulted in severe or fatal VOC (Abboud et al. 1998; Adler et al. 2001). In another case, a patient with stage II invasive ductal breast carcinoma and sickle cell/β^{+} thalassemia received chemotherapy followed by G-CSF treatment to correct neutropenia. Shortly after the G-CSF treatment, the patient developed severe sickle cell crisis leading to life-threatening multi-organ failure (Grigg 2001). In a more recent report, a patient was identified to have a rare co-existence of sickle cell disease and severe congenital neutropenia associated with a mutation in ELANE, which resulted in significantly reduced sickle cell complications compared to his siblings. The patient received G-CSF treatment to correct his neutropenia, which markedly worsened the course of disease (Wali et al. 2012).

These reports suggest an important role of myeloid cells in the pathogenesis of sickle cell VOC, given that G-CSF and GM-CSF are potent inducers of myeloid cell expansion and activation (Hamilton 2008; Hakansson et al. 1997; Khajah et al. 2011). These findings also raise important issues on the management of sickle cell disease that myeloid growth factors are contraindications for homozygous or compound heterozygous sickle cell patients, and their usage should be carefully evaluated.

5.2.3 *Reduction in Neutrophil Count Benefits SCD*

Hydroxyurea is the most commonly used drug that has shown clinical efficacy for both SCD adults and children (Hankins et al. 2005; Charache et al. 1995; Steinberg et al. 2003). In the MSH study, hydroxyurea treatment resulted in a marked decrease in the frequency of painful crises and ACS, and a reduction in transfusion requirements and hospitalizations in patients with moderate to severe SCD (Charache et al. 1995). Hydroxyurea has been shown to be a potent fetal hemoglobin inducer (Cokic et al. 2003; Letvin et al. 1984), but also with many other effects that may benefit SCD. For example, hydroxyurea treatment could decrease the expression level of soluble VCAM-1 and reduce the adhesion of sickle RBCs to the endothelium (Saleh et al. 1999; Bridges et al. 1996). Currently it is still not entirely clear how much of the clinical benefit from hydroxyurea can be attributed to its effect on fetal hemoglobin levels compared with its other activities. Interestingly, hydroxyurea was also found to suppress neutrophils numbers while inducing fetal hemoglobin expression in SCD patients (Charache et al. 1996). In fact, hydroxyurea treatment shows beneficial effects even in some patients with no detectable rise of fetal hemoglobin, whereas all patients who respond well to hydroxyurea treatment have a decrease in neutrophil count (Charache 1997; Charache et al. 1995).

Neutrophils from patients with SCD also show an activated phenotype with lower expression level of L-selectin (CD62L) and higher level of CD11b (Lard et al. 1999). These neutrophils exhibited increased adhesive properties that could be reversed by inhibiting stimulating NO/cyclic guanosine monophosphate (cGMP)-dependent signaling (Canalli et al. 2008). In patients treated with hydroxyurea, abnormalities in these neutrophil activation markers are corrected, suggesting that neutrophils are an important target of this drug (Benkerrou et al. 2002). Further studies suggest that hydroxyurea treatment has immediate benefits on acute VOC with a mechanism probably involving the formation of intravascular nitric oxide and the amplification of NO/cGMP-dependent signaling (Almeida et al. 2012). These findings suggest a pivotal role of leukocytes, especially neutrophils, in the pathophysiology of SCD.

5.3 Adherent Leukocytes in the Vaso-Occlusive Process

5.3.1 *Adherent Leukocytes Interact with Sickle RBCs*

Sickle RBCs were initially thought to obstruct mechanically the blood vessels due to their rigidity and decreased capability to pass through the capillaries. In a rat mesocecum ex vivo perfusion model, sickle RBCs were found to interact with post-capillary and collecting venules (Kaul et al. 1989). The adhesion of sickle RBCs was also found to be density class-dependent, with young RBCs most adherent to the endothelium (Kaul et al. 1989). Following these observations, a model was proposed that young RBCs adhere in post-capillary venules, resulting in secondary trapping of dense cells followed by vaso-occlusion. However, the post-capillary venule is also the primary site for leukocyte adhesion and transmigration during their recruitment to tissues (Ley et al. 2007), raising the possibility that the vaso-occlusive process involves complicated interactions between sickle RBCs, leukocytes and the endothelium.

The first clue that leukocytes may directly participate in the vaso-occlusive process came from observations that neutrophils bind sickle RBCs in vitro. In contrast to the interactions with the endothelium, the dense cell fraction that includes irreversibly sickled RBCs was found to be the most adherent (Hofstra et al. 1996). In vivo evidence for this phenomenon was first reported in SCD mice that exclusively express human sickle hemoglobin (Paszty et al. 1997), where dynamic interactions between circulating blood cells and the endothelium in the cremasteric microcirculation was analyzed using intravital microscopy (Turhan et al. 2002). Although occasional interactions between sickle RBCs with the endothelium were observed in this model, sickle RBCs were found to predominantly interact with adherent leukocytes. The interactions were induced by surgical trauma, enhanced and then sustained by TNF-α administration, resulting in a lethal VOC. Mice deficient in both P- and E-selectin were prevented from recruiting leukocytes to the endothelium, and were protected from VOC in this model. These findings suggest that recruitment of leukocytes to the activated endothelium is a necessary step in the vaso-occlusive process.

5.3.2 *Neutrophil Microdomains Mediate Heterotypic Interactions*

The development of high-speed multichannel fluorescence intravital microscopy (MFIM) allows the identification of cellular and molecular mediators for the heterotypic interactions between sickle RBCs and adherent leukocytes (Chiang et al. 2007). In TNF-α stimulated SCD mice, $Gr\text{-}1^+$ neutrophils are robustly recruited to and comprise ~80 % of the leukocytes that adhere to the cremasteric venular endothelium. These adherent neutrophils are not stationary but actively migrate on the endothelium, and exhibit marked polarization of surface adhesion receptors, including P-selectin glycoprotein ligand-1 (PSGL-1), L-selectin and activated $\alpha_M\beta_2$ integrin (CD11b/CD18 or Mac-1). Heterotypic interactions between sickle RBCs and adherent neutrophils have been found to be predominantly on the leading edge, suggesting a potential role of these polarized microdomains in mediating heterotypic interactions (Hidalgo et al. 2009; Chiang et al. 2007).

Although selectins are best known to mediate leukocyte rolling, they can also trigger "inside-out" signals that lead to integrin activation, allowing leukocytes to firmly adhere to the endothelium (Zarbock et al. 2007a; Hidalgo et al. 2007; Simon et al. 2000; Lo et al. 1991). For example, engagement of E-selectin on adherent neutrophils generates a secondary wave of activating signals, transduced specifically by E-selectin ligand-1 (ESL-1), that induce polarized, activated $\alpha_M\beta_2$ integrin clusters on the leading edge of adherent neutrophils, allowing the capture of circulating RBCs and platelets (Hidalgo et al. 2009). In SCD mice, the capture of sickle RBCs by $\alpha_M\beta_2$ integrin microdomains leads to acute lethal VOC. Inactivation of E-selectin and $\alpha_M\beta_2$ integrin by either genetic deficiency or antibody blocking prevents heterotypic interactions, leading to increased blood flow and prolonged survival of SCD mice during VOC. In addition, ESL-1-mediated signaling involves Src family kinases, since inhibition of Src kinases, but not p38 MAPK or spleen tyrosine kinase (Syk), reduces RBC-neutrophil interactions. Mice deficient in the C3 complement protein, a ligand for $\alpha_M\beta_2$ integrin, have a partial reduction in RBC-neutrophil interactions, suggesting a role of complement opsonization in heterotypic interactions. Although the responsible receptors on RBCs remain to be determined, potential candidates include complement (Wang et al. 1993) and ICAM-4 (Zennadi et al. 2008).

Activated $\alpha_M\beta_2$ integrin microdomains also promote heterotypic interactions between platelets and adherent neutrophils (Hidalgo et al. 2009). Heterotypic interactions between platelets and neutrophils promote neutrophil activation in inflammation (Zarbock et al. 2007b; Caudrillier et al. 2012). In SCD patients, the circulating levels of platelet-monocyte and platelet-neutrophil aggregates are significantly higher compare to healthy controls (Frelinger et al. 2014). Platelets have also been found to participate in 20–50 % of neutrophil-RBC aggregates (Dominical et al. 2014). However, direct evidence for a role of platelet-neutrophil interactions in sickle cell vaso-occlusion is still lacking.

5.3.3 A Multistep and Multicellular Model of Sickle Cell VOC

Direct observations in SCD mice suggest that sickle cell VOC may arise from a complex multistep and multicellular process that involves heterotypic interactions between adherent neutrophils and sickle RBCs (Manwani and Frenette 2013; Frenette 2002). A direct role of neutrophils in the vaso-occlusive process is supported by clinical observations that high neutrophil count correlates with severe disease outcome. Although the exact mechanisms remain incompletely elucidated, the following model has been proposed (Fig. 5.1).

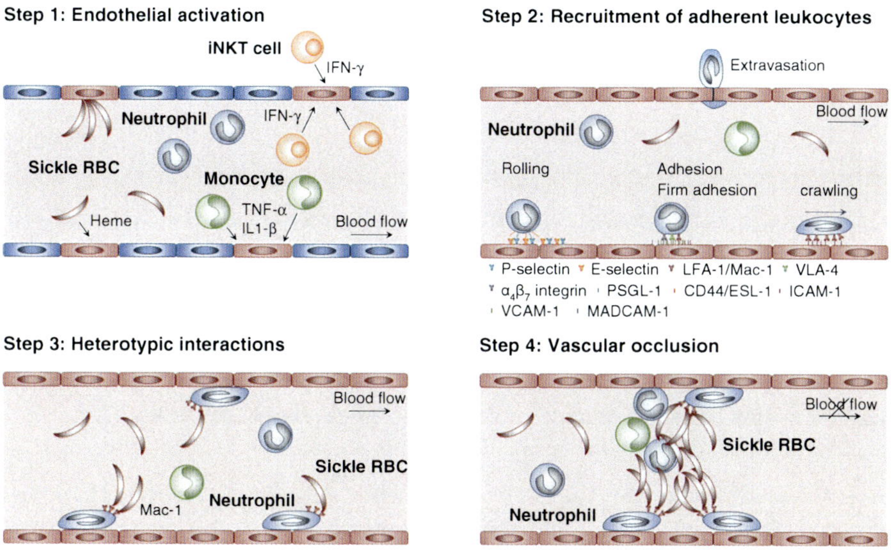

Fig. 5.1 The multistep and multicellular model for sickle cell vaso-occlusion. Sickle cell vaso-occlusion involves complex interactions between endothelial cells, leukocytes and sickle RBCs. In steady state, monocytes, iNKT cells and sickle RBCs contribute to a persistent inflammatory condition that leads to sporadic endothelial activation. In the presence of a triggering event that enables full endothelial activation, the recruitment of adherent leukocytes occurs, leading to heterotypic interactions between sickle RBCs and adherent neutrophils. Repeated interactions result in clogging of post-capillary venules by heterotypic cell–cell aggregates, leading to irreversible vascular occlusion

Step 1: Endothelial Activation SCD is associated with a chronic inflammatory condition that predisposes to sickle cell VOC. Perturbations in the plasma membrane of sickle RBCs expose molecules such as phosphatidylserine (PS) and sulfated glycolipids, which could activate endothelial cells and leukocytes (Setty et al. 2002; Barabino et al. 1999). Enhanced hemolysis of sickle RBCs can also activate endothelial cells and leukocytes by the release of heme and the activation of the TLR4-mediated signaling pathway (Chen et al. 2014; Belcher et al. 2014). Leukocyte populations, including monocytes and iNKT cells, exhibit activated phenotypes and secret pro-inflammatory cytokines including TNF-α, IL-1β and IFN-γ (Wallace et al. 2009; Perelman et al. 2003; Belcher et al. 2000). Higher levels of cytokines in the circulation of SCD patients result in systemic endothelial cell activation (Solovey et al. 1997), allowing recruitment of neutrophils to the endothelium in post-capillary venules. Interplay of all these factors, in the presence of a "second hit", can lead to VOC.

Step 2: Recruitment of Adherent Leukocytes Under inflammatory conditions, leukocytes are robustly recruited to the endothelial vessel wall by a well-defined cascade of adhesive events (Ley et al. 2007). Due to their size and rigidity, an adherent leukocyte may reduce the blood flow to a greater extent than the adhesion of a sickle RBC. The largest leukocytes, monocytes, have diameters of 14–20 μm, about threefold larger than those of RBCs (6–8 μm). Lymphocytes (6–14 μm) and neutrophils (12–14 μm) are also larger than RBCs. Therefore, the hemodynamics in blood vessels containing large numbers of adherent leukocytes may be proportionally reduced. Further, adhesion of leukocytes also enables their interactions with other blood components, leading to further occlusion in the microvasculature.

Step 3: Interactions of Sickle RBCs with Adherent Neutrophils Direct observations from intravital microscopy studies suggest that sickle RBCs predominantly interact with adherent neutrophils in TNF-α stimulated post-capillary venules. These interactions are mediated by activated $\alpha_M\beta_2$ integrin microdomains on the leading edge of adherent neutrophils. Heterotypic interactions are enhanced in SCD mice and lead to lethal VOC. Inactivation of E-selectin or $\alpha_M\beta_2$ integrin prevents neutrophil-RBC interactions and protects SCD mice from acute VOC. These findings highlight a key role of adherent neutrophils in the vaso-occlusive process.

Step 4: Vascular Clogging by Heterotypic Cell–Cell Aggregates Repeated interactions between sickle RBCs and adherent neutrophils cause accumulation of heterotypic cell–cell aggregates, followed by non-specific secondary trapping of additional sickle RBCs, resulting in transient or prolonged obstruction of venular blood flow. The obstruction of blood flow increases the transit time of RBCs and produces ischemia, which exacerbates the situation by activating the endothelium, increasing leukocyte recruitment and enhancing RBC sickling. All these steps contribute to a vicious circle that culminates in an acute VOC, leading to tissue damage and life-threatening complications.

5.4 Targeting Vaso-Occlusion

5.4.1 Targeting Inflammation

Regadenoson As activated iNKT cells express high levels of adenosine A_{2A} receptor ($A_{2A}R$), they become highly sensitive to inhibition by $A_{2A}R$ agonist. Regadenoson, an $A_{2A}R$ agonist in phase 1 trial, has been reported to reduce iNKT activation to levels similar to control and steady-state SCD patients (Field et al. 2013; Nathan et al. 2012). Patients at steady state (n=21) and during VOC (n=6) were examined in this trial. No toxicities were noted for the infusion of Regadenoson at 1.44 μg/kg/h. Based on these results, a randomized, placebo-controlled phase 2 trial is currently ongoing to determine whether administration of Regadenoson with a 48-h constant infusion induces faster remission in VOC and ACS. Notably, iNKT cell activation was found to be associated with increased phosphorylation of NFκB p65, increased expression of $A_{2A}R$ and higher levels of IFN-γ. Although NFκB p65 phosphorylation was reduced to baseline levels, the reduction in $A_{2A}R$ expression and IFN-γ levels did not reach baseline (Field et al. 2013).

5.4.2 Targeting Adhesion

Rivipansel (GMI-1070) Rivipansel, a synthetic pan-selectin inhibitor, has been shown to predominantly inhibit E-selectin-mediated leukocyte adhesion and dramatically reduce RBC-leukocyte interactions, leading to improved blood flow and prolonged survival in SCD mice during VOC (Chang et al. 2010). In a phase 1 clinical trial, GMI-1070 was well tolerated without significant adverse effects. SCD patients receiving GMI-1070 exhibited a modest increase in total peripheral white blood cell count without clinical symptoms (Wun et al. 2014). Recently a phase 2 randomized, double-blinded study has examined the efficacy, safety and pharmacokinetics of rivipansel in hospitalized sickle cell disease patients experiencing VOC. In this study, GlycoMimetics successfully enrolled 76 patients of 12–60 years of age at 22 trial sites in the United States and Canada. Patients treated with rivipansel experienced clinically meaningful reductions in time to reach resolution of VOC, in length of hospital stay and in use of opioid analgesics for pain management, in each case as compared to patients receiving placebo (Telen et al. 2015). Currently a Phase 3 study of GMI-1070 (rivipansel) has been registered.

Tinzaparin Heparins are capable of binding endothelial P-selectin and leukocyte Mac-1 integrin (Peter et al. 1999; Nelson et al. 1993). Administration of heparin leads to inhibitory effects on leukocyte rolling and firm adhesion in vivo (Xie et al. 1997). Tinzaparin, a low-molecular-weight heparin (LMWH), was studied in a randomized, double-blind clinical trial. In this trial, 253 patients with acute painful crisis but with no other complications of SCD were randomized to treatment or control groups. The group of patients that received tinzaparin treatment showed a statistically significant reduction in the duration of painful crisis with no severe bleeding complications, as compared to the group of patients that received placebo (Qari et al. 2007).

Pentosan Polysulfate Sodium (PPS) Pentosan Polysulfate Sodium (PPS) is an orally absorbable semisynthetic heparin analog with less anticoagulant activity compared to heparin, but with one order of magnitude greater potency in blocking P-selectin. In a phase 1 clinical trial, a single oral dose of 300 mg PPS was found to be safe, but with a relatively short half-life. In a phase 2 clinical trial, daily oral doses of PPS administered for 8 weeks tended to improve the microvascular blood flow in SCD patients. The phase 2 trial was prematurely terminated due to economic reasons (Kutlar et al. 2012).

SelG1 SelG1 is a humanized monoclonal antibody specifically against P-selectin. Single and multiple doses of SelG1 were found safe and well tolerated in a phase 1 clinical study conducted by Selexys Pharmaceuticals. Currently a phase 2 multicenter, randomized, placebo-controlled, double-blind clinical trial has been initiated to assess safety and efficacy of SelG1 with or without hydroxyurea therapy in sickle cell disease patients with sickle cell-related pain crises.

5.4.3 *Targeting Neutrophil Activation*

Hydroxyurea Hydroxyurea is a well-established agent that induces fetal hemoglobin expression in SCD patients and requires long-term treatment. However, hydroxyurea administration also shows immediate beneficial effects including reduced leukocyte rolling and adhesion, decreased heterotypic RBC-leukocyte interactions, and prolonged survival. These benefits are mechanistically associated with decreased endothelial adhesion molecule expression, diminished neutrophil $\alpha_M\beta_2$ integrin activation and amplified NO/cGMP-dependent-signaling (Almeida et al. 2012).

Intravenous Immunoglobulin (IVIG) Intravenous immunoglobulin (IVIG) can reverse acute VOC by rapidly inhibiting neutrophil adhesion to the endothelium and abrogating RBC-neutrophil interactions (Chang et al. 2008; Turhan et al. 2004). IVIG signaling is mediated by FcγRIII receptors, the only Fc receptor expressed on murine neutrophils, resulting in the recruitment of Src homology 2-containing tyrosine phosphatase-1 (SHP-1) and the inhibition of adhesion and $\alpha_M\beta_2$ integrin activation. The protective effects of IVIG are abrogated in SHP-1 deficient mice, suggesting an important role of SHP-1 signaling in regulating neutrophil adhesion and activation (Jang et al. 2012). The efficacy of IVIG in SCD patients with acute VOC is being investigated in phase 1 and 2 studies via a dose-escalation strategy.

5.5 Conclusion

In summary, the vaso-occlusive process in SCD involves complex interactions between endothelial cells, leukocytes and sickle RBCs. Adherent leukocytes, especially neutrophils, play an important role in promoting vaso-occlusion. The observation of heterotypic interactions between adherent neutrophils and sickle RBCs has led to a multistep and multicellular model for vaso-occlusion, which has triggered several exciting clinical trials targeting its major driving pathways. Currently the mechanisms that regulate the pro-inflammatory activities of neutrophils and their capacity of interacting with sickle RBCs remain to be elucidated. Further understanding of these mechanisms may provide novel therapeutic targets and strategies for sickle cell vaso-occlusion. Recent studies have also suggested that the levels of heme are elevated during VOC in SCD patients and mice, leading to the formation of NETs in the pulmonary vasculature and causing acute lung injury (Chen et al. 2014). Administration of exogenous heme or hemin can also trigger VOC or ACS in SCD mice (Belcher et al. 2014; Ghosh et al. 2013). These findings suggest that targeting heme or NETs may benefit SCD and its major acute complications. It will be exciting to see whether any of the ongoing early phase trials will bring forth the first targeted therapy against sickle cell vaso-occlusion.

References

Abboud M, Laver J, Blau CA (1998) Granulocytosis causing sickle-cell crisis. Lancet 351(9107):959. doi:10.1016/S0140-6736(05)60614-9

Adler BK, Salzman DE, Carabasi MH, Vaughan WP, Reddy VV, Prchal JT (2001) Fatal sickle cell crisis after granulocyte colony-stimulating factor administration. Blood 97(10):3313–3314

Ahmed SG (2011) The role of infection in the pathogenesis of vaso-occlusive crisis in patients with sickle cell disease. Mediterr J Hematol Infect Dis 3(1):e2011028. doi:10.4084/MJHID.2011.028

Almeida CB, Scheiermann C, Jang JE, Prophete C, Costa FF, Conran N, Frenette PS (2012) Hydroxyurea and a cGMP-amplifying agent have immediate benefits on acute vaso-occlusive events in sickle cell disease mice. Blood 120(14):2879–2888. doi:10.1182/blood-2012-02-409524

Anyaegbu CC, Okpala IE, Akren'Ova YA, Salimonu LS (1998) Peripheral blood neutrophil count and candidacidal activity correlate with the clinical severity of sickle cell anaemia (SCA). Eur J Haematol 60(4):267–268

Barabino GA, Liu XD, Ewenstein BM, Kaul DK (1999) Anionic polysaccharides inhibit adhesion of sickle erythrocytes to the vascular endothelium and result in improved hemodynamic behavior. Blood 93(4):1422–1429

Belcher JD, Marker PH, Weber JP, Hebbel RP, Vercellotti GM (2000) Activated monocytes in sickle cell disease: potential role in the activation of vascular endothelium and vaso-occlusion. Blood 96(7):2451–2459

Belcher JD, Mahaseth H, Welch TE, Vilback AE, Sonbol KM, Kalambur VS, Bowlin PR, Bischof JC, Hebbel RP, Vercellotti GM (2005) Critical role of endothelial cell activation in hypoxia-induced vasoocclusion in transgenic sickle mice. Am J Physiol Heart Circ Physiol 288(6):H2715–H2725. doi:10.1152/ajpheart.00986.2004

Belcher JD, Chen C, Nguyen J, Milbauer L, Abdulla F, Alayash AI, Smith A, Nath KA, Hebbel RP, Vercellotti GM (2014) Heme triggers TLR4 signaling leading to endothelial cell activation and vaso-occlusion in murine sickle cell disease. Blood 123(3):377–390. doi:10.1182/blood-2013-04-495887

Benkerrou M, Delarche C, Brahimi L, Fay M, Vilmer E, Elion J, Gougerot-Pocidalo MA, Elbim C (2002) Hydroxyurea corrects the dysregulated L-selectin expression and increased H(2)O(2) production of polymorphonuclear neutrophils from patients with sickle cell anemia. Blood 99(7):2297–2303

Bridges KR, Barabino GD, Brugnara C, Cho MR, Christoph GW, Dover G, Ewenstein BM, Golan DE, Guttmann CR, Hofrichter J, Mulkern RV, Zhang B, Eaton WA (1996) A multiparameter analysis of sickle erythrocytes in patients undergoing hydroxyurea therapy. Blood 88(12):4701–4710

Canalli AA, Franco-Penteado CF, Saad ST, Conran N, Costa FF (2008) Increased adhesive properties of neutrophils in sickle cell disease may be reversed by pharmacological nitric oxide donation. Haematologica 93(4):605–609. doi:10.3324/haematol.12119

Castro O, Brambilla DJ, Thorington B, Reindorf CA, Scott RB, Gillette P, Vera JC, Levy PS (1994) The acute chest syndrome in sickle cell disease: incidence and risk factors. The Cooperative Study of Sickle Cell Disease. Blood 84(2):643–649

Caudrillier A, Kessenbrock K, Gilliss BM, Nguyen JX, Marques MB, Monestier M, Toy P, Werb Z, Looney MR (2012) Platelets induce neutrophil extracellular traps in transfusion-related acute lung injury. J Clin Invest 122(7):2661–2671. doi:10.1172/JCI61303

Chang J, Shi PA, Chiang EY, Frenette PS (2008) Intravenous immunoglobulins reverse acute vaso-occlusive crises in sickle cell mice through rapid inhibition of neutrophil adhesion. Blood 111(2):915–923. doi:10.1182/blood-2007-04-084061

Chang J, Patton JT, Sarkar A, Ernst B, Magnani JL, Frenette PS (2010) GMI-1070, a novel pan-selectin antagonist, reverses acute vascular occlusions in sickle cell mice. Blood 116(10):1779–1786. doi:10.1182/blood-2009-12-260513

Charache S (1997) Mechanism of action of hydroxyurea in the management of sickle cell anemia in adults. Semin Hematol 34(3 Suppl 3):15–21

Charache S, Terrin ML, Moore RD, Dover GJ, Barton FB, Eckert SV, McMahon RP, Bonds DR (1995) Effect of hydroxyurea on the frequency of painful crises in sickle cell anemia. Investigators of the Multicenter Study of Hydroxyurea in Sickle Cell Anemia. N Engl J Med 332(20):1317–1322. doi:10.1056/NEJM199505183322001

Charache S, Barton FB, Moore RD, Terrin ML, Steinberg MH, Dover GJ, Ballas SK, McMahon RP, Castro O, Orringer EP (1996) Hydroxyurea and sickle cell anemia. Clinical utility of a myelosuppressive "switching" agent. The Multicenter Study of Hydroxyurea in Sickle Cell Anemia. Medicine 75(6):300–326

Chen G, Zhang D, Fuchs TA, Manwani D, Wagner DD, Frenette PS (2014) Heme-induced neutrophil extracellular traps contribute to the pathogenesis of sickle cell disease. Blood 123(24):3818–3827. doi:10.1182/blood-2013-10-529982

Chiang EY, Hidalgo A, Chang J, Frenette PS (2007) Imaging receptor microdomains on leukocyte subsets in live mice. Nat Methods 4(3):219–222, doi:nmeth1018 [pii]10.1038/nmeth1018

Cokic VP, Smith RD, Beleslin-Cokic BB, Njoroge JM, Miller JL, Gladwin MT, Schechter AN (2003) Hydroxyurea induces fetal hemoglobin by the nitric oxide-dependent activation of soluble guanylyl cyclase. J Clin Invest 111(2):231–239. doi:10.1172/JCI16672

Croizat H (1994) Circulating cytokines in sickle cell patients during steady state. Br J Haematol 87(3):592–597

Dominical VM, Samsel L, Nichols JS, Costa FF, McCoy JP Jr, Conran N, Kato GJ (2014) Prominent role of platelets in the formation of circulating neutrophil-red cell heterocellular aggregates in sickle cell anemia. Haematologica 99(11):e214–e217. doi:10.3324/haematol.2014.108555

Field JJ, Lin G, Okam MM, Majerus E, Keefer J, Onyekwere O, Ross A, Campigotto F, Neuberg D, Linden J, Nathan DG (2013) Sickle cell vaso-occlusion causes activation of iNKT cells that is decreased by the adenosine A2A receptor agonist regadenoson. Blood 121(17):3329–3334. doi:10.1182/blood-2012-11-465963

Francis RB Jr, Haywood LJ (1992) Elevated immunoreactive tumor necrosis factor and interleukin-1 in sickle cell disease. J Natl Med Assoc 84(7):611–615

Frelinger AL 3rd, Jakubowski JA, Brooks JK, Carmichael SL, Berny-Lang MA, Barnard MR, Heeney MM, Michelson AD (2014) Platelet activation and inhibition in sickle cell disease (pains) study. Platelets 25(1):27–35. doi:10.3109/09537104.2013.770136

Frenette PS (2002) Sickle cell vaso-occlusion: multistep and multicellular paradigm. Curr Opin Hematol 9(2):101–106

Ghosh S, Adisa OA, Chappa P, Tan F, Jackson KA, Archer DR, Ofori-Acquah SF (2013) Extracellular hemin crisis triggers acute chest syndrome in sickle mice. J Clin Invest 123(11):4809–4820. doi:10.1172/JCI64578

Graido-Gonzalez E, Doherty JC, Bergreen EW, Organ G, Telfer M, McMillen MA (1998) Plasma endothelin-1, cytokine, and prostaglandin E2 levels in sickle cell disease and acute vaso-occlusive sickle crisis. Blood 92(7):2551–2555

Griffin TC, McIntire D, Buchanan GR (1994) High-dose intravenous methylprednisolone therapy for pain in children and adolescents with sickle cell disease. N Engl J Med 330(11):733–737. doi:10.1056/NEJM199403173301101

Grigg AP (2001) Granulocyte colony-stimulating factor-induced sickle cell crisis and multiorgan dysfunction in a patient with compound heterozygous sickle cell/beta + thalassemia. Blood 97(12):3998–3999

Hakansson L, Hoglund M, Jonsson UB, Torsteinsdottir I, Xu X, Venge P (1997) Effects of in vivo administration of G-CSF on neutrophil and eosinophil adhesion. Br J Haematol 98(3):603–611

Hamilton JA (2008) Colony-stimulating factors in inflammation and autoimmunity. Nat Rev Immunol 8(7):533–544. doi:10.1038/nri2356

Hankins JS, Ware RE, Rogers ZR, Wynn LW, Lane PA, Scott JP, Wang WC (2005) Long-term hydroxyurea therapy for infants with sickle cell anemia: the HUSOFT extension study. Blood 106(7):2269–2275. doi:10.1182/Blood-2004-12-4973

Hebbel RP, Eaton JW, Balasingam M, Steinberg MH (1982) Spontaneous oxygen radical generation by sickle erythrocytes. J Clin Invest 70(6):1253–1259

Hidalgo A, Peired AJ, Wild MK, Vestweber D, Frenette PS (2007) Complete identification of E-selectin ligands on neutrophils reveals distinct functions of PSGL-1, ESL-1, and CD44. Immunity 26(4):477–489

Hidalgo A, Chang J, Jang JE, Peired AJ, Chiang EY, Frenette PS (2009) Heterotypic interactions enabled by polarized neutrophil microdomains mediate thromboinflammatory injury. Nat Med 15(4):384–391

Hofstra TC, Kalra VK, Meiselman HJ, Coates TD (1996) Sickle erythrocytes adhere to polymorphonuclear neutrophils and activate the neutrophil respiratory burst. Blood 87(10):4440–4447

Jang JE, Hod EA, Spitalnik SL, Frenette PS (2011) CXCL1 and its receptor, CXCR2, mediate murine sickle cell vaso-occlusion during hemolytic transfusion reactions. J Clin Invest 121(4):1397–1401

Jang JE, Hidalgo A, Frenette PS (2012) Intravenous immunoglobulins modulate neutrophil activation and vascular injury through FcgammaRIII and SHP-1. Circ Res 110(8):1057–1066

Kaul DK, Hebbel RP (2000) Hypoxia/reoxygenation causes inflammatory response in transgenic sickle mice but not in normal mice. J Clin Invest 106(3):411–420

Kaul DK, Fabry ME, Nagel RL (1989) Microvascular sites and characteristics of sickle cell adhesion to vascular endothelium in shear flow conditions: pathophysiological implications. Proc Natl Acad Sci U S A 86(9):3356–3360

Kaul DK, Liu XD, Choong S, Belcher JD, Vercellotti GM, Hebbel RP (2004) Anti-inflammatory therapy ameliorates leukocyte adhesion and microvascular flow abnormalities in transgenic sickle mice. Am J Physiol Heart Circ Physiol 287(1):H293–H301

Kaul DK, Finnegan E, Barabino GA (2009) Sickle red cell-endothelium interactions. Microcirculation 16(1):97–111

Khajah M, Millen B, Cara DC, Waterhouse C, McCafferty DM (2011) Granulocyte-macrophage colony-stimulating factor (GM-CSF): a chemoattractive agent for murine leukocytes in vivo. J Leukoc Biol 89(6):945–953

Kinney TR, Sleeper LA, Wang WC, Zimmerman RA, Pegelow CH, Ohene-Frempong K, Wethers DL, Bello JA, Vichinsky EP, Moser FG, Gallagher DM, DeBaun MR, Platt OS, Miller ST (1999) Silent cerebral infarcts in sickle cell anemia: a risk factor analysis. The Cooperative Study of Sickle Cell Disease. Pediatrics 103(3):640–645

Kutlar A, Ataga KI, McMahon L, Howard J, Galacteros F, Hagar W, Vichinsky E, Cheung AT, Matsui N, Embury SH (2012) A potent oral P-selectin blocking agent improves microcirculatory blood flow and a marker of endothelial cell injury in patients with sickle cell disease. Am J Hematol 87(5):536–539

Lard LR, Mul FP, de Haas M, Roos D, Duits AJ (1999) Neutrophil activation in sickle cell disease. J Leukoc Biol 66(3):411–415

Letvin NL, Linch DC, Beardsley GP, McIntyre KW, Nathan DG (1984) Augmentation of fetal-hemoglobin production in anemic monkeys by hydroxyurea. N Engl J Med 310(14): 869–873

Ley K, Laudanna C, Cybulsky MI, Nourshargh S (2007) Getting to the site of inflammation: the leukocyte adhesion cascade updated. Nat Rev Immunol 7(9):678–689

Lin G, Field JJ, Yu JC, Ken R, Neuberg D, Nathan DG, Linden J (2013) NF-kappaB is activated in CD4+ iNKT cells by sickle cell disease and mediates rapid induction of adenosine A2A receptors. PLoS One 8(10):e74664

Lo SK, Lee S, Ramos RA, Lobb R, Rosa M, Chi-Rosso G, Wright SD (1991) Endothelial-leukocyte adhesion molecule 1 stimulates the adhesive activity of leukocyte integrin CR3 (CD11b/CD18, Mac-1, alpha m beta 2) on human neutrophils. J Exp Med 173(6):1493–1500

Malave I, Perdomo Y, Escalona E, Rodriguez E, Anchustegui M, Malave H, Arends T (1993) Levels of tumor necrosis factor alpha/cachectin (TNF alpha) in sera from patients with sickle cell disease. Acta Haematol 90(4):172–176

Manwani D, Frenette PS (2013) Vaso-occlusion in sickle cell disease: pathophysiology and novel targeted therapies. Blood 122(24):3892–3898

Miller ST, Sleeper LA, Pegelow CH, Enos LE, Wang WC, Weiner SJ, Wethers DL, Smith J, Kinney TR (2000) Prediction of adverse outcomes in children with sickle cell disease. N Engl J Med 342(2):83–89

Nathan DG, Field J, Lin G, Neuberg D, Majerus E, Onyekwere O, Keefer J, Okam M, Ross A, Linden J (2012) Sickle cell disease (SCD), iNKT cells, and regadenoson infusion. Trans Am Clin Climatol Assoc 123:312–317

Nelson RM, Cecconi O, Roberts WG, Aruffo A, Linhardt RJ, Bevilacqua MP (1993) Heparin oligosaccharides bind L- and P-selectin and inhibit acute inflammation. Blood 82(11): 3253–3258

Paszty C, Brion CM, Manci E, Witkowska HE, Stevens ME, Mohandas N, Rubin EM (1997) Transgenic knockout mice with exclusively human sickle hemoglobin and sickle cell disease. Science 278(5339):876–878

Perelman N, Selvaraj SK, Batra S, Luck LR, Erdreich-Epstein A, Coates TD, Kalra VK, Malik P (2003) Placenta growth factor activates monocytes and correlates with sickle cell disease severity. Blood 102(4):1506–1514

Peter K, Schwarz M, Conradt C, Nordt T, Moser M, Kubler W, Bode C (1999) Heparin inhibits ligand binding to the leukocyte integrin Mac-1 (CD11b/CD18). Circulation 100(14):1533–1539

Pieters RC, Rojer RA, Saleh AW, Saleh AE, Duits AJ (1995) Molgramostim to treat SS-sickle cell leg ulcers. Lancet 345(8948):528

Platt OS, Thorington BD, Brambilla DJ, Milner PF, Rosse WF, Vichinsky E, Kinney TR (1991) Pain in sickle cell disease. Rates and risk factors. N Engl J Med 325(1):11–16

Platt OS, Brambilla DJ, Rosse WF, Milner PF, Castro O, Steinberg MH, Klug PP (1994) Mortality in sickle cell disease. Life expectancy and risk factors for early death. N Engl J Med 330(23):1639–1644

Qari MH, Aljaouni SK, Alardawi MS, Fatani H, Alsayes FM, Zografos P, Alsaigh M, Alalfi A, Alamin M, Gadi A, Mousa SA (2007) Reduction of painful vaso-occlusive crisis of sickle cell anaemia by tinzaparin in a double-blind randomized trial. Thromb Haemost 98(2):392–396

Safaya S, Steinberg MH, Klings ES (2012) Monocytes from sickle cell disease patients induce differential pulmonary endothelial gene expression via activation of NF-kappaB signaling pathway. Mol Immunol 50(1–2):117–123

Saleh AW, Hillen HF, Duits AJ (1999) Levels of endothelial, neutrophil and platelet-specific factors in sickle cell anemia patients during hydroxyurea therapy. Acta Haematol 102(1):31–37

Schaer DJ, Buehler PW, Alayash AI, Belcher JD, Vercellotti GM (2013) Hemolysis and free hemoglobin revisited: exploring hemoglobin and hemin scavengers as a novel class of therapeutic proteins. Blood 121(8):1276–1284

Setty BN, Kulkarni S, Stuart MJ (2002) Role of erythrocyte phosphatidylserine in sickle red cell-endothelial adhesion. Blood 99(5):1564–1571

Simon SI, Hu Y, Vestweber D, Smith CW (2000) Neutrophil tethering on E-selectin activates beta 2 integrin binding to ICAM-1 through a mitogen-activated protein kinase signal transduction pathway. J Immunol 164(8):4348–4358

Solovey A, Lin Y, Browne P, Choong S, Wayner E, Hebbel RP (1997) Circulating activated endothelial cells in sickle cell anemia. N Engl J Med 337(22):1584–1590

Solovey AA, Solovey AN, Harkness J, Hebbel RP (2001) Modulation of endothelial cell activation in sickle cell disease: a pilot study. Blood 97(7):1937–1941

Steinberg MH, Barton F, Castro O et al (2003) Effect of hydroxyurea on mortality and morbidity in adult sickle cell anemia: risks and benefits up to 9 years of treatment. JAMA 289(13): 1645–1651

Sultana C, Shen Y, Rattan V, Johnson C, Kalra VK (1998) Interaction of sickle erythrocytes with endothelial cells in the presence of endothelial cell conditioned medium induces oxidant stress leading to transendothelial migration of monocytes. Blood 92(10):3924–3935

Telen MJ, Wun T, McCavit TL et al (2015) Randomized phase 2 study of GMI-1070 in SCD: reduction in time to resolution of vaso-occlusive events and decreased opioid use. Blood. doi:10.1182/blood-2014-06-583351

Thomas PW, Higgs DR, Serjeant GR (1997) Benign clinical course in homozygous sickle cell disease: a search for predictors. J Clin Epidemiol 50(2):121–126

Turhan A, Weiss LA, Mohandas N, Coller BS, Frenette PS (2002) Primary role for adherent leukocytes in sickle cell vascular occlusion: a new paradigm. Proc Natl Acad Sci U S A 99(5):3047–3051

Turhan A, Jenab P, Bruhns P, Ravetch JV, Coller BS, Frenette PS (2004) Intravenous immune globulin prevents venular vaso-occlusion in sickle cell mice by inhibiting leukocyte adhesion and the interactions between sickle erythrocytes and adherent leukocytes. Blood 103(6):2397–2400

Wagener FA, Eggert A, Boerman OC, Oyen WJ, Verhofstad A, Abraham NG, Adema G, van Kooyk Y, de Witte T, Figdor CG (2001) Heme is a potent inducer of inflammation in mice and is counteracted by heme oxygenase. Blood 98(6):1802–1811

Wali Y, Beshlawi I, Fawaz N, Alkhayat A, Zalabany M, Elshinawy M, Al-Kindi S, Al-Rawas AH, Klein C (2012) Coexistence of sickle cell disease and severe congenital neutropenia: first impressions can be deceiving. Eur J Haematol 89(3):245–249

Wallace KL, Linden J (2010) Adenosine A2A receptors induced on iNKT and NK cells reduce pulmonary inflammation and injury in mice with sickle cell disease. Blood 116(23):5010–5020

Wallace KL, Marshall MA, Ramos SI, Lannigan JA, Field JJ, Strieter RM, Linden J (2009) NKT cells mediate pulmonary inflammation and dysfunction in murine sickle cell disease through production of IFN-gamma and CXCR3 chemokines. Blood 114(3):667–676

Wang RH, Phillips G Jr, Medof ME, Mold C (1993) Activation of the alternative complement pathway by exposure of phosphatidylethanolamine and phosphatidylserine on erythrocytes from sickle cell disease patients. J Clin Invest 92(3):1326–1335

Wun T, Styles L, DeCastro L, Telen MJ, Kuypers F, Cheung A, Kramer W, Flanner H, Rhee S, Magnani JL, Thackray H (2014) Phase 1 study of the E-selectin inhibitor GMI 1070 in patients with sickle cell anemia. PLoS One 9(7):e101301

Xie X, Thorlacius H, Raud J, Hedqvist P, Lindbom L (1997) Inhibitory effect of locally administered heparin on leukocyte rolling and chemoattractant-induced firm adhesion in rat mesenteric venules in vivo. Br J Pharmacol 122(5):906–910

Zarbock A, Lowell CA, Ley K (2007a) Spleen tyrosine kinase Syk is necessary for E-selectin-induced alpha(L)beta(2) integrin-mediated rolling on intercellular adhesion molecule-1. Immunity 26(6):773–783

Zarbock A, Polanowska-Grabowska RK, Ley K (2007b) Platelet-neutrophil-interactions: linking hemostasis and inflammation. Blood Rev 21(2):99–111

Zennadi R, De Castro L, Eyler C, Xu K, Ko M, Telen MJ (2008) Role and regulation of sickle red cell interactions with other cells: ICAM-4 and other adhesion receptors. Transfus Clin Biol 15(1–2):23–28

Chapter 6
Hypercoagulability and Sickle Cell Disease

Marina Pereira Colella, Erich Vinicius de Paula, Margareth Castro Ozelo, and Fabiola Traina

Abstract Thrombotic complications have always been recognized as one of the hallmarks of sickle cell disease (SCD). Epidemiological data demonstrate that stroke and venous thromboembolism are much more frequent in these patients. Furthermore, hypercoagulability has been implicated in the pathogenesis of other complications of SCD such as acute chest syndrome. In the last two decades, robust experimental data have demonstrated that almost every element of hemostasis, both protein and cellular, is altered in a way that shifts the hemostatic balance towards a procoagulant state in SCD. During recent years, exciting new data have shed light on the mechanisms responsible for these alterations, such as inflammation, endothelial activation, and intravascular hemolysis. In this chapter, we discuss the clinical and laboratory evidence supporting the concept that SCD is associated with a significant hypercoagulable state, as well as the potential mechanisms responsible for these alterations. We also discuss old, current and future therapeutic strategies aimed to modulate the risk of thrombosis in SCD.

Keywords Sickle cell anemia • Thromboembolism • Hemolysis

6.1 Association between Hemoglobin S and Thromboembolic Events

There is abundant clinical evidence indicating the existence of an hypercoagulable state in sickle cell anemia (SCA), which is best illustrated by the increased rates of venous and arterial thrombotic events in these patients. Ischemic stroke is a major

M.P. Colella (✉) • E.V. de Paula • M.C. Ozelo
Hematology Center, School of Medical Sciences, University of Campinas-Unicamp, Rua Carlos Chagas, 480, Campinas, São Paulo, CEP 13083-878, Brazil
e-mail: marinasp@unicamp.br; erich@unicamp.br; margaret@unicamp.br

F. Traina
Department of Internal Medicine, University of São Paulo at Ribeirão Preto Medical School, Avenida Bandeirantes, 3900, Ribeirão Preto, São Paulo CEP 14049-900, Brazil
e-mail: ftraina@fmrp.usp.br

© Springer International Publishing Switzerland 2016
F.F. Costa, N. Conran (eds.), *Sickle Cell Anemia*,
DOI 10.1007/978-3-319-06713-1_6

cause of morbidity and mortality in adults and children with SCA, reaching a prevalence of almost 10 % at 50 years (Ohene-Frempong et al. 1998). Children with SCA have the highest rates of ischemic stroke in infants, with an incidence of approximately 240 cases per 100,000 per year (Earley et al. 1998) compared to the incidence of 2.3 per 100,000 in normal children (Fullerton et al. 2003). Magnetic resonance imaging studies show that at least 25 % of children with SCA present silent brain infarcts (without clinical manifestations) at 6 years of age, and this prevalence reaches 37 % at 14 years (Bernaudin et al. 2005; Kwiatkowski et al. 2009). Interestingly, the main risk factors for the occurrence of silent brain infarcts in SCA children are high blood pressure and lower levels of hemoglobin, suggesting that patients with higher hemolytic activity are at increased risk of ischemic stroke (DeBaun et al. 2012).

Pulmonary embolism is another important clinical complication of SCA, and is considered the leading cause of death associated with acute chest syndrome (Vichinsky et al. 2000). Venous thromboembolic events, especially pulmonary thromboembolism, also have an increased incidence in patients with SCA. Early autopsy studies identified new and old thrombi in the pulmonary circulation of 25–60 % of patients with SCA (Oppenheimer and Esterly 1971; Manci et al. 2003). Moreover, the prevalence of pulmonary thromboembolism in hospitalized patients with sickle cell disease (SCD) was reported to be four times higher, compared to the prevalence in other African-American patients (Stein et al. 2006); during the observation period (1979–2003), the prevalence of pulmonary thromboembolism in patients with SCD under 40 years of age was 0.44 %, compared with 0.12 % in age-matched patients of African descent. Interestingly, the prevalence of deep vein thrombosis (DVT) was similar in both groups. Similar findings were observed in another study, in which the incidence of pulmonary thromboembolism was 50–100 times higher in the hospitalized USA population with SCD compared with the general population (Novelli et al. 2012). SCA is also considered a significant risk factor for the occurrence of thromboembolism associated with pregnancy, with an odds ratio of 6.7 (James et al. 2006). More recently, data from the Cooperative Study of Sickle Cell Disease (CSSCD) confirmed a higher risk of venous thromboembolism (VTE) in SCD. The incidence rate for first VTE from ages 15–30 years was 6.7 events/1000 person-years, which is nearly four times higher than reported rates for factor V Leiden carriers of the same age. Again, the incidence of pulmonary embolism was around twofold higher than the incidence of DVT, although this difference was not statistically significant (Naik et al. 2014).

Interestingly, studies of individuals with sickle cell trait also support the concept that SCA is associated with a hypercoagulable state. In the early 2000s, a study demonstrated that sickle cell trait is associated with higher levels of several laboratory markers of coagulation activation (Westerman et al. 2002). This observation was followed by epidemiological data showing that the incidence of VTE was twofold higher in African-Americans with sickle cell trait, compared to a control group of hospitalized African-Americans without sickle cell trait (odds ratio 1.8, 95 % confidence interval [CI] 1.2–2.9) (Austin et al. 2007). The risk of pulmonary thromboembolism was four times higher in sickle cell trait (odds ratio 3.9; 95 % CI 2.2–6.9), but the risk of DVT did not significantly differ between the two groups. Overall, the proportion of

VTE in African-American patients attributable to sickle cell trait was about 7 % (Austin et al. 2007), which is higher than the prothrombotic effect of prothrombin G20210A and factor V Leiden mutations in caucasians. Accordingly, the MEGA case-control study, a large Dutch population study of VTE risk factors, identified that the presence of sickle cell trait was associated with an odds ratio of 3.9 for pulmonary thromboembolism, compared with an odds ratio of 1.7 for factor V Leiden and 2.3 for prothrombin mutation (van Langevelde et al. 2012). These data were recently confirmed in a prospective study that evaluated 268 sickle cell trait individuals, compared with 3748 non-sickle cell trait individuals during 24 years of follow up, for the incidence of pulmonary thromboembolism and DVT (Folsom et al. 2015). The authors confirmed that sickle cell trait in African Americans carries a twofold increased risk of pulmonary thromboembolism (hazard ratio 2.05, 95 % 1.12–3.16), while the risk for DVT was not significantly increased (hazard ratio 1.15, 95 % 0.58–2.27). The major implication of these findings is the recognition that the sickle cell trait is an important form of inherited thrombophilia in the African-descendent population.

In addition to the increased incidence of thrombotic events, it is also believed that the hypercoagulable state in SCA contributes to a spectrum of disorders related to hemolysis and endothelial dysfunction, such as pulmonary hypertension, priapism and leg ulcers (Morris 2008). There seems to be a relationship between hemostatic activation and the development of vasculopathy leading to pulmonary hypertension, a major cause of mortality in SCA (Ataga et al. 2008). There is also evidence of associations between levels of procoagulant markers and retinopathy and ischemic stroke (Ataga et al. 2012). Painful crises are associated with increased levels of hypercoagulability markers, which suggests a possible role of hypercoagulability in the development of vaso-occlusion (van Beers et al. 2009).

SC hemoglobinopathy (HbSC) is the second most prevalent hemoglobinopathy after SCA (Weatherall 2010). Studies have shown an increased risk of thromboembolic events in HbSC, but HbSC patients are only the minority of patients included in larger cohorts of SCD (Stein et al. 2006; Novelli et al. 2012). Autopsy studies show that pulmonary thromboembolism is the second leading cause of mortality in these patients, accounting for 13.6 % of deaths, an increased frequency compared to SCA patients (Manci et al. 2003). The incidence of ischemic stroke in childhood is also increased, being approximately 100 times greater than for the general population (Powars et al. 1990). With regard to the relative frequency of VTE in HbSC patients, compared with SS patients, conflicting results have emerged from two recent studies. In a retrospective analysis of 404 patients with SCD, the prevalence of non-catheter related VTE was significantly higher in the subgroup of patients with sickle cell variants, of which 67.2 % (84 out of 125 patients) had HbSC, compared to SS patients (Naik et al. 2013). In contrast, patients with HbSC from the CSSCD presented a lower frequency of VTE than SS patients, a difference that was partially attributed to the lower age of the latter cohort (Folsom et al. 2015).

Recently, our group performed a cross-sectional observational study evaluating coagulation activation markers in 56 adult HbSC patients, in comparison with 39 SCA patients and 27 healthy controls. We found that HbSC patients present a hypercoagulable state, as evidenced by increased expression of the gene encoding tissue factor (TF), thrombin-antithrombin complex and D-dimer, compared with healthy subjects, although this manifestation was not as intense as that seen in SCA. Hemostatic activation was associated with two very prevalent chronic complications seen in SC disease; retinopathy and osteonecrosis (Colella et al. 2015).

6.2 The Hemostatic Balance in SCA

The hemostatic balance depends on the equilibrium between several procoagulant and anticoagulant factors and on the restriction of the coagulation process on cell surfaces. Alterations in this balance can lead to bleeding and thrombosis. The endothelium is the central player in maintaining this balance, in that it separates cells expressing tissue factor, the physiological initiator of coagulation, from platelets and coagulation factors, and also regulates blood cell adhesion to the vascular wall.

Tissue factor is a transmembrane protein found in several sub-endothelium cells (Furie and Furie 2008). Under normal conditions, TF is expressed on cells of the adventitial layer of the vessel wall, being exposed in the flow after the occurrence of vascular lesions, and then triggering the activation of coagulation. TF forms a complex with activated factor VII, which is present in small quantities in the circulation. This TF/FVIIa complex activates factor X, which converts prothrombin into thrombin. Markers of thrombin generation and fibrinolysis may be assessed in the plasma; thrombin-antithrombin complex (TAT), protrombin fragment 1+2 (F1+2) and D-dimer (DD) (Fig. 6.1).

In various pathological conditions, especially in proinflammatory states, TF expression is upregulated in monocytes and in circulating microparticles (MPs) (Mackman 2009; Geddings and Mackman 2014). Previous studies in SCA have

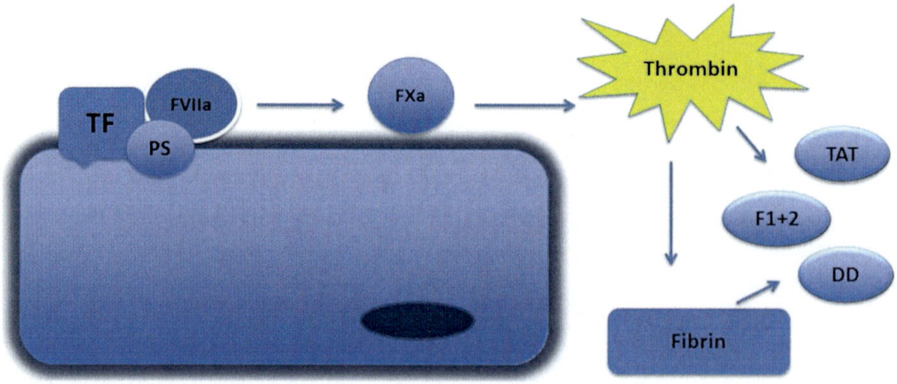

Fig. 6.1 Illustrative diagram of thrombin generation. Tissue factor (TF) is the main physiological initiator of coagulation in vivo. TF is the cellular receptor and cofactor of factor VII. The formation of the TF: FVIIa complex on surfaces presenting phosphatidylserine (PS) leads to factor X activation, initiating a cascade of enzymatic reactions that culminate in the formation of thrombin and fibrin thrombi. The generation and degradation of thrombin and fibrin is measured by thrombin-antithrombin complex (TAT), protrombin fragment 1+2 (F1+2) and D-dimer (DD)

Table 6.1 Hemostatic alterations observed in sickle cell anemia

Component	Alterations
Endothelium	• Expression of TF on pulmonary veinsa • High levels of CECs with TF expression • Increased expression of proadhesive molecules: ICAM-1, VCAM-1, E-selectin • Elevation of soluble thrombomodulin levels • Release of high amounts of high molecular weight VWF multimers • High levels of endothelium-derived MPs with TF expression • NO consumption
Platelets	• Increased activation • Liberation of MPs
Leukocytes	• Elevation of monocyte levels with expression of functionally-active TF • Release of monocyte-derived MPs expressing TF • Increased adhesion properties
Red blood cells	• Exposure of PS on membrane surface • Liberation of MPs • Increased adhesive properties • Heme release and subsequent TF activation and NET formation[a]
Coagulation factors	• Increased TF expression and activity • Consumption of coagulation factors • Increased thrombin generation and fibrinolysis markers: TAT, F1+2, D-dimer
Natural anticoagulants	• Reduction of levels of protein C and protein S

TF tissue factor, *CECs* circulating endothelial cells, *ICAM-1* intercellular adhesion molecule1, *VCAM-1* vascular cell adhesion molecule 1, *VWF* von Willebrand factor, *MPs* microparticles, *NO* nitric oxide, *PS* phosphatidylserine, *NET* neutrophil extracellular trap, *TAT* thrombin-antithrombin complex, *F1+2* protrombin fragment 1+2

[a]This data was demonstrated in SCD-mouse-models

shown increased TF procoagulant activity in mononuclear cells (Key et al. 1998) and TF expression on microparticles (MPs) (Shet et al. 2003), monocytes (Setty et al. 2012) and on circulating endothelial cells (CECs) (Solovey et al. 1998). Importantly, in a sickle cell disease (SCD)-mouse-model, TF was shown to be the main factor responsible for coagulation activation, since inhibition of TF expression reduced TAT levels to normal values (Chantrathammachart et al. 2012).

It is not only TF expression that seems to be upregulated in SCA. In fact, practically every element of the hemostatic balance is altered in the pro-coagulant direction in SCA, leading to the recognition of this condition as a "hypercoagulable state" (Table 6.1). In general, these coagulation abnormalities are present in steady state, and are further increased during painful crisis.

6.3 Global Hemostasis Assays in SCA

Given the interaction of erythrocytes, platelets, leukocytes and plasma proteins in coagulation activation, and the limitation of classical hemostasis assays in evaluating this interaction, there has been recent interest in the so-called "global hemostasis assays" for the evaluation of the hypercoagulable state found in SCA (Lim et al. 2013). Among these, thromboelastometry (TEM) and the thrombin generation test (TGT) are the most well-studied. TEM evaluates the viscoelastic properties of whole blood, taking into account the role of platelets, erythrocytes and leukocytes (Nair et al. 2010). The TGT is an assay that measures the magnitude and kinetics of thrombin generation over time, which represent critical biomarkers of clot quality and hemostasis activation (Ten Cate 2012). Patients with increased risk of thromboembolic events present higher levels of thrombin generation (Hron et al. 2006). Both tests have been used to assess the presence of hypercoagulability in SCA (reviewed in Lim et al. 2013). In 2005, Yee and colleagues demonstrated that patients with SCA present a TEM pattern suggestive of a hypercoagulable state, which was even more evident during acute crisis (Yee et al. 2005). A much larger number of studies have used the TGT to evaluate hemostatic changes in SCA. Noubouossie et al., found increased thrombin generation compared to age-matched controls, but no differences were observed between patients with and without acute crisis (Noubouossie et al. 2012). In contrast, Shah et al., found significant differences suggestive of hypercoagulability in SCA patients during acute crisis (Shah et al. 2012). With a somewhat different experimental protocol, characterized by the use of higher doses of TF for initiation of thrombin generation, Gerotziafas et al. also found evidence of faster and stronger thrombin generation in patients with SCA (Gerotziafas et al. 2012). In contrast, Betal et al. (2009) and Wolberg et al. (2009) did not find evidence of increased thrombin generation in SCA. Despite this variability, most of these studies demonstrate a trend towards an increase in thrombin generation in patients with SCA. More recent data confirm this impression, by demonstrating an increased capacity of SS red blood cells to contribute to the generation of thrombin, when compared with red blood cells from control individuals (Whelihan et al. 2013). It should be noted that, despite the importance of these tests in providing relevant information about the pathophysiology of hypercoagulability in SCA, there is currently no indication to perform any of these tests in the clinical management of SCA.

6.4 Mechanisms That Lead to Hypercoagulability in Sickle Cell Anemia

Robust evidence demonstrates that endothelial dysfunction, inflammation, exposure of phosphatidylserine (PS) on the surface of red blood cells (RBC) and intravascular hemolysis are among the most important factors contributing to the development of hypercoagulability in SCA. Unfortunately, the relative importance, and the hierarchical organization, of each of these factors to the development of a hypercoagulable state in SCA remain to be determined. Indeed, while the discussion of these factors will be presented separately in this chapter, complex feedback mechanisms involving all of these mechanisms should be considered the most likely explanation for the increased risk of thrombotic events in SCA.

6.4.1 Endothelial Dysfunction and Activation

An abnormally activated proadhesive and procoagulant endothelium is a hallmark of SCA. Several biomarkers of endothelial activation are increased in SCA patients (Kato et al. 2005). In addition, higher numbers of circulating endothelial cells (CECs) are observed in SCA patients, which further increase during vaso-occlusive crises (Solovey et al. 1997). These CECs present an increased expression of adhesion molecules, such as intercellular adhesion molecule1 (ICAM-1), vascular cell adhesion molecule 1 (VCAM-1) and E-selectin, and can also express surface TF (Solovey et al. 1998). A higher percentage of CECs from SCA patients express TF, compared with those of normal subjects (78 vs. 10 %), and TF expression is higher during vaso-occlusive episodes, compared to steady state (83 vs. 66 %). Immunofluorescence analysis of CECs expressing TF showed that these cells also carry factors VII/VIIa, which are able to activate factor X, a finding that could be associated with the lower factor VII plasma half-life observed in these patients (Kurantsin-Mills et al. 1992). Von Willebrand factor (vWF), another marker of endothelial activation, is secreted by endothelial cells and involved in platelet adhesion. Larger amounts of high molecular weight VWF multimers, as well as increased VWF activity, were observed in patients with SCA, suggesting a role for hyperreactive VWF in the pathogenesis of SCA (Chen et al. 2011).

In addition, several lines of evidence demonstrate the increased adhesive properties of the endothelium in SCA (Conran et al. 2009), as described in more detail in Chap. 7.

6.4.2 Inflammation

SCA is recognized as a chronic proinflammatory state with increased inflammatory cytokines, increased total leukocyte counts, monocyte and functional changes of leukocytes (Platt 2000). The association of inflammation and coagulation activation observed in SCA should be of no surprise, since hemostasis and innate immunity evolved together during at least 450 million years (Opal and Esmon 2003). Accordingly, coagulation activation is a hallmark of several inflammatory processes such as sepsis (van der Poll and Herwald 2014). Patients with SCA have increased numbers of circulating monocytes. These monocytes are activated and, in turn, are able to activate endothelial cells, thereby contributing to vascular inflammation and activation of coagulation. In in vitro experiments, the incubation of mononuclear leukocytes of patients with SCA with human umbilical vein endothelial cells (HUVECS) resulted in an increased expression of TF by HUVECS (Belcher et al. 2000). In a SCD-mouse-model, vessels of the pulmonary circulation presented increased TF expression, which was further increased after episodes of hypoxia/reoxygenation (Solovey et al. 2004). In addition to activating TF expression by endothelial cells, monocytes in SCA can also express TF themselves. The total procoagulant activity of TF, measured using whole blood coagulation assays is increased in SCA. In such coagulation assays, the entire TF procoagulant activity was concentrated in the fraction of mononuclear cells isolated from patients with SCA, demonstrating that monocytes are capable of expressing functional TF (Solovey et al. 1998).

The interaction between pro-inflammatory and pro-coagulant pathways is bidirectional. As these inflammatory changes lead to increased expression of TF, the opposite is also true. There seems to be a role for TF in triggering or feeding the pro-inflammatory state in SCA (Sparkenbaugh and Pawlinski 2013). Studies in SCD-mouse-models have demonstrated that TF inhibition with an anti-TF antibody led to the decrease in plasma levels of proinflammatory markers and a reduction in neutrophil pulmonary infiltration (Chantrathammachart et al. 2012). As previously mentioned, although several proinflammatory and procoagulant changes have been identified in clinical and non-clinical models of SCA, the key triggers and perpetuators of inflammation that ultimately lead to the increased thrombotic risk observed in these patients are yet to be determined.

6.4.3 *Exposure of Phosphatidylserine in Sickle RBC*

In normal RBC, procoagulant phospholipids such as phosphatidylserine (PS) are almost restricted to the inner face of the cell membrane (Connor and Schroit 1991). It has been shown that repeated cycles of sickling and unsickling in SCA result in the loss of this asymmetry, and in the exposure of PS to the outer RBC leaflet. Surface PS facilitates the docking and assembly of coagulation factors on the RBC membrane, thereby contributing to thrombin generation and coagulation activation (Whelihan et al. 2012).

6.4.4 *Intravascular Hemolysis*

The most compelling evidence that intravascular hemolysis is associated with a hypercoagulable state stems from the observation that different hemolytic anemias, with distinct pathogenic mechanisms, share with SCA the common finding of an increased risk for arterial and/or venous thrombotic events. Accordingly, an increased risk of thrombotic events is a hallmark of both thalassemia major and intermedia (Cappellini et al. 2000), hereditary spherocytosis (Schilling 1997), and paroxysmal nocturnal hemoglobinuria (PNH) (Hillmen et al. 1995), in which thrombosis represents the most important cause of death. In PNH, thrombosis is directly associated with hemolytic activity, as indicated by LDH levels (Schrezenmeier et al. 2014). In the context of SCA, this association between hemolysis and coagulation activation is further corroborated by studies in which coagulation activation markers, such as D-dimer and thrombin-antithrombin complexes, correlated with hemolysis markers in independent patient cohorts (Ataga et al. 2012; Setty et al. 2012).

Based on currently available evidence, the association between intravascular hemolysis and hypercoagulability in SCA is caused by the constant release of free hemoglobin (Hb) and free heme from hemolysed RBC, which leads to nitric oxide (NO) depletion and innate immunity activation respectively. Nitric oxide (NO) is a well-known regulator of endothelial homeostasis, acting in the physiological down-regulation of several important elements of hemostasis such as vasoconstriction, platelet activation, inflammatory cell attachment to the endothelium, and procoagulant factors expression (Kato and Taylor 2010). It has been shown that intravascular hemolysis results in decreased bioavailability of NO, due to NO consumption and reduction by hemoglobin released from the cytoplasm of hemolysed RBC (Reiter et al. 2002). This state of NO deficiency is further aggravated by the release of RBC arginase during hemolysis, which reduces the bioavailability of arginine, an important substrate for NO synthesis. NO depletion leads to a hyperadhesive endothelium, platelet activation, among others (Conran et al. 2009). Accordingly, impairment of the broad anti-coagulant functions of NO is regarded as an important contributor to the shift of the hemostatic balance towards a hypercoagulable state in patients with SCA.

Another important procoagulant mechanism is the release of free heme. It has been known for almost 50 years that patients with SCA present higher levels of heme in plasma, associated with lower levels of the most important heme-binding protein, hemopexin (Muller-Eberhard et al. 1968). Unbound extracellular heme exerts toxic effects on cells and tissues by two different mechanisms. Directly, via generation of reactive oxygen species (ROS), and indirectly, through the activation of innate immunity (Dutra and Bozza 2014). The latter effect was confirmed in 2007, by the demonstration that heme can activate TLR4 (Figueiredo et al. 2007), acting as a "danger-associated molecular pattern", thereby triggering proinflammatory pathways similar to those activated in sepsis and in other conditions of sterile inflammation. Besides these mechanistic rationales, both epidemiological and non-clinical experimental data support the association of plasma free heme with inflammation and coagulation activation in SCA. In a study of 942 children with SCD, a polymorphism in the Heme-oxygenase-1 gene promoter region was associated with a significantly lower risk of acute chest syndrome (ACS) (Bean et al. 2012). Similarly, plasma free heme levels were independently associated with the risk of vaso-occlusive crisis and ACS in a study with 81 children (Adisa et al. 2013). Besides these clinical data, a growing number of studies in animal models implicate free heme as a relevant activator of innate immunity in SCD. In animal models of SCA, heme was shown to induce an acute lung injury that resembles ACS (Ghosh et al. 2013) as well as vaso-occlusive events (Belcher et al. 2014). In these two latter studies, the effect of heme was reversed by the use of hemopexin, and by a TLR-4 inhibitor, reinforcing the idea that free heme acts through the activation of innate immunity, rather than by ROS-mediated cell damage.

Tissue factor expression is one of the consequences of innate immune activation in several inflammatory conditions. Heme has been shown to induce TF expression in endothelial cells (Setty et al. 2008), and TF expression correlated with markers of hemolysis in a small cohort of children with SCD (Setty et al. 2012). More recently, heme infusion was directly implicated in the expression of TF and coagulation activation in mice (Sparkenbaugh et al. 2015). The complex roles of heme in the interplay between coagulation activation and inflammation in SCD are illustrated by the recent demonstration that in a SCD-mouse-model, heme was capable of inducing neutrophil extracellular trap (NET) formation (Chen et al. 2014), which appears to have an important role in the development of DVT (Fuchs et al. 2012).

Together, these data suggest that free Hb and free extracellular heme released during intravascular hemolysis act in concert in several compartments of hemostasis, shifting the hemostatic balance towards a prothrombotic state.

6.5 Treatment Strategies for Hypercoagulability in Sickle Cell Anemia

6.5.1 Antiplatelet Agents

Despite the quantity of evidence demonstrating the existence of a hypercoagulable state in SCA, the potential benefit of modulating these hemostatic abnormalities is not yet clear. For many years, authors attempted to use anticoagulants and antiplatelet agents in SCA patients (reviewed in Ataga and Key 2007). Given that aspirin is not only an antiplatelet agent, but also is an anti-inflammatory agent, it is fair to hypothesize that this therapy could bring benefits to these patients. Unfortunately, no correlations between the antiplatelet effects of aspirin and clinical benefits have been demonstrated in the few clinical studies performed so far (Chaplin et al. 1980; Osamo et al. 1981; Greenberg et al. 1983; Zago et al. 1984). More recently, a double-blinded randomized trial compared the use of the antiplatelet agent, prasugrel, versus placebo in SCA patients (Wun et al. 2013). There was a reduction in platelet activation biomarkers and a non-significant decrease in painful events in the group taking prasugrel. Therapy with aspirin is recommended in adults with SCA and previous stroke, as a secondary prevention of this complication (Kernan et al. 2014).

6.5.2 Anticoagulants

The evaluation of the use of oral anticoagulants in SCA has been made in a few studies involving a small number of patients and/or non-randomized trials (reviewed in Ataga and Key 2007). The use of warfarin was associated with a modest decrease in pain episodes (Salvaggio et al. 1963) and a reduction in D-dimer levels (Ahmed et al. 2004).

The chronic use of unfractionated heparin in mini-doses occasioned a reduction in the frequency and severity of vaso-occlusive crises (Chaplin et al. 1989). A more recent randomized, placebo-controlled study showed that the use of a low molecular weight heparin, tinzaparin, in SCA patients with painful crises was able to reduce the number of hospitalization days and decrease the intensity and duration of the painful crisis (Qari et al. 2007).

Despite studies performed over a number of years, it is not yet clear what the benefit that these drugs may have on SCA. Although some have reported an apparent trend towards an improvement in painful crises, there is still no evidence that the use of antiplatelet agents or anticoagulants can reduce the occurrence of thromboembolic complications or other chronic complications in SCA. The American College of Chest Physicians' evidence-based clinical guideline lists no specific recommendations regarding the use of prophylactic anticoagulation in SCA patients for the prevention of thromboembolic events in nonsurgical or surgical situations (Gould et al. 2012; Kahn et al. 2012). However, many authors agree that, in special risk situations, thrombophrophylaxis should be considered, especially in painful crisis. Likewise, there are no formal recommendations as to the duration of anticoagulant treatment in SCA patients that present a venous thromboembolic event.

6.5.3 Hydroxyurea

Considering the role of intravascular hemolysis in SCD-associated hypercoagulability, it is expected that measures that reduce hemolysis can have a beneficial effect on the prevention of thrombotic complications. One of the pillars of SCA treatment is the use of hydroxyurea, a drug that reduces hemolysis and presents several well-defined beneficial effects that could contribute to an inhibition of the hypercoagulability state in SCA. These include; a reduction in PS exposure by RBCs (Setty et al. 2000; Nébor et al. 2013), a reduction in the adhesive properties of RBCs and leukocytes, reductions in endothelial activation and NO depletion, and reductions in platelet activation and adhesion (Styles et al. 1997; Gladwin et al. 2002; Conran et al. 2004; Gambero et al. 2007; Cokic et al. 2008; Canalli et al. 2008).

Considering these beneficial consequences of HbF elevation, our group hypothesized that hydroxyurea could modulate the hypercoagulable state observed in SCA, and evaluated its effects on activation of coagulation in a cohort of SCA patients. Hydroxyurea therapy was associated with an important inhibition of TF expression, associated with lower levels of TAT and F1+2, reflecting a down-regulation of thrombin generation. These potential beneficial changes were associated with a significant decrease in levels of markers of endothelial activation and inflammation (Fig. 6.2). Thrombin-antithrombin complex and F1+2 levels showed significant positive correlations with LDH levels, which suggests that the beneficial effects of hydroxyurea on the hypercoagulability state were at least partially associated with decreased hemolysis (Colella et al. 2012). Our results are in agreement

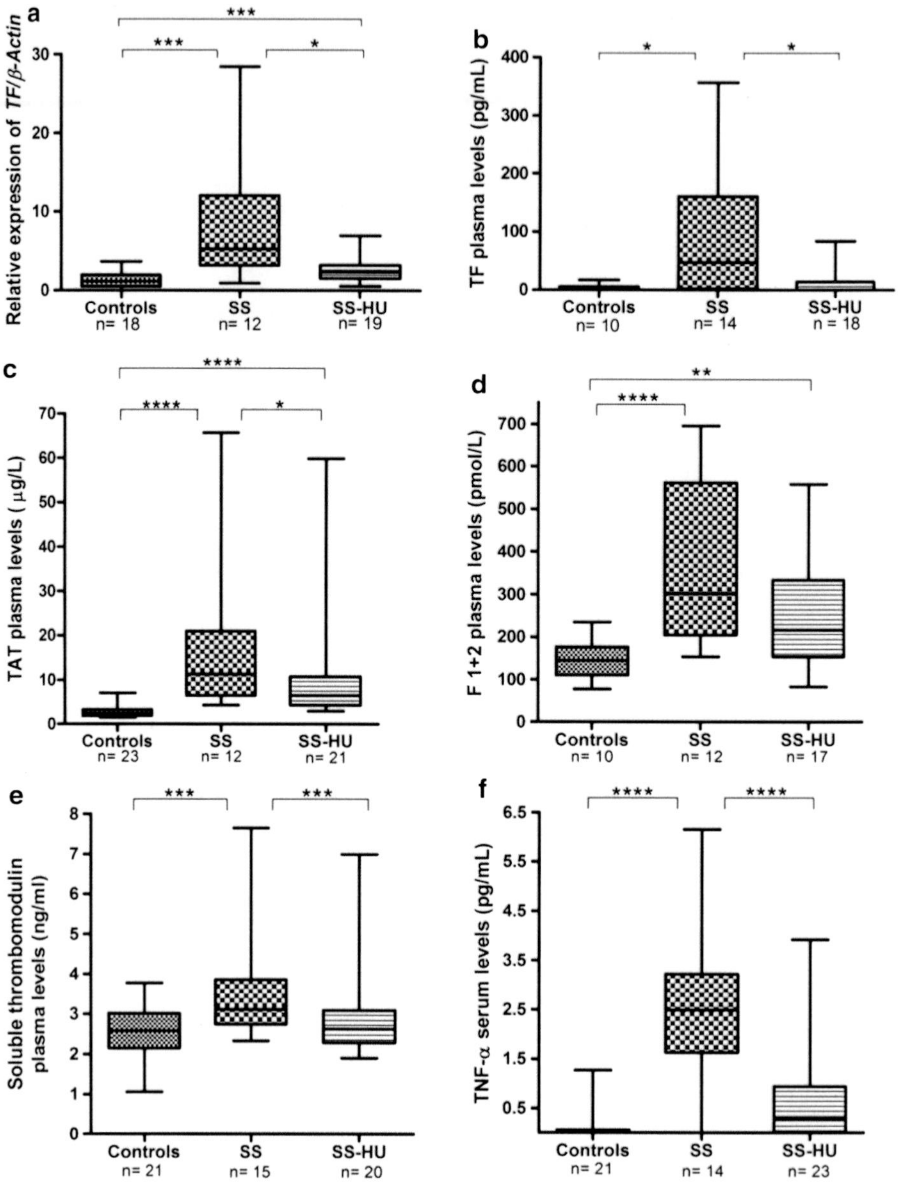

Fig. 6.2 Hydroxyurea therapy is associated with reduced levels of TF expression, TAT, F1+2, soluble thrombomodulin and TNF-α. Tissue factor (TF) mRNA relative expression (**a**), plasma levels of TF (**b**), thrombin-antithrombin complex (TAT) (**c**), prothrombin fragment F1+2 (F1+2) (**d**), soluble thrombomodulin (**e**) and serum levels of tumor necrosis factor-alpha (TNF-α) (**f**) were all measured in controls and SCA patients not on hydroxyurea (SS) and on hydroxyurea (SS-HU). *TF* expression was analysed by real-time quantitative PCR assays (qPCR) from total leukocyte mRNA. ELISA kits were used to measure plasma levels of TF, soluble thrombomodulin, TAT, F1+2, and serum levels of TNF-α. The numbers of patients studied are indicated in each panel. P-values resulting from the comparison of two groups (indicated with *bars*) are shown in the figure; $*p \leq 0.05$, $**p \leq 0.01$, $***p \leq 0.001$, $****p < 0.0001$ (Mann–Whitney U-test or Fisher's exact test). Reproduced with permission from (Colella et al. 2012)

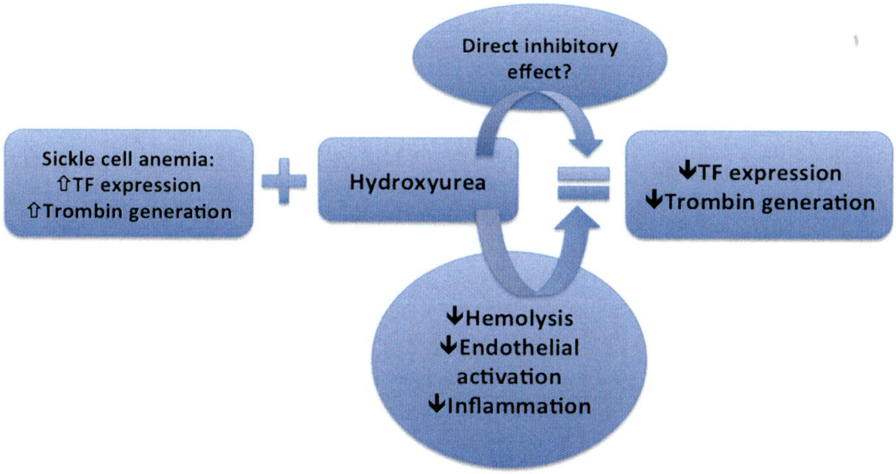

Fig. 6.3 Potential model for the beneficial effect of hydroxyurea on the hypercoagulability state of sickle cell anemia

with a study in children with SCD that also showed a significant association of TF activity and TAT with markers of hemolysis (reticulocyte count and LDH levels) (Setty et al. 2012). The authors suggested that these findings support a role for the early use of agents such as hydroxyurea to reduce hemolytic activity and minimize pro-thrombotic alterations, as was demonstrated in our study.

Hemolysis, endothelial activation and inflammation are closely connected pathways, all of which are associated with coagulation activation, and modulated by hydroxyurea. In our study, despite the findings of bivariate associations between coagulation activation markers and hemolysis markers, in a multiple regression analysis, hydroxyurea was an independent factor associated with TF expression and TAT levels. This finding could imply that hydroxyurea may have an additional inhibitory effect on coagulation activation, independently of its classical effects (Fig. 6.3). Although HbF induction is thought to mediate the principal mechanism of its action, hydroxyurea has many pleiotropic effects, which are not all clearly defined and could modulate numerous emerging therapeutic targets. Whatever the mechanism, the benefits of hydroxyurea on SCA hypercoagulability are suggested by clinical data. Hydroxyurea has been associated with a reduction in stroke recurrence in children with SCA (Ware and Helms 2012) and also reduces the prevalence of pulmonary hypertension in adults with SCA (Ataga et al. 2006), a clinical complication associated with pro-coagulant alterations. Future longitudinal prospective studies including a large number of patients and longer follow-up are needed to verify whether this biological effect of hydroxyurea may result in a decreased incidence of thrombotic complications in SCA patients.

6.6 Future Perspectives

During recent years, increasing evidence suggests extracellular hemoglobin and heme as triggers of several adverse clinical outcomes in SCA patients. Therefore, investigators have been considering hemoglobin and heme scavengers as new possible therapeutic agents (Schaer and Buehler 2013). Hemopexin and TLR4 inhibitors have been tested in animal models, incurring a reduction in the pathological effects of free heme. As yet, there has been no clinical experience with the use of these agents in SCA. Finally, considering the potential of heme in the induction of NET formation, the inhibition of the peptidylarginine deaminase 4 (PADI4), a central enzyme in NET formation, may also be a novel therapeutic strategy (L'Acqua and Hod 2014). These are potential agents that could prevent and/or revert all of the pathological effects of intravascular hemolysis, including the pro-thrombotic complications. In parallel, there are ongoing clinical trials with new anticoagulant and antiplatelet agents in SCA patients that can also bring new potential beneficial effects on the pro-coagulant state seen in these patients.

References

Adisa OA, Hu Y, Ghosh S et al (2013) Association between plasma free haem and incidence of vaso-occlusive episodes and acute chest syndrome in children with sickle cell disease. Br J Haematol 162:702–705. doi:10.1111/bjh.12445

Ahmed S, Siddiqui AK, Iqbal U et al (2004) Effect of low-dose warfarin on D-dimer levels during sickle cell vaso-occlusive crisis: a brief report. Eur J Haematol 72:213–216. doi:10.1111/j.0902-4441.2003.00209.x

Ataga KI, Key NS (2007) Hypercoagulability in sickle cell disease: new approaches to an old problem. Hematology Am Soc Hematol Educ Program 91–6. doi:10.1182/asheducation-2007.1.91

Ataga KI, Moore CG, Jones S et al (2006) Pulmonary hypertension in patients with sickle cell disease: a longitudinal study. Br J Haematol 134:109–115. doi:10.1111/j.1365-2141.2006.06110.x

Ataga KI, Moore CG, Hillery CA et al (2008) Coagulation activation and inflammation in sickle cell disease-associated pulmonary hypertension. Haematologica 93:20–26. doi:10.3324/haematol.11763

Ataga KI, Brittain JE, Desai P et al (2012) Association of coagulation activation with clinical complications in sickle cell disease. PLoS One 7:e29786. doi:10.1371/journal.pone.0029786

Austin H, Key NS, Benson JM et al (2007) Sickle cell trait and the risk of venous thromboembolism among blacks. Blood 110:908–912. doi:10.1182/blood-2006-11-057604

Bean CJ, Boulet SL, Ellingsen D et al (2012) Heme oxygenase-1 gene promoter polymorphism is associated with reduced incidence of acute chest syndrome among children with sickle cell disease. Blood 120:3822–3828. doi:10.1182/blood-2011-06-361642

Belcher JD, Marker PH, Weber JP et al (2000) Activated monocytes in sickle cell disease: potential role in the activation of vascular endothelium and vaso-occlusion. Blood 96:2451–2459

Belcher JD, Chen C, Nguyen J et al (2014) Heme triggers TLR4 signaling leading to endothelial cell activation and vaso-occlusion in murine sickle cell disease. Blood 123:377–390. doi:10.1182/blood-2013-04-495887

Bernaudin F, Verlhac S, Coïc L et al (2005) Long-term follow-up of pediatric sickle cell disease patients with abnormal high velocities on transcranial Doppler. Pediatr Radiol 35:242–248. doi:10.1007/s00247-005-1419-5

Betal SG, Kato GJ, Lawrence MP, et al. (2009) Thrombin generation in sickle cell disease: insights from computerized automated thrombography. Blood 114: 2587.

Canalli AA, Franco-Penteado CF, Saad STO et al (2008) Increased adhesive properties of neutrophils in sickle cell disease may be reversed by pharmacological nitric oxide donation. Haematologica 93:605–609. doi:10.3324/haematol.12119

Cappellini MD, Robbiolo L, Bottasso BM et al (2000) Venous thromboembolism and hypercoagulability in splenectomized patients with thalassaemia intermedia. Br J Haematol 111:467–473

Chantrathammachart P, Mackman N, Sparkenbaugh E et al (2012) Tissue factor promotes activation of coagulation and inflammation in a mouse model of sickle cell disease. Blood 120:636–646. doi:10.1182/blood-2012-04-424143

Chaplin H, Alkjaersig N, Fletcher AP et al (1980) Aspirin-dipyridamole prophylaxis of sickle cell disease pain crises. Thromb Haemost 43:218–221

Chaplin H, Monroe MC, Malecek AC et al (1989) Preliminary trial of minidose heparin prophylaxis for painful sickle cell crises. East Afr Med J 66:574–584

Chen J, Hobbs WE, Le J et al (2011) The rate of hemolysis in sickle cell disease correlates with the quantity of active von Willebrand factor in the plasma. Blood 117:3680–3683. doi:10.1182/blood-2010-08-302539

Chen G, Zhang D, Fuchs TA et al (2014) Heme-induced neutrophil extracellular traps contribute to the pathogenesis of sickle cell disease. Blood. doi:10.1182/blood-2013-10-529982

Cokic VP, Andric SA, Stojilkovic SS et al (2008) Hydroxyurea nitrosylates and activates soluble guanylyl cyclase in human erythroid cells. Blood 111:1117–1123. doi:10.1182/blood-2007-05-088732

Colella MP, De Paula EV, Conran N et al (2012) Hydroxyurea is associated with reductions in hypercoagulability markers in sickle cell anemia. J Thromb Haemost 10:1967–1970. doi:10.1111/j.1538-7836.2012.04861.x

Colella MP, de Paula EV, Machado-Neto JA et al (2015) Elevated hypercoagulability markers in hemoglobin SC disease. Haematologica. doi:10.3324/haematol.2014.114587

Connor J, Schroit AJ (1991) Transbilayer movement of phosphatidylserine in erythrocytes. Inhibitors of aminophospholipid transport block the association of photolabeled lipid to its transporter. Biochim Biophys Acta 1066:37–42

Conran N, Fattori A, Saad STO, Costa FF (2004) Increased levels of soluble ICAM-1 in the plasma of sickle cell patients are reversed by hydroxyurea. Am J Hematol 76:343–347. doi:10.1002/ajh.20129

Conran N, Franco-Penteado CF, Costa FF (2009) Newer aspects of the pathophysiology of sickle cell disease vaso-occlusion. Hemoglobin 33:1–16. doi:10.1080/03630260802625709

DeBaun MR, Sarnaik SA, Rodeghier MJ et al (2012) Associated risk factors for silent cerebral infarcts in sickle cell anemia: low baseline hemoglobin, sex, and relative high systolic blood pressure. Blood 119:3684–3690. doi:10.1182/blood-2011-05-349621

Dutra FF, Bozza MT (2014) Heme on innate immunity and inflammation. Front Pharmacol 5:115. doi:10.3389/fphar.2014.00115

Earley CJ, Kittner SJ, Feeser BR et al (1998) Stroke in children and sickle-cell disease: Baltimore-Washington Cooperative Young Stroke Study. Neurology 51:169–176

Figueiredo RT, Fernandez PL, Mourao-Sa DS et al (2007) Characterization of heme as activator of Toll-like receptor 4. J Biol Chem 282:20221–20229. doi:10.1074/jbc.M610737200

Folsom AR, Tang W, Roetker NS et al (2015) Prospective study of sickle cell trait and venous thromboembolism incidence. J Thromb Haemost 13:2–9. doi:10.1111/jth.12787

Fuchs TA, Brill A, Wagner DD (2012) Neutrophil extracellular trap (NET) impact on deep vein thrombosis. Arterioscler Thromb Vasc Biol 32:1777–1783. doi:10.1161/ATVBAHA.111.242859

Fullerton HJ, Wu YW, Zhao S, Johnston SC (2003) Risk of stroke in children: ethnic and gender disparities. Neurology 61:189–194

Furie B, Furie BC (2008) Mechanisms of thrombus formation. N Engl J Med 359:938–949. doi:10.1056/NEJMra0801082

Gambero S, Canalli AA, Traina F et al (2007) Therapy with hydroxyurea is associated with reduced adhesion molecule gene and protein expression in sickle red cells with a concomitant reduction in adhesive properties. Eur J Haematol 78:144–151. doi:10.1111/j.1600-0609.2006.00788.x

Geddings JE, Mackman N (2014) New players in haemostasis and thrombosis. Thromb Haemost 111:570–574. doi:10.1160/TH13-10-0812

Gerotziafas GT, Van Dreden P, Chaari M et al (2012) The acceleration of the propagation phase of thrombin generation in patients with steady-state sickle cell disease is associated with circulating erythrocyte-derived microparticles. Thromb Haemost 107:1044–1052. doi:10.1160/TH11-10-0689

Ghosh S, Adisa OA, Chappa P et al (2013) Extracellular hemin crisis triggers acute chest syndrome in sickle mice. J Clin Invest 123:4809–4820. doi:10.1172/JCI64578

Gladwin MT, Shelhamer JH, Ognibene FP et al (2002) Nitric oxide donor properties of hydroxyurea in patients with sickle cell disease. Br J Haematol 116:436–444

Gould MK, Garcia DA, Wren SM et al (2012) Prevention of VTE in nonorthopedic surgical patients: Antithrombotic Therapy and Prevention of Thrombosis, 9th ed: American College of Chest Physicians Evidence-Based Clinical Practice Guidelines. Chest 141:e227S–e277S. doi:10.1378/chest.11-2297

Greenberg J, Ohene-Frempong K, Halus J et al (1983) Trial of low doses of aspirin as prophylaxis in sickle cell disease. J Pediatr 102:781–784

Hillmen P, Lewis SM, Bessler M et al (1995) Natural history of paroxysmal nocturnal hemoglobinuria. N Engl J Med 333:1253–1258. doi:10.1056/NEJM199511093331904

Hron G, Kollars M, Binder BR et al (2006) Identification of patients at low risk for recurrent venous thromboembolism by measuring thrombin generation. JAMA 296:397–402. doi:10.1001/jama.296.4.397

James AH, Jamison MG, Brancazio LR, Myers ER (2006) Venous thromboembolism during pregnancy and the postpartum period: incidence, risk factors, and mortality. Am J Obstet Gynecol 194:1311–1315. doi:10.1016/j.ajog.2005.11.008

Kahn SR, Lim W, Dunn AS et al (2012) Prevention of VTE in nonsurgical patients: Antithrombotic Therapy and Prevention of Thrombosis, 9th ed: American College of Chest Physicians Evidence-Based Clinical Practice Guidelines. Chest 141:e195S–e226S. doi:10.1378/chest.11-2296

Kato GJ, Taylor JG (2010) Pleiotropic effects of intravascular haemolysis on vascular homeostasis. Br J Haematol 148:690–701. doi:10.1111/j.1365-2141.2009.08004.x

Kato GJ, Martyr S, Blackwelder WC et al (2005) Levels of soluble endothelium-derived adhesion molecules in patients with sickle cell disease are associated with pulmonary hypertension, organ dysfunction, and mortality. Br J Haematol 130:943–953. doi:10.1111/j.1365-2141.2005.05701.x

Kernan WN, Ovbiagele B, Black HR et al (2014) Guidelines for the prevention of stroke in patients with stroke and transient ischemic attack: a guideline for healthcare professionals from the American Heart Association/American Stroke Association. Stroke 45:2160–2236. doi:10.1161/STR.0000000000000024

Key NS, Slungaard A, Dandelet L et al (1998) Whole blood tissue factor procoagulant activity is elevated in patients with sickle cell disease. Blood 91:4216–4223

Kurantsin-Mills J, Ofosu FA, Safa TK et al (1992) Plasma factor VII and thrombin-antithrombin III levels indicate increased tissue factor activity in sickle cell patients. Br J Haematol 81:539–544

Kwiatkowski JL, Zimmerman RA, Pollock AN et al (2009) Silent infarcts in young children with sickle cell disease. Br J Haematol 146:300–305. doi:10.1111/j.1365-2141.2009.07753.x

L'Acqua C, Hod E (2014) New perspectives on the thrombotic complications of haemolysis. Br J Haematol 168:175–185. doi:10.1111/bjh.13183

Lim MY, Ataga KI, Key NS (2013) Hemostatic abnormalities in sickle cell disease. Curr Opin Hematol 20:472–477. doi:10.1097/MOH.0b013e328363442f

Mackman N (2009) The many faces of tissue factor. J Thromb Haemost 7(Suppl 1):136–139. doi:10.1111/j.1538-7836.2009.03368.x

Manci EA, Culberson DE, Yang Y-M et al (2003) Causes of death in sickle cell disease: an autopsy study. Br J Haematol 123:359–365
Morris CR (2008) Mechanisms of vasculopathy in sickle cell disease and thalassemia. Hematology Am Soc Hematol Educ Program 177–85. doi:10.1182/asheducation-2008.1.177
Muller-Eberhard U, Javid J, Liem HH et al (1968) Plasma concentrations of hemopexin, haptoglobin and heme in patients with various hemolytic diseases. Blood 32:811–815
Naik RP, Streiff MB, Haywood C et al (2013) Venous thromboembolism in adults with sickle cell disease: a serious and under-recognized complication. Am J Med 126:443–449. doi:10.1016/j.amjmed.2012.12.016
Naik RP, Streiff MB, Haywood C et al (2014) Venous thromboembolism incidence in the Cooperative Study of Sickle Cell Disease. J Thromb Haemost 12:2010-6. doi:10.1111/jth.12744
Nair SC, Dargaud Y, Chitlur M, Srivastava A (2010) Tests of global haemostasis and their applications in bleeding disorders. Haemophilia 16(Suppl5):85–92. doi:10.1111/j.1365-2516.2010.02304.x
Nébor D, Romana M, Santiago R et al (2013) Fetal hemoglobin and hydroxycarbamide moduate both plasma concentration and cellular origin of circulating microparticles in sickle cell anemia children. Haematologica 98:862–867. doi:10.3324/haematol.2012.073619
Noubouossie DF, Lê PQ, Corazza F et al (2012) Thrombin generation reveals high procoagulant potential in the plasma of sickle cell disease children. Am J Hematol 87:145–149. doi:10.1002/ajh.22206
Novelli EM, Huynh C, Gladwin MT et al (2012) Pulmonary embolism in sickle cell disease: a case-control study. J Thromb Haemost 10:760–766. doi:10.1111/j.1538-7836.2012.04697.x
Ohene-Frempong K, Weiner SJ, Sleeper LA et al (1998) Cerebrovascular accidents in sickle cell disease: rates and risk factors. Blood 91:288–294
Opal SM, Esmon CT (2003) Bench-to-bedside review: functional relationships between coagulation and the innate immune response and their respective roles in the pathogenesis of sepsis. Crit Care 7:23–38
Oppenheimer EH, Esterly JR (1971) Pulmonary changes in sickle cell disease. Am Rev Respir Dis 103:858–859
Osamo NO, Photiades DP, Famodu AA (1981) Therapeutic effect of aspirin in sickle cell anaemia. Acta Haematol 66:102–107
Platt OS (2000) Sickle cell anemia as an inflammatory disease. J Clin Invest 106:337–338. doi:10.1172/JCI10726
Powars D, Chan LS, Schroeder WA (1990) The variable expression of sickle cell disease is genetically determined. Semin Hematol 27:360–376
Qari MH, Aljaouni SK, Alardawi MS et al (2007) Reduction of painful vaso-occlusive crisis of sickle cell anaemia by tinzaparin in a double-blind randomized trial. Thromb Haemost 98:392–396
Reiter CD, Wang X, Tanus-Santos JE et al (2002) Cell-free hemoglobin limits nitric oxide bioavailability in sickle-cell disease. Nat Med 8:1383–1389. doi:10.1038/nm799
Salvaggio JE, Arnold CA, Banov CH (1963) Long-term anti-coagulation in sickle-cell disease. A clinical study. N Engl J Med 269:182–186. doi:10.1056/NEJM196307252690403
Schaer DJ, Buehler PW (2013) Cell-free hemoglobin and its scavenger proteins: new disease models leading the way to targeted therapies. Cold Spring Harb Perspect Med. doi:10.1101/cshperspect.a013433
Schilling RF (1997) Spherocytosis, splenectomy, strokes, and heat attacks. Lancet 350:1677–1678
Schrezenmeier H, Muus P, Socié G et al (2014) Baseline characteristics and disease burden in patients in the International Paroxysmal Nocturnal Hemoglobinuria Registry. Haematologica 99:922–929. doi:10.3324/haematol.2013.093161
Setty BN, Kulkarni S, Rao AK, Stuart MJ (2000) Fetal hemoglobin in sickle cell disease: relationship to erythrocyte phosphatidylserine exposure and coagulation activation. Blood 96:1119–1124
Setty BNY, Betal SG, Zhang J, Stuart MJ (2008) Heme induces endothelial tissue factor expression: potential role in hemostatic activation in patients with hemolytic anemia. J Thromb Haemost 6:2202–2209. doi:10.1111/j.1538-7836.2008.03177.x

Setty BNY, Key NS, Rao AK et al (2012) Tissue factor-positive monocytes in children with sickle cell disease: correlation with biomarkers of haemolysis. Br J Haematol 157:370–380. doi:10.1111/j.1365-2141.2012.09065.x

Shah N, Thornburg C, Telen MJ, Ortel TL (2012) Characterization of the hypercoagulable state in patients with sickle cell disease. Thromb Res 130:e241–e245. doi:10.1016/j.thromres.2012.08.307

Shet AS, Aras O, Gupta K et al (2003) Sickle blood contains tissue factor-positive microparticles derived from endothelial cells and monocytes. Blood 102:2678–2683. doi:10.1182/blood-2003-03-0693

Solovey A, Lin Y, Browne P et al (1997) Circulating activated endothelial cells in sickle cell anemia. N Engl J Med 337:1584–1590. doi:10.1056/NEJM199711273372203

Solovey A, Gui L, Key NS, Hebbel RP (1998) Tissue factor expression by endothelial cells in sickle cell anemia. J Clin Invest 101:1899–1904. doi:10.1172/JCI1932

Solovey A, Kollander R, Shet A et al (2004) Endothelial cell expression of tissue factor in sickle mice is augmented by hypoxia/reoxygenation and inhibited by lovastatin. Blood 104:840–846. doi:10.1182/blood-2003-10-3719

Sparkenbaugh E, Pawlinski R (2013) Interplay between coagulation and vascular inflammation in sickle cell disease. Br J Haematol 162:3–14. doi:10.1111/bjh.12336

Sparkenbaugh EM, Chantrathammachart P, Wang S et al (2015) Excess of heme induces tissue factor-dependent activation of coagulation in mice. Haematologica. doi:10.3324/haematol.2014.114728

Stein PD, Beemath A, Meyers FA et al (2006) Deep venous thrombosis and pulmonary embolism in hospitalized patients with sickle cell disease. Am J Med 119:897.e7–11. doi:10.1016/j.amjmed.2006.08.015

Styles LA, Lubin B, Vichinsky E et al (1997) Decrease of very late activation antigen-4 and CD36 on reticulocytes in sickle cell patients treated with hydroxyurea. Blood 89:2554–2559

Ten Cate H (2012) Thrombin generation in clinical conditions. Thromb Res 129:367–370. doi:10.1016/j.thromres.2011.10.017

Van Beers EJ, Schaap MCL, Berckmans RJ et al (2009) Circulating erythrocyte-derived microparticles are associated with coagulation activation in sickle cell disease. Haematologica 94:1513–1519. doi:10.3324/haematol.2009.008938

Van der Poll T, Herwald H (2014) The coagulation system and its function in early immune defense. Thromb Haemost. doi:10.1160/TH14-01-0053

Van Langevelde K, Flinterman LE, van Hylckama Vlieg A et al (2012) Broadening the factor V Leiden paradox: pulmonary embolism and deep-vein thrombosis as 2 sides of the spectrum. Blood 120:933–946. doi:10.1182/blood-2012-02-407551

Vichinsky EP, Neumayr LD, Earles AN et al (2000) Causes and outcomes of the acute chest syndrome in sickle cell disease. National Acute Chest Syndrome Study Group. N Engl J Med 342:1855–1865. doi:10.1056/NEJM200006223422502

Ware RE, Helms RW (2012) Stroke With Transfusions Changing to Hydroxyurea (SWiTCH). Blood 119:3925–3932. doi:10.1182/blood-2011-11-392340

Weatherall DJ (2010) The inherited diseases of hemoglobin are an emerging global health burden. Blood 115:4331–4336. doi:10.1182/blood-2010-01-251348

Westerman MP, Green D, Gilman-Sachs A et al (2002) Coagulation changes in individuals with sickle cell trait. Am J Hematol 69:89–94

Whelihan MF, Zachary V, Orfeo T, Mann KG (2012) Prothrombin activation in blood coagulation: the erythrocyte contribution to thrombin generation. Blood 120:3837–3845. doi:10.1182/blood-2012-05-427856

Whelihan MF, Mooberry MJ, Zachary V et al (2013) The contribution of red blood cells to thrombin generation in sickle cell disease: meizothrombin generation on sickled red blood cells. J Thromb Haemost 11:2187–2189. doi:10.1111/jth.12423

Wolberg AG, Amin C, Adam S, et al. (2009) Thrombin generation and fibrin clot formation in patients with sickle cell disease. J Thromb Haemost 7: PP-TH-655

Wun T, Soulieres D, Frelinger AL et al (2013) A double-blind, randomized, multicenter phase 2 study of prasugrel versus placebo in adult patients with sickle cell disease. J Hematol Oncol 6:17. doi:10.1186/1756-8722-6-17

Yee DL, Edwards RM, Mueller BU, Teruya J (2005) Thromboelastographic and hemostatic characteristics in pediatric patients with sickle cell disease. Arch Pathol Lab Med 129:760–765. doi:10.1043/1543-2165(2005)129[760:TAHCIP]2.0.CO;2

Zago MA, Costa FF, Ismael SJ et al (1984) Treatment of sickle cell diseases with aspirin. Acta Haematol 72:61–64

Chapter 7
Cardiovascular Adaptations to Anemia and the Vascular Endothelium in Sickle Cell Disease Pathophysiology

Lydia H. Pecker and Hans C. Ackerman

Abstract The vascular endothelium is a heterogenous collection of cells whose actions contribute significantly to sickle cell disease pathophysiology. At the cellular level, the endothelium elaborates vasoactive, adhesive, and inflammatory signals that drive acute and chronic injury causing ultimately irreversible organ damage. The endothelium is also fundamentally involved in the cardiovascular adaptations to anemia. Vasodilation lowers systemic vascular resistance and allows higher cardiac output to maintain oxygen transport in an anemic state. Cardiovascular adaptations to anemia and hypoxia may play a role in the pathogenesis of sickle cell disease. Some measures of endothelium-dependent vasodilation appear to be impaired in people with sickle cell disease, but this may be due in part to the effects of chronic anemia. Endothelium-derived vasoactive molecules, such as endothelin-1 and nitric oxide, appear dysregulated and may also contribute to the vascular complications of sickle cell disease. The therapeutic potential of pharmacologically manipulating these molecules has not yet been achieved; however, evidence from patients treated with hydroxyurea and hematopoietic stem cell transplant shows that although it may be difficult to reverse pre-existing injury, effective therapies for sickle cell disease do change endothelial behavior. Ongoing investigations will determine how best to exploit our understanding of endothelial biology and pathobiology to develop new treatments for people with sickle cell disease.

Keywords Adhesion • Anemia • Blood pressure • Vascular endothelium • Vascular smooth muscle

---

L.H. Pecker, M.D.
Center for Cancer and Blood Disorders, Children's National Medical Center, 111 Michigan Ave, NW, Washington, DC 20010, USA

Physiology Section, Sickle Cell Branch, National Heart, Lung, and Blood Institute, 10 Center Drive, Bethesda, MD 20892, USA
e-mail: peckerlh@nhlbi.nih.gov

H.C. Ackerman, M.D., D.Phil. (✉)
Physiology Section, Sickle Cell Branch, National Heart, Lung, and Blood Institute, 10 Center Drive, Bethesda, MD 20892, USA
e-mail: ackermanh@nhlbi.nih.gov

© Springer International Publishing Switzerland 2016

F.F. Costa, N. Conran (eds.), *Sickle Cell Anemia*,
DOI 10.1007/978-3-319-06713-1_7

7.1 Introduction

7.1.1 *Erythrocyte–Endothelium Interactions Give Rise to Sickle Cell Disease Pathophysiology*

The observation that sickled erythrocytes adhere abnormally to endothelial cells first implicated the vascular endothelium as the red cell's co-conspirator in sickle cell disease pathophysiology (Hebbel et al. 1980; Hoover et al. 1979). These observations coincided with evolving understandings of the endothelial contributions to vascular reactivity (Furchgott and Zawadzki 1980) and coagulation (Bunting et al. 1977). The endothelium is no longer regarded simply as an inert lining of the blood vessels, but as an active participant in inflammation, adhesion, permeability, coagulation, blood flow regulation and new vessel growth.

Sickle cell disease is a vascular disease driven by interactions between the endothelium and the circulating components of blood: sickled, hemolyzed and/or immature erythrocytes, leukocytes, activated platelets, coagulation factors and inflammatory proteins. These interactions cause episodic, progressive and cumulative organ injury. Most people with sickle cell disease do not have classic risk factors for vascular disease. The prevalence of hypercholesterolemia, hyperglycemia and hypertension is lower among individuals with sickle cell disease, although these factors still affect vascular function and modify the risks of vascular disease (Pegelow et al. 1997; Rodgers et al. 1993; Yuditskaya et al. 2009). Endothelial interactions with the cellular components of blood may trigger many of the complications of sickle cell disease and help explain why a disease that originates from a single molecular defect can have such profound phenotypic variability.

7.1.2 *The Healthy Endothelium Participates in Multiple Homeostatic Mechanisms*

In 1865, the Swiss anatomist Wilhelm His first used the term endothelium to describe the internal lining of blood vessels, lymphatics and mesothelial-lined cavities. Today the term refers only to the linings of blood and lymphatic vessels. The endothelium covers an astonishing 350 m^2 surface area, and encompasses a heterogeneous group of cells that participate in trans- and paracellular communication to coordinate local and systemic activities (Aird 2007a, b, c). Endothelial cells within and across vascular beds can be structurally and functionally distinct. They may be continuous or discontinuous and fenestrated or non-fenestrated. Arterial and venous endothelial cells differ in shape and alignment, reflecting differences in flow and function for each vessel type and the organ they serve. The single label "endothelium" oversimplifies the structural and functional diversity of this thin cell layer.

Endothelial cells are challenging to study because of their functional and anatomical heterogeneity and their sensitivity to their environment. For example, measurements performed on accessible vascular beds, like those in the skin, eye, or skeletal muscle, may lead to different conclusions about endothelial function than measurements made in brain, or kidney vascular beds. In vitro studies may not reflect in vivo endothelial cell behavior; ex vivo studies must be interpreted cautiously with careful controls because endothelial cell phenotype can change even after brief removal from a specific environment (Durr et al. 2004). Despite these challenges, we continue to learn more about the endothelium in sickle cell disease through studies involving human patients, animal models of sickle cell disease, in vitro experiments, and computer modeling. Over the next four sections of this chapter, we will explore the systemic cardiovascular adaptations to anemia (Sect. 7.2), the damaging interactions between sickle cell erythrocytes and the endothelium (Sect. 7.3), and the endothelial response to hypoxia, shear stress, and vasoactive molecules in patients with sickle cell disease (Sects. 7.4 and 7.5).

7.2 Chronic Anemia Causes Systemic Cardiovascular Changes

Changes in vascular resistance and cardiac output that accompany anemia are examples of how the endothelium integrates local signals to effect a systemic change in cardiovascular function. The cardiovascular changes in patients with sickle cell disease reflect physiologic adaptations to chronic anemia and pathologic responses to recurrent ischemia-reperfusion injury triggered by blood cell adhesion and small vessel obstruction. Few studies directly compare cardiovascular function in patients with sickle cell disease to other forms of anemia, making it difficult to distinguish the cardiovascular changes that are adaptations to anemia per se versus those caused by sickle cell disease-specific mechanisms. In this section, we review the cardiovascular changes associated with non-hemolytic anemia and compare these changes to those seen in people with sickle cell disease. This background is necessary to interpret studies of endothelial function in sickle cell disease, especially endothelial responses to hypoxia, shear stress and vasoactive molecules in patients with sickle cell disease (Sect. 7.4). Assessment of vascular function in sickle cell disease must also account for the ways anemic states affect vascular function.

7.2.1 In Chronic Anemia, Systemic Vascular Resistance Falls to Raise Cardiac Output and Maintain Oxygen Transport

Anemia is a state of low oxygen carrying capacity (see Text Box 7.1) (Fig. 7.1). When oxygen carrying capacity is low, oxygen transport to tissues can be maintained by increasing cardiac output and/or increasing oxygen extraction. Increasing cardiac output raises oxygen saturations in the venous circulation, but raises the oxygen and energy demands of the heart muscle. Over time, cardiomegaly develops as the heart works to maintain high cardiac output. Increasing oxygen extraction in tissues lowers the venous blood oxygen saturation, but allows more oxygen to be delivered without raising cardiac output.

Text Box 7.1

Oxygen content in blood is determined by the oxygen saturation of hemoglobin times the hemoglobin concentration times the oxygen binding capacity of hemoglobin (1.34 mL/g) plus the usually insignificant fraction of oxygen dissolved in blood:

$$O_2\,\text{content}\,(\text{mL}\,O_2\,/\,100\,\text{mL blood}) = 1.34\,(\text{mL}\,/\,\text{g}) \times \text{Hb}\,(\text{g}\,/\,\text{dL}) \times \text{Oxygen Saturation}\,(\%) + 0.003 \times PaO_2\,(\text{mmHg})$$

Hemoglobin concentration and the oxygen saturation of hemoglobin are the main determinants of oxygen carrying capacity. For example, someone with a hemoglobin of 15 g/dL and an oxygen saturation of 100 % carries 20.1 mL/100 mL of oxygen on hemoglobin and 0.3 mL/100 mL of dissolved oxygen in arterial blood. This small amount of dissolved oxygen in blood can become important in patients with very severe anemia (Fig. 7.1).

The amount of oxygen that is ultimately extracted by tissues can be determined from the cardiac output and the difference in oxygen content between arterial and venous blood:

$$\text{Oxygen extracted}\,(\text{mL}) = \text{arterial}\,O_2\,\text{content}\,(\text{mL}\,/\,\text{dL}) \times \text{cardiac output}\,(\text{L}\,/\,\text{min}) \times 10\,\text{dL}\,/\,\text{L} \times (\text{arterial}\,O_2\,\text{content} - \text{venous}\,O_2\,\text{content})\,/\,(\text{arterial}\,O_2\,\text{content})$$

For example, if the cardiac output is 5 L/min, and the oxygen content is 20 mL/100 mL, then 1000 mL of oxygen is transported in arterial blood each minute. If oxygen saturation falls from 100 % in the artery to 75 % in the vein, then oxygen content falls from approximately 20 mL/100 mL in the artery to approximately 15 mL/100 mL in the vein, a difference of 5 mL/100 mL and an extraction fraction of 25 %. At a cardiac output of 5 L/min, 250 mL of oxygen is extracted each minute. In some anemic states, the oxygen extraction fraction can increase to extract more oxygen from blood, desaturating venous blood to a greater extent. In adults with sickle cell disease, venous oxygen saturation tends to be higher than expected, suggesting incomplete oxygen extraction or shunting.

Evidence from chronically anemic patients shows that when the oxygen carrying capacity of blood is low, the cardiac output increases to maintain oxygen transport (Fig. 7.2). In patients with chronic anemia of blood loss from intestinal parasites,

Fig. 7.2 (continued) cells in the kidney, signal via erythropoietin (**Epo**) to increase the production of red blood cells and raise the oxygen carrying capacity of blood. As the concentration of red blood cells increases, the **viscosity** of blood also increases. More viscous blood has a greater resistance to flow, lowering vascular conductance. (More viscous blood also exerts a greater shear stress on the vessel wall, which triggers vasodilation). Anemia primarily lowers systemic vascular resistance by hypoxia- and shear stress-mediated vasodilation, by new vessel growth, and by the effects of lower viscosity of blood. The fall in systemic vascular resistance allows larger stroke volumes and a greater cardiac output, which raises oxygen transport to meet the oxygen demands of tissues

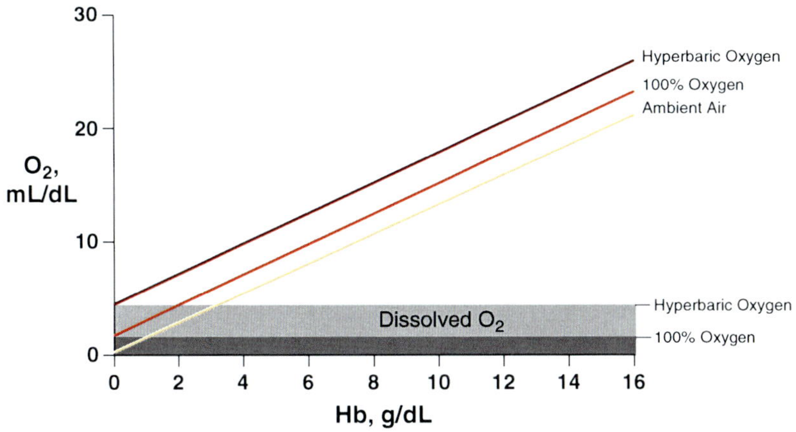

Fig. 7.1 The oxygen content of blood is primarily determined by the concentration of hemoglobin. Blood carries both hemoglobin-bound and dissolved oxygen. The *diagonal lines* represent the total oxygen (mL) in a deciliter (100 mL) of blood. Changing the partial pressure of inspired oxygen (ambient air, 100 % oxygen, or hyperbaric oxygen) has small effects on the oxygen content of blood, but changing the hemoglobin concentration has large effects on the oxygen content of blood. At very low hemoglobin levels, dissolved oxygen becomes a more substantial fraction of the total oxygen in blood. This illustration assumes normal lung function

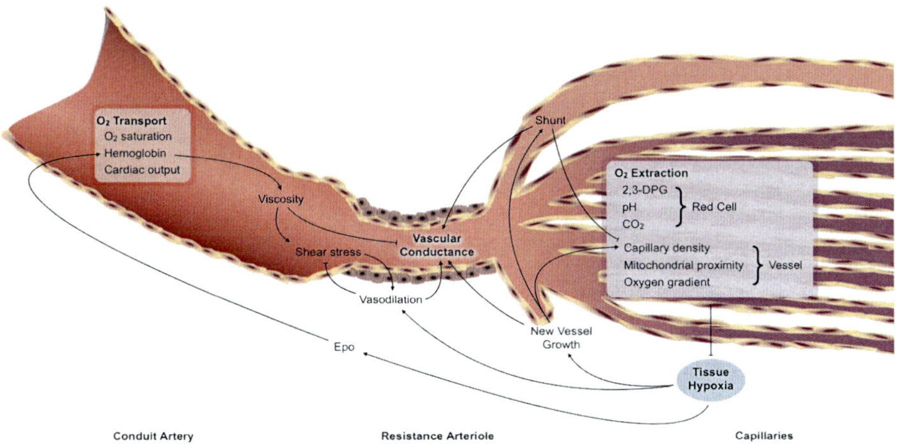

Fig. 7.2 Cardiovascular responses to anemia. Oxygen transport is primarily determined by the oxygen saturation of hemoglobin, the concentration of hemoglobin, and the cardiac output (*left panel*). **Oxygen extraction** in the capillary beds of tissues is determined by red cell factors that alter the affinity of hemoglobin for oxygen (such as 2,3-DPG, pH, and CO_2) and by vessel and tissue factors such as the oxygen gradient, and the proximity of red blood cells to mitochondria. When the oxygen demand of tissues exceeds the supply of oxygen, **tissue hypoxia** develops. Hypoxia triggers local responses such as **vasodilation** to increase blood flow to the hypoxic tissue and **new vessel growth** to increase the density of vessels where gas exchange can take place. Vasodilation increases **vascular conductance** (i.e., lowers vascular resistance), which increases local blood flow. When this occurs over a large region, systemic vascular resistance falls, and cardiac stroke volume and cardiac output increase. New vessel growth increases the vascular cross-sectional area, and can increase vascular conductance when new resistance arteries form. A new vessel can also form a **shunt** that bypasses capillary beds; a shunt can lower vascular resistance but doesn't participate in oxygen delivery. Resistance arterioles dilate in response to vessel wall **shear stress**, preventing turbulent blood flow and mechanical injury to endothelial cells. Specialized oxygen-sensing cells, such as the juxta-glomerular

cardiac index was elevated in proportion to the severity of anemia (Roy et al. 1963). In chronic anemia, high cardiac output is sustained by a larger stroke volume, not by an increase in heart rate or an increase in preload (Escobar et al. 1966). Stroke volume increases primarily through a fall in systemic vascular resistance (Varat et al. 1972). In patients with anemia, the fall in systemic vascular resistance is mediated by three important changes in the vasculature and blood:

1. *Vasodilation of resistance arterioles.* Vasodilation is triggered by endothelial responses to tissue hypoxia and shear stress and is the primary mechanism for lowering systemic vascular resistance.
2. *Perfusion of new vessels.* The total cross-sectional area of the vasculature increases initially by perfusion of previously unused vessels such as those in skin and muscle, and over time through hypoxia-triggered new vessel growth.
3. *Lowering of blood viscosity.* Blood viscosity is proportional to the concentration of red blood cells. Blood that has a lower viscosity is less resistant to flow.

Additional mechanisms account for cardiovascular changes in patients with sickle cell disease. Cardiac index rises as systemic vascular resistance falls (Table 7.1 and Fig. 7.3a). In patients with sickle cell disease, the increase in cardiac index and fall in systemic vascular resistance are greater than expected for the degree of anemia (Fig. 7.3b, c). This suggests that in sickle cell disease, additional factors, perhaps hemolysis-induced inflammation or ischemia-induced new vessel growth, contribute to the lower vascular resistance. Whatever the cause, elevated cardiac output and left ventricular volume overload contribute to sickle cell disease pathophysiology and may specifically contribute to the cardiopulmonary hemodynamic abnormalities observed in people with sickle cell disease (Mushemi-Blake et al. 2015).

7.2.2 Hemodynamic and Structural Changes Induced by Anemia Are Reversible

Studies of the hemodynamic effects of treating anemia help to establish the relationship between oxygen carrying capacity and cardiac output. Transfusion of patients who had chronic anemia from helminth infection raises the systemic vascular resistance and lowers the cardiac index to normal (Roy et al. 1963). In patients treated for iron deficiency anemia, raising the mean hemoglobin from 5.8 to 12.5 g/dL normalized their previously elevated cardiac index and stroke volume, and reversed cardiac structural changes. In addition, left ventricular diameter and left ventricular mass index decreased significantly towards normal (Cho et al. 2014).

The cardiac abnormalities associated with sickle cell disease are dynamic, reversible, and partly dependent on the hemoglobin or percentage of hemoglobin S. Like people with other chronic anemias, people with sickle cell disease develop cardiomegaly with an increased left ventricular end-diastolic diameter and left ventricular mass index (Fig. 7.4) (Balfour et al. 1984; Caldas et al. 2008; Lester et al. 1990;

Table 7.1 Hemodynamic measurements in people with anemia at rest and during exercise

	Healthy, non-anemic[a]		Mild anemia[a]		Severe anemia[a]		Sickle Cell Disease[b]	
Number	11		9		18		11	
Hemoglobin (g/dL)	13.5 ± 0.5		9.4 ± 0.4		5.2 ± 0.3		7.9 ± 1.6	
	Rest	Exercise	Rest	Exercise	Rest	Exercise	Rest	Exercise
Systemic vascular resistance (dyne-sec-cm^{-5})	1526 ± 125	1141 ± 83	1392 ± 121	1000 ± 89	930 ± 59	714 ± 66	734 ± 134	601 ± 103
Cardiac index (L/min/m^2)	3.2 ± 0.2	4.4 ± 0.3	3.4 ± 0.2	5.8 ± 0.6	4.8 ± 0.3	7.3 ± 0.5	6.1 ± 0.8	8.1 ± 1.3
Oxygen extraction (%)	22.7 ± 1.9	32.7 ± 1.9	31.5 ± 1.7	40.7 ± 3.9	43.2 ± 1.6	46.1 ± 1.9	26.8 ± 6.0	33.6 ± 4.6

Source:
[a]Graettinger et al. (1963)
[b]Leight et al. (1954)

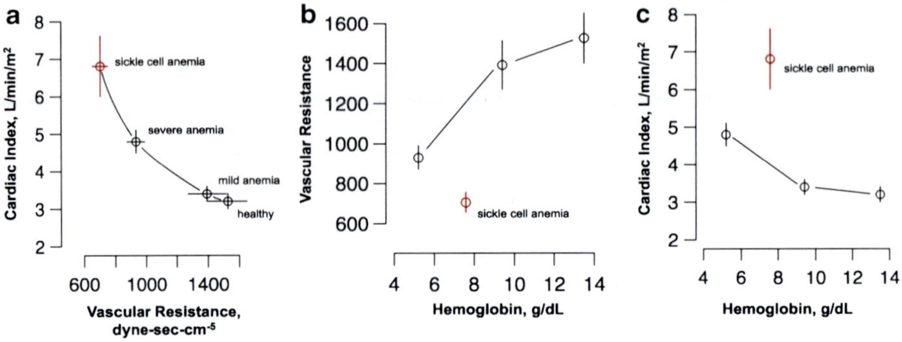

Fig. 7.3 Anemia is associated with low vascular resistance and high cardiac output. (**a**) Cardiac index has a reciprocal relationship with vascular resistance (flow = (pressure$_2$ – pressure$_1$)/resistance). This is represented by data from four different groups of patients: healthy, mild anemia, severe anemia, and sickle cell anemia, whose cardiac indices increase as vascular resistances fall (shown as mean +/– standard error). (**b**) Vascular resistance falls with the severity of anemia, indicated here as the hemoglobin concentration. Patients with sickle cell disease have a lower vascular resistance than expected given the severity of anemia. (**c**) Cardiac index increases with the severity of anemia. Patients with sickle cell disease have a greater cardiac index than expected given the severity of anemia. Data calculated from tables presented in Graettinger et al. (1963) and Leight et al. (1954)

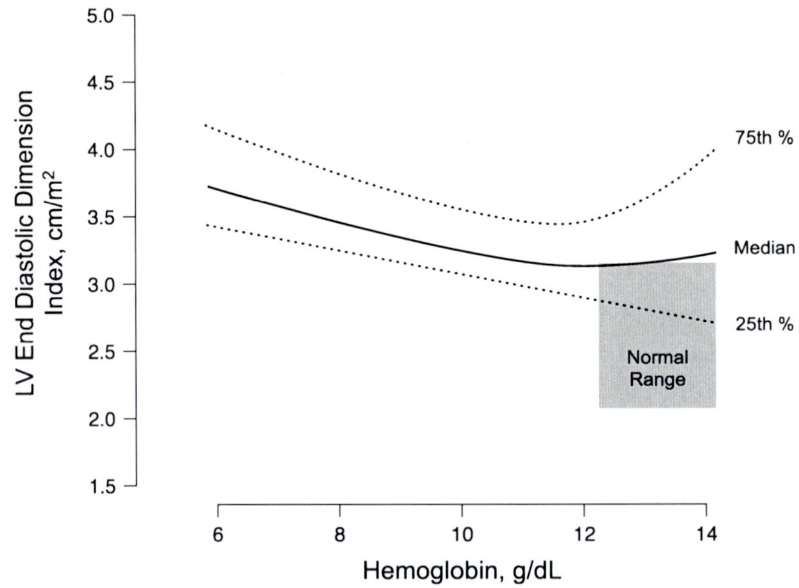

Fig. 7.4 The left ventricle of the heart is enlarged in people with sickle cell disease and related to the severity of anemia. Left ventricular end diastolic dimension (LVEDD) was measured by ultrasound in 191 people with sickle cell disease, aged 13 years or older (mean age: 25.9 ± 8.8 years) at four centers participating in the cardiac sub-study of the Cooperative Study of Sickle Cell Disease. The LVEDD index was calculated by dividing the LVEDD by body surface area. *Solid line* depicts the median for patients with sickle cell disease, and the *dotted lines* are the 25th and 75th percentiles. Patients with lower hemoglobin values had greater LVEDD indices. The *shaded area* represents normal values. Adapted from Covitz et al. (1995). Normal LVEDD index range values are from Feigenbaum, *Echocardiography* 3rd Ed

Lindsay et al. 1974). Circulating blood volume is not elevated in sickle cell disease (Gross and Godel 1971). In men with sickle cell disease, blood transfusion lowered stroke volume (−10.8 ± 4.9 mL) and cardiac index (−0.5 ± 0.2 L/min/m^2). In contrast, women with sickle cell disease who received transfusion increased their stroke volume (+3.2 ± 3.6 mL), suggesting that anemia limited their myocardial performance. Of note, other differences in the vascular behavior of men versus women with sickle cell disease have been described (Gladwin et al. 2003b), but are not completely explained.

In most studies of patients with sickle cell disease, the left ventricular systolic ejection fraction is normal or elevated. Although there does not appear to be a functional cardiomyopathy associated with sickle cell disease, lower velocity of circumferential myocardial muscle fiber shortening (Covitz et al. 1995), and other worse measures of cardiac systolic function may occur more frequently in sickle cell disease than in other anemias (Bahl et al. 1992; Bosi et al. 2003). Unfortunately, the measurements used in these studies are not directly comparable. Patients with sickle cell disease have impaired left ventricle relaxation (Balfour et al. 1988; Şan et al. 1998). Diastolic dysfunction is reported in patients with sickle cell disease (Caldas et al. 2008) and is associated with a 3.5-fold increase in mortality (Sachdev et al. 2007).

Blood pressure is lower in people with sickle cell disease, compared to age- and sex- matched African American controls. This difference widens with age (Fig. 7.5). Patients with sickle cell disease have higher blood pressures than patients with beta-thalassemia major, despite having lower hematocrit. This may be explained by increased blood viscosity in sickle cell disease, or progression of renal or vascular injury (Rodgers et al. 1993). Even at the 90th percentile for blood pressure, a

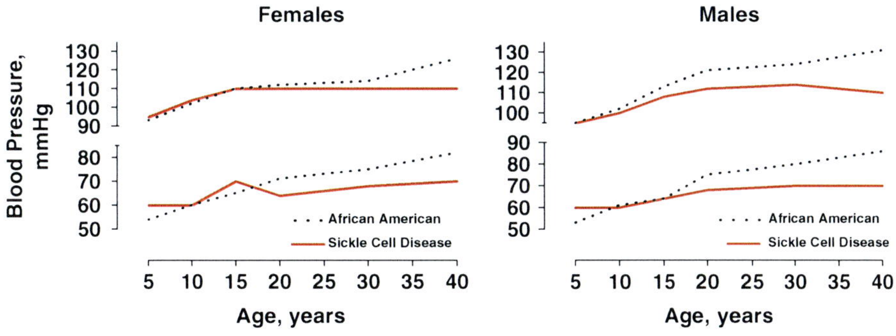

Fig. 7.5 Blood pressure is lower in people with sickle cell disease compared to non-anemic African Americans. Average blood pressures of different age groups are presented for approximately 4000 people with sickle cell disease from the Cooperative Study of Sickle Cell Disease, 1978–1988 (*solid orange lines*). Average blood pressures of African Americans who participated in the National Health and Nutrition Examination Survey II, 1976–1980 are provided for comparison (*dotted lines*). Figure adapted from Rodgers et al. (1993)

measure within the normal range for people without sickle cell disease, patients with sickle cell disease have increased risk of stroke and death (Pegelow et al. 1997). Sickle cell-specific normal blood pressure ranges are necessary to evaluate blood pressure in patients with sickle cell disease.

7.2.3 Hypoxia and Shear Stress Regulate Vessel Diameter

Hypoxia stimulates endothelium to release vasodilators that increase blood flow locally. Endothelial nitric oxide synthesis is central to hypoxia-mediated vasodilation (Meredith et al. 1996; Schrage et al. 2004). The vasodilatory response to hypoxia also involves endothelial release of adenosine and prostaglandins (Crecelius et al. 2011; Marshall 2001). In response to hypoxia, autonomic nerve endings in muscle vascular beds release the vasoconstrictor norepinephrine to maintain blood pressure. This systemic vasoconstriction helps redirect blood to hypoxic areas (Heistad et al. 1980; Joyner and Casey 2014).

Red blood cells also contribute to hypoxic vasodilation. Deoxyhemoglobin in red blood cells catalyzes the conversion of nitrite to nitric oxide, selectively releasing this vasodilator in hypoxic tissues (Cosby et al. 2003; Crawford et al. 2006). Erythrocytes also express a functional nitric oxide synthase that can produce nitric oxide and lowers blood pressure (Cortese-Krott and Kelm 2014; Kleinbongard et al. 2006; Wood et al. 2013). ATP released from hypoxic red blood cells also affects vasodilation (Ellsworth et al. 2009). Whether the release of nitric oxide from S-nitrosylated hemoglobin contributes to hypoxia-mediated vasodilation is debated (Gladwin et al. 2003a; Isbell et al. 2008; Kulandavelu et al. 2015; Zhang et al. 2015).

Endothelium maintains shear stress by regulating vessel diameter in response to changes in blood velocity. Ex vivo and in vivo studies demonstrated that chronic exposure to high blood flow caused endothelium to produce more vasodilatory nitric oxide (Miller et al. 1986; Miller and Vanhoutte 1988). The relationship between anemia and shear stress is complex. Anemia is associated with high blood flow that would raise shear stress; however, the lower viscosity of anemic blood would lower shear stress.

In patients with anemia, who have decreased oxygen carrying capacity and high blood flow, endothelial nitric oxide production is enhanced. Inhibiting nitric oxide synthesis in anemic patients exerted a stronger vasoconstricting effect than in non-anemic controls, showing that increased nitric oxide synthesis is involved in the vasodilatory response to anemia (Anand et al. 1995). After correction of anemia, nitric oxide inhibition had less effect on forearm blood flow.

In sickle cell disease, low SVR and high cardiac output suggest that the anemia-associated vasodilatory responses to hypoxia and shear stress are active. In Sect. 7.4 we examine the question of whether patients with sickle cell disease have specific impairments in the vasodilatory responses to shear stress and hypoxia.

7.2.4 *Lower Blood Viscosity in Anemic States Helps Increase Stroke Volume and Cardiac Output*

Blood flows through a vessel in concentric layers. The fastest moving layer is in the center of the vessel, and the slowest layer is in contact with the endothelium. The extent to which one layer adheres to the next is described by the blood's viscosity. Because blood is a mixture of cells and macromolecules in water, its viscosity is more complex than the viscosity of a pure liquid like oil. The primary determinant of blood viscosity is the concentration of red blood cells. In anemic states, lower viscosity increases cardiac stroke volume and cardiac output (Fowler and Holmes 1975; Murray and Escobar 1968).

As in other anemic states, people with sickle cell disease have lower blood viscosity than non-anemic individuals (Fig. 7.6) (Chien et al. 1970). But the viscosity of sickle cell blood is higher than normal blood when they are compared at the same hematocrit (Usami et al. 1975). Sickle red blood cells are less deformable and more likely to form aggregates. When deoxygenated, hemoglobin polymerization leads to a dramatic increase in viscosity. But even at normal oxygen tensions, sickle cell blood viscosity adversely affects tissue perfusion. This leads to decreased oxygen transport effectiveness as demonstrated by the theoretical oxygen carrying capacity to viscosity ratio (Fig. 7.6). When transfusing patients with sickle cell disease, the potentially harmful effects of increased blood viscosity must be balanced against the beneficial effect of increasing oxygen carrying capacity (Alexy et al. 2006; Detterich et al. 2013).

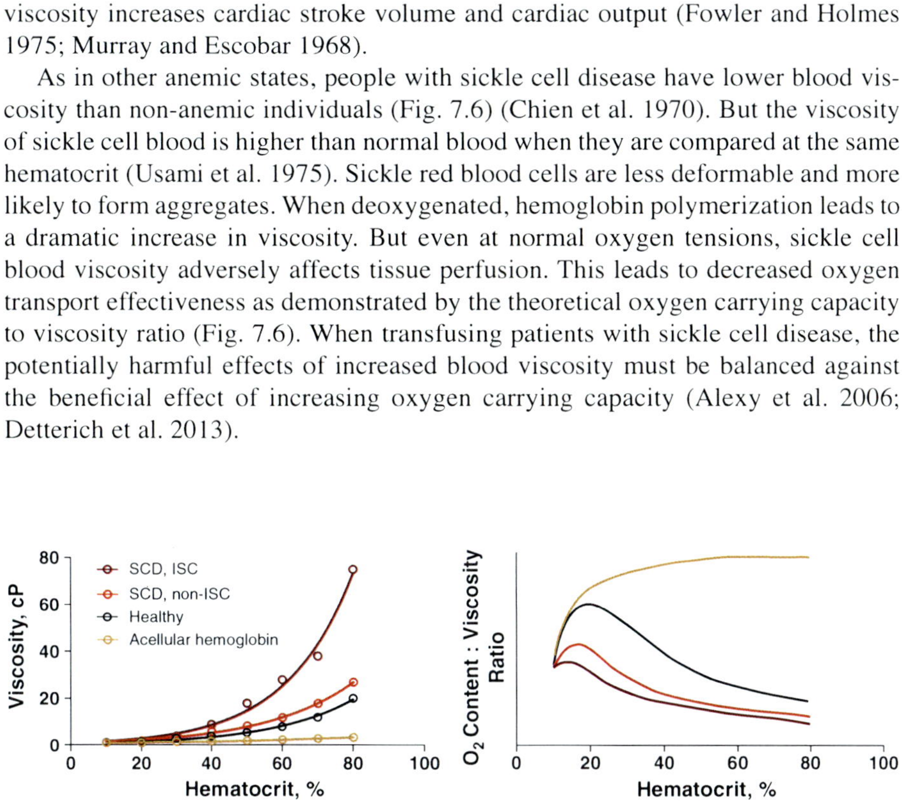

Fig. 7.6 Blood viscosity increases with hematocrit. *Left*: Blood from patients with sickle cell disease (*orange* or *red lines*) has a higher viscosity than blood from healthy individuals (*black line*), at any given hematocrit. Irreversibly sickled cells (ISC) are more viscous than non-irreversibly sickled cells (non-ISC). Acellular hemoglobin (*tan line*) is much less viscous than equivalent concentrations of hemoglobin in red blood cells. Viscosity was measured at a shear rate of 0.052 s^{-1}; data are from Chien et al. (1970). *Right*: As hematocrit rises, oxygen carrying capacity increases, but viscosity also increases. The trade-off between oxygen content and blood viscosity is illustrated here as the oxygen content divided by the viscosity

7.2.5 *Oxygen Extraction Is Impaired in Sickle Cell Disease*

In anemic states, the rightward shift of the hemoglobin-oxygen dissociation curve maintains oxygen delivery to tissues. This shift favors oxygen unloading in hypoxic tissues at the expense of reoxygenation in the lungs. Increased 2,3-diphosphoglycerate (2,3-DPG) concentration decreases hemoglobin oxygen affinity and facilitates oxygen unloading in hypoxic tissues (Benesch and Benesch 1969; Delivoria-Papadopoulos et al. 1969). Sickle erythrocytes have particularly high 2,3-DPG levels favoring the low oxygen affinity T state conformation of hemoglobin that is prone to polymerization. Sickle erythrocytes also have high sphingosine-1-phosphate (S-1-P) levels that may further lower sickle hemoglobin oxygen affinity (Zhang et al. 2014).

Despite elevated 2,3-DPG levels, adults with sickle cell disease do not seem to extract oxygen as effectively as patients with chronic anemia. Table 7.1 compares oxygen extraction fractions in patients with sickle cell disease to patients with other anemic conditions and shows that adults with sickle cell disease have lower oxygen extraction (Graettinger et al. 1963; Leight et al. 1954). During exercise, adults with sickle cell disease did not increase oxygen extraction as much as healthy adults did (sickle cell: increased from 24% to 39%; healthy adults: increased from 25% to 50%) despite being anemic. Instead, adults with sickle cell disease increased cardiac output to a much greater extent (sickle cell: fourfold; healthy adults: twofold) (Lonsdorfer et al. 1983). In contrast, adults with chronic blood loss anemia were able to extract as much as 80 % of the oxygen from arterial blood (Roy et al. 1963). Impaired oxygen extraction in sickle cell disease may be due to loss of functional capillaries, increased capillary wall thickness, more artery-to-vein shunts, or reduced capillary transit time. The observation that children with sickle cell disease have appropriate oxygen extraction (Pianosi et al. 1991) suggests that changes in oxygen extraction may be age-related.

Anti-sickling drugs are under investigation that counteract the effect of high intra-erythrocytic 2,3-DPG and S-1-P and stabilize hemoglobin in its R state (Safo and Kato 2014). Although increasing the affinity of hemoglobin for oxygen may limit tissue oxygen extraction, reduced hemoglobin polymerization and improved erythrocyte rheology may improve overall tissue perfusion and therefore oxygen delivery. No anti-sickling agent is yet available, but several early phase trials are promising (Kuypers 2014).

7.2.6 *People with Sickle Cell Disease Have Exercise-Induced Myocardial Ischemia in the Absence of Atherosclerosis*

While atherosclerotic disease of the coronary arteries is notably rare in sickle cell disease, there is evidence of cardiac vessel dysfunction (Gerry Jr. et al. 1978). Indeed, although usually attributed to pulmonary, musculoskeletal, or vaso-occlusive causes, chest pain in sickle cell disease can be caused by myocardial infarction and exercise testing can elicit myocardial ischemia. In one study, 47 children with sickle cell disease aged 5–18 years (mean 10.3 years) performed exercise with electrocardiographic (EKG) monitoring. During exercise, seven (16 %) had definite ischemia and 16 (34 %) had equivocal ischemia. In contrast, among 170 healthy African American children, five (less than 3 %) had equivocal ischemia and none had definite ischemia (Alpert et al. 1981). Among the children with sickle cell disease, those with ischemia were more anemic than those without ischemia (hemoglobin 7.2 vs 8.2 g/dL). Follow-up radionuclide perfusion studies found that those with ischemic EKG changes had wall motion abnormalities and were unable to increase cardiac output during exercise (Covitz et al. 1983). More recently, 22 children with sickle cell disease and chest pain or with concern for ischemia on EKG or echocardiographic (ECHO) underwent thallium-201 single photon emission computed tomography to assess myocardial perfusion. Fourteen (64 %) had perfusion defects. In nine children, exercise or pharmacologic stress elicited the defects. The remaining five children had fixed perfusion defects that were present both at rest and during stress. Chest pain in patients with sickle cell disease should be evaluated by EKG, troponin-I, and functional imaging as indicated, and treatment of myocardial infarction should begin with exchange transfusion (Voskaridou et al. 2012).

Myocardial ischemia in sickle cell disease may be primarily due to anemia, and in some cases to vascular stenosis. Intima-medial proliferation, rather than atherosclerotic plaque may cause these changes. Myocardial vessels appear to be generally spared from sickling or adhesion of red blood cells, which is surprising given the low oxygen tension in myocardial venules. In the laboratory, expression of human sickle beta globin protects ApoE-deficient mice from atherosclerosis and thrombosis by a mechanism that is dependent in part on hemoxygenase activity (Wang et al. 2013). Maybe high hemoxygenase activity, a source of anti-inflammatory carbon monoxide (Sylvester et al. 2004), explains the paucity of atherosclerotic lesions in people with sickle cell disease.

7.2.7 *Hypoxia, New Vessel Growth, and Arterio-Venous Shunting*

Severe anemia triggers new vessel growth that lowers systemic vascular resistance. In sheep, severe anemia led to the development of larger capillary diameters, greater myocardial capillary density and greater coronary blood flow (Davis et al. 1996; Martin et al. 1998). These changes were associated with increased myocardial expression of hypoxia inducible factor-1 (HIF-1) and vascular endothelial growth factor (VEGF). Anemia also stimulated the formation of interarterial coronary anastomoses that regressed after the anemia resolved (Eckstein 1955; Rakusan et al. 2001; Zoll et al. 1952). In a post-mortem angiographic analysis of structurally normal human hearts without coronary disease, anemia was associated with a higher prevalence of collateral vessels connecting coronary arteries (35 % versus 9 %) (Zoll et al. 1951).

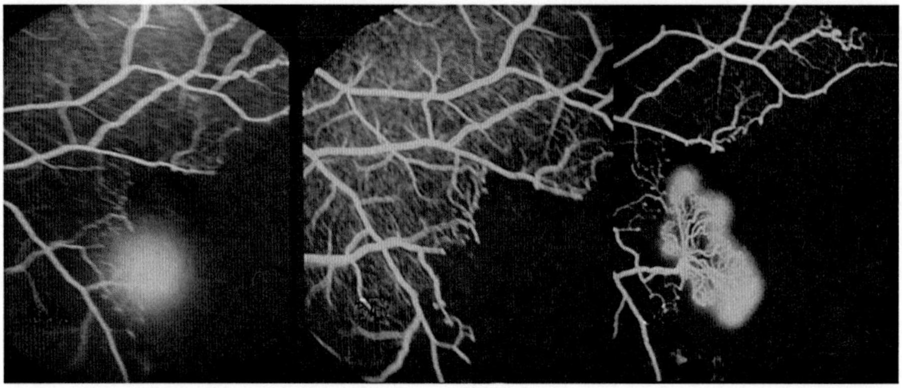

Fig. 7.7 Proliferative vascular changes in response to hypoxia in patients with sickle cell disease. This is a series of fluorescein angiograms of retinal vessels in an eight and a half year old boy with sickle cell disease. Initially, leakage was identified from a proliferative lesion in an area with little capillary perfusion (*left*); eight days later, the proliferative lesion and surrounding area were not perfused at all (*middle*); one year later, a proliferation of new vessels appeared in this previously ischemic area (*right*). Images are reprinted from Downes et al. (2005) with permission

In sickle cell disease, key angiogenic molecules are highly expressed, likely stimulated by hypoxia (Lopes et al. 2015). Arteriovenous shunts form following ischemic cerebral stroke due to in situ thrombosis and proliferative arteriopathy. The most severe form is moyamoya disease ("puff of smoke" in Japanese). When present, moyamoya disease increases the risk of hemorrhagic stroke (Dobson et al. 2002; Fasano et al. 2014; Kassim and DeBaun 2013; Seeler et al. 1978). Retinal vessel proliferation is also common and associated with hemorrhage among patients with sickle cell disease (Figs. 7.7 and 12.6). High oxygen saturation in peripheral venous blood has been observed in SCD at rest and during vaso-occlusive crisis, suggesting that arteriovenous shunts have formed in response to chronic hypoxia or microvascular occlusion (Manfredi et al. 1960; Nahavandi et al. 2002; Sproule et al. 1958; Wyche et al. 2003). These peripheral arterio-venous formations would bypass small resistance vessels and capillaries, thereby decreasing systemic vascular resistance, increasing cardiac output, and increasing venous oxygenation level, but at the expense of tissue perfusion. Overall, these vascular proliferations may be a maladaptive response to tissue hypoxia.

7.2.8 Summary

In anemia, cardiovascular adaptations help maintain oxygen delivery in the setting of the reduced blood oxygen carrying capacity. These adaptations include larger cardiac stroke volume, lower blood viscosity and increased oxygen extraction. In people with sickle cell disease, these adaptations may be incomplete or dysfunctional. Although patients with sickle cell disease maintain a low systemic vascular resistance and a high cardiac output, the viscosity of blood is high relative to the hematocrit, and in adults, oxygen extraction is inefficient. The increased stiffness of individual erythrocytes shifts the hematocrit to viscosity relationship. New vessel growth may lead to shunts that raise venous blood oxygen saturation but compromise tissue perfusion (Fig. 7.2). The pathophysiology of sickle cell disease arises from the reduced oxygen carrying capacity of blood and from the altered rheological and adhesive properties of blood cells, leading to small vessel occlusion, ischemia, and repetitive and cumulative tissue injury.

7.3 Interactions between Erythrocytes and Endothelial Cells Cause Sickle Cell Pathology

In this section, we discuss how erythrocyte sickling, adhesion, and lysis contribute to endothelial activation and injury in sickle cell disease. Sickling and adhesion are discussed in greater detail in Chaps. 3 and 4.

7.3.1 Erythrocyte Sickling Activates the Vascular Endothelium Promoting Adhesion and Vascular Occlusion

Abnormal hemoglobin polymerization in sickle cell disease drives the pathologic interactions between erythrocytes and the vascular endothelium (Kaul et al. 1995). Hemoglobin polymerization causes red cells to take their eponymous sickle shape with impaired deformability and altered expression of red cell surface membrane proteins. Poorly deformable red cells clog the microvasculature, irritate the endothelium and, when lysed, release plasma free hemoglobin and heme, stimulating the production of inflammatory, pro-coagulant and vasoactive molecules and contributing to the activation and recruitment of leukocytes and platelets (Frei et al. 2008).

Microvascular congestion slows blood flow and increases the opportunity for interactions between blood cells, plasma proteins and the endothelium. Sickle erythrocytes' adherence to the endothelial wall is central to erythrocyte–endothelium interactions in sickle cell disease (Hebbel et al. 1980; Hoover et al. 1979). Reticulocytes, immature erythrocytes that are abundant in anemic states, are a particularly adherent and injurious subpopulation of erythrocytes. Among children in the Cooperative Study of Sickle Cell Disease, increased reticulocyte count was associated with mortality (Meier et al. 2014). Whether reticulocytes have a causal role in sickle cell pathology or simply reflect the severity of anemia and hemolysis is unclear; regardless, their presence is damaging (Sakamoto et al. 2013). Sickle reticulocytes have increased surface adhesion receptors, including CD36 (Joneckis et al. 1993), very late activation antigen 4 (VLA-4) and sulfate glycolipids (Brousse et al. 2014). Mature sickle erythrocytes also have increased surface adhesion receptors including Lutheran blood group antigen (also called basal cell adhesion molecule/Lu, BCAM/Lu or CD239), integrin associated protein (CD47), CD147 and intercellular adhesion molecule-4 (ICAM-4) (Johnson and Telen 2008; Telen 2014). In addition, red cell phosphatidylserine exposure is increased and binds with endothelial matrix proteins, especially thrombospondin (Manodori et al. 2000; Setty et al. 2002; Wautier et al. 2011). Finally, red cell microparticles may also contribute to abnormal red cell adhesion (Camus et al. 2012, 2015; Kasar et al. 2014).

Endothelial cells exposed to sickle blood have increased expression of endothelial cell adhesion molecules such as vascular endothelial adhesion molecule 1 (VCAM-1), intercellular adhesion molecule 1 (ICAM-1) and E-selectin (Brown et al. 2001; Gee and Platt 1995). The P-, E-, and L-selectins mediate cytoadhesion and are critical facilitators of leukocyte rolling in sickle cell disease (Kutlar and Embury 2014; Matsui 2001). Platelet activation contributes to the thrombophilia of sickle cell disease (Franceschi et al. 2011; Wun et al. 1998). Finally, leukocytes are increased in number and interact with adhesion molecules to form aggregates and adhere to the endothelium (Polanowska-Grabowska et al. 2010; Turhan et al. 2002).

Recognition that leukocytes, platelets, extracellular matrix proteins and endothelial cell surface proteins also contribute to vaso-occlusion has led to the identification of a novel set of therapeutic targets (Hoppe 2011; Johnson and Telen 2008). Therapies that target pathological cell adhesion are covered in Chap. 16. In addition to a host of agents in early phase trials, hydroxyurea is also recognized as affecting the adhesion of reticulocytes, platelets and leukocytes to endothelium (Chaar et al. 2014). Specifically, hydroxyurea downregulates the expression of pro-adhesion molecules such as CD36, CD49d and CD29, leading to decreased interaction between sickle erythrocytes and the subendothelial matrix proteins thrombospondin and laminin (Gambero et al. 2007; Hillery et al. 2000; Styles et al. 1997). Hydroxyurea has also been found to correct dysregulated L-selectin expression (Benkerrou 2002), reduce phosphatidylserine expression (Covas et al. 2004), and reduce soluble ICAM-1 (Conran et al. 2004). The anti-adhesive effects of hydroxyurea might augment the primary anti-sickling effect of the drug and help to decrease the frequency of painful crises (Charache et al. 1995).

7.3.2 Erythrocyte–Endothelial Cell Interactions Cause Ischemia and Reperfusion Injury

Ischemia and reperfusion injury is a central pathophysiologic process driving organ injury in sickle cell disease (Conran et al. 2009). The process of ischemia and reperfusion injury distinguishes sickle cell anemia from other chronic anemic states. In ischemia and reperfusion injury, obstructed blood flow causes ischemic changes to downstream tissues. With resolution of the obstruction, activated inflammatory cascades cause local injury that may rapidly evolve into overwhelming systemic inflammation, damaging organs remote from the initial site of obstruction (Eltzschig and Eckle 2011; Schwartz et al. 2011). This process has the potential to culminate in life-threatening multi-organ injury or failure (Park et al. 2011).

Some aspects of ischemia and reperfusion injury in sickle cell disease are inferred from other ischemia and reperfusion injury models, but sickle cell disease mouse models support the importance of ischemia and reperfusion injury in sickle cell disease (Hebbel 2014). Under hypoxic conditions and at baseline, sickle cell mice have evidence of ischemia and reperfusion injury (Osarogiagbon et al. 2000).

In sickle cell disease, initial cellular damage in ischemia and reperfusion injury is precipitated by vaso-occlusion leading to local tissue hypoxia. Deprived of oxygen, cells are unable to perform aerobic respiration and become adenosine triphosphate (ATP) deplete. Intracellular hypercalcemia develops in association with mitochondrial dysfunction and the cells swell and die (Hotchkiss et al. 2009). Cell death is associated with immune system activation, platelet activation and aggregation (Eltzschig and Eckle 2011) and with pro-inflammatory NF-kappaB pathway activation (Cummins et al. 2006). These mechanisms are relevant to sickle cell disease (Belcher et al. 2003; Davila et al. 2014; Kaul et al. 2000). Other mediators of adhesion, inflammation and coagulation relevant to ischemia and reperfusion injury in sickle cell disease include monocyte chemoatractant protein 1 (MCP-1), vascular endothelial growth factor (VEGF), and platelet activating factor (PAF) (Aufradet et al. 2013; Kaul and Hebbel 2000; Solovey et al. 2001, 2004; Vinchi et al. 2013).

The model of microvascular dysfunction described in ischemia-reperfusion injury recapitulates the microvascular pathophysiology of sickle cell disease specifically. These hallmark changes include increased microvascular permeability, pro-inflammatory and pro-coagulable endothelial cell activation, alterations in the levels of vasoactive mediators and generation of reactive oxygen species. As cells become hypoxic and necrose, hypoxanthine levels increase. Hypoxia also causes capillary xanthine dehydrogenase to become xanthine oxidase via both irreversible and reversible mechanisms. The ischemia-induced accumulation of xanthine oxidase and hypoxanthine becomes toxic when blood flow is re-established and oxygen delivery resumes (Osarogiagbon et al. 2000; Ou et al. 2003; Pritchard Jr. et al. 2004). Nitric oxide deficiency also develops. Usually, nitric oxide exerts anti-inflammatory and anti-thrombotic effects on endothelial cells. The generation of superoxides and increased activity of NADPH oxidase leads to decreased endothelial nitric oxide synthase activity. Ferrous hemoglobin released from red blood cells can rapidly oxygenate nitric oxide, converting it to nitrate, shortening its half-life, and limiting its ability to diffuse across cell membranes. Loss of nitric oxide signaling activates platelets and leukocytes, activates NF-kappaB, and leads to the release of P-selectin and von Willebrand factor from Weibel-Palade bodies (Lowenstein et al. 2005).

Persistent, episodic microvascular occlusions chronically damage vascular beds, but organs seem to have different propensities to damage. Animal studies suggest that the brain, heart and kidney are more vulnerable to local ischemia and reperfusion injury than intestine, liver, skeletal muscle or lung (Hebbel 2014), but ultimately all are injured by the systemic effects of ischemia and reperfusion injury.

7.3.3 *Hemolysis Contributes to Endothelial Pathobiology in Sickle Cell Disease*

Up to 10 % of circulating erythrocytes can be lysed per day in a patient with sickle cell disease, releasing 30 g of hemoglobin. Although most red cell turnover occurs in a controlled fashion involving macrophages and the reticulo-endothelial system, an estimated 30 % of erythrocyte lysis occurs in the vasculature (Crosby 1955) where the release of hemoglobin can exceed the capacity of endogenous hemoglobin sequestration and recycling mechanisms. At normal physiologic levels of hemolysis, serum haptoglobin efficiently binds to hemoglobin and macrophages and other cells take up the hemoglobin-haptoglobin via the CD163 receptor. Intracellularly, hemoxygenase processes the hemoglobin, releasing biliverdin, iron, and carbon monoxide. Free heme, dissociated from the hemoglobin protein, is bound by serum hemopexin, and taken up by liver cells via the low-density lipoprotein receptor-related protein CD91 (Nielsen et al. 2010). However, during massive hemolysis such as occurs in many patients with sickle cell disease, both of these recycling pathways become saturated, haptoglobin and hemopexin are depleted, and extracellular hemoglobin and heme circulate in plasma (Muller-Eberhard et al. 1968).

In sickle cell mice, free heme functions as a danger signal by stimulating toll-like receptor-4 (TLR4) and activating an innate inflammatory response (Belcher et al. 2014; Buehler et al. 2012; Ghosh et al. 2013; Gladwin and Ofori-Acquah 2014). TLR4 and members of the inflammasome pathway are highly expressed by peripheral blood mononuclear cells, a process that may be induced by intracellular iron (van Beers et al. 2015). Heme also induces neutrophils to release DNA NETs (strands of DNA and histones that are intended to trap bacteria) in the pulmonary circulation of sickle mice and this mechanism may contribute to vascular occlusion (Chen et al. 2014).

Free heme is found at higher levels in children with sickle cell disease who have suffered acute chest syndrome, supporting a potential clinical role for heme-associated acute pulmonary vasculopathy in sickle cell disease patients (Adisa et al. 2013). Sickle cell patients with high free hemoglobin levels have impaired vasodilation responses to nitroprusside, a nitric oxide donor, and to shear stress—in vivo evidence that free hemoglobin is related to the development of vascular dysfunction. Circulating heme and hemoglobin promote oxidative stress and compromise nitric oxide bioavailability; these concepts are explored further in Sect. 7.5.1.

7.3.4 *Endothelial Progenitors and Neovascularization in Sickle Cell Disease*

Neovascularization in sickle cell disease is an adaptive response to microvascular obstruction caused by sickled erythrocytes, overabundance of adhesion molecules, chronic inflammation, and hypercoagulation. This process is ultimately pathologic and is exemplified by clinical complications of proliferative retinopathy, cerebral neovascularization in moyamoya syndrome, pulmonary hypertension and leg ulcers (Anjum et al. 2012; Dobson et al. 2002; Downes et al. 2005; Elagouz et al. 2010; Minniti et al. 2014; Mohan 2005; Niu et al. 2009). Gradual, pathologic neovascularization epitomizes the chronic, progressive vascular damage in sickle cell disease (Cheung et al. 2010) and highlights both phenotypic and genotypic disease variability. For example, although the exact incidence is unknown, only some patients with sickle cell disease develop moyamoya syndrome (Dobson et al. 2002) and proliferative retinopathy is more common in HbSC than HbSS disease (Downes et al. 2005; Gill and Lam 2008). Differences in the frequency of proliferative retinopathy in HbSC and HbSS are attributed to differences in retinal vasculature occlusion rates. In HbSS, vascular obstruction inhibits de novo revascularization whereas in, HbSC, hyperviscosity leads to indolent hypoxia that stimulates angiogenesis. Thrombospondin levels are elevated in HbSS disease but not HbSC and counteract circulating angiogenic factors (Elagouz et al. 2010).

In early development, vasculogenesis is supported by the endoderm while angiogenesis is supported by both ectoderm and endoderm. Endothelial cells participate in the molecular events associated with this process by producing vascular endothelial derived growth factor (VEGF) and placenta derived growth factor (PIGF). Both growth factors direct endothelial cell proliferation and migration. Because of the endothelium's clear role in stimulating new vessel formation, it is fundamentally implicated in pathologic collateral vasculature formation in sickle cell disease. Indeed, circulating angiogenic factors VEGF, angiopoietin-1 and -2, placental growth factor, and erythropoietin are stimulated by hypoxia and endothelial injury and are elevated in sickle cell disease (Brittain et al. 2010; Cruz et al. 2014; Duits et al. 2006; Landburg et al. 2009; Lopes et al. 2015; Niu et al. 2009).

The collateral vessels that develop in the retinal and cerebral circulations are prone to bleeding. Moyamoya syndrome is sometimes managed surgically using encephaloduroarteriosynagiosis (EDAS) to redirect cerebral blood flow, circumventing areas of stenosis and collateralization (Arias et al. 2014). In sickle cell retinopathy, laser and targeted anti-VEGF therapies are understudied but case reports suggest they may lead to regression of severe sickle retinopathy (Mitropoulos et al. 2014; Shaikh 2008; Siqueira et al. 2006). The long-term impact of these agents on the prognosis of proliferative retinopathy is unknown (Elagouz et al. 2010). The impact of systemic sickle cell disease therapies, hydroxyurea and hematopoietic stem cell transplant, on inhibiting or reversing pathologic vasculogenesis is under investigation and discussed below.

7.4 Endothelial Regulation of Blood Flow in Sickle Cell Disease

The endothelium integrates information about shear stress, oxygen tension, temperature and metabolic factors into a signal for vascular smooth muscle to relax or contract to regulate blood flow. One measure of endothelial function is its ability to induce vasodilation in response to experimentally induced changes in shear stress, tissue oxygenation, or other factors. This approach, originally developed to study atherosclerosis, has been applied to patients with sickle cell disease to determine whether they have impaired endothelium-dependent vasodilation.

7.4.1 Endothelial Regulation of Blood Flow in the Skin Microcirculation

In sickle cell disease, compromised microcirculatory function is thought to contribute to painful crises and end-organ injury. Five studies comparing patients with sickle cell disease to non-anemic controls have examined microcirculatory blood flow responses after transient arterial occlusion (Table 7.2). Compared to control subjects, baseline microcirculatory blood flow was the same or higher in patients with sickle cell disease (Bachir et al. 1993; Lipowsky et al. 1987; Mohan et al. 2011; Tharaux et al. 2002). After a brief period of ischemia to induce endothelium-dependent vasodilation, patients with sickle cell disease had greater hyperemic blood flow than controls (Mohan et al. 2011; Rodgers et al. 1990; Tharaux et al. 2002). In two studies, patients with sickle cell disease had significant prolongation of the hyperemic period, a response that is nitric oxide dependent (Bachir et al. 1993; Rodgers et al. 1990). These studies suggest that, in sickle cell disease, endothelium-dependent vasodilation in the skin is intact or even enhanced. This may be attributable to anemia, inflammation or shunting of blood to the skin surface. Unfortunately, measures of microcirculatory blood flow do not capture information about functional capillary density. If capillary density falls, blood flow velocity in the remaining functional capillaries would increase. High flow might not be appropriate compensation and may instead represent a pathologic or maladapted state.

Two studies examined sickle cell patients' microcirculatory response to temperature changes. They found that sickle cell patients had impaired microcirculatory vasodilation responses to heat (Tharaux et al. 2002) and enhanced microcirculatory vasoconstrictor responses to cold (Bachir et al. 1993). This may explain the poor cold tolerance often reported by patients with sickle cell disease.

7.4.2 Endothelial Regulation of Blood Flow in the Upper Limb

Endothelium-dependent vasodilation has been studied in patients with sickle cell disease using ultrasound measurements of the brachial artery, a technique originally used to study atherosclerosis. In this approach, the brachial artery is occluded for 3–5 min causing hypoxia and vasodilation in the small resistance vessels in forearm skeletal muscle. With release of the occlusion, brachial artery blood flow accelerates and shear stress increases. Healthy endothelium senses this increased shear stress

Table 7.2 Microvascular blood flow and reactivity in sickle cell disease patients in steady state compared to healthy non-anemic individuals

Baseline flow	Maximum hyperemic flow	Maximum/baseline flow	Time to reach maximum flow	Measurement location	Occlusion duration	Reference
Same	Same	Same	Same	Fingernail bed	60 s	Lipowsky et al. (1987)
–	–	Higher in SCD	Longer in SCD	Forearm skin	60 s	Rodgers et al. (1990)
Same	Lower in SCD	Same	Longer in SCD	Finger	180 s	Bachir et al. (1993)
Higher in SCD	Higher in SCD	Same	–	Foot dorsum	240 s	Tharaux et al. (2002)
Same	Same	–	–	Finger	ACh stimulation	Mohan et al. (2011)
Higher in SCD	Higher in SCD	–	–	Forearm skin	ACh stimulation	Mohan et al. (2011)

–, not reported

and elaborates signals such as nitric oxide and prostaglandins that relax vascular smooth muscle and dilate the vessel. The percent increase in brachial artery diameter after occlusive cuff release, flow mediated dilation, is a measure of vascular health. In people without sickle cell disease, the extent of flow mediated dilation correlates with atherosclerotic risk factors and coronary vasodilation responses (Anderson et al. 1995; Celermajer et al. 1992; Deanfield et al. 2007). In this section, we examine the change in blood flow elicited by transient forearm hypoxia, and the subsequent change in brachial artery diameter that occurs in response to changes in shear stress.

The increase in blood flow triggered by transient occlusion of the brachial artery appears to be intact or even enhanced in patients with sickle cell disease. Compared to non-anemic subjects, baseline forearm blood flows were twice as high in patients with sickle cell disease (Table 7.3). As discussed in Sect. 7.2.1, this is consistent with the lower systemic vascular resistance and higher cardiac output in people with anemia. When measured as maximum flow or absolute change in flow, blood flow increased to a higher level in patients with sickle cell disease compared to controls after brachial artery occlusion release. The percentage increase in blood flow from baseline was similar in the sickle cell and the healthy control group.

Both baseline and maximum brachial artery diameter were greater in patients with sickle cell disease compared to controls (Table 7.4). However, among patients with sickle cell disease, the absolute change in diameter between baseline and maximum, and the percentage change in diameter were both less. Multiple studies agree that patients with sickle cell disease have a low percentage increase in brachial artery diameter after a transient brachial artery occlusion (Table 7.5). Was the low percentage change due to a specific defect in endothelial response to shear stress, or was it due to the larger baseline brachial artery diameter observed in patients with

Table 7.3 Blood flow in the brachial artery before and after transient occlusion

	Belhassen et al. (2001)		Eberhardt et al. (2003)		Aessopos et al. (2007)	
	Healthy	Sickle cell	Healthy	Sickle cell	Healthy	Sickle cell (SS/B^0)
Number	15	16	41	17	40	47
Baseline flow (mL/min)	47 ± 12	89 ± 22*	104 ± 75	179 ± 61*	113 ± 82	196 ± 96*
Maximum flow (mL/min)	132 ± 24	219 ± 32*	686 ± 317	1121 ± 324*	553[a]	990[a]
Flow change (mL/min)	85[a]	130[a]	582[a]	942[a]	440[a]	794[a]
Flow change (%)	234	193	771 ± 486	579 ± 238	389 ± 185	405 ± 201

*$p < 0.001$ compared to healthy non-anemic control group

[a]Inferred from the published mean or percentage change. Published values have been rounded

Table 7.4 Diameter of the brachial artery before and after transient occlusion

	Belhassen et al. (2001)		Eberhardt et al. (2003)		Aessopos et al. (2007)		Scoffone et al. (2013)
	Healthy	Sickle cell	Healthy	Sickle cell	Healthy	Sickle cell (SS/B^0)	Sickle cell
Number	15	16	41	17	40	47	25
Baseline diameter (mm)	4.3±0.1	4.6±0.2*	3.5±0.8	3.7±0.4	3.2±0.9	3.9±0.4*	3.5±0.1
Maximum diameter (mm)	4.5±0.1	4.7±0.2*	4.0±0.8	4.1±0.5	3.5[a]	4.1[a]	3.8±0.1
Diameter change (mm)	0.2[a]	0.08[a]	0.46±0.2	0.33±0.17*	0.3[a]	0.2[a]	0.3±0.04
Diameter change (%)	4.0±0.2	1.7±0.4*	13.7±7.2	8.9±4.2*	9.2±3.8	4.2±2.9*	9.0±1.0

*$p<0.05$ compared to healthy, non-anemic controls. Healthy subjects were not studied in Scoffone et al. (2013)
[a]Inferred from the published mean or percentage change. Published values have been rounded

Table 7.5 Flow mediated dilation of the brachial artery after transient occlusion

Brachial artery diameter (% change from baseline)		
Healthy	Sickle cell	Reference
4.0±0.2	1.7±0.4*	Belhassen et al. (2001)
13.7±7.2	8.9±4.2*	Eberhardt et al. (2003)
11.6±7.7	4.6±4.1*	Blum et al. (2005)
16.9±1.1	6.2±0.9*	Zawar et al. (2005)
9.2±3.8	4.2±2.9*	Aessopos et al. (2007)
8.0±0.2	5.6±0.2*	De Montalembert et al. (2007) (children)
–	9.0±1.0	Scoffone et al. (2013)
8.2±5.0	9.3±4.2	Hadeed et al. (2014) (children)
7.9±1.6	5.5±2.5*	Detterich et al. (2015)

*$p<0.05$

sickle cell disease? Eberhardt et al. (2003) used analysis of covariance to account for different baseline brachial artery diameters and found sickle cell disease status was still associated with a lower percentage change in vessel diameter. Belhassen et al. (2001) used blood viscosity, vessel diameter and flow to calculate the wall shear stress in the brachial artery. Calculated shear stress was higher in sickle cell patients at baseline and at maximum flow, but elicited a smaller vasodilation response. These studies imply that patients with sickle cell disease have impaired endothelium-dependent vasodilation responses to shear stress. Future studies should include subjects with chronic non-hemolytic anemia as comparison groups to determine whether the impaired vasodilation is related to anemia or to a more specific sickle cell-related pathology such as hemolysis.

Table 7.6 Nitroglycerin-induced vasodilation of the brachial artery.

	Brachial artery dilation (% change from baseline)	
Reference	Healthy	Sickle cell
Eberhardt et al. (2003)	24.0 ± 10.7	17.6 ± 6.8*
Zawar et al. (2005)	26.1 ± 1.6	25.1 ± 1.5
de Montalembert et al. (2007) (children)	21 ± 8	20 ± 8

Brachial artery diameters were measured by ultrasound before and after a systemic dose of nitroglycerin in healthy, non-anemic controls and in patients with sickle cell disease. The percentage change relative to baseline is presented

*In Eberhardt et al., the percentage change from baseline was lower in patients with sickle cell disease; however, the absolute change in diameter (mm) was not different in healthy vs sickle cell, respectively: baseline, 3.63 ± 0.90 vs 3.85 ± 0.41, p = 0.38; post-NTG, 4.42 ± 0.79 vs 4.51 ± 0.44, p = 0.68; absolute change in diameter, 0.79 ± 0.25 vs 0.67 ± 0.23, p = 0.11

Endothelium-independent vasodilation, assessed by change in brachial artery diameter after a single dose of the nitric oxide donor nitroglycerin, was normal in most studies of sickle cell disease (Table 7.6) (Eberhardt et al. 2003; de Montalembert et al. 2007; Zawar et al. 2005), indicating that sickle cell patients are not maximally dilated at baseline and that the smooth muscle response to nitric oxide is intact. However, this observation is inconsistent with the impaired vasodilatory response to intra-arterial sodium nitroprusside, another nitric oxide donor, discussed in the next section.

7.4.3 Forearm Blood Flow Responses to Pharmacological Vasodilators and Vasoconstrictors in Patients with Sickle Cell Disease

Another way to assess endothelial function is by measuring forearm blood flow response to vasoactive drug infusions. To measure forearm blood flow, an upper arm pneumatic cuff is briefly inflated to occlude venous return but not arterial inflow. A stretch gauge around the forearm measures the rate of forearm expansion, which is proportional to arterial inflow (Hokanson et al. 1975). Measures of arterial inflow are taken before and during infusions that either stimulate endothelial muscarinic receptors (acetylcholine), inhibit endothelial nitric oxide synthase (L-NMMA or L-NAME) or donate nitric oxide independent of the endothelium (sodium nitroprusside). These drugs and their expected effects are summarized in Table 7.7. Forearm blood flow responses from multiple studies of patients with sickle cell disease, non-hemolytic anemia, and healthy controls are tabulated in Table 7.8.

Baseline forearm blood flow was elevated in sickle cell patients compared to non-anemic controls (Table 7.8), consistent with the Doppler ultrasound measures

Table 7.7 Drugs used to test vascular reactivity.

Vasoactive agent	Mechanism	Expected effect
Acetylcholine	Endothelial muscarinic receptor stimulation	Vasodilation via nitric oxide, prostaglandins, and endothelium-derived hyperpolarizing factor
L-NMMA or L-NAME	Endothelial nitric oxide synthase inhibition	Vasoconstriction via inhibition of nitric oxide synthase
Sodium nitroprusside	Direct nitric oxide release	Vasodilation via diffusion of nitric oxide from blood to smooth muscle

of forearm blood flow in the brachial artery discussed earlier. Acetylcholine-stimulated blood flow (an endothelium-dependent response) was also greater among sickle cell patients compared to healthy individuals whether expressed as maximum flow (Belhassen et al. 2001; Eberhardt et al. 2003; Gladwin et al. 2003b) or as percentage increase from baseline (Belhassen et al. 2001; Gladwin et al. 2003b), suggesting that endothelium-dependent vasodilation to acetylcholine is intact or even enhanced in patients with sickle cell disease.

Further evidence that endothelial function is intact in patients with sickle cell disease is provided by the observation of enhanced vasoconstriction to L-NMMA, a measure of the contribution of endothelial nitric oxide synthase to basal vasodilation. In three studies, patients with sickle cell disease had greater L-NMMA-induced decrements in forearm blood flow than non-anemic controls (Belhassen et al. 2001; Bereal-Williams et al. 2012; Eberhardt et al. 2003); in a fourth study, the responses to L-NMMA were the same (Gladwin et al. 2003b). Overall, endothelial nitric oxide synthase signaling appears to be not only intact, but also enhanced in people with sickle cell disease, a finding that is consistent with the response to L-NMMA observed in patients with non-hemolytic anemia (Anand et al. 1995). One study evaluated the contribution of nitric oxide synthase to the acetylcholine-induced increase in blood flow. L-NMMA reduced acetylcholine-stimulated blood flow by significantly more in healthy controls than in patients with sickle cell disease (Eberhardt et al. 2003), suggesting that in sickle cell disease the acetylcholine response may be mediated by non-nitric oxide vasodilating mechanisms, such as prostaglandins.

Sodium nitroprusside, a nitric oxide donor, tests smooth muscle dilation independent of the endothelium. Sodium nitroprusside infusion into the brachial artery increased forearm blood flow of patients with sickle cell disease to a higher level and by a larger amount than controls but the patients with sickle cell disease had a smaller percentage increase from baseline (Belhassen et al. 2001; Eberhardt et al. 2003). This lower percentage change from baseline was also observed in patients with non-hemolytic anemia (Anand et al. 1995). The smaller percentage increase in blood flow may be explained by the high baseline blood flow. This affects the calculation of percentage change and reduces the effective dose of the drug being infused into the artery.

Table 7.8 Forearm blood flow in patients with sickle cell disease.

	Anand et al. (1995)			Belhassen et al. (2001)		Cardillo et al. (1999)	Gladwin et al. (2003b)	Eberhardt et al. (2003)		Gorbach et al. (2012)
	Healthy controls	Anemia, pre-transfusion	Anemia, post-transfusion	Healthy	Sickle cell	Healthy	Sickle cell	Healthy	Sickle cell	Sickle cell
Number	6	8	6	15	16	18	21	11	8	25
Hb, g/dL	13.0 ± 0.5	4.8 ± 0.7	9.6 ± 0.7	14.0 ± 0.3	8.6 ± 0.3	–	9.2 [a]	13.5 ± 1.3	8.4 ± 1.1	8.8 ± 1.2
Baseline FBF, mL/min/100 mL	2.8 ± 0.7	6.5 ± 1.2	3.5 ± 1.1	1.6 ± 0.2	2.5 ± 0.3	3.0 ± 0.3	6.3 ± 0.7	2.6 ± 1.1	7.9 ± 3.0	6.0 ± 0.4
Acetylcholine FBF, mL/min/100 mL	14.4 ± 6.6	19.7 ± 5.5	18.6 ± 5.6	2.5 ± 1.5	9.7 ± 2.9	7.2 ± 1.1	15.9[a]	21.4[a]	24.6[a]	25.9 ± 2.3
% Change	+414[a]	+203[a]	+431[a]	+56	+388	+134 ± 24	+252 ± 37	+723[a]	+278[a]	+365 ± 51
L-NMMA FBF, mL/min/100 mL	1.8 ± 0.4	3.6 ± 0.8	2.5 ± 0.9	1.1[a]	1.6[a]	2.3[a]	4.7[a]	2[a]	5[a]	5.4 ± 0.4
% Change	−36[a]	−55[a]	−29[a]	−34 ± 4	−51 ± 5	−24 ± 5	−25 ± 4	−23[a]	−37[a]	−22 ± 4
SNP FBF, mL/min/100 mL	13.5 ± 4.7	12.6 ± 4.0	18.0 ± 5.9	4.9[a]	5.5[a]	8.2 ± 1.1	–	15.4[a]	28.8[a]	15.1 ± 0.9
SNP, % Change	+382[a]	+94[a]	+414[a]	+206[a]	+120[a]	–	–	+492[a]	+264[a]	+149 ± 20

FBF forearm blood flow, *SNP* sodium nitroprusside

–, not reported

[a]Inferred from the published mean or percentage change

7.5 Endothelium-Derived Vasomodulators Nitric Oxide, Eicosanoids, and Endothelin-1 in the Pathophysiology of Sickle Cell Disease

Under physiologic conditions, vasoactive peptides help maintain vascular tone, directing the local and systemic vascular response to maintain blood pressure and meet the body's metabolic demands. Endothelial cells produce the major vasoactive substances that direct vascular smooth muscle contraction and relaxation. Between 1978 and 1988, the discovery of prostacyclin (Weksler et al. 1977), nitric oxide (NO) (Furchgott and Zawadzki 1980; Palmer et al. 1987), platelet-derived growth factor (PDGF) (Berk et al. 1986) and endothelin-1 (ET-1) (Yanagisawa et al. 1988) established the critical endothelium-derived mediators of vascular tone. Identification of the vasodilatory effects of NO and prostacyclin, and the vasoconstricting effects of ET-1 and PDGF enabled studies of these substances' dynamic contributions to physiologic vascular muscle response, coagulation, vascular remodeling and vascular injury. Vasoactive peptides are both constitutively and episodically released. They contribute to physiologic maintenance of vascular tone and are integral to the endothelial response to vascular injury, shear stress, inflammatory or angiogenic stimuli. Vasoactive peptides are implicated in acute and chronic complications of sickle cell disease.

7.5.1 Endothelial Nitric Oxide Signaling and Vascular Inflammation

Nitric oxide was discovered to be the endothelium-derived relaxing factor in Brooklyn in 1980; in 1998 the three scientists primarily responsible for this discovery shared the Nobel Prize for Medicine and Physiology (SoRelle 1998). This history reflects the evolving recognition that nitric oxide is central to the physiology and pathophysiology of the cardiovascular system. Several excellent texts describe the role of nitric oxide in the vascular endothelium (Aird 2007a; Moncada and Higgs 2006a). Here we focus on aspects most important to sickle cell disease pathophysiology.

Nitric oxide plays several important roles in the vascular endothelium (Fig. 7.8). First, endothelial nitric oxide regulates blood flow by relaxing vascular smooth muscle and dilating vessels. Second, nitric oxide modulates platelet adhesion and aggregation and platelet-derived nitric oxide helps regulate clot formation. Third, nitric oxide modulates microcirculatory leukocyte adhesion by down-regulating endothelial adhesion molecules and by maintaining endothelial barrier integrity. Fourth, nitric oxide inhibits vascular smooth muscle proliferation. Finally, nitric oxide interacts with vascular endothelial growth factor to promote angiogenesis (Moncada and Higgs 2006b).

Nitric oxide synthase catalyzes the reaction of molecular oxygen with L-arginine to form nitric oxide and L-citrulline (Palmer et al. 1988). The three major nitric

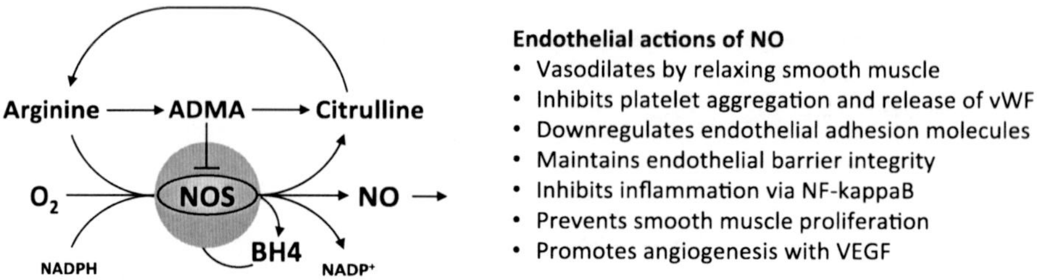

Fig. 7.8 Nitric oxide synthesis and activities in the vascular endothelium. Nitric oxide (NO) is formed from molecular oxygen and arginine. The reaction is catalyzed by nitric oxide synthase (NOS) and requires the reducing equivalent provided by NADPH, as well as the cofactor tetrahydrobiopterin (BH4), which is not consumed. The reaction product citrulline can be recycled to arginine via the enzymes ASS1 and ASL (not pictured). Asymmetric dimethylarginine (ADMA) is an endogenous inhibitor of NOS that is metabolized by the enzyme DDAH (not pictured). Nitric oxide has pleiotropic effects on cells in the vasculature, generally maintaining endothelial quiescence. Figure adapted from Matthew Alkaitis, *Biochemical Determinants of Nitric Oxide Synthesis in Severe Malaria*, D. Phil. Thesis, University of Oxford, 2014, and used with permission of the author

oxide synthase isoforms are endothelial nitric oxide synthase, neurologic nitric oxide synthase and inducible nitric oxide synthase. Endothelial nitric oxide synthase is constitutively active in the endothelium, and can be stimulated by endothelial exposure to high shear stress (Uematsu et al. 1995), vascular endothelial growth factor (Bouloumié et al. 1999), chronic exercise (Kojda et al. 2001) and statins (Hernández-Perera et al. 1998). In patients with sickle cell disease, there are conflicting data describing nitric oxide bioavailability. Compared with healthy African Americans, patients with sickle cell disease have low systemic vascular resistance, high baseline forearm blood flow, and pronounced vasoconstrictive responses to the nitric oxide synthase inhibitor, L-NMMA—implying that a high level of constitutive endothelial nitric oxide synthesis maintains a vasodilated state. However, among patients with sickle cell disease, those with higher plasma hemoglobin tend to have diminished vasodilation responses to nitric oxide and to shear stress, and higher estimates of pulmonary vasoconstriction (Detterich et al. 2015; Reiter et al. 2002). Sickle cell mice show a similar blunting of vasodilatory response to nitric oxide donors that is proportional to cell-free hemoglobin plasma concentration (Kaul et al. 2008).

Cell-free hemoglobin can cause vasoconstriction directly by reacting with nitric oxide (Reiter et al. 2002) or indirectly by producing reactive oxygen species that react with nitric oxide (Huie and Padmaja 1993) or by downregulating endothelial nitric oxide synthesis. Cell-free hemoglobin causes vasoconstriction and blunts the effects of nitric oxide in a canine model of intravascular hemolysis (Minneci et al. 2005). Continuous infusion of cell-free hemoglobin accelerates hypoxia-induced pulmonary hypertension and can be prevented by co-infusion of haptoglobin (Irwin et al. 2015). Free heme released from denatured or oxidized hemoglobin can stimulate reactive oxygen species production, impair nitric oxide synthase activity, and upregulate the expression of endothelial adhesion molecules—effects that are partially reversed by administering exogenous hemopexin, the heme scavenger (Vinchi et al. 2013).

Hemolysis is also associated with changes in the substrates, inhibitors and co-factors involved in nitric oxide synthesis. In sickle cell disease, arginase activity is elevated, and associated with arginine deficiency and an elevated ratio of ornithine to arginine, which together could potentially limit nitric oxide synthesis from arginine (Omodeo-Sale et al. 2010; Schnog et al. 2004). Plasma arginase is associated with elevated estimated pulmonary artery pressures and early mortality in sickle cell disease (Morris et al. 2005). Arginine deficiency can also lead to nitric oxide synthase uncoupling, allowing the production of the free radical superoxide instead of nitric oxide (Antoniades et al. 2009; Kim et al. 2009).

Deficiency of tetrahydrobiopterin, a nitric oxide synthase co-factor, also causes uncoupling and superoxide production (Guzik et al. 2002). A trial of sepiapterin to raise tetrahydrobiopterin levels improved endothelium-dependent vasodilation among patients with sickle cell disease who had impaired vasodilation at baseline (Hsu et al. 2008). Variants in the gene encoding GTP cyclohydrolase, a gene involved in synthesis of tetrahydrobiopterin, are associated with altered endothelial-dependent blood flow in women with sickle cell disease (Belfer et al. 2014).

Asymmetric dimethylarginine, an endogenous nitric oxide synthase inhibitor, is abundant in erythrocytes and released upon proteolysis of erythrocyte proteins (D'Alecy and Billecke 2010; Billecke 2006; Davids et al. 2012). Patients with sickle cell disease have elevated ADMA that is associated with higher estimated pulmonary artery pressure (Kato et al. 2009; Landburg et al. 2008, 2010; Schnog et al. 2004; El-Shanshory et al. 2013).

Hemolysis has the potential to limit nitric oxide signaling via direct nitric oxide consumption and by altering the biochemistry of nitric oxide synthesis. The concepts of hemolysis-associated nitric oxide deficiency have recently been reviewed in detail (Potoka and Gladwin 2015; Schaer et al. 2014). The extent to which hemolysis and impaired nitric oxide signaling explain the pathophysiology of sickle cell disease in humans needs to be determined. Studies of haptoglobin or hemopexin infusions in people with sickle cell disease may help define the importance of extra-erythrocytic hemoglobin in sickle cell disease, while efforts to restore the balance of arginine, ADMA, and tertrahydrobiopterin may highlight the importance of impaired nitric oxide synthesis in sickle cell pathophysiology (see Sect. 7.5.4 for a discussion of therapeutic manipulation of nitric oxide).

7.5.2 Eicosanoids Play a Mixed Role in SCD Pathophysiology

Endothelial eicosanoids are synthesized in endothelial cells and have diverse biologic actions including influencing vascular tone, modulating platelet and leukocyte behavior and maintaining vascular wall integrity. Eicosanoids are synthesized from arachadonic acid via three enzymatic pathways: the cyclooxygenase (COX), cytochrome p450 (CYP), and lipoxygenase (LOX) pathways. The major products of the COX pathway are prostacyclin (PGI_2), which inhibits platelet aggregation and relaxes vascular smooth muscle cells, prostaglandins (PGE_2 and PGD_2), which are involved in pain pathways, and thromboxane (TXA2), a vasoconstricting substance released by platelets. The LOX pathway synthesizes leukotrienes A_4-D_4. Finally, the CYP pathway produces epoxy eicosatetranoic acids (EETs). Overviews of the physiologic function of eicosanoids are available (Aird 2007a; Moncada and Higgs 2006b). The eicosanoids contribute to sickle cell disease's inter-related pathologies of endothelial activation, vascular remodeling and inflammation (Hoppe 2014).

In sickle cell disease, PGI_2 contributes to vascular tone modulation and inhibits platelet aggregation. PGI_2 is synthesized via COX-1 and COX-2 mediated pathways, most prominently produced in endothelial cells and vascular smooth muscle cells (Moncada et al. 1976, 1977). In vitro and in vivo studies of PGI_2 activity in sickle cell disease have produced contradictory results. In vivo measurements of PGI_2 levels and the prostacyclin metabolite 6-keto-prostaglandin are variable in patients with sickle cell disease (Buchanan and Holtkamp 1985; Longenecker and Mankad 1983; Mehta and Albiol 1982). In contrast, studies of the effects of sickled red cells and shear stress on cultured endothelial cells indicate that these interactions increase endothelial PGI_2 production under static (Sowemimo-Coker et al. 1992) and flow conditions (Shiu et al. 2002). These inconsistencies may reflect variability in PGI_2 production via the constitutively active COX-1 pathway and the induction of the COX-2 pathway under stress and at sites of inflammation and may be further complicated by organ specific regulation of COX enzyme activity. Increases in PGI_2 in vivo may be accompanied by the production of other eicosanoids that contribute to sickle cell pathophysiology such as leukotrienes, TXA_2 and prostaglandins. As PGI_2 is the major TXA_2 antagonist, increases in PGI_2 in sickle cell disease may represent a physiologic regulatory response to increased TXA_2 production.

7.5.3 *Endothelin Is Elevated in Sickle Cell Disease*

Endothelin-1 (ET-1), the most potent vasoconstrictor known, acts on large arteries and veins, resistance arterioles and postcapillary venules. ET-1 stimulates inflammation (Huribal et al. 1994; McMillen and Sumpio 1995), and up-regulates adhesion molecules (McCarron et al. 1993), while in the kidney it stimulates natriuresis (Nambi et al. 1992). ET-1 is constitutively produced by endothelial cells to help maintain vascular tone. Weibel-Palade bodies release ET-1 in response to signals of vascular distress such as circulating transforming growth factor-β, shear stress, hypoxia and the adhesion of sickled erythrocytes (Phelan et al. 1995). ET-1 effects are mediated through endothelin receptor-a (ET_A) and -b (ET_B); ET_A receptors predominate in vascular beds and their stimulation causes vasoconstriction. ET_B receptors are expressed in lung and kidney tissue and perform a counter-regulatory function; by clearing ET-1 from the circulation, they inhibit vasoconstriction.

ET-1 may be involved in several aspects of sickle cell pathophysiology. ET-1 is elevated in sickle cell patients at steady state, and is further elevated during crisis (Rybicki and Benjamin 1998) and in acute chest syndrome (Hammerman et al. 1997). These elevations may exacerbate microvasculature occlusion and may be at least partially compensated for by elevations in PGE_2 (Graido-Gonzalez et al. 1998). An endothelin-converting enzyme mutation is associated with stroke in sickle cell disease (Sebastiani et al. 2005) and, in adults without sickle cell disease, ET-1 is implicated in subarachnoid hemorrhage-associated cerebral vasospasm (Mascia et al. 2001). The endothelin-converting enzyme gene is expressed in peripheral blood mononuclear cells at 50-fold higher levels in adults with SCD than healthy controls (van Beers et al. 2015). Finally, red cell exposure to ET-1 may exacerbate sickling. Acting through the ET_B receptor, ET-1 modulates Gardos channels and causes erythrocyte dehydration and increased intracellular hemoglobin concentration, factors that favor sickle hemoglobin polymerization (Rivera et al. 1999, 2002).

Pulmonary hypertension in SCD appears to involve high levels of ET-1, a final common pathway in many forms of pulmonary hypertension. High plasma levels of ET-1 are associated with high pulmonary artery pressure estimated by echocardiography in adults with SCD (Sundaram et al. 2010) and ET-1 levels correlate with plasma levels of the VEGF family member, placenta growth factor (PlGF) (Patel et al. 2008). In mice, experimental overexpression of PlGF induces high levels of ET-1 and a pulmonary hypertension phenotype at necropsy, documenting a cause and effect relationship (Sundaram et al. 2010); PlGF is secreted by proerythroblasts under erythropoietin stimulation (Gonsalves et al. 2015; Perelman et al. 2003; Tordjman et al. 2001) and increased by free heme released by hemolysis (Wang et al. 2014).

Endothelin may also play an important role in the evolution of sickle cell kidney disease. Systemic ET-1 is degraded in the kidney and ET-1 excreted in the urine is of renal origin (Janas et al. 2000). Young adults with SCD secrete four times more urinary ET-1 than age- and ethnicity-matched controls (Tharaux 2005). This finding may be a function of the chronic ischemic injury to sickle cell kidneys, as in experimental models of chronic ischemic nephropathies ET-1 is also increased (Oishi et al. 1991). ET-1 promotes free water clearance and counters the effects of antidiuretic hormone, contributing to the classic finding of hyposthenuria in patients with sickle cell disease (Ge et al. 2005; Nadler et al. 1992; Oishi et al. 1991). Finally, albumin stimulates ET-1 production, but whether reductions in albuminuria modify ET-1 production is unknown.

7.5.4 *Therapeutic Promise of Modulating Nitric Oxide, Prostacyclin or Endothelin-1*

Because changes in nitric oxide bioavailability, prostacyclin synthesis and endothelin-1 synthesis have likely pathophysiologic roles in the evolution of sickle cell vascular disease, they are therapeutic targets whose potential is as of yet unrealized.

Despite promising pre-clinical studies (Hataishi et al. 2006; Lang et al. 2007; Mack et al. 2008; Mathru et al. 2007), in a multicenter study of 150 patients with sickle cell disease presenting to the hospital with painful crisis, treatment with inhaled nitric oxide gas versus placebo showed no difference in length of painful crisis, pain scores, opioid use or rate of acute chest syndrome (Gladwin et al. 2011). Treatment with sildenafil, a phosphodiesterase-5 inhibitor that prolongs the half-life of cyclic GMP, the second messenger of NO in smooth muscle, did not improve exercise capacity or estimates of pulmonary pressure (Machado et al. 2011). Patients treated with sildenafil had a higher rate of hospitalization for pain compared to placebo.

Promoting endogenous nitric oxide production pathways has also shown initial promise. Because the nitric oxide precursor arginine is depleted in patients with sickle cell disease, especially during painful crisis, and the inhibitor asymmetric dimethylarginine is elevated (Lopez et al. 2003; Morris et al. 2005; Schnog et al. 2004, 2005), arginine therapy is of interest in sickle cell disease (Morris et al. 2000). Arginine supplementation in sickle cell mice increased nitric oxide metabolites, decreased prostaglandin (PGE2) levels, improved oxidative stress, and restored nitric oxide-mediated vasoreactivity (Dasgupta et al. 2006; Kaul et al. 2008). A study of arginine supplementation in children with sickle cell disease did not meet primary end points (length of stay), but opiate use in treated patients decreased by over 50 % (Morris et al. 2013). Arginine has also been used in the treatment of leg ulcers (Sher and Olivieri 1994). Arginine therapy may also be beneficial to patients with sickle cell disease by changing erythrocyte Gardos channel activity (Romero et al. 2002) and by reducing erythrocyte fragility and oxidative stress (Kehinde et al. 2015).

Hydroxyurea can act as a nitric oxide donor, an additional mechanism through which hydroxyurea may be beneficial to patients with sickle cell disease (Almeida et al. 2012, 2015; Gladwin et al. 2002; Glover et al. 1999; Nahavandi et al. 2000). Although the importance of this pathway is debated, recent evidence suggests that this is a plausible mechanism. After inducing hemolysis and acute inflammation in C57Bl/6 wild-type mice, treatment with hydroxyurea improved leukocyte function. However, administration of hydroxyurea with nitric oxide scavengers abrogated this response. These results suggest that hydroxyurea changes leukocyte activation by stimulating nitric oxide production (Almeida et al. 2015), though L-NMMA could have harmful effects independent of hydroxyurea.

Although PGI_2 analogues are used to treat pulmonary hypertension, they have not been specifically evaluated for the management of pulmonary hypertension in patients with sickle cell disease (Klings et al. 2014). In one case report, Iloprost worked as analgesia in a sickle cell patient with severe bone pain (Disch et al. 2004). Although use of selective COX-2 inhibitors was promising in one small study of children with sickle cell disease (Edwards et al. 2004), they are no longer in use due to cardiovascular toxicity attributed to the selective inhibition of prostacyclin production.

Unfortunately, the therapeutic promise of endothelin-1 receptor antagonists has yet to be demonstrated for sickle cell disease. Bosentan, an ET-1 receptor antagonist, prevented death in mice exposed to hypoxic conditions (Sabaa et al. 2008), and decreased ET-1 production in the kidneys of sickle mice (Tharaux 2005). Bosentan improved the six-minute walk distance of patients with sickle cell disease and pulmonary hypertension (Barst et al. 2010; Minniti et al. 2009). ET-1 antagonism may also have a role in the treatment of patients with intractable leg ulcers (Lionnet et al. 2008).

7.5.5 *Sickle Cell-Directed Therapies Ameliorate Endothelial Injury*

Clinical evidence suggests that hydroxyurea and hematopoietic stem cell transplant (HSCT) mitigate vascular complications of sickle cell disease. Hydroxyurea changes many serologic measures associated with endothelial abnormalities of sickle cell disease (Table 7.9). Hydroxyurea not only increases fetal hemoglobin (HbF), but also decreases platelet, reticulocyte and leukocyte counts, decreases inflammatory markers, has anti-angiogenic effects (Lopes et al. 2014, 2015), alters

Table 7.9 Hydroxyurea changes mediators of endothelial activity

Mediator	Effect of hydroxyurea	In vivo/ in vitro
Adhesion		
Reticulocytes	Decreased adhesion to endothelial cells (Bridges et al. 1996) Decreases expression of VLA-4 and CD36 (Styles et al. 1997)	In vivo
Phosphatidylserine	Decreases erythrocyte expression (Covas et al. 2004)	
Neutrophils	Decreases absolute count Reduces H_2O_2 production (Benkerrou 2002)	In vivo
L-selectin	Normalizes neutrophil surface expression (Benkerrou 2002)	In vivo
Vascular Cell Adhesion Molecule-1 (VCAM-1)	Soluble levels decreased (Conran et al. 2004)	In vivo
Inducible Cell Adhesion Molecule-1	Soluble levels decreased (Conran et al. 2004)	In vivo
Angiogenesis		
Hypoxia-inducible factor-1	Decreased expression (Lopes et al. 2014)	In vitro
Vascular endothelial growth factor-D	Decreased (Lopes et al. 2015)	In vivo
Angiotensin-1	Decreased (Lopes et al. 2015)	In vivo
Platelet derived growth factor-AA, -BB	Decreased (Lopes et al. 2015)	In vivo
Vasoactive mediators		
Nitric oxide bioavailability	Increased (Almeida et al. 2015)	In vivo
Endothelin-1	Decreased (Brun et al. 2003)	In vitro
Arginase	Decreased (Moreira et al. 2015)	In vivo

reticulocyte-endothelial adhesion (Chaar et al. 2014) and down regulates ET-1 expression (Brun et al. 2003). Plasma arginase levels are also lower after hydroxyurea therapy (Iyamu et al. 2005).

Long-term follow-up after HSCT in children is increasingly available and suggests that many sickle cell complications are reversed following curative treatment. In a study of 22 children (ages 11 ± 3.9 years) receiving matched related donor HSCT, peri-transplant cerebrovascular complications occurred, but five years after transplant, some abnormalities resolved and no patients experienced stroke or cerebrovascular disease progression. The same cohort demonstrated post-transplant improvements in splenic function, suggesting improved splenic vascular circulation. In a cohort study of children with abnormal transcranial Doppler velocities who received either chronic transfusion therapy or HSCT, the group receiving HSCT had significantly greater decreases in their transcranial Doppler velocities, compared to the chronically transfused children (Bernaudin et al. 2014). In a meta-analysis of four cohorts of sickle cell disease patients receiving HSCT, 81 of 196 patients had pre-transplant neuroimaging demonstrating cerebrovascular anomalies; 16 % of these patients continued to worsen post-transplant (Bodas and Rotz 2014). Progression of cerebral vasculopathy, even after sickled erythrocytes have been replaced by typical erythrocytes, implies that vascular injury may resolve slowly if at all (Fasano et al. 2014).

7.6 Summary

The role of the vascular endothelium in sickle cell disease is complex and must be interpreted with attention to how the cardiovascular system responds to anemia, communication between blood cells and the endothelium and the acute and chronic endothelial response to the conditions precipitated by erythrocyte sickling. Endothelial heterogeneity demands that researchers resist the temptation to generalize findings from one vascular bed to others. Approaches to study organ-specific endothelial abnormalities are especially needed to understand the devastating cerebral, cardio-pulmonary, renal and hepatic complications sickle cell disease. Drugs that ameliorate sickling and reduce ischemia-reperfusion injury may protect the vascular endothelium in patients with sickle cell disease. In the future, cell-based therapies may be available that improve sickle cell vasculopathy by regenerating blood vessels' lining with new, undamaged endothelium.

References

Adisa OA, Hu Y, Ghosh S, Aryee D, Osunkwo I, Ofori-Acquah SF (2013) Association between plasma free haem and incidence of vaso-occlusive episodes and acute chest syndrome in children with sickle cell disease. Br J Haematol 162(5):702–705

Aessopos A, Farmakis D, Tsironi M, Diamanti-Kandarakis E, Matzourani M, Fragodimiri C et al (2007) Endothelial function and arterial stiffness in sickle-thalassemia patients. Atherosclerosis 191(2):427–432

Aird WC (2007a) Endothelial biomedicine, 1st edn. Cambridge University Press, Cambridge

Aird WC (2007b) Phenotypic heterogeneity of the endothelium: II. Representative vascular beds. Circ Res 100(2):174–190

Aird WC (2007c) Phenotypic heterogeneity of the endothelium: I. Structure, function, and mechanisms. Circ Res 100(2):158–173

Alexy T, Pais E, Armstrong JK, Meiselman HJ, Johnson CS, Fisher TC (2006) Rheologic behavior of sickle and normal red blood cell mixtures in sickle plasma: implications for transfusion therapy. Transfusion 46(6):912–918

Almeida CB, Scheiermann C, Jang JE et al (2012) Hydroxyurea and a cGMP-amplifying agent have immediate benefits on acute vaso-occlusive events in sickle cell disease mice. Blood 120(14):2879–2888

Almeida CB, Souza LEB, Leonardo FC et al (2015) Acute hemolytic vascular inflammatory processes are prevented by nitric oxide replacement or a single dose of hydroxyurea. Blood 126(6):711–720

Alpert BS, Gilman PA, Strong WB et al (1981) Hemodynamic and ECG responses to exercise in children with sickle cell anemia. Am J Dis Child 135(4):362–366

Anand IS, Chandrashekhar Y, Wander GS, Chawla LS (1995) Endothelium-derived relaxing factor is important in mediating the high output state in chronic severe anemia. J Am Coll Cardiol 25(6):1402–1407

Anderson TJ, Uehata A, Gerhard MD et al (1995) Close relation of endothelial function in the human coronary and peripheral circulations. J Am Coll Cardiol 26(5):1235–1241

Anjum F, Lazar J, Zein J, Jamaleddine G, Demetis S, Wadgaonkar R (2012) Characterization of altered patterns of endothelial progenitor cells in sickle cell disease related pulmonary arterial hypertension. Pulm Circ 2(1):54–60

Antoniades C, Shirodaria C, Leeson P et al (2009) Association of plasma asymmetrical dimethylarginine (ADMA) with elevated vascular superoxide production and endothelial nitric oxide synthase uncoupling: implications for endothelial function in human atherosclerosis. Eur Heart J 30(9):1142–1150

Arias EJ, Derdeyn CP, Dacey RG, Zipfel GJ (2014) Advances and surgical considerations in the treatment of moyamoya disease. Neurosurgery 74(Suppl 1):S116–S125

Aufradet E, Desouza G, Bourgeaux V et al (2013) Hypoxia/reoxygenation stress increases markers of vaso-occlusive crisis in sickle SAD mice. Clin Hemorheol Microcirc 54(3):297–312

Bachir D, Maurel A, Portos JL, Galacteros F (1993) Comparative evaluation of laser Doppler flux metering, bulbar conjunctival angioscopy, and nail fold capillaroscopy in sickle cell disease. Microvasc Res 45(1):20–32

Bahl VK, Malhotra OP, Kumar D et al (1992) Noninvasive assessment of systolic and diastolic left ventricular function in patients with chronic severe anemia: a combined M-mode, two-dimensional, and Doppler echocardiographic study. Am Heart J 124(6):1516–1523

Balfour IC, Covitz W, Davis H, Rao PS, Strong WB, Alpert BS (1984) Cardiac size and function in children with sickle cell anemia. Am Heart J 108(2):345–350

Balfour IC, Covitz W, Arensman FW, Eubig C, Garrido M, Jones C (1988) Left ventricular filling in sickle cell anemia. Am J Cardiol 61(4):395–399

Barst RJ, Mubarak KK, Machado RF et al (2010) Exercise capacity and haemodynamics in patients with sickle cell disease with pulmonary hypertension treated with bosentan: results of the ASSET studies. Br J Haematol 149(3):426–435

Belcher JD, Bryant CJ, Nguyen J et al (2003) Transgenic sickle mice have vascular inflammation. Blood 101(10):3953–3959

Belcher JD, Chen C, Nguyen J et al (2014) Heme triggers TLR4 signaling leading to endothelial cell activation and vaso-occlusion in murine sickle cell disease. Blood 123(3):377–390

Belfer I, Youngblood V, Darbari DS, Wang Z, Diaw L, Freeman L et al (2014) A GCH1 haplotype confers sex-specific susceptibility to pain crises and altered endothelial function in adults with sickle cell anemia. Am J Hematol 89(2):187–193

Belhassen L, Pelle G, Sediame S, Bachir D, Carville C, Bucherer C et al (2001) Endothelial dysfunction in patients with sickle cell disease is related to selective impairment of shear stress–mediated vasodilation. Blood 97(6):1584–1589

Benesch R, Benesch RE (1969) Intracellular organic phosphates as regulators of oxygen release by haemoglobin. Nature 221(5181):618–622

Benkerrou M (2002) Hydroxyurea corrects the dysregulated L-selectin expression and increased H2O2 production of polymorphonuclear neutrophils from patients with sickle cell anemia. Blood 99(7):2297–2303

Bereal-Williams C, Machado RF, McGowan V, Chi A, Hunter CJ, Kato GJ et al (2012) Atorvastatin reduces serum cholesterol and triglycerides with limited improvement in vascular function in adults with sickle cell anemia. Haematologica 97(11):1768–1770

Berk BC, Alexander RW, Brock TA, Gimbrone MA, Webb RC (1986) Vasoconstriction: a new activity for platelet-derived growth factor. Science 232(4746):87–90

Bernaudin F, Verlhac S, Delatour RP et al (2014) Cerebral arterial velocities in SCA-children with abnormal doppler are reduced and normalized more frequently after transplantation than after transfusion program (French national trial "drepagreffe" AP-HP N°: NCT 01340404). Blood 124(21):561

Billecke SS (2006) Contribution of whole blood to the control of plasma asymmetrical dimethylarginine. Am J Physiol Heart Circ Physiol 291(4):H1788–H1796

Blum A, Yeganeh S, Peleg A et al (2005) Endothelial function in patients with sickle cell anemia during and after sickle cell crises. J Thromb Thrombolysis 19(2):83–86

Bodas P, Rotz S (2014) Cerebral vascular abnormalities in pediatric patients with sickle cell disease after hematopoietic cell transplant. J Pediatr Hematol Oncol 36(3):190–193

Bosi G, Crepaz R, Gamberini MR et al (2003) Left ventricular remodelling, and systolic and diastolic function in young adults with β thalassaemia major: a Doppler echocardiographic assessment and correlation with haematological data. Heart 89(7):762–766

Bouloumié A, Schini-Kerth VB, Busse R (1999) Vascular endothelial growth factor up-regulates nitric oxide synthase expression in endothelial cells. Cardiovasc Res 41(3):773–780

Bridges KR, Barabino GD, Brugnara C et al (1996) A multiparameter analysis of sickle erythrocytes in patients undergoing hydroxyurea therapy. Blood 88(12):4701–4710

Brittain JE, Hulkower B, Jones SK et al (2010) Placenta growth factor in sickle cell disease: association with hemolysis and inflammation. Blood 115(10):2014–2020

Brousse V, Colin Y, Pereira C et al (2014) Erythroid adhesion molecules in sickle cell anaemia infants: insights into early pathophysiology. EBioMedicine 2(2):154–157

Brown MD, Wick TM, Eckman JR (2001) Activation of vascular endothelial cell adhesion molecule expression by sickle blood cells. Pediatr Pathol Mol Med 20(1):47–72

Brun M, Bourdoulous S, Couraud PO, Elion J, Krishnamoorthy R, Lapoumeroulie C (2003) Hydroxyurea downregulates endothelin-1 gene expression and upregulates ICAM-1 gene expression in cultured human endothelial cells. Pharmacogenomics J 3(4):215–226

Buchanan GR, Holtkamp CA (1985) Plasma levels of platelet and vascular prostaglandin derivatives in children with sickle cell anaemia. Thromb Haemost 54(2):394–396

Buehler PW, Baek JH, Lisk C et al (2012) Free hemoglobin induction of pulmonary vascular disease: evidence for an inflammatory mechanism. Am J Physiol Lung Cell Mol Physiol 303(4):L312–L326

Bunting S, Moncada S, Vane JR (1977) Antithrombotic properties of vascular endothelium. Lancet 310(8047):1075–1076

Caldas MC, Meira ZA, Barbosa MM (2008) Evaluation of 107 patients with sickle cell anemia through tissue Doppler and myocardial performance index. J Am Soc Echocardiogr 21(10):1163–1167

Camus SM, Gausserès B, Bonnin P et al (2012) Erythrocyte microparticles can induce kidney vaso-occlusions in a murine model of sickle cell disease. Blood 120(25):5050–5058

Camus SM, Moraes JAD, Bonnin P et al (2015) Circulating cell membrane microparticles transfer heme to endothelial cells and trigger vaso-occlusions in sickle cell disease. Blood 25(24):3805–3814

Cardillo C, Kilcoyne CM, Cannon RO 3rd, Panza JA (1999) Attenuation of cyclic nucleotide-mediated smooth muscle relaxation in blacks as a cause of racial differences in vasodilator function. Circulation 99(1):90–95

Celermajer D, Sorensen K, Gooch V et al (1992) Non-invasive detection of endothelial dysfunction in children and adults at risk of atherosclerosis. Lancet 340(8828):1111–1115

Chaar V, Laurance S, Lapoumeroulie C et al (2014) Hydroxycarbamide decreases sickle reticulocyte adhesion to resting endothelium by inhibiting endothelial lutheran/basal cell adhesion molecule (Lu/BCAM) through phosphodiesterase 4A activation. J Biol Chem 289(16): 11512–11521

Charache S, Terrin ML, Moore RD et al (1995) Effect of hydroxyurea on the frequency of painful crises in sickle cell anemia. N Engl J Med 332(20):1317–1322

Chen G, Zhang D, Fuchs TA, Manwani D, Wagner DD, Frenette PS (2014) Heme-induced neutrophil extracellular traps contribute to the pathogenesis of sickle cell disease. Blood 123(24):3818–3827

Cheung ATW, Miller JW, Craig SM et al (2010) Comparison of real-time microvascular abnormalities in pediatric and adult sickle cell anemia patients. Am J Hematol 85(11):899–901

Chien S, Usami S, Bertles JF (1970) Abnormal rheology of oxygenated blood in sickle cell anemia. J Clin Invest 49(4):623–634

Cho I-J, Mun YC, Kwon KH, Shin GJ (2014) Effect of anemia correction on left ventricular structure and filling pressure in anemic patients without overt heart disease. Korean J Intern Med 29(4):445–453

Conran N, Fattori A, Saad STO, Costa FF (2004) Increased levels of soluble ICAM-1 in the plasma of sickle cell patients are reversed by hydroxyurea. Am J Hematol 76(4):343–347

Conran N, Franco-Penteado CF, Costa FF (2009) Newer aspects of the pathophysiology of sickle cell disease vaso-occlusion. Hemoglobin 33(1):1–16

Cortese-Krott MM, Kelm M (2014) Endothelial nitric oxide synthase in red blood cells: key to a new erythrocrine function? Redox Biol 2:251–258

Cosby K, Partovi K, Crawford J et al (2003) Nitrite reduction to nitric oxide by deoxyhemoglobin vasodilates the human circulation. Nat Med 9(12):1498–1505

Covas DT, de Lucena Angulo I, Vianna Bonini Palma P, Zago MA (2004) Effects of hydroxyurea on the membrane of erythrocytes and platelets in sickle cell anemia. Haematologica 89(3):273–280

Covitz W, Eubig C, Balfour IC et al (1983) Exercise-induced cardiac dysfunction in sickle cell anemia: a radionuclide study. Am J Cardiol 51(3):570–575

Covitz W, Espeland M, Gallagher D, Hellenbrand W, Leff S, Talner N (1995) The heart in sickle cell anemia: the cooperative study of sickle cell disease (CSSCD). Chest 108(5):1214–1219

Crawford JH, Isbell TS, Huang Z et al (2006) Hypoxia, red blood cells, and nitrite regulate NO-dependent hypoxic vasodilation. Blood 107(2):566–574

Crecelius AR, Kirby BS, Voyles WF, Dinenno FA (2011) Augmented skeletal muscle hyperaemia during hypoxic exercise in humans is blunted by combined inhibition of nitric oxide and vasodilating prostaglandins. J Physiol 589(14):3671–3683

Crosby WH (1955) The metabolism of hemoglobin and bile pigment in hemolytic disease. Am J Med 18(1):112–122

Cruz PRS, Lira RPC, Pereira Filho SAC et al (2014) Increased circulating PEDF and low sICAM-1 are associated with sickle cell retinopathy. Blood Cells Mol Dis 54(1):33–37

Cummins EP, Berra E, Comerford KM et al (2006) Prolyl hydroxylase-1 negatively regulates IκB kinase-β, giving insight into hypoxia-induced NFκB activity. Proc Natl Acad Sci U S A 103(48):18154–18159

D'Alecy LG, Billecke SS (2010) Massive quantities of asymmetric dimethylarginine (ADMA) are incorporated in red blood cell proteins and may be released by proteolysis following hemolytic stress. Blood Cells Mol Dis 45(1):40

Dasgupta T, Hebbel RP, Kaul DK (2006) Protective effect of arginine on oxidative stress in transgenic sickle mouse models. Free Radic Biol Med 41(12):1771–1780

Davids M, van Hell AJ, Visser M, Nijveldt RJ, van Leeuwen PAM, Teerlink T (2012) Role of the human erythrocyte in generation and storage of asymmetric dimethylarginine. Am J Physiol Heart Circ Physiol 302(8):H1762–H1770

Davila J, Manwani D, Vasovic L et al (2014) A novel inflammatory role for platelets in sickle cell disease. Platelets 24:1–4

Davis LE, Hohimer AR, Giraud GD, Reller MD, Morton MJ (1996) Right ventricular function in chronically anemic fetal lambs. Am J Obstet Gynecol 174(4):1289–1294

de Montalembert M, Aggoun Y, Niakate A, Szezepanski I, Bonnet D (2007) Endothelial-dependent vasodilation is impaired in children with sickle cell disease. Haematologica 92(12): 1709–1710

Deanfield JE, Halcox JP, Rabelink TJ (2007) Endothelial function and dysfunction testing and clinical relevance. Circulation 115(10):1285–1295

Delivoria-Papadopoulos M, Oski FA, Gottlieb AJ (1969) Oxygen-hemoglobulin dissociation curves: effect of inherited enzyme defects of the red cell. Science 165(3893):601–602

Detterich J, Alexy T, Rabai M et al (2013) Low-shear red blood cell oxygen transport effectiveness is adversely affected by transfusion and further worsened by deoxygenation in sickle cell disease patients on chronic transfusion therapy. Transfusion 53(2):297–305

Detterich JA, Kato RM, Rabai M, Meiselman HJ, Coates TD, Wood JC (2015) Chronic transfusion therapy improves but does not normalize systemic and pulmonary vasculopathy in sickle cell disease. Blood 126(6):703–710

Disch AC, Matziolis G, Reinke P, Perka C (2004) Intravenous Iloprost treatment for severe bone pain caused by sickle cell crisis. Thromb Haemost 91(5):1047–1049

Dobson SR, Holden KR, Nietert PJ et al (2002) Moyamoya syndrome in childhood sickle cell disease: a predictive factor for recurrent cerebrovascular events. Blood 99(9):3144–3150

Downes SM, Hambleton IR, Chuang EL, Lois N, Serjeant GR, Bird AC (2005) Incidence and natural history of proliferative sickle cell retinopathy. Ophthalmology 112(11):1869–1875

Duits AJ, Rodriguez T, Schnog J-JB, the CURAMA Study Group (2006) Serum levels of angiogenic factors indicate a pro-angiogenic state in adults with sickle cell disease. Br J Haematol 134(1):116–119

Durr E, Yu J, Krasinska KM et al (2004) Direct proteomic mapping of the lung microvascular endothelial cell surface in vivo and in cell culture. Nat Biotechnol 22(8):985–992

Eberhardt RT, McMahon L, Duffy SJ et al (2003) Sickle cell anemia is associated with reduced nitric oxide bioactivity in peripheral conduit and resistance vessels. Am J Hematol 74(2):104–111

Eckstein RW (1955) Development of interarterial coronary anastomoses by chronic anemia; disappearance following correction of anemia. Circ Res 3(3):306–310

Edwards DJ, Prescilla RP, Fratarelli DA, Haritos D, Aranda JV (2004) Pharmacokinetics of rofecoxib in children. Clin Pharmacol Ther 75(2):P73

Elagouz M, Jyothi S, Gupta B, Sivaprasad S (2010) Sickle cell disease and the eye: old and new concepts. Surv Ophthalmol 55(4):359–377

Ellsworth ML, Ellis CG, Goldman D, Stephenson AH, Dietrich HH, Sprague RS (2009) Erythrocytes: oxygen sensors and modulators of vascular tone. Physiology (Bethesda) 24(2):107–116

El-Shanshory M, Badraia I, Donia A, Abd El-Hameed F, Mabrouk M (2013) Asymmetric dimethylarginine levels in children with sickle cell disease and its correlation to tricuspid regurgitant jet velocity. Eur J Haematol 91(1):55–61

Eltzschig HK, Eckle T (2011) Ischemia and reperfusion—from mechanism to translation. Nat Med 17(11):1391–1401

Escobar E, Jones NL, Rapaport E, Murray JF (1966) Ventricular performance in acute normovolemic anemia and effects of beta blockade. Am J Physiol 211(4):877–884

Fasano RM, Meier ER, Hulbert ML (2014) Cerebral vasculopathy in children with sickle cell anemia. Blood Cells Mol Dis doi:10.1016/j.bcmd.2014.08.007

Fowler NO, Holmes JC (1975) Blood viscosity and cardiac output in acute experimental anemia. J Appl Physiol 39(3):453–456

Franceschi L, Cappellini M, Olivieri O (2011) Thrombosis and sickle cell disease. Semin Thromb Hemost 37(03):226–236

Frei AC, Guo Y, Jones DW et al (2008) Vascular dysfunction in a murine model of severe hemolysis. Blood 12(2):398–405

Furchgott RF, Zawadzki JV (1980) The obligatory role of endothelial cells in the relaxation of arterial smooth muscle by acetylcholine. Nature 288(5789):373–376

Gambero S, Canalli AA, Traina F et al (2007) Therapy with hydroxyurea is associated with reduced adhesion molecule gene and protein expression in sickle red cells with a concomitant reduction in adhesive properties. Eur J Haematol 78(2):144–151

Ge Y, Ahn D, Stricklett PK et al (2005) Collecting duct-specific knockout of endothelin-1 alters vasopressin regulation of urine osmolality. Am J Physiol Renal Physiol 288(5):F912–F920

Gee BE, Platt OS (1995) Sickle reticulocytes adhere to VCAM-1. Blood 85(1):268–274

Gerry JL Jr, Bulkley BH, Hutchins GM (1978) Clinicopathologic analysis of cardiac dysfunction in 52 patients with sickle cell anemia. Am J Cardiol 42(2):211–216

Ghosh S, Adisa OA, Chappa P et al (2013) Extracellular hemin crisis triggers acute chest syndrome in sickle mice. J Clin Invest 123(11):4809–4820

Gill HS, Lam WC (2008) A screening strategy for the detection of sickle cell retinopathy in pediatric patients. Can J Ophthalmol 43(2):188–191

Gladwin MT, Ofori-Acquah SF (2014) Erythroid DAMPs drive inflammation in SCD. Blood 123(24):3689–3690

Gladwin MT, Shelhamer JH, Ognibene FP et al (2002) Nitric oxide donor properties of hydroxyurea in patients with sickle cell disease. Br J Haematol 116(2):436–444

Gladwin MT, Lancaster JR, Freeman BA, Schechter AN (2003a) Nitric oxide's reactions with hemoglobin: a view through the SNO-storm. Nat Med 9(5):496–500

Gladwin MT, Schechter AN, Ognibene FP et al (2003b) Divergent nitric oxide bioavailability in men and women with sickle cell disease. Circulation 107(2):271–278

Gladwin MT, Kato GJ, Weiner D et al (2011) Nitric oxide for inhalation in the acute treatment of sickle cell pain crisis: a randomized controlled trial. JAMA 305(9):893–902

Glover RE, Ivy ED, Orringer EP, Maeda H, Mason RP (1999) Detection of nitrosyl hemoglobin in venous blood in the treatment of sickle cell anemia with hydroxyurea. Mol Pharmacol 55(6):1006–1010

Gonsalves CS, Li C, Mpollo MS et al (2015) Erythropoietin mediated expression of placenta growth factor is regulated via activation of hypoxia inducible factor-1α and post-transcriptionally by mir214 in sickle cell disease. Biochem J 468(3):409–423

Gorbach AM, Ackerman HC, Liu WM et al (2012) Infrared imaging of nitric oxide-mediated blood flow in human sickle cell disease. Microvasc Res 84(3):262–269

Graettinger JS, Parsons RL, Campbell JA (1963) A correlation of clinical and hemodynamic studies in patients with mild and severe anemia with and without congestive failure. Ann Intern Med 58:617–626

Graido-Gonzalez E, Doherty JC, Bergreen EW, Organ G, Telfer M, McMillen MA (1998) Plasma endothelin-1, cytokine, and prostaglandin E2 levels in sickle cell disease and acute vaso-occlusive sickle crisis. Blood 92(7):2551–2555

Gross S, Godel JC (1971) Comparative studies of height and weight as a blood volume reference standard in normal children and children with sickle cell anemia. Am J Clin Pathol 155(6):662–670

Guzik TJ, Mussa S, Gastaldi D et al (2002) Mechanisms of increased vascular superoxide production in human diabetes mellitus: role of NAD(P)H oxidase and endothelial nitric oxide synthase. Circulation 105:1656–1662

Hadeed K, Hascoet S, Castex M-P, Munzer C, Acar P, Dulac Y (2014) Endothelial function and vascular properties in children with sickle cell disease. Echocardiography doi:10.1111/echo.12851

Hammerman SI, Kourembanas S, Conca TJ, Tucci M, Brauer M, Farber HW (1997) Endothelin-1 production during the acute chest syndrome in sickle cell disease. Am J Respir Crit Care Med 156(1):280–285

Hataishi R, Rodrigues AC, Neilan TG et al (2006) Inhaled nitric oxide decreases infarction size and improves left ventricular function in a murine model of myocardial ischemia-reperfusion injury. Am J Physiol Heart Circ Physiol 291(1):H379–H384

Hebbel RP (2014) Ischemia-reperfusion injury in sickle cell anemia. Hematol Oncol Clin North Am 28(2):181–198

Hebbel RP, Yamada O, Moldow CF, Jacob HS, White JG, Eaton JW (1980) Abnormal adherence of sickle erythrocytes to cultured vascular endothelium. J Clin Invest 65(1):154–160

Heistad DD, Abboud FM, Dickinson W (1980) Richards lecture: circulatory adjustments to hypoxia. Circulation 61(3):463–470

Hernández-Perera O, Pérez-Sala D, Navarro-Antolín J et al (1998) Effects of the 3-hydroxy-3-methylglutaryl-CoA reductase inhibitors, atorvastatin and simvastatin, on the expression of endothelin-1 and endothelial nitric oxide synthase in vascular endothelial cells. J Clin Invest 1101(12):2711–2719

Hillery CA, Du MC, Wang WC, Scott JP (2000) Hydroxyurea therapy decreases the in vitro adhesion of sickle erythrocytes to thrombospondin and laminin. Br J Haematol 109(2):322–327

Hokanson D, Sumner D, Strandness D (1975) An electrically calibrated plethysmograph for direct measurement of limb blood flow. IEEE Trans Biomed Eng 22(1):25–29

Hoover R, Rubin R, Wise G, Warren R (1979) Adhesion of normal and sickle erythrocytes to endothelial monolayer cultures. Blood 54(4):872–876

Hoppe CC (2011) Novel therapies targeting the endothelium in sickle cell disease. Hemoglobin 35(5–6):530–546

Hoppe CC (2014) Inflammatory mediators of endothelial injury in sickle cell disease. Hematol Oncol Clin North Am 28(2):265–286

Hotchkiss RS, Strasser A, McDunn JE, Swanson PE (2009) Cell death. N Engl J Med 361(16):1570–1583

Hsu L, Ataga KI, Gordeuk VR et al (2008) Tetrahydrobiopterin (6R-BH4): novel therapy for endothelial dysfunction in sickle cell disease. Blood 112(11):LB-5 (Abstract)

Huie R, Padmaja S (1993) The reaction of NO with superoxide. Free Radic Res Commun 18(4):195–199

Huribal M, Kumar R, Cunningham ME, Sumpio BE, McMillen MA (1994) Endothelin-stimulated monocyte supernatants enhance neutrophil superoxide production. Shock 1(3):184–187

Irwin DC, Baek JH, Hassell K et al (2015) Hemoglobin-induced lung vascular oxidation, inflammation, and remodeling contribute to the progression of hypoxic pulmonary hypertension and is attenuated in rats with repeated-dose haptoglobin administration. Free Radic Biol Med 82:50–62

Isbell TS, Sun CW, Wu C et al (2008) SNO-hemoglobin is not essential for red blood cell-dependent hypoxic vasodilation. Nat Med 14(7):773–777

Iyamu EW, Cecil R, Parkin L, Woods G, Ohene-Frempong K, Asakura T (2005) Modulation of erythrocyte arginase activity in sickle cell disease patients during hydroxyurea therapy. Br J Haematol 131(3):389–394

Janas J, Sitkiewicz D, Januszewicz A, Szczesniak C, Grenda R, Janas RM (2000) Endothelin-1 inactivating peptidase in the human kidney and urine. J Hypertens 18(4):475–483

Johnson C, Telen MJ (2008) Adhesion molecules and hydroxyurea in the pathophysiology of sickle cell disease. Haematologica 93(4):481–485

Joneckis CC, Ackley RL, Orringer EP, Wayner EA, Parise LV (1993) Integrin alpha 4 beta 1 and glycoprotein IV (CD36) are expressed on circulating reticulocytes in sickle cell anemia. Blood 82(12):3548–3555

Joyner MJ, Casey DP (2014) Muscle blood flow, hypoxia, and hypoperfusion. J Appl Physiol 2116(7):852–857

Kasar M, Boğa C, Yeral M, Asma S, Kozanoglu I, Ozdogu H (2014) Clinical significance of circulating blood and endothelial cell microparticles in sickle-cell disease. J Thromb Thrombolysis 38(2):167–175

Kassim AA, DeBaun MR (2013) Sickle cell disease, vasculopathy, and therapeutics. Annu Rev Med 64:451–466

Kato GJ, Wang Z, Machado RF, Blackwelder WC, Taylor JG, Hazen SL (2009) Endogenous nitric oxide synthase inhibitors in sickle cell disease: abnormal levels and correlations with pulmonary hypertension, desaturation, haemolysis, organ dysfunction and death. Br J Haematol 145(4):506–513.

Kato GJ (2015) Defective nitric oxide metabolism in sickle cell disease. Pediatr Blood Cancer 62(3):373–374

Kaul DK, Hebbel RP (2000) Hypoxia/reoxygenation causes inflammatory response in transgenic sickle mice but not in normal mice. J Clin Invest 106(3):411

Kaul DK, Fabry ME, Costantini F, Rubin EM, Nagel RL (1995) In vivo demonstration of red cell-endothelial interaction, sickling and altered microvascular response to oxygen in the sickle transgenic mouse. J Clin Invest 96(6):2845–2853

Kaul DK, Liu X-D, Fabry ME, Nagel RL (2000) Impaired nitric oxide-mediated vasodilation in transgenic sickle mouse. Am J Physiol Heart Circ Physiol 278(6):H1799–H1806

Kaul DK, Zhang X, Dasgupta T, Fabry ME (2008) Arginine therapy of transgenic-knockout sickle mice improves microvascular function by reducing non-nitric oxide vasodilators, hemolysis, and oxidative stress. Am J Physiol Heart Circ Physiol 295(1):H39–H47

Kehinde MO, Ogungbemi SI, Anigbogu CN, Jaja SI (2015) l-Arginine supplementation enhances antioxidant activity and erythrocyte integrity in sickle cell anaemia subjects. Pathophysiology 22(3):137–142

Kim JH, Bugaj LJ, Oh YJ et al (2009) Arginase inhibition restores NOS coupling and reverses endothelial dysfunction and vascular stiffness in old rats. J Appl Physiol (1985) 107(4): 1249–1257

Kleinbongard P, Schulz R, Rassaf T et al (2006) Red blood cells express a functional endothelial nitric oxide synthase. Blood 107:2943–2951

Klings ES, Machado RF, Barst RJ et al (2014) An official American thoracic society clinical practice guideline: diagnosis, risk stratification, and management of pulmonary hypertension of sickle cell disease. Am J Respir Crit Care Med 189(6):727–740

Kojda G, Cheng YC, Burchfield J, Harrison DG (2001) Dysfunctional regulation of endothelial nitric oxide synthase (eNOS) expression in response to exercise in mice lacking one eNOS gene. Circulation 103(23):2839–2844

Kulandavelu S, Balkan W, Hare JM (2015) Regulation of oxygen delivery to the body via hypoxic vasodilation. Proc Natl Acad Sci U S A 112(20):6254–6255

Kutlar A, Embury SH (2014) Cellular adhesion and the endothelium: P-selectin. Hematol Oncol Clin North Am 28(2):323–339

Kuypers FA (2014) Hemoglobin s polymerization and red cell membrane changes. Hematol Oncol Clin North Am 28(2):155–179

Landburg PP, Teerlink T, Muskiet FAJ, Duits AJ, Schnog J-JB, CURAMA study group (2008) Plasma concentrations of asymmetric dimethylarginine, an endogenous nitric oxide synthase inhibitor, are elevated in sickle cell patients but do not increase further during painful crisis. Am J Hematol 83(7):577–579

Landburg PP, Nur E, Maria N et al (2009) Elevated circulating stromal-derived factor-1 levels in sickle cell disease. Acta Haematol 122(1):64–69

Landburg PP, Teerlink T, Biemond BJ et al (2010) Plasma asymmetric dimethylarginine concentrations in sickle cell disease are related to the hemolytic phenotype. Blood Cells Mol Dis 44(4):229–232

Lang JD, Teng X, Chumley P et al (2007) Inhaled NO accelerates restoration of liver function in adults following orthotopic liver transplantation. J Clin Invest 117(9):2583–2591

Leight L, Snider TH, Clifford GO, Hellems HK (1954) Hemodynamic studies in sickle cell anemia. Circulation 10(5):653–662

Lester LA, Sodt PC, Hutcheon N, Arcilla RA (1990) Cardiac abnormalities in children with sickle cell anemia. Chest 98(5):1169–1174

Lindsay J Jr, Meshel JC, Patterson RH (1974) The cardiovascular manifestations of sickle cell disease. Arch Intern Med 133(4):643–651

Lionnet F, Bachmeyer C, Stankovic K, Tharaux PL, Girot R, Aractingi S (2008) Efficacy of the endothelin receptor blocker bosentan for refractory sickle cell leg ulcers. Br J Haematol 142(6):991–992
Lipowsky HH, Sheikh NU, Katz DM (1987) Intravital microscopy of capillary hemodynamics in sickle cell disease. J Clin Invest 80(1):117–127
Longenecker GL, Mankad V (1983) Decreased prostacyclin levels in sickle cell disease. Pediatrics 71(5):860–861
Lonsdorfer J, Bogui P, Otayeck A, Bursaux E, Poyart C, Cabannes R (1983) Cardiorespiratory adjustments in chronic sickle cell anemia. Bull Eur Physiopathol Respir 19(4):339–344
Lopes FCM, Ferreira R, Albuquerque DM et al (2014) In vitro and in vivo anti-angiogenic effects of hydroxyurea. Microvasc Res 94:106–113
Lopes FCM, Traina F, Almeida CB et al (2015) Key endothelial cell angiogenic mechanisms are stimulated by the circulating milieu in sickle cell disease and attenuated by hydroxyurea. Haematologica 100(6):730–739
Lopez BL, Kreshak AA, Morris CR, Davis-Moon L, Ballas SK, Ma XL (2003) L-arginine levels are diminished in adult acute vaso-occlusive sickle cell crisis in the emergency department. Br J Haematol 120(3):532–534
Lowenstein CJ, Morrell CN, Yamakuchi M (2005) Regulation of Weibel–Palade body exocytosis. Trends Cardiovasc Med 15(8):302–308
Machado RF, Barst RJ, Yovetich NA et al (2011) Hospitalization for pain in patients with sickle cell disease treated with sildenafil for elevated TRV and low exercise capacity. Blood 118(4):855–864
Mack AK, McGowan Ii VR, Tremonti CK et al (2008) Sodium nitrite promotes regional blood flow in patients with sickle cell disease: a phase I/II study. Br J Haematol 142(6):971–978
Manfredi F, Spoto AP, Saltzman HA, Sieker HO (1960) Studies of peripheral circulation during sickle-cell crisis. Circulation 22(4):602–607
Manodori AB, Barabino GA, Lubin BH, Kuypers FA (2000) Adherence of phosphatidylserine-exposing erythrocytes to endothelial matrix thrombospondin. Blood 95(4):1293–1300
Marshall JM (2001) Roles of adenosine and nitric oxide in skeletal muscle in acute and chronic hypoxia. Adv Exp Med Biol 502:349–363
Martin C, Yu AY, Jiang BH et al (1998) Cardiac hypertrophy in chronically anemic fetal sheep: Increased vascularization is associated with increased myocardial expression of vascular endothelial growth factor and hypoxia-inducible factor 1. Am J Obstet Gynecol 178(3):527–534
Mascia L, Fedorko L, Stewart DJ et al (2001) Temporal relationship between endothelin-1 concentrations and cerebral vasospasm in patients with aneurysmal subarachnoid hemorrhage. Stroke 32(5):1185–1190
Mathru M, Huda R, Solanki DR, Hays S, Lang JD (2007) Inhaled nitric oxide attenuates reperfusion inflammatory responses in humans. Anesthesiology 106(2):275–282
Matsui NM, Borsig L, Rosen SD, Yaghmai M, Varki A, Embury SH (2001) P-selectin mediates the adhesion of sickle erythrocytes to the endothelium. Blood 98(6):1955–1962
McCarron RM, Wang L, Stanimirovic DB, Spatz M (1993) Endothelin induction of adhesion molecule expression on human brain microvascular endothelial cells. Neurosci Lett 156(1–2): 31–34
McMillen MA, Sumpio BE (1995) Endothelins: polyfunctional cytokines. J Am Coll Surg 180(5):621–637
Mehta P, Albiol L (1982) Prostacyclin and platelet aggregation in sickle cell disease. Pediatrics 70(3):354–359
Meier ER, Wright EC, Miller JL (2014) Reticulocytosis and anemia are associated with an increased risk of death and stroke in the newborn cohort of the cooperative study of sickle cell disease. Am J Hematol 89(9):904–906
Meredith IT, Currie KE, Anderson TJ, Roddy MA, Ganz P, Creager MA (1996) Postischemic vasodilation in human forearm is dependent on endothelium-derived nitric oxide. Am J Physiol Heart Circ Physiol 270(4):H1435–H1440

Miller VM, Vanhoutte PM (1988) Enhanced release of endothelium-derived factor(s) by chronic increases in blood flow. Am J Physiol Heart Circ Physiol 255(3):H446–H451

Miller VM, Aarhus LL, Vanhoutte PM (1986) Modulation of endothelium-dependent responses by chronic alterations of blood flow. Am J Physiol Heart Circ Physiol 251(3):H520–H527

Minneci PC, Deans KJ, Zhi H et al (2005) Hemolysis-associated endothelial dysfunction mediated by accelerated NO inactivation by decompartmentalized oxyhemoglobin. J Clin Invest 115(12):3409–3417

Minniti CP, Machado RF, Coles WA, Sachdev V, Gladwin MT, Kato GJ (2009) Endothelin receptor antagonists for pulmonary hypertension in adult patients with sickle cell disease. Br J Haematol 147(5):737–743

Minniti CP, Delaney KM, Gorbach AM et al (2014) Vasculopathy, inflammation, and blood flow in leg ulcers of patients with sickle cell anemia. Am J Hematol 89(1):1–6

Mitropoulos PG, Chatziralli IP, Parikakis EA, Peponis VG, Amariotakis GA, Moschos MM (2014) Intravitreal ranibizumab for stage IV proliferative sickle cell retinopathy: a first case report. Case Rep Ophthalmol Med 2014:1–6

Mohan JS (2005) The angiopoietin/Tie-2 system in proliferative sickle retinopathy: relation to vascular endothelial growth factor, its soluble receptor Flt-1 and von Willebrand factor, and to the effects of laser treatment. Br J Ophthalmol 89(7):815–819

Mohan JS, Lip GYH, Blann AD, Bareford D, Marshall JM (2011) Endothelium-dependent and endothelium-independent vasodilatation of the cutaneous circulation in sickle cell disease. Eur J Clin Invest 41(5):546–551

Moncada S, Higgs A (2006a) The vascular endothelium II. Springer

Moncada S, Higgs A (2006b) The vascular endothelium I. Springer

Moncada S, Gryglewski R, Bunting S, Vane JR (1976) An enzyme isolated from arteries transforms prostaglandin endoperoxides to an unstable substance that inhibits platelet aggregation. Nature 263(5579):663–665

Moncada S, Vane JR, Whittle BJ (1977) Relative potency of prostacyclin, prostaglandin E1 and D2 as inhibitors of platelet aggregation in several species. J Physiol 273(2):2P–4P

Moreira JA, Laurentino MR, Machado RPG et al (2015) Pattern of hemolysis parameters and association with fetal hemoglobin in sickle cell anemia patients in steady state. Rev Bras Hematol Hemoter 37(3):167–171

Morris CR, Kuypers FA, Larkin S et al (2000) Arginine therapy: a novel strategy to induce nitric oxide production in sickle cell disease. Br J Haematol 111(2):498–500

Morris C, Kato G, Poljakovic M et al (2005) Dysregulated arginine metabolism, hemolysis-associated pulmonary hypertension, and mortality in sickle cell disease. JAMA 294(1):81–90

Morris CR, Kuypers FA, Lavrisha L et al (2013) A randomized, placebo-controlled trial of arginine therapy for the treatment of children with sickle cell disease hospitalized with vaso-occlusive pain episodes. Haematologica 98(9):1375–1382

Muller-Eberhard U, Javid J, Liem HH, Hanstein A, Hanna M (1968) Brief report: plasma concentrations of hemopexin, haptoglobin and heme in patients with various hemolytic diseases. Blood 32(5):811–815

Murray JF, Escobar E (1968) Circulatory effects of blood viscosity: comparison of methemoglobinemia and anemia. J Appl Physiol 25(5):594–599

Mushemi-Blake S, Melikian N, Drasar E et al (2015) Pulmonary haemodynamics in sickle cell disease are driven predominantly by a high-output state rather than elevated pulmonary vascular resistance: a prospective 3-dimensional echocardiography/Doppler study. PLoS One 10(8), e0135472

Nadler SP, Zimpelmann JA, Hebert RL (1992) Endothelin inhibits vasopressin-stimulated water permeability in rat terminal inner medullary collecting duct. J Clin Invest 90(4):1458

Nahavandi M, Wyche MQ, Perlin E, Tavakkoli F, Castro O (2000) Nitric oxide metabolites in sickle cell anemia patients after oral administration of hydroxyurea; hemoglobinopathy. Hematology 5(4):335–339

Nahavandi M, Millis RM, Tavakkoli F et al (2002) Arterialization of peripheral venous blood in sickle cell disease. J Natl Med Assoc 94(5):320–326

Nambi P, Pullen M, Wu HL, Aiyar N, Ohlstein EH, Edwards RM (1992) Identification of endothelin receptor subtypes in human renal cortex and medulla using subtype-selective ligands. Endocrinology 131(3):1081–1086

Nielsen MJ, Møller HJ, Moestrup SK (2010) Hemoglobin and heme scavenger receptors. Antioxid Redox Signal 12(2):261–273

Niu X, Nouraie M, Campbell A et al (2009) Angiogenic and inflammatory markers of cardiopulmonary changes in children and adolescents with sickle cell disease. PLoS One 4(11):e7956

Oishi R, Nonoguchi H, Tomita K, Marumo F (1991) Endothelin-1 inhibits AVP-stimulated osmotic water permeability in rat inner medullary collecting duct. Am J Physiol 261(6):F951–F956

Omodeo-Sale F, Cortelezzi L, Vommaro Z, Scaccabarozzi D, Dondorp AM (2010) Dysregulation of L-arginine metabolism and bioavailability associated to free plasma heme. Am J Physiol Cell Physiol 299:C148–C154

Osarogiagbon UR, Choong S, Belcher JD, Vercellotti GM, Paller MS, Hebbel RP (2000) Reperfusion injury pathophysiology in sickle transgenic mice. Blood 96(1):314–320

Ou J, Ou Z, Jones DW et al (2003) L-4 F, an apolipoprotein A-1 mimetic, dramatically improves vasodilation in hypercholesterolemia and sickle cell disease. Circulation 107(18):2337–2341

Palmer RM, Ferrige AG, Moncada S (1987) Nitric oxide release accounts for the biological activity of endothelium-derived relaxing factor. Nature 327:524–526

Palmer RM, Rees DD, Ashton DS, Moncada S (1988) L-arginine is the physiological precursor for the formation of nitric oxide in endothelium-dependent relaxation. Biochem Biophys Res Commun 153:1251–1256

Park SW, Kim M, Brown KM, D'Agati VD, Lee HT (2011) Paneth cell-derived interleukin-17A causes multiorgan dysfunction after hepatic ischemia and reperfusion injury. Hepatology 53(5):1662–1675

Patel N, Gonsalves CS, Malik P, Kalra VK (2008) Placenta growth factor augments endothelin-1 and endothelin-B receptor expression via hypoxia-inducible factor-1 alpha. Blood 112(3): 856–865

Pegelow CH, Colangelo L, Steinberg M, Wright EC, Smith J, Phillips G, Vichinsky E (1997) Natural history of blood pressure in sickle cell disease: risks for stroke and death associated with relative hypertension in sickle cell anemia. Am J Med 102(2):171–177

Perelman N, Selvaraj SK, Batra S et al (2003) Placenta growth factor activates monocytes and correlates with sickle cell disease severity. Blood 102(4):1506–1514

Phelan M, Perrine SP, Brauer M, Faller DV (1995) Sickle erythrocytes, after sickling, regulate the expression of the endothelin-1 gene and protein in human endothelial cells in culture. J Clin Invest 96(2):1145–1151

Pianosi P, D'souza SJA, Charge TD, Béland MJ, Esseltine DW, Coates AL (1991) Cardiac output and oxygen delivery during exercise in sickle cell anemia. Am Rev Respir Dis 143(2):231–235

Polanowska-Grabowska R, Wallace K, Field JJ et al (2010) P-selectin–mediated platelet-neutrophil aggregate formation activates neutrophils in mouse and human sickle cell disease. Arterioscler Thromb Vasc Biol 30(12):2392–2399

Potoka KP, Gladwin MT (2015) Vasculopathy and pulmonary hypertension in sickle cell disease. Am J Physiol Lung Cell Mol Physiol 308(4):L314–L324

Pritchard KA Jr, Ou J, Ou Z et al (2004) Hypoxia-induced acute lung injury in murine models of sickle cell disease. Am J Physiol Lung Cell Mol Physiol 286(4):L705–L714

Rakusan K, Cicutti N, Kolar F (2001) Effect of anemia on cardiac function, microvascular structure, and capillary hematocrit in rat hearts. Am J Physiol Heart Circ Physiol 280(3):H1407–H1414

Reiter CD, Wang X, Tanus-Santos JE et al (2002) Cell-free hemoglobin limits nitric oxide bioavailability in sickle-cell disease. Nat Med 8(12):1383–1389

Rivera A, Rotter MA, Brugnara C (1999) Endothelins activate Ca(2+)-gated K(+) channels via endothelin B receptors in CD-1 mouse erythrocytes. Am J Physiol Cell Physiol 277(4): C746–C754

Rivera A, Jarolim P, Brugnara C (2002) Modulation of Gardos channel activity by cytokines in sickle erythrocytes. Blood 99(1):357–363

Rodgers GP, Schechter AN, Noguchi CT, Klein HG, Nienhuis AW, Bonner RF (1990) Microcirculatory adaptations in sickle cell anemia: reactive hyperemia response. Am J Physiol Heart Circ Physiol 258(1):H113–H120

Rodgers GP, Walker EC, Podgor MJ (1993) Is "relative" hypertension a risk factor for vaso-occlusive complications in sickle cell disease? Am J Med Sci 305(3):150–156

Romero JR, Suzuka SM, Nagel RL, Fabry ME (2002) Arginine supplementation of sickle transgenic mice reduces red cell density and Gardos channel activity. Blood 99(4):1103–1108

Roy SB, Bhatia ML, Mathur VS, Virmani S (1963) Hemodynamic effects of chronic severe anemia. Circulation 28(3):346–356

Rybicki AC, Benjamin LJ (1998) Increased levels of endothelin-1 in plasma of sickle cell anemia patients. Blood 92(7):2594–2596

Sabaa N, de Franceschi L, Bonnin P et al (2008) Endothelin receptor antagonism prevents hypoxia-induced mortality and morbidity in a mouse model of sickle-cell disease. J Clin Invest 118(5):1924–1933

Sachdev V, Machado R, Shizukuda Y et al (2007) Diastolic dysfunction is an independent risk factor for death in patients with sickle cell disease. J Am Coll Cardiol 49(4):472–479

Safo MK, Kato GJ (2014) Therapeutic strategies to alter the oxygen affinity of sickle hemoglobin. Hematol Oncol Clin North Am 28(2):217–231

Sakamoto TM, Canalli AA, Traina F et al (2013) Altered red cell and platelet adhesion in hemolytic diseases: hereditary spherocytosis, paroxysmal nocturnal hemoglobinuria and sickle cell disease. Clin Biochem 46(18):1798–1803

Şan M, Demirtaş M, Burgut R, Birand A, Başlamişh F (1998) Left ventricular systolic and diastolic functions in patients with sickle cell anemia. Int J Angiol 7(3):185–187

Schaer DJ, Vinchi F, Ingoglia G, Tolosano E, Buehler PW (2014) Haptoglobin, hemopexin, and related defense pathways-basic science, clinical perspectives, and drug development. Front Physiol 5:415

Schnog JB, Jager EH, van der Dijs FPL et al (2004) Evidence for a metabolic shift of arginine metabolism in sickle cell disease. Ann Hematol 83(6):371–375

Schnog JB, Teerlink T, van der Dijs FPL, Duits AJ, Muskiet FA, CURAMA Study Group (2005) Plasma levels of asymmetric dimethylarginine (ADMA), an endogenous nitric oxide synthase inhibitor, are elevated in sickle cell disease. Ann Hematol 84(5):282–286

Schrage WG, Joyner MJ, Dinenno FA (2004) Local inhibition of nitric oxide and prostaglandins independently reduces forearm exercise hyperaemia in humans. J Physiol 557(2):599–611

Schwartz RS, Eltzschig HK, Carmeliet P (2011) Hypoxia and inflammation. N Engl J Med 364(7):656–665

Scoffone HM, Krajewski M, Zorca S et al (2013) Effect of extended-release niacin on serum lipids and on endothelial function in adults with sickle cell anemia and low high-density lipoprotein cholesterol levels. Am J Cardiol 112(9):1499–1504

Sebastiani P, Ramoni MF, Nolan V, Baldwin CT, Steinberg MH (2005) Genetic dissection and prognostic modeling of overt stroke in sickle cell anemia. Nat Genet 37(4):435–440

Seeler RA, Royal JE, Powe L, Goldberg HR (1978) Moyamoya in children with sickle cell anemia and cerebrovascular occlusion. J Pediatr 193(5):808–810

Setty BNY, Kulkarni S, Stuart MJ (2002) Role of erythrocyte phosphatidylserine in sickle red cell-endothelial adhesion. Blood 99(5):1564–1571

Shaikh S (2008) Intravitreal bevacizumab (Avastin) for the treatment of proliferative sickle retinopathy. Indian J Ophthalmol 56(3):259

Sher GD, Olivieri NF (1994) Rapid healing of chronic leg ulcers during arginine butyrate therapy in patients with sickle cell disease and thalassemia. Blood 84(7):2378–2380

Shiu YT, McIntire LV, Udden MM (2002) Sickle erythrocytes increase prostacyclin and endothelin-1 production by cultured human endothelial cells under flow conditions. Eur J Haematol 68(3):163–169

Siqueira RC, Costa RA, Scott IU, Cintra LP, Jorge R (2006) Intravitreal bevacizumab (Avastin) injection associated with regression of retinal neovascularization caused by sickle cell retinopathy. Acta Ophthalmol Scand 84(6):834–835

Solovey AA, Solovey AN, Harkness J, Hebbel RP (2001) Modulation of endothelial cell activation in sickle cell disease: a pilot study. Blood 97(7):1937–1941

Solovey A, Kollander R, Shet A et al (2004) Endothelial cell expression of tissue factor in sickle mice is augmented by hypoxia/reoxygenation and inhibited by lovastatin. Blood 104(3):840–846

SoRelle R (1998) Nobel prize awarded to scientists for nitric oxide discoveries. Circulation 98(22):2365–2366

Sowemimo-Coker SO, Haywood LJ, Meiselman HJ, Francis RB (1992) Effects of normal and sickle erythrocytes on prostacyclin release by perfused human umbilical cord veins. Am J Hematol 40(4):276–282

Sproule BJ, Halden ER, Miller WF (1958) A study of cardiopulmonary alterations in patients with sickle cell disease and its variants. J Clin Invest 37(3):486–495

Styles LA, Lubin B, Vichinsky E et al (1997) Decrease of very late activation antigen-4 and CD36 on reticulocytes in sickle cell patients treated with hydroxyurea. Blood 89(7):2554–2559

Sundaram N, Tailor A, Mendelsohn L et al (2010) High levels of placenta growth factor in sickle cell disease promote pulmonary hypertension. Blood 116(1):109–112

Sylvester KP, Patey RA, Rafferty GF, Rees D, Thein SL, Greenough A (2004) Exhaled carbon monoxide levels in children with sickle cell disease. Eur J Pediatr 164(3):162–165

Telen MJ (2014) Cellular adhesion and the endothelium. Hematol Oncol Clin North Am 28(2):341–354

Tharaux PL, Hagège I, Placier S et al (2005) Urinary endothelin-1 as a marker of renal damage in sickle cell disease. Nephrol Dial Transplant 20(11):2408–2413

Tharaux PL, Girot R, Kanfer A et al (2002) Cutaneous microvascular blood flow and reactivity in patients with homozygous sickle cell anaemia. Eur J Haematol 68(6):327–331

Tordjman R, Delaire S, Plouët J et al (2001) Erythroblasts are a source of angiogenic factors. Blood 97(7):1968–1974

Turhan A, Weiss LA, Mohandas N, Coller BS, Frenette PS (2002) Primary role for adherent leukocytes in sickle cell vascular occlusion: a new paradigm. Proc Natl Acad Sci U S A 99(5):3047–3051

Uematsu M, Ohara Y, Navas JP et al (1995) Regulation of endothelial cell nitric oxide synthase mRNA expression by shear stress. Am J Physiol 269(6 Pt 1):C1371–C1378

Usami S, Chien S, Scholtz PM, Bertles JF (1975) Effect of deoxygenation on blood rheology in sickle cell disease. Microvasc Res 9(3):324–334

van Beers EJ, Yang Y, Raghavachari N et al (2015) Iron, inflammation, and early death in adults with sickle cell disease. Circ Res 116(2):298–306

Varat MA, Adolph RJ, Fowler NO (1972) Cardiovascular effects of anemia. Am Heart J 83(3):415–426

Vinchi F, De Franceschi L, Ghigo A et al (2013) Hemopexin therapy improves cardiovascular function by preventing heme-induced endothelial toxicity in mouse models of hemolytic diseases. Circulation 127(12):1317–1329

Voskaridou E, Christoulas D, Terpos E (2012) Sickle-cell disease and the heart: review of the current literature. Br J Haematol 157(6):664–673

Wang H, Luo W, Wang J et al (2013) Paradoxical protection from atherosclerosis and thrombosis in a mouse model of sickle cell disease. Br J Haematol 162(1):120–129

Wang X, Mendelsohn L, Rogers H et al (2014) Heme-bound iron activates placenta growth factor in erythroid cells via erythroid Krüppel-like factor. Blood 124(6):946–954

Wautier MP, HéRon E, Picot J, Colin Y, Hermine O, Wautier JL (2011) Red blood cell phosphatidylserine exposure is responsible for increased erythrocyte adhesion to endothelium in central retinal vein occlusion: central retinal vein occlusion and RBC adhesion. J Thromb Haemost 9(5):1049–1055

Weksler BB, Marcus AJ, Jaffe EA (1977) Synthesis of prostaglandin I2 (prostacyclin) by cultured human and bovine endothelial cells. Proc Natl Acad Sci U S A 74(9):3922–3926

Wood KC, Cortese-Krott MM, Kovacic JC et al (2013) Circulating blood endothelial nitric oxide synthase contributes to the regulation of systemic blood pressure and nitrite homeostasis. Arterioscler Thromb Vasc Biol 33(8):1861–1871

Wun T, Paglieroni T, Rangaswami A et al (1998) Platelet activation in patients with sickle cell disease. Br J Haematol 100(4):741–749

Wyche MQ, Perlin E, Millis RM, Nahavandi M, Tavakkoli F (2003) Arterialization of venous blood for differentiation of sickle cell subjects in vaso-occlusive crisis. Hematology 8(6):421–428

Yanagisawa M, Kurihara H, Kimura S et al (1988) A novel potent vasoconstrictor peptide produced by vascular endothelial cells. Nature 332(6163):411–415

Yuditskaya S, Tumblin A, Hoehn G et al (2009) Proteomic identification of altered apolipoprotein patterns in pulmonary hypertension and vasculopathy of sickle cell disease. Blood 113(5):1122–1128

Zawar SD, Vyawahare MA, Nerkar M, Jawahirani AR (2005) Non-invasive detection of endothelial dysfunction in sickle cell disease by Doppler ultrasonography. J Assoc Physicians India 53:677–680

Zhang Y, Berka V, Song A et al (2014) Elevated sphingosine-1-phosphate promotes sickling and sickle cell disease progression. J Clin Invest 124(6):2750–2761

Zhang R, Hess DT, Qian Z et al (2015) Hemoglobin βCys93 is essential for cardiovascular function and integrated response to hypoxia. Proc Natl Acad Sci U S A 112(20):6425–6430

Zoll PM, Wessler S, Schlesinger MJ (1951) Interarterial coronary anastomoses in the human heart, with particular reference to anemia and relative cardiac anoxia. Circulation 4(6):797–815

Zoll PM, Norman LR, Cassin S (1952) The effects of vasomotor drugs and of anemia upon interarterial coronary anastomoses. Circulation 6(6):832–842

Chapter 8
Inflammation and Sickle Cell Anemia

Camila Bononi de Almeida, Gregory J. Kato, and Nicola Conran

Abstract Inflammatory processes play a key role in the initiation of the acute painful vaso-occlusive crises that constitute the main cause of hospitalization in individuals with sickle cell anemia, as well as many of its numerous complications, including autosplenectomy, pulmonary hypertension, acute chest syndrome, leg ulcers, nephropathy and stroke. Ischemia-reperfusion injury (due to microvascular and macrovascular occlusions), membrane alterations of the sickle red blood cell, and hemolysis may all trigger endogenous proinflammatory signals (damage-associated molecular patterns-DAMPs) that lead to the vicious circle of pan-cellular activation, inflammatory mediator release, leukocyte recruitment and occlusive mechanisms that result in the chronic inflammatory state that is associated with sickle cell anemia. We, herein, review the probable primary inflammatory triggers that initiate inflammatory mechanisms in the disease and postulate the cells and molecules that may contribute to establish chronic inflammation. The anti-inflammatory effects of hydroxyurea are discussed, as are novel anti-inflammatory approaches currently under study.

Keywords Cytokine • DAMPs • Endothelium • Ischemia-reperfusion • Leukocytes

---

C.B. de Almeida
Instituto Israelita de Ensino e Pesquisa Albert Einstein, Hospital Israelita Albert Einstein, São Paulo, São Paulo, Brazil
e-mail: camilalmeida@hotmail.com

G.J. Kato
Sickle Cell Center of Excellence, University of Pittsburgh Medical Center, Pittsburgh, PA 15261, USA
e-mail: katogj@upmc.edu

N. Conran (✉)
Hematology Center, School of Medical Science, University of Campinas – UNICAMP, Campinas, São Paulo, Brazil
e-mail: conran@unicamp.br

© Springer International Publishing Switzerland 2016

F.F. Costa, N. Conran (eds.), *Sickle Cell Anemia*,
DOI 10.1007/978-3-319-06713-1_8

8.1 Introduction

Inflammation constitutes the adaptive response of the cells of an organism to a stimulus, such as infection or tissue injury, that has the objective of restoring organ function and homeostasis. While the inflammatory response to invasion by pathogens has long been characterized, non-microbial activators also trigger inflammatory mechanisms in processes of sterile inflammation (Shen et al. 2013). Sterile inflammation occurs during acute conditions of tissue injury and following events such as ischemia-reperfusion injury, as well as manifesting as chronic inflammation in certain diseases, such as atherosclerosis and sickle cell anemia (SCA) (Chen and Nunez 2010).

Tissue stress or injury can lead to the release of endogenous molecules that act as damage-associated molecular patterns (DAMPs), setting inflammatory processes in motion (Bianchi 2007). Although inflammatory responses are important for repairing tissue and eliminating harmful molecules, unresolved inflammation, due to constant tissue damage and the failure to remove harmful inflammatory stimuli, can be detrimental to the organism and result in tissue destruction (Chen and Nunez 2010). In the case of sickle cell anemia, ischemia-reperfusion injury (due to microvascular and macrovascular occlusions and their consequent resolution), red blood cell membrane alterations, and hemolysis may all trigger proinflammatory signals that lead to the vicious circle of pan-cellular activation and occlusive mechanisms that result in the chronic inflammatory state associated with SCA. These inflammatory processes play a key role in the initiation of the acute painful crises that represent the main cause of hospitalization in individuals with the disease (Ballas and Lusardi 2005) and many of its numerous manifestations, including autosplenectomy (Brousse et al. 2014), pulmonary hypertension (Brittain et al. 2010; Ataga et al. 2008), acute chest syndrome (Hebbel 2014), leg ulcers (Minniti et al. 2014), nephropathy (Nath and Hebbel 2015), impaired cognitive function (Andreotti et al. 2014) and stroke (De Montalembert and Wang 2013).

8.2 Orchestration of Sterile Inflammatory Responses

Endogenous inflammatory triggers, or DAMPs, released by apoptotic or necrotic cells, following injury, or by erythrocytes undergoing hemolytic processes, can be detected by inflammatory cells such as monocytes, T-cells, neutrophils, macrophages and dendritic cells (van Golen et al. 2012). Necrotic cells release a range of DAMPs, including high-mobility group box 1 (HMGB1) and purine metabolites such as ATP, while ruptured erythrocytes liberate cell-free hemoglobin; furthermore, damage to the extracellular matrix during tissue injury results in the release of molecules such as small leucine-rich proteoglycans (SLRPs) and hyaluronan fragments (Moreth et al. 2012). Intracellular stores of pro-inflammatory cytokines, such as IL-1α and IL-33, can also be released by necrotic cells, together with reactive oxygen species (ROS) and activated proteases, all of which can stimulate sterile inflammatory pathways (Chen and Nunez 2010).

Once released, these DAMPs and sterile inflammatory stimuli, in turn, activate cells via interactions with a range of membrane surface receptors that include the toll-like receptors (TLR)-2,-4 and -9, receptor for advanced glycation end products (RAGE) and the purinergic $P2X_7$ receptor, as well as intracellular receptors, such as NOD-like receptor pyrin domain containing 3 (NLRP3) (Lister et al. 2007; Shen et al. 2013; Weber et al. 2015). Activation of these receptors results in gene transcription and the production of inflammatory cytokines. In some cases, DAMP release induces the assembly of cytosolic molecular complexes, termed inflammasomes, in the inflammatory cells; the most characterized being the NLRP3 inflammasome. These complexes contain a pattern recognition receptor (PRR), typically NLRP3, which once activated recruits the adapter protein ASC (apoptosis-related speck-like protein containing a caspase recruitment domain) and pro-caspase-1. Pro-caspase-1 is then cleaved into its activated form, which then cleaves pro-interleukin (IL)-1β and pro-IL-18 into their biologically active forms (Ozaki et al. 2015). As a consequence of the release of proinflammatory cytokines, whether due to inflammasome formation or the activation of other intracellular pathways, leukocyte recruitment occurs together with further oxidative stress and inflammatory molecule production.

The cellular response to sterile inflammation, and its resolution, are similar to those of microbial inflammation. One of the first cells to be recruited to the site of injury are the neutrophils, which have a short half-life (in the range of hours when non-stimulated) and make up about 70 % of circulating human leukocytes, with numbers that can rapidly increase to propagate inflammatory responses (Kolaczkowska and Kubes 2013). Neutrophils migrate to the inflamed tissue in response to chemokine production and, in turn, stimulate the recruitment of monocytes and macrophages to the site, potentiating the inflammatory response. Leukocyte recruitment to the blood vessel wall involves a multi-step cascade, whereby adhesion molecules (namely selectins and integrins) mediate their tethering and subsequent rolling along the endothelium, followed by their arrest and transmigration into inflamed tissues (Leick et al. 2014). Activated and infiltrated neutrophils and macrophages, in addition to assisting in dead cell and debris removal, secrete chemokines and cytokines, such as TNF-α, IL-1 and IL-6, leading to endothelial activation and further immune cell recruitment (Medzhitov 2008; Shen et al. 2013). Lymphocytes, including invariant natural killer T (iNKT) cells, platelets and dendritic cells are also recruited to inflammatory sites, where they amplify endothelial and leukocyte activation, aggravating the inflammatory response due to interactions with other cells and the release of proinflammatory molecules, such as interferon (IFN)s and CD40L (Van Kaer et al. 2013; Gros et al. 2015; Chistiakov et al. 2014). Activation of inflammatory cells and their signaling pathways, in turn, leads to the production and secretion of a plethora of molecules, including proteases, growth factors and leukotrienes (Serhan et al. 2014; Shen et al. 2013; Chen and Nunez 2010).

Effective resolution of inflammation constitutes the conclusion of the recruitment of immune cells to the inflammatory site and their clearance by apoptosis or other cell death pathways (McCracken and Allen 2014). Neutrophils often undergo apoptosis following their recruitment and action at the inflammatory site, while macrophages ingest apoptotic neutrophils. Simultaneously, abrogation of chemokine signaling inhibits continued neutrophil tissue inflammation (Ortega-Gomez et al. 2013). However, in chronic diseases, such as sickle cell anemia, constant hemolytic and ischemia-reperfusion processes lead to the continuous generation of DAMPs and inflammatory stimuli that make resolution of inflammation processes difficult, if not impossible.

8.3 The Chronic Inflammatory State and Sickle Cell Disease

8.3.1 Primary Inflammatory Triggers in SCA

Multiple and complex mechanisms mediated by diverse cell types are involved in the establishment of the chronic inflammatory state in SCA, making it difficult to pinpoint specific mechanisms that trigger the initial inflammatory processes leading to chronic inflammation in the disease. It would, however, seem reasonable to assume that four primary events in sickle cell anemia pathophysiology instigate the initial processes that result in a chronic inflammatory state (see Box 8.1, Table 8.1 and Fig. 8.1).

Box 8.1: Primary Inflammatory Triggers in SCA

- Hemolytic events
- Abnormalities in the sickle red blood cell membrane (phosphatidylserine exposure, adhesion molecule expression etc.)
- Ischemia-reperfusion processes
- Oxidative stress

Table 8.1 DAMPs and primary sterile inflammatory stimuli reported in SCA

DAMPs/sterile inflammatory stimuli	Source	Event
Hemoglobin/heme	Erythrocytes	Hemolysis
HMGB1	Injured/necrotic cells	Ischemia
Extracellular heat shock proteins (HSP-70)	Injured/necrotic cells	Ischemia
ATP	Injured/necrotic cells	Hemolysis/ischemia
Circulating DNA	Injured/necrotic cells	Ischemia
IL-1α	Injured/necrotic cells	Ischemia

ATP adenosine triphosphate, *HMGB1* high mobility group box B1 protein, *IL-1α* interleukin-1α

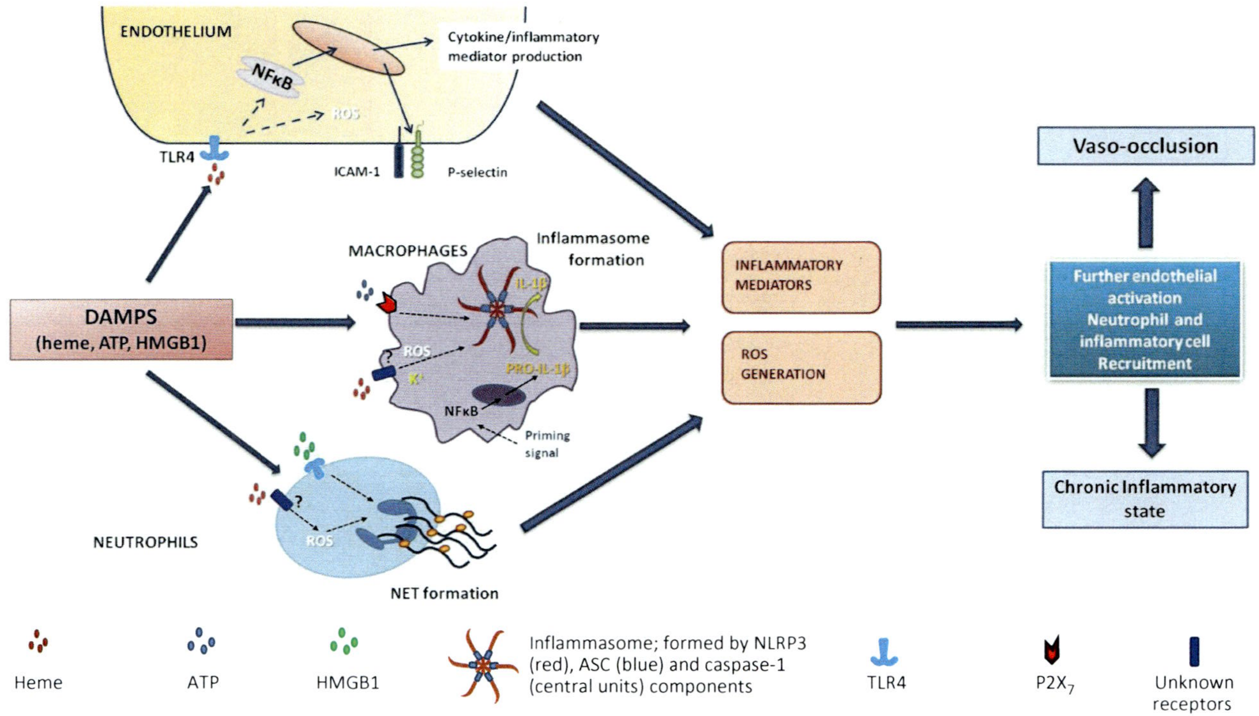

Fig. 8.1 Inflammatory stimuli in sickle cell disease. Damage-associated molecular patterns (DAMPs) are released from injured cells, due to hemolysis and ischemic injury. In turn, DAMPs such as heme, ATP and high-mobility group box 1 (HMGB1) activate endothelial cells, macrophages and leukocytes via interaction with membrane receptors such as toll-like receptor 4 (TLR4) or $P2X_7$, respectively, or other unknown receptors. In the endothelium, heme-mediated TLR4 signaling leads to reactive oxygen species (ROS) production and activates the NFκB transcription factor, resulting in the upregulation of surface adhesion molecules and inflammatory mediator production. Macrophages are previously primed, by lipopolysaccharide or cytokines such as TNF-α (or possibly by the binding of heme to TLR4), to produce Pro-IL-1β and other inflammasome components. Subsequent DAMP interaction induces the assembly of inflammasomes formed by the NLRP3 pattern recognition receptor, ASC and caspase-1. Pro-IL-1β is then cleaved by caspase-1 to form IL-1β. In neutrophils, heme and high-mobility group box 1 (HMGB1) can activate and promote NET formation, the former via ROS generation and the latter via TLR4 binding. Subsequent inflammatory mediator production and ROS generation leads to further endothelial activation and leukocyte recruitment in the blood vessel, with ensuing amplification of inflammatory molecule release and, under certain circumstances, triggering of vaso-occlusive processes

Hemolysis Hemolysis represents a major trigger of inflammation in sickle cell disease. Polymerization of HbS in red blood cells (RBC), under deoxygenated conditions, causes RBC sickling and makes the cells more rigid and less deformable leaving them more susceptible to rupture in the circulation. Ensuing intravascular hemolysis results in the release of cell-free Hb (CFHb) from the red cells, which has numerous and significant pathophysiological consequences (Kato et al. 2007; Schaer et al. 2013). Sickle cell disease hemolysis and its consequences are described in detail in other chapters of this book (Chaps. 4 and 7), but in summary, upon RBC lysis, liberation of CFHb into the blood stream results in rapid consumption of endothelium-derived nitric oxide (NO) (Reiter et al. 2002). NO produced by endothelial nitric oxide synthase (Tsoumani et al. 2012) has important anti-inflammatory effects, reducing leukocyte activation, leukocyte-endothelial interactions and oxidative stress, as well as inhibiting platelet aggregation and modulating the production of endothelin-converting enzyme-1 and some inflammatory mediators, such as tissue factor and TNF-α (Arndt et al. 1993; Hossain et al. 2012; Rubanyi et al. 1991; Wallace 2005; Kuruppu et al. 2014; Bzowska et al. 2009; Walley et al. 1999; Solovey et al. 2010). In addition to local endothelium-derived NO depletion by CFHb, in its oxidized Hb-Fe^{3+} form, Hb can release the toxic hemoglobin product, hemin. The hydrophobic hemin (also denominated heme in some reports) molecule can then bind to and oxidize proteins or lipids, generating reactive molecules, including oxidized low-density lipoprotein and reactive oxygen species (ROS), which can have potent and inflammatory and damaging effects (Schaer et al. 2013; Dutra and Bozza 2014), and cause further endothelial activation (Belcher et al. 2014). Heme-laden erythrocyte microparticles have recently been reported to be generated in sickle cell disease (SCD), and these microparticles can adhere to and transfer heme to endothelial cells, inducing oxidative stress and apoptosis (Camus et al. 2015). Additionally, heme/hemin can act as a DAMP, interacting with a number of cell surface receptors, including toll-like receptor 4 (TLR4) (Gladwin and Ofori-Acquah 2014). In SCD mice, heme/hemin administration triggers acute chest syndrome and induces vaso-occlusion via interaction with endothelial TLR4 and consequent NFκB (nuclear factor kappa B) activation, leading to the expression of adhesion molecules such as intercellular adhesion molecule (ICAM)-1 and P-selectin on the endothelial cell surface (Belcher et al. 2014; Dutra and Bozza 2014; Ghosh et al. 2013) (see Fig. 8.1). Furthermore, heme/hemin administration to SCD mice induces the release of NETs from activated neutrophils; these NETs have anti-microbial activity and consist of decondensed chromatin and granular enzymes and are likely pathogenic in the SCD setting (Chen et al. 2014). In addition to binding to cell surface receptors, heme/hemin is also a major regulator of redox-sensitive gene expression, modulating the expressions of heme oxygenase-1 (HO-1), ferritin, thioredoxin, Hsp70, c-fos and Egr-1, a regulator ofcell proliferation and apoptosis (Iwasaki et al. 2006; Hasan and Schafer 2008). New data also indicate a role for heme/hemin in inflammasome formation in lipopolysaccharide-primed macrophages, promoting NLRP3-dependent processing of interleukin (IL)-1β (Dutra et al. 2014), where such inflammasome formation probably makes an important contribution to the chronic inflammatory state in SCD (van Beers et al. 2015).

In addition to the release of CFHb, hemolysis is also accompanied by the release of ATP from the erythrocytes (Sikora et al. 2014). Extracellular ATP functions predominantly as a signaling molecule via the activation of purinergic P2 receptors (Idzko et al. 2014a); binding of ATP to the $P2X_7$ receptor, for example, leads to K^+ efflux via ATP-gated cation channel opening and may contribute to NLRP3 activation and inflammasome formation (Idzko et al. 2014b). Furthermore, extracellular ATP is rapidly converted to adenosine by ectonucleotidases; while interaction of adenosine with the Adora2a adenosine receptor may have anti-inflammatory effects by selectively inhibiting the iNKT cells, adenosine signaling through the Adora2b adenosine receptor on the RBC membrane may contribute to erythrocyte sickling in SCD (Field et al. 2014; Zhang et al. 2011).

Red Blood Cell Membrane Alterations Mature erythrocytes, under normal physiological conditions, do not adhere to other cells and present a very low-level surface adhesion molecule expression (Colin et al. 2014). However, in SCA, increased RBC turnover and physical alterations in the erythrocyte, such as dehydration, give rise to alterations in the expression of molecules on the cell surface (Kaul et al. 2009; Wood et al. 1996). RBC of SCA (SSRBC) individuals demonstrate an augmented expression of a number of adhesion molecules, including integrin $\alpha_4\beta_1$ (CD49d/CD29; very-late antigen-4), CD36, ICAM-4 and Lutheran/basal cell adhesion molecule (Lu/BCAM) (Joneckis et al. 1993; Colin et al. 2014), which facilitate their interaction with and adhesion to other cells. Adhesive interactions of SSRBC, in addition to participating in occlusive mechanisms, may induce endothelial oxidative stress and activation, upregulating the expression of surface endothelial adhesion molecules (Shiu et al. 2000; Sultana et al. 1998). Additionally, dehydrated and dense sickle red cells expose negatively-charged phosphatidylserine on their plasma membrane. In addition to interacting with phosphatidylserine receptors on the endothelial surface, these exposed glycoproteins are capable of activating the coagulation cascade, promoting further inflammation via the generation of tissue factor (Yasin et al. 2003; Setty and Betal 2008; Franck et al. 1985; Chantrathammachart et al. 2012).

Ischemia-Reperfusion Injury Ischemia-reperfusion tissue injury occurs as the result of the interruption of blood supply followed by resolution and subsequent reperfusion of the tissue (Kalogeris et al. 2012). In SCA, vaso-occlusive processes cause ischemia-induced tissue injury. Injured cells undergoing cell death mechanisms release DAMPs such as HMGB1 and heat shock proteins, known to be increased in sickle cell disease (Xu et al. 2014; Adewoye et al. 2005), and display cytosolic calcium accumulation, mitochondrial dysfunction, and cell swelling (Kalogeris et al. 2012; Hebbel 2014). HMGB1 can promote NET formation in neutrophils via a TLR4-signaling pathway, while ATP release from necrotic cells also has direct inflammatory effects, as mentioned above (Idzko et al. 2014b; Tadie et al. 2013) (Fig. 8.1). If blood flow is then restored following ischemic processes and the tissue reperfused, further damage occurs upon the reoxygenation of damaged tissues, due to the production of ROS and calcium overload (Kalogeris et al. 2012).

Ischemia-reperfusion injury can activate iNKT cells in SCA, which may subsequently contribute to the inflammatory cascade by involving IFN-γ and INF-γ-inducible chemokines (Field et al. 2011).

Oxidative Stress The production of ROS (unstable oxygen containing molecules with a tendency to easily form radicals) is augmented by a number of mechanisms in SCA. The activities of enzymes such as NADPH oxidase and xanthine oxidase are augmented as a result of leukocytosis and endothelial activation, respectively (Wood et al. 2005; Aslan et al. 2001); additionally, HbS can auto-oxidate in the presence of oxygen to produce superoxide and hydroxyl radicals (Hebbel et al. 1982) and, as mentioned above, processes of ischemia-reperfusion lead to the production of further oxygen radicals (Aslan et al. 2000). Asymmetric dimethylarginine (ADMA) formation and resulting hyperhomocysteinaemia in SCA may also lead to ROS generation and nitric oxide synthase may produce superoxide rather than NO, in the absence of L-arginine (Xia et al. 1996; Wood and Granger 2007). On the other hand, endogenous anti-oxidant defense mechanisms are altered in SCA, as individuals demonstrate a reduction in levels of important enzymatic antioxidants, including glutathione peroxidase and superoxide dismutase, and low levels of non-enzymatic antioxidants such as vitamins A, C and E (Amer et al. 2006; Natta et al. 1990; Schacter et al. 1988).

In turn, ROS can act as important secondary messengers for signaling pathways associated with cell death, damage, endothelial activation and inflammation (Bondeva and Wolf 2014). There is some evidence to suggest that ROS may activate NLRP3 and, therefore, mediate inflammasome activation, under certain circumstances (Abais et al. 2014; van Golen et al. 2012); furthermore, ROS formation has been shown to participate in heme-induced NET release from neutrophils in mice with SCD (Chen et al. 2014) (see Fig. 8.1).

8.3.2 Propagation of the Chronic Inflammatory State in SCA

In vivo imaging studies using a sickle cell mouse model demonstrate that systemic inflammation in these mice is significantly greater than that of wild type mice, as demonstrated by generalized bioluminescence visualized in these animals following their injection with a chemiluminescent probe that reacts with myeloperoxidase produced by neutrophils and phagocytes (Almeida et al. 2015). Such data exemplify the chronic inflammatory state that is known to accompany sickle cell anemia.

Following the incidence of initial inflammatory triggering mechanisms in SCA, it is probable that the consequent release of inflammatory mediators and ROS primes the endothelium, leukocytes and platelets. As previously proposed in Chap. 5, secondary inflammatory triggers (or a "second hit"), possibly consisting of an infectious or another acute inflammatory stimulus, may then be able to induce vaso-occlusive processes in the microcirculation. Given the evidence that leukocyte and inflammatory cell recruitment to the endothelium appears to constitute a key step in the initiation of the vaso-occlusive process (Turhan et al. 2002, 2004), it seems reasonable to suggest that the inflammatory state associated with SCA, comprising cellular activation and the production of inflammatory molecules, is the driving force behind the vaso-occlusive process. In turn, repeated vaso-occlusions, leading to further activation of the endothelium and leukocytes, together with ischemia result in a vicious circle of occlusive mechanisms, pancellular activation and escalating inflammatory mediator production that propagate the chronic inflammatory state associated with SCA.

8.4 Cellular Contribution to Inflammation in SCA

8.4.1 Endothelium

As described in more detail in Chap. 7, the endothelium controls vascular homeostasis, modulates local inflammation and participates in key steps of the angiogenic process (Huang and Vita 2006). Intact, non-activated endothelium usually inhibits the adhesion of inflammatory cells to the vessel wall using inhibitory and modulating mechanisms such as the production and release of NO and prostacyclin (Tsoumani et al. 2012). Reduced endothelium-derived NO bioavailability in SCD, due to hemolysis, and uncoupling of endothelial nitric oxide synthase, resulting from endothelial dysfunction (Kato et al. 2007; Reiter et al. 2002), conceivably contributes significantly to chronic inflammation in SCD, augmenting leukocyte and platelet activity, increasing endothelial interactions and amplifying inflammatory mediator production (Canalli et al. 2008).

Once activated, in addition to expressing adhesion molecules on the endothelial surface, including VCAM-1, ICAM-1 and E-selectin (Duits et al. 1996), the endothelium produces and releases a number of potent inflammatory molecules, such as IL-8, IL-6, GM-CSF, PAI-1 (plasminogen activator inhibitor-1), MCP-1 (monocyte chemotactic protein-1), IL-1α, RANTES and further IL-1β (Table 8.2) (Proenca-Ferreira et al. 2014; Sakamoto et al. 2013; Pathare et al. 2004; Conran et al. 2007a; Zachlederova and Jarolim 2000; Patel et al. 2010; Almeida et al. 2015). These potent inflammatory mediators contribute to the chronic inflammatory state in SCD, while the expression of adhesion molecules on the endothelial surface can result in the tethering of leukocytes, red cells and platelets to the endothelium.

8.4.2 Leukocytes

As mentioned, leukocytes are key protagonists in inflammatory processes via events that are controlled by a range of extracellular molecular regulators, including cytokines and chemokines, which mediate both cell recruitment and intracellular signaling inflammatory control mechanisms (Turner et al. 2014). Leukocytosis is a

Table 8.2 Elevation of inflammatory mediators in SCD during VOC and steady state

Inflammatory mediator	Steady-state/ VOC	Major source cells	Major target cells	Major effects	References
Cytokines					
TNF-α	Stst/VOC	Monocytes/macrophages, other leukocytes	ECs, leukocytes	Cellular activation (via NFκB and MAPK pathways); stimulation of cell adhesion and ROS production; downregulates eNOS expression; modulation of apoptotic pathways	Lanaro et al. (2009), Pathare et al. (2004), Qari et al. (2012), and Keikhaei et al. (2013)
TNFSF14 (TNF superfamily member 14; LIGHT)	Stst	Platelets, also activated T cells, monocytes, granulocytes	ECs, leukocytes	Pro-inflammatory and prothrombotic cytokine; mediates platelet adhesion to ECs. Activates ECs, inducing ICAM-1, VCAM-1, and IL-8 expression. Activates monocytes, inducing MCP-1 and IL-8 production	Garrido et al. (2012)
CD40L (CD40 ligand; CD154)	Stst; further increased in VOC	Platelets, presentation on T-lymphocytes and other leukocytes	ECs, leukocytes	Prothrombotic properties; binds to and activates platelet integrin GPIIb/IIIa; upregulates tissue factor production from monocytes. Pro-inflammatory properties; interacts with wide variety of cells via ligation with CD40 receptor; activates ECs, induces B-cell proliferation and activates macrophages	Lee et al. (2006) and Garrido et al. (2012)
IL-1α	Stst/VOC	Multiple; macrophages and other leukocytes, epithelial cells, ECs	Multiple; ECs, leukocytes	Primary inflammatory trigger, induces leukocyte recruitment, activates endothelial cells and induces IL-6, G-CSF and prostaglandin production	Driss et al. (2012) and Francis and Haywood (1992)

IL-1β	Stst/VOC	Macrophages, monocytes, also platelets, other leukocytes, ECs	ECs, leukocytes	Stimulates cell activation, adhesion molecule expression and release of IL-6/IL-17	Qari et al. (2012), Asare et al. (2010), Wun et al. (2002), Proenca-Ferreira et al. (2014), and Davila et al. (2015)
IL-17	Stst/VOC	Lymphocytes (Th17)	Multiple, fibroblasts, ECs, keratinocytes, leukocytes	Induces a neutrophil-dominant inflammatory response by stimulating the production of cyto/chemokines, such as IL-1, IL-6, IL-8, TNF-α	Keikhaei et al. (2013)
IL-3	Stst	Basophils, T and B lymphocytes	Myeloid cells	Stimulates myeloid cell proliferation and differentiation; amplifies acute inflammation	Rodrigues et al. (2006) and Conran et al. (2007b)
IL-6	Stst; further increased during VOC	ECs, osteoblasts, leukocytes (macrophages, T cells)	ECs, VSMCs, hepatocytes	Pro-inflammatory effects: Stimulates acute phase protein synthesis, e.g. CRP. Activates ECs and VSMCs, resulting in chemokine release. Amplifies TLR-mediated cytokine production Modulator of hematopoiesis Anti-inflammatory effects: Inhibition of TNF-α, upregulation of IL-10	Sakamoto et al. (2013), Pathare et al. (2004), Keikhaei et al. (2013), and Qari et al. (2012)
IL-18	Stst; further increased in VOC	Macrophages, monocytes, other leukocytes, ECs	VSMCs, leukocytes	Stimulates proliferation and migration of VSMC and production of IFNγ, IL-2, IL-12	Cerqueira et al. (2011) and Keikhaei et al. (2013)

(continued)

Table 8.2 (continued)

Inflammatory mediator	Steady-state/ VOC	Major source cells	Major target cells	Major effects	References
IFN-γ	Stst	Multiple; T lymphocytes, NK cells, macrophages	Multiple	Induces the production of cytokines and the expression of class I and II MHC antigens and leukocyte adhesion molecules. Modulates macrophage effector functions and enhances T helper cell expansion	Pathare et al. (2004)
Chemokines					
IL-8 (CXCL8)	Stst; further increased in VOC	Multiple; ECs, leukocytes, T cells, platelets, keratinocytes, hepatocytes, chondrocytes	Principally neutrophils, but also ECs, macrophages, amongst others	Potent chemotactic factor for neutrophils; also induces neutrophil adhesion, cell shape changes and generation of ROS among other effects	Qari et al. (2012), Keikhaei et al. (2013), and Lanaro et al. (2009)
MCP-1 (CCL2)	Stst/VOC	Multiple; ECs, fibroblasts, epithelial, VSMCs	Monocytes, NK cells and other leukocytes, VSMCs, ECs	Recruits monocytes/macrophages amongst other cells to sites of inflammation. Stimulates histamine/ leukotriene release from mast cells/ basophils. May play a role in inflammatory lung disorders	Qari et al. (2012)
RANTES (CCL5)	Stst	Multiple; ECs, platelets, VSMCs, T cells	Leukocytes	Recruitment of eosinophils, amongst other leukocytes. Role in angiogenesis	Pallis et al. (2014)
PF4 (CXCL4)	Stst/VOC	Platelets	Leukocytes, ECs	Chemotactic for neutrophils, fibroblasts and monocytes. Inhibits EC proliferation and migration, thereby reducing angiogenesis	Papadimitriou et al. (1993) and Westwick et al. (1983)
Eotaxin-1 (CCL11)	Stst	Multiple; ECs, fibroblasts, VSMCs, epithelial cells	Leukocytes, especially eosinophils	Recruitment of eosinophils, as well as basophils and T cells to sites of inflammation. Associated with allergic inflammation and asthma	Pallis et al. (2014)

MIP-1α (CCL3)	Stst/VOC	Multiple; macrophages, dendritic cells, lymphocytes and other leukocytes; also platelets, osteoblasts	Leukocytes, esp. monocytes, NK cells, dendritic cells	Recruitment of inflammatory cells to sites of inflammation. Inhibits hematopoietic stem cell proliferation. Also induces Ca^{2+} release, upregulation of activation markers and release of proinflammatory mediators	Qari et al. (2012) and Croizat and Nagel (1999)
Peptides/proteins					
Plasminogen activator inhibitor (PAI-1; SERPINE1)	Stst/VOC	ECs, platelets, hepatocytes and fibroblasts		Inhibits fibrinolysis, and the activity of matrix metalloproteins. Also promotes cell migration. Elevated PAI-1 levels have been associated with diminished lung function	Dos Santos et al. (unpublished data), Patel et al. (2010), and Nsiri et al. (1996)
Tissue factor (TF)	Stst	Fibroblasts, VSMCs: Under inflammatory conditions; EC, leukocytes		Activates the extrinsic coagulation pathway, promoting thrombin generation. Also stimulates fibrin deposition, platelet activation (via thrombin generation), activation of certain integrins, cell migration and inhibits apoptotic pathways	Key et al. (1998)
Endothelin-1	Stst/VOC	ECs	VSMCs	Powerful vasoconstrictor and involved in vascular remodeling	Werdehoff et al. (1998) and Graido-Gonzalez et al. (1998)
Substance P	Stst; further increased in VOC	Mast cells, nerve endings, also ECs, eosinophils, macrophages	Multiple; mast cells, neutrophils, eosinophils, fibroblasts, ECs	Promotes neurogenic inflammation, increases vascular leakage and amplifies inflammatory responses. Also has a role in wound healing	Michaels et al. (1998)

(continued)

Table 8.2 (continued)

Inflammatory mediator	Steady-state/VOC	Major source cells	Major target cells	Major effects	References
C-reactive protein (CRP)	Stst; further increased in VOC	Hepatocytes, also macrophages and VSMCs	ECs, monocytes	Acute phase protein. Directly inhibits endothelial NO production and stimulates IL-6/endothelin-1 production, can also activate complement pathway. May represent a marker for VOC onset	Nur et al. (2011)
Pentraxin-3 (PTX3)	VOC	Multiple; ECs, mononuclear cells, neutrophils, fibroblasts, dendritic cells	ECs, monocytes	Acute phase protein, amplifies inflammatory response. Activates complement pathway. Possible marker of endothelial dysfunction. Complexes with neutrophil extracellular trap (NET) component proteins. May play a protective/anti-inflammatory role	Elshazly et al. (2014) and Nur et al. (2011)
Eicosanoids					
PGI_2 (prostacyclin)	Stst	ECs, VSMCs, endothelial progenitor cells	Multiple; VSMCs, platelets, fibroblasts	Vasodilator, induces edema and pain during acute inflammatory processes. Amplification of cytokine production	Mehta and Albiol (1982) and Buchanan and Holtkamp (1985)
PGE_2	Stst	Multiple	Multiple; T cells, dendritic cells, ECs	Induction of pain, fever, redness, edema. Amplification of cytokine and chemokine production (may contribute to chronic inflammation establishment). Modulation of tissue remodeling and T cell differentiation	Conran et al. (2007a) and Graido-Gonzalez et al. (1998)

Leukotriene B4 (LTB4)	Stst; further increased in VOC	Leukocytes, epithelial cells, fibroblasts	Multiple, particularly leukocytes	Chemoattractant for neutrophils and other leukocytes. Also enhances inflammatory mediator production from leukocytes	Setty and Stuart (2002)
Growth factors					
GM-CSF	Stst	Multiple; EC, macrophages, T cells, mast cells, NK cells, fibroblasts	Multiple; leukocytes, progenitor cells, erythroid cells	Stimulates the proliferation of granulocytes and macrophages from bone marrow precursor cells. Modulates leukocyte numbers and fetal hemoglobin production in SCD. Also enhances pro-inflammatory cytokine production and promotes leukocyte adhesion and migration	Conran et al. (2007b) and Croizat and Nagel (1999)
M-CSF	Stst	Multiple; fibroblasts, ECs, monocytes/macrophages, marrow stromal cells, B and T cells, osteoblasts	Progenitor cells, monocytes	Stimulates differentiation of progenitor cells to mature monocytes. Also stimulates production of various cytokines by priming monocytes	Conran et al. (2007b)
Transforming growth factor-β (TGF-β)	Stst/VOC	Multiple; macrophages, fibroblasts, ECs, epithelial cells, platelets, VSMCs	Multiple; progenitor cells, fibroblasts, lymphocytes, macrophages, and neutrophils	Negative regulation of hematopoietic stem cell and progenitor cell proliferation and differentiation. Potent chemotactic and important for tissue repair. Has been implicated in renal fibrosis	Keikhaei et al. (2013)

(continued)

Table 8.2 (continued)

Inflammatory mediator	Steady-state/ VOC	Major source cells	Major target cells	Major effects	References
VEGF	Stst/VOC	Multiple	ECs, progenitor ECs, also macrophages, monocytes	Key regulator of angiogenesis (induces EC proliferation, sprouting and capillary formation) and progenitor EC differentiation. Potent vasopermeability activity	Niu et al. (2009), Qari et al. (2012), and Lopes et al. (2015)
VEGF D	Stst	Multiple	ECs	Upregulated during hypoxia, regulates EC-mediated angiogenic processes	Lopes et al. (2015)
Angiopoietin-1	Stst	Multiple; VSMCs, pericytes, astrocytes	ECs, early hematopoietic cells	Induces vascular remodeling by organizing angiogenesis and tightening EC junctions	Mohan et al. (2005) and Lopes et al. (2015)
Angiopoietin-2	Stst/VOC	ECs, macrophages	Ecs, early hematopoietic cells, monocytes, neutrophils	Both an agonist and antagonist of angiopoietin-1 and is expressed during vascular remodeling. Inflammatory role; induces IL-8 production by neutrophils and neutrophil/monocyte adhesion	Mohan et al. (2005) and Duits et al. (2006)
Basic FGF (bFGF; FGF2)	Stst/VOC	Multiple; ECs, VSMCs, Adipocytes, neutrophils	Multiple; ECs, VSMCs, stem cells	Released from extracellular matrix during wound healing. Induces inflammatory mediator production in ECs and adhesion molecule expression	Qari et al. (2012) and Niu et al. (2009)
Pigment epithelium-derived factor (PEDF)	Stst	Multiple; epithelial cells	Stem/progenitor cells	Anti-angiogenic and anti-inflammatory properties, may represent a marker for retinopathy in SCD. Also exerts anti-vasopermeability, anti-tumor, antioxidant and neuroprotective activities	Cruz et al. (2015)

Placenta growth factor (PlGF)	Stst/VOC	Sickle RBC, bone marrow stromal cells	Multiple; ECs, fibroblasts, macrophages, dendritic cells	Enhances VEGF-stimulated angiogenesis under pathological conditions. Induces PAI-1 expression	Brittain et al. (2010) and Duits et al. (2006)
Other molecules					
Neopterin	Stst	Monocytes/macrophages		Metabolite of guanosine triphosphate, produced following monocyte/macrophage activation. Decreases erythropoietin gene expression. Biomarker of inflammation and oxidative stress	Rodrigues et al. (2006)

ECs endothelial cells, *eNOS* endothelial nitric oxide synthase, *IL* interleukin, *GM-CSF* granulocyte macrophage-colony stimulating factor, *M-CSF* macrophage-colony stimulating factor, *PG* prostaglandin, *ROS* reactive oxygen species, *TNF* tumor necrosis factor, *VEGF* vascular endothelial growth factor, *VSMCs* vascular smooth muscle cells

common characteristic of sickle cell anemia, where increased leukocyte counts have been associated with increased mortality, acute chest syndrome and stroke (Platt et al. 1991), probably due to the role that these cells play in the initiation of vaso-occlusive processes and their innate ability to contribute to processes of oxidative stress and inflammatory mechanisms.

8.4.3 Platelets

In addition to their role in hemostasis, platelets also contribute to both physiological and pathological inflammatory processes (Garraud and Cognasse 2015). Platelets, when activated, can interact with and adhere to other cells, in turn activating or priming these cells (McGregor et al. 2006). Platelet-neutrophil complexes, for example, form during inflammatory processes and are known to enhance leukocyte recruitment to sites of inflammation and tissue injury (Page and Pitchford 2013). Augmented platelet-leukocyte aggregate formation has been well documented in SCD (Jakubowski et al. 2014; Lee et al. 2006; Wun et al. 2002) and may contribute to the up regulation of leukocyte recruitment to vessel walls. Furthermore, the adhesion of platelets to endothelial cells leads to their activation and expression of the endothelial adhesion molecules, ICAM-1 and E-selectin, and IL-8 secretion via an NFκB-dependent pathway (Proenca-Ferreira et al. 2014), probably due to the release of potent platelet-derived inflammatory mediators such as IL-1β, CD40 ligand, TNFSF14 (LIGHT) and IL-6 (Lee et al. 2006; Proenca-Ferreira et al. 2014; Garrido et al. 2012; Davila et al. 2015). Interestingly platelets may also mediate the adhesion of erythrocytes to neutrophils in SCD (Dominical et al. 2014), indicating a role for platelets in the recruitment of RBC to the vessel wall and, therefore, in the initiation of vaso-occlusive processes.

8.5 Molecular Mediators in SCA Inflammation

Inflammation is controlled by a huge array of extracellular mediators including cytokines, chemokines, growth factors, eicosanoids and peptides, which in turn orchestrate intracellular signaling mechanisms that activate inflammatory cells and regulate their function and interactions with other cells. Several cell types produce these inflammatory mediators and the chronic inflammatory state associated with SCA propagates continual inflammatory cell activation that results in the excessive production of many of these molecules (see Table 8.2).

Cytokines are significant modulators of inflammation and the production of a large number of these proteins is augmented in SCA (see Table 8.2). Interleukin (IL)-1 family cytokine levels are modulated in SCA (Driss et al. 2012; Asare et al. 2010; Keikhaei et al. 2013; Francis and Haywood 1992), where elevated IL-1β and IL-18 in SCA (Cerqueira et al. 2011; Keikhaei et al. 2013; Qari et al. 2012) may be indicative of the formation of inflammasomes, even during steady-state SCA.

Tumor necrosis factor-α (TNF-α) has been consistently demonstrated to be elevated in steady-state SCA and during VOC (Lanaro et al. 2009; Pathare et al. 2004; Qari et al. 2012), presumably as the result of the activation of monocytes and macrophages (Safaya et al. 2012; Wun et al. 2002). Given that this potent cytokine plays a key role in the inflammatory response, causing endothelial activation, lipid mediator expression and activation of leukocytes (Turner et al. 2014) as well as modulating cell survival, differentiation and proliferation (Bradley 2008), it is reasonable to assume that this molecule plays a major role in the inflammatory state in SCA. TNF-α interacts with two receptors, denominated TNFR1 and TNFR2, which are differentially expressed on cells and tissues; TNFR1 is widely expressed while TNFR2 is produced predominantly on the surface of leukocytes and endothelial cells (Sedger and McDermott 2014). TNFR1 expression has been correlated with disease severity in SCA (Dworkis et al. 2011) and the importance of TNF-α in inflammatory signaling in SCA can be illustrated by the fact that well-established mice models of SCD inflammatory vaso-occlusion employ TNF-α to stimulate leukocyte recruitment, resulting in widespread vaso-occlusion of the microcirculation and, generally, leading to the death of the mouse within hours (Turhan et al. 2002, 2004).

Elevated plasma levels of IL-6 have been reported in steady-state SCA patients and in transgenic SCD mice models (Pathare et al. 2004; Hibbert et al. 2005). Furthermore, there is evidence to suggest that IL-6 concentrations further increase during VOC (Pathare et al. 2004; Qari et al. 2012) and that augmented mononuclear IL-6 production may be associated with hemolysis in SCA (da Silva et al. 2014), with increased plasma IL-6 correlating with a higher risk for developing pulmonary hypertension (Niu et al. 2009). Numerous inflammatory cell types express IL-6, including neutrophils and monocytes/macrophages, upon stimulation of Toll-like receptors. IL-6 can modulate hematopoiesis and is critical for the maturation of B-cells into plasma cells and, therefore, antibody production. Stimulation of endothelial and smooth-muscle cells by IL-6 leads to chemokine release, which can result in the recruitment of more immune cells (Calabrese and Rose-John 2014). Furthermore, IL-6 stimulation of hepatocytes in the liver results in the synthesis of acute-phase proteins including, C-reactive protein (CRP), a principal marker of both acute and chronic inflammation (Heinrich et al. 1990). Other cytokines known to be elevated in sickle cell disease include IL-3, IL-17 and interferon (IFN)-γ (Pathare et al. 2004; Rodrigues et al. 2006; Keikhaei et al. 2013) (Table 8.2).

Chemokines are small chemotactic cytokines that regulate leukocyte trafficking, although they also play roles in angiogenesis, embryonic development and cell homeostasis (Koenen and Weber 2011). Currently, over 40 chemokines have been identified and these are grouped in four distinct families (C, CC, CXC and CX3C) (Lira and Furtado 2012), a number of which have been reported as augmented in SCA (see Table 8.2). IL-8 (CXCL8) is a potent chemotactic factor, principally for neutrophils, but also induces neutrophil adhesive properties, shape change, lysosomal enzyme release and the generation of ROS and of bioactive lipids (Mukaida et al. 1998). Circulating IL-8 levels are reported as augmented in SCA both during steady state and VOC (Keikhaei et al. 2013; Qari et al. 2012; Niu et al. 2009; Lanaro et al. 2009) and, given the initiating role that neutrophils may play in inflammatory vascular occlusion (Turhan et al. 2002), it is probable that this chemokine is important for SCA pathophysiology. Other circulating chemokines known to be elevated in SCA include MCP-1 (monocyte chemoattractant protein-1; CCL2), eotaxin-1 (CCL11) and RANTES (CCL5) (Qari et al. 2012; Pallis et al. 2014). MCP-1 and KC (CXCL1) expressions are increased in the liver and lungs of SCD mice, and blood outgrowth endothelial cells (BOEC), when proliferated from the peripheral blood of SCA individuals, secrete higher concentrations of IL-8 and MCP-1 (Sakamoto et al. 2013). In addition, cultured endothelial cells produce MCP-1 and IL-8 following stimulation with hemoglobin products (Almeida et al. 2015), indicating a role for hemolysis in chemokine production. Platelets are an important source of chemokines, and the activation of platelets in SCA leads to the release of a number of platelet-derived chemokines, including platelet factor-4 (PF4; CXCL4) (Tomer et al. 2001; Adamides et al. 1990; Papadimitriou et al. 1993) that has important anti-angiogenic properties, as well having a role in hemostasis/thrombosis and in macrophage differentiation (Kowalska et al. 2010).

Growth Factors constitute a group of molecules that can stimulate cellular growth, proliferation, healing, and cellular differentiation. Of the many growth factors, some regulate hematopoiesis (hematopoietic growth factors), others regulate neurogenesis (neurotrophins) and a number of these molecules also play roles in angiogenic processes.

The hematopoietic growth factors, granulocyte colony-stimulating factor (G-CSF), granulocyte-macrophage colony-stimulating factor (GM-CSF), erythropoietin (O'Donnell et al. 2009), stem cell factor (SCF), growth differentiation factor-15 (GDF-15), and stromal-derived factor-1 (SDF-1) (Landburg et al. 2009; Tantawy et al. 2014; Conran et al. 2007b; Croizat and Nagel 1999) have all been reported as augmented in sickle cell disease. GM-CSF may play a role in regulating both leukocyte numbers and fetal hemoglobin expression in SCA (Ikuta et al. 2011; Conran et al. 2007b) and may promote mast cell activation and proliferation, possibly contributing to hyperalgesia in the disease (Vincent et al. 2013). On the other hand, increases in the neurotrophin, brain-derived neurotrophic factor (BDNF), may be associated with elevated transcranial Doppler velocities and stroke in SCA (Lance et al. 2014; Hyacinth et al. 2012).

A number of angiogenic growth factors are also known to be augmented in sickle cell disease, including vascular endothelial growth factor (VEGF), VEGF-D, placenta growth factor (PlGF), angiopoietin-1, angiopoietin-2, basic fibroblast GF (bFGF) and the anti-angiogenic pigment epithelium derived factor (PEGF) (Duits et al. 2006; Landburg et al. 2009; Brittain et al. 2010; Niu et al. 2009; Lopes et al. 2015; Cruz et al. 2015). Angiogenic factors regulate the formation of new blood capillaries and are essential for processes of development, reproduction and wound repair (Lopes et al. 2015). Alterations in angiogenic factors have been associated with the incidence of pulmonary hypertension and retinopathy in SCD (Landburg et al. 2009; Sundaram et al. 2010; Niu et al. 2009; Cruz et al. 2015; Lopes et al. 2015). PlGF, for example, is released at high concentrations from sickle red blood cells and has been shown to induce hypoxia-inducible factor-1α (HIF-1) activity in endothelial cells, activate monocytes, and may have a role in pulmonary hypertension due to the induction of endothelin-1 expression (Patel and Kalra 2010; Perelman et al. 2003; Sundaram et al. 2010; Patel et al. 2008). PlGF can also induce plasminogen activator inhibitor-1 (PAI-1) expression, in endothelial cells and monocytes, with possible effects on fibrinolysis and lung injury (Patel et al. 2010).

Eicosanoids are biologically-active lipids that are generated at sites of inflammation and mediate their effects through specific receptors to coordinate specific cellular responses to inflammation (Capra et al. 2013). The prostanoids, formed by the prostaglandins and thromboxane A_2 (TxA_2), are synthesized by the cyclooxygenase pathway from arachidonic acid, while leukotrienes and lipoxins are generated from the lipoxygenase pathway. TxA_2, produced by activated platelets, has pro-thrombotic properties that can be balanced by the anti-aggregating and vasodilating effects of prostacyclin (or prostaglandin (PG)I_2), produced by the endothelium (Capra et al. 2013). Elevations in TxA_2 and prostaglandins, such as prostacyclin and the pro-inflammatory PGE_2, or their metabolites, have been reported in sickle cell disease (Graido-Gonzalez et al. 1998; Lanaro et al. 2009; Conran et al. 2007a; Buchanan and Holtkamp 1985; Mehta and Albiol 1982). Furthermore, sickle erythrocytes have been shown to induce prostaglandin (PGI_2 and PGE_2) and TxA_2 production in isolated perfused rat lungs (Ibe et al. 1997) and to induce PGI_2 synthesis by endothelial cells (Shiu et al. 2000). Prostaglandins, such as PGI_2 and PGE_2 induce the classic signals of inflammation; redness, swelling and pain and have been recently implicated in the modulation of both anti-inflammatory mechanisms (PGI_2 may augment IL-10 production from T helper 2 cells) and pro-inflammatory pathways due to the amplification of cytokine and chemokine production, as well as contributing to tissue remodeling (Aoki and Narumiya 2012; Ricciotti and FitzGerald 2011).

Leukotriene (LT) B_4 and cysteinyl leukotrienes (CystLTs), such as LTC_4, are produced in the lungs during hypoxia and their production has been associated with the induction of pulmonary hypertension (Morganroth et al. 1984; Opene et al. 2014). Of the leukotrienes, LTB_4 has been reported as elevated in steady state SCA and further increased during vaso-occlusive crisis and acute chest syndrome (Setty and Stuart 2002), while elevated urinary LTE_4 levels have been associated with pain and an increased risk for acute chest syndrome in sickle cell disease (Field et al. 2009; Jennings et al. 2008). Sickle erythrocytes and activated platelets have been shown to increase LTC_4 when perfused over rat lungs (Opene et al. 2014), while erythrocyte-derived PlGF can upregulate the expression of 5-lipoxygenase and, therefore, leukotriene production in monocytes (Patel et al. 2009).

Inflammatory Peptides and Proteins Endothelin-1 (ET-1) is a vasoconstrictor peptide, synthesized principally by the endothelial cells, that plays a role in the regulation of vascular function (Pernow et al. 2012). ET-1 expression is upregulated during endothelial dysfunction and in response to inducers that include angiotensin II, cytokines such as PlGF and hypoxia. Plasma ET-1 has been reported as elevated in SCA both during steady state and vaso-occlusive crisis (Werdehoff et al. 1998; Graido-Gonzalez et al. 1998) and has been implicated in the development of acute chest syndrome and pulmonary hypertension (Hammerman et al. 1997; Patel et al. 2008; Werdehoff et al. 1998).

Plasminogen activator factor -1 (PAI-1) is a protein synthesized by a number of cell types including endothelial cells, hepatocytes, platelets and fibroblasts. In addition to being modulated by PlGF, PAI-1 production is also induced by hypoxia and oxidative stress via activation of the transcription factors HIF-1α and AP-1, respectively. PAI-1 is an inhibitor of fibrinolysis, modulating fibrinolysis and cellular responses to vascular remodeling and may contribute to the development of lung injury and fibrosis, as well as angiogenic processes in SCA and, therefore, in pulmonary hypertension (Patel et al. 2010; Diebold et al. 2008). High levels of PAI-1 have been observed in the pulmonary endothelial cells, alveolar macrophages and bronchial epithelial cells of sickle mice (Patel et al. 2010) and elevated plasma concentrations of this protein have also been observed in steady state SCA patients (Dos Santos unpublished data; Nsiri et al. 1996; Patel et al. 2010).

C-reactive protein (CRP) is a stable acute-phase protein, synthesized in the liver, which is rapidly synthesized in response to inflammation. Levels of CRP have been consistently found to be augmented in the plasma of SCD patients during steady state and further increased during vaso-occlusive crisis, with some authors postulating the use of CRP as a marker of VOC onset (Krishnan et al. 2010; Mohammed et al. 2010; Nur et al. 2011; Okocha et al. 2014; Akinlade et al. 2013; Kanavaki et al. 2012; Rowley et al. 2014). Another acute phase protein implicated in sickle cell inflammation and reportedly increased during VOC is pentraxin-3 (PTX3) (Nur et al. 2011; Elshazly et al. 2014), while Substance P, a neuropeptide released from activated mast cells, is thought to contribute to neuroinflammation in SCA (Vincent et al. 2013; Michaels et al. 1998).

Anti-Inflammatory Molecules IL-10 is a class 2 cytokine that can modulate innate and adaptive immune responses, limiting the production of pro-inflammatory cytokines, including IFNγ, TNF-α, IL-1β and IL-6, in order to prevent tissue damage. IL-10 is ubiquitously expressed, but major producers of this cytokine include macrophages, T and B lymphocytes, natural killer cells and monocytes (Walter 2014; Hofmann et al. 2012). Levels of IL-10 have been reported as elevated in steady-state SCD (Lanaro et al. 2009; Niu et al. 2009), but reduced (compared to steady state) in patients in vaso-occlusive crisis (Sarray et al. 2015).

Heme oxygenase-1 (HO-1) is an anti-inflammatory protein, whose expression is upregulated by heme as well as oxidative signals. HO-1 catalyzes the degradation of heme to carbon monoxide, free iron, and biliverdin. HO-1 gene expression is reportedly up-regulated in SCD, presumably as a consequence of hemolytic events (Lanaro et al. 2009; Nath et al. 2001), while gene delivery of HO-1 to the liver has been shown to benefit SCD mice, inhibiting local hypoxia-induced stasis (Belcher et al. 2010). An important consequence of HO-1-mediated heme degradation may be the release of carbon monoxide (CO), also known to have anti-inflammatory and anti-sickling properties. Reports have described effects of CO on increasing RBC survival and decreasing leukocytosis and NFκB activation and in the upregulation of anti-inflammatory signaling pathways in SCD (Beutler 1975; Beckman et al. 2009; Belcher et al. 2013).

8.6 Cross Talk Between Inflammation and Coagulation

Inflammation and hemolysis both contribute to induce a state of hypercoagulability in SCA (Sparkenbaugh and Pawlinski 2013). Activation of the endothelium and leukocytes, particularly monocytes, in SCA leads to upregulation of tissue factor (TF), a cell surface receptor for factor VII/VIIa and the primary activator of the extrinsic coagulation pathway (Setty et al. 2012; Solovey et al. 1998; Key et al. 1998). Additionally, the hemolytic product, heme, can also induce TF expression in leukocytes (Sparkenbaugh et al. 2015). Augmented TF can, in turn, promote thrombin generation, fibrin deposition and platelet activation, as can be observed in SCA (Colella et al. 2012; Proenca-Ferreira et al. 2010; Westwick et al. 1983; Shah et al. 2012; Francis 1989).

As previously mentioned, repeated cycles of RBC sickling results in phosphatidylserine exposure on the cell surface (Lubin et al. 1981), further contributing to procoagulant activity and thrombin generation (Franck et al. 1985). Thrombin and fibrin generation can also be promoted by circulating microparticles released from erythrocytes and activated platelets, endothelial cells and monocytes, amongst other cells, in SCA (Shet et al. 2003; Sparkenbaugh and Pawlinski 2013). Additionally, ultralarge von Willebrand factor multimers are expressed on the endothelium, when activated, and these may mediate the binding of erythrocytes, platelets, as well as coagulation proteins, to the endothelial surface (Dong et al. 2002; Sultana et al. 1998; Belcher et al. 2014; Kaul et al. 1993). Subsequent thrombotic events can participate in ischemia-reperfusion processes in SCA and the production of potent inflammatory mediators from activated platelets, such as CD40L and TNFSF14 (Lee et al. 2006; Garrido et al. 2012), may further amplify the inflammation associated with the disease (Sparkenbaugh and Pawlinski 2013).

8.7 Anti-inflammatory Effects of Hydroxyurea in Sickle Cell Anemia

Currently the only drug approved by the FDA for SCA therapy, hydroxyurea (or hydroxycarbamide), is a cytostatic agent that significantly improves the disease's clinical course, improving mortality rates and reducing hospitalization for vaso-occlusive crisis, the incidence of acute chest syndrome, as well as the necessity for transfusions. The reader is referred to Chaps. 10 and 12 for further information regarding the clinical effects of hydroxyurea (Charache et al. 1995; Platt et al. 1984; Steinberg et al. 2003). One of the principal effects of hydroxyurea is the induction of fetal hemoglobin (HbF) production in erythrocyte lineage cells, which inhibits the polymerization of HbS, reducing hemolysis and red cell sickling (Charache et al. 1995; McGann and Ware 2011). However, it is becoming increasingly clear that hydroxyurea has major anti-inflammatory properties, which probably also make an important contribution to its therapeutic benefits.

Longer-term anti-inflammatory effects of hydroxyurea include a significant reduction in leukocyte counts, which are often observed before HbF elevation (Charache et al. 1996) and this effect certainly reduces the amplitude of inflammatory responses in SCA. Hydroxyurea therapy also reduces adhesion molecule expression and activity on the surface of red cells, leukocytes and the endothelium, probably via indirect anti-inflammatory mechanisms (Chaar et al. 2014; Bartolucci et al. 2010; Cartron and Elion 2008; Proenca-Ferreira et al. 2010; Canalli et al. 2007; Gambero et al. 2007). Furthermore, hydroxyurea therapy has been associated with decreases in the production and expression numerous of the inflammatory mediators thought to contribute to the inflammatory state, including endothelin-1, TNF-α, IL-1β, IL-17, TF and GM-CSF (Brun et al. 2003; Lapoumeroulie et al. 2005; Lanaro et al. 2009; Conran et al. 2007b; Colella et al. 2012; Keikhaei et al. 2013), in addition to increasing the expressions of the anti-inflammatory proteins, IL-10 and HO-1 (Lanaro et al. 2009). Potent anti-angiogenic effects of hydroxyurea on endothelial cell function have also been reported both in vivo and in vitro (Lopes et al. 2014) and this drug appears to reduce angiogenic mediator production in sickle cell disease (Lopes et al. 2015). These anti-angiogenic effects may enable hydroxyurea to halt or decelerate manifestations of the disease in which upregulated angiogenesis may play a role, such as retinopathy and pulmonary hypertension.

Emerging evidence indicates that hydroxyurea may have important acute and immediate effects that are independent of the drug's ability to elevate HbF production. Hydroxyurea may release nitric oxide, in vivo (King 2003), and it is becoming apparent that this nitric oxide donating property may have significant anti-inflammatory effects. The administration of a single dose of hydroxyurea has been shown to decrease leukocyte recruitment to the vasculature in SCD mice following an inflammatory stimulus. Furthermore, a single dose of hydroxyurea synergistically augmented the effects of a phosphodiesterase 9 inhibitor, in this same model, by amplifying nitric oxide-cyclic guanosine monophosphate (cGMP)-signaling, resulting in the inhibition of vaso-occlusive processes and prolonged animal survival following inflammatory stimulation (Almeida et al. 2012). Similarly, results from a recent study (Almeida et al. 2015) demonstrate that a single dose of hydroxyurea is able to abolish the effects of a hemolytic insult on systemic inflammation and on leukocyte recruitment in the microcirculation. As such, the anti-inflammatory properties of hydroxyurea are extensive and may represent a major mechanism by which this drug exerts its effects.

8.8 Other Prospective Anti-inflammatory Approaches for SCA

A number of anti-inflammatory drugs are currently under investigation as potential therapeutic approaches for SCA (the reader is referred to Chap. 16 for a more in depth review). Various drugs aiming to reduce leukocyte adhesion to the blood vessel wall and, therefore, diminish the initiation of vaso-occlusive processes are currently in clinical trials for use in SCA (Wun et al. 2014; Manwani et al. 2014; Cheung et al. 2004; Okpala 2015). Statins and TNF-α antagonists are also potential approaches for diminishing endothelial activation (Hoppe et al. 2011), while iNKT cell depletants and A2AR agonists in development could be useful for decreasing iNKT cell numbers and activation and, therefore, reduce inflammation (Field et al. 2013, 2014). To reduce the inflammatory effects of hypoxia, pegylated hemoglobin carbon monoxide carriers are under investigation, as carbon monoxide delivery may impart significant anti-inflammatory and cytoprotective effects in SCA (Belcher et al. 2013).

8.9 Conclusions

Evidence gleaned over recent years has revealed the primary and driving role that inflammation plays in the induction of the vaso-occlusive process and primary complications of sickle cell anemia. Major triggers of inflammation in sickle cell anemia appear to be alterations in the red cell itself and ensuing hemolytic and hypoxic processes. Of the plethora of inflammatory mediators that are upregulated in sickle cell anemia, it is difficult to identify any one of these proteins as being of more significance to the inflammatory response and, therefore, representing a more significant therapeutic target in the disease. Rather, approaches to reduce hemoglobin S polymerization, and consequent red cell sickling, and to limit the effects of hemolysis and ischemia-reperfusion, as well to reduce cellular activation in a pan-cellular manner may be more effective for reducing inflammation and therefore vaso-occlusive processes in the disease. Optimizing the manner in which hydroxyurea is used and administered in the disease may also be key to taking full advantage of its nitric oxide donating and anti-inflammatory properties.

References

Abais JM, Xia M, Li G et al (2014) Contribution of endogenously produced reactive oxygen species to the activation of podocyte NLRP3 inflammasomes in hyperhomocysteinemia. Free Radic Biol Med 67:211–220

Adamides S, Konstantopoulos K, Toumbis M et al (1990) A study of beta-thromboglobulin and platelet factor-4 plasma levels in steady state sickle cell patients. Blut 61(4):245–247

Adewoye AH, Klings ES, Farber HW et al (2005) Sickle cell vaso-occlusive crisis induces the release of circulating serum heat shock protein-70. Am J Hematol 78(3):240–242

Akinlade KS, Atere AD, Rahamon SK, Olaniyi JA (2013) Serum levels of copeptin, C-reactive protein and cortisol in different severity groups of sickle cell anaemia. Niger J Physiol Sci 28(2):159–164

Almeida CB, Scheiermann C, Jang JE et al (2012) Hydroxyurea and a cGMP-amplifying agent have immediate benefits on acute vaso-occlusive events in sickle cell disease mice. Blood 120(14):2879–2888

Almeida CB, Souza LE, Leonardo FC et al (2015) Acute hemolytic vascular inflammatory processes are prevented by nitric oxide replacement or a single dose of hydroxyurea. Blood

Amer J, Ghoti H, Rachmilewitz E et al (2006) Red blood cells, platelets and polymorphonuclear neutrophils of patients with sickle cell disease exhibit oxidative stress that can be ameliorated by antioxidants. Br J Haematol 132(1):108–113

Andreotti C, King AA, Macy E, Compas BE, DeBaun MR (2014) The association of cytokine levels with cognitive function in children with sickle cell disease and normal MRI studies of the brain. J Child Neurol 30(10):1349–1353

Aoki T, Narumiya S (2012) Prostaglandins and chronic inflammation. Trends Pharmacol Sci 33(6):304–311

Arndt H, Russell JB, Kurose I, Kubes P, Granger DN (1993) Mediators of leukocyte adhesion in rat mesenteric venules elicited by inhibition of nitric oxide synthesis. Gastroenterology 105(3):675–680

Asare K, Gee BE, Stiles JK et al (2010) Plasma interleukin-1beta concentration is associated with stroke in sickle cell disease. Cytokine 49(1):39–44

Aslan M, Thornley-Brown D, Freeman BA (2000) Reactive species in sickle cell disease. Ann N Y Acad Sci 899:375–391

Aslan M, Ryan TM, Adler B et al (2001) Oxygen radical inhibition of nitric oxide-dependent vascular function in sickle cell disease. Proc Natl Acad Sci U S A 98(26):15215–15220

Ataga KI, Moore CG, Hillery CA et al (2008) Coagulation activation and inflammation in sickle cell disease-associated pulmonary hypertension. Haematologica 93(1):20–26

Ballas SK, Lusardi M (2005) Hospital readmission for adult acute sickle cell painful episodes: frequency, etiology, and prognostic significance. Am J Hematol 79(1):17–25

Bartolucci P, Chaar V, Picot J et al (2010) Decreased sickle red blood cell adhesion to laminin by hydroxyurea is associated with inhibition of Lu/BCAM protein phosphorylation. Blood 116(12):2152–2159

Beckman JD, Belcher JD, Vineyard JV et al (2009) Inhaled carbon monoxide reduces leukocytosis in a murine model of sickle cell disease. Am J Physiol Heart Circ Physiol 297(4):H1243–H1253

Belcher JD, Vineyard JV, Bruzzone CM et al (2010) Heme oxygenase-1 gene delivery by Sleeping Beauty inhibits vascular stasis in a murine model of sickle cell disease. J Mol Med (Berl) 88(7):665–675

Belcher JD, Young M, Chen C et al (2013) MP4CO, a pegylated hemoglobin saturated with carbon monoxide, is a modulator of HO-1, inflammation, and vaso-occlusion in transgenic sickle mice. Blood 122(15):2757–2764

Belcher JD, Chen C, Nguyen J et al (2014) Heme triggers TLR4 signaling leading to endothelial cell activation and vaso-occlusion in murine sickle cell disease. Blood 123(3):377–390

Beutler E (1975) The effect of carbon monoxide on red cell life span in sickle cell disease. Blood 46(2):253–259

Bianchi ME (2007) DAMPs, PAMPs and alarmins: all we need to know about danger. J Leukoc Biol 81(1):1–5

Bondeva T, Wolf G (2014) Reactive oxygen species in diabetic nephropathy: friend or foe? Nephrol Dial Transplant 29(11):1998–2003

Bradley JR (2008) TNF-mediated inflammatory disease. J Pathol 214(2):149–160

Brittain JE, Hulkower B, Jones SK et al (2010) Placenta growth factor in sickle cell disease: association with hemolysis and inflammation. Blood 115(10):2014–2020

Brousse V, Buffet P, Rees D (2014) The spleen and sickle cell disease: the sick(led) spleen. Br J Haematol 166(2):165–176

Brun M, Bourdoulous S, Couraud PO et al (2003) Hydroxyurea downregulates endothelin-1 gene expression and upregulates ICAM-1 gene expression in cultured human endothelial cells. Pharmacogenomics J 3(4):215–226

Buchanan GR, Holtkamp CA (1985) Plasma levels of platelet and vascular prostaglandin derivatives in children with sickle cell anaemia. Thromb Haemost 54(2):394–396

Bzowska M, Stalinska K, Mezyk-Kopec R et al (2009) Exogenous nitric oxide inhibits shedding of ADAM17 substrates. Acta Biochim Pol 56(2):325–335

Calabrese LH, Rose-John S (2014) IL-6 biology: implications for clinical targeting in rheumatic disease. Nat Rev Rheumatol 10(12):720–727

Camus SM, De Moraes JA, Bonnin P et al (2015) Circulating cell membrane microparticles transfer heme to endothelial cells and trigger vaso-occlusions in sickle cell disease. Blood 125(24):3805–3814

Canalli AA, Franco-Penteado CF, Traina F et al (2007) Role for cAMP-protein kinase A signalling in augmented neutrophil adhesion and chemotaxis in sickle cell disease. Eur J Haematol 79(4):330–337

Canalli AA, Franco-Penteado CF, Saad ST, Conran N, Costa FF (2008) Increased adhesive properties of neutrophils in sickle cell disease may be reversed by pharmacological nitric oxide donation. Haematologica 93(4):605–609

Capra V, Back M, Barbieri SS et al (2013) Eicosanoids and their drugs in cardiovascular diseases: focus on atherosclerosis and stroke. Med Res Rev 33(2):364–438

Cartron JP, Elion J (2008) Erythroid adhesion molecules in sickle cell disease: effect of hydroxyurea. Transfus Clin Biol 15(1–2):39–50

Cerqueira BA, Boas WV, Zanette AD, Reis MG, Goncalves MS (2011) Increased concentrations of IL-18 and uric acid in sickle cell anemia: contribution of hemolysis, endothelial activation and the inflammasome. Cytokine 56(2):471–476

Chaar V, Laurance S, Lapoumeroulie C et al (2014) Hydroxycarbamide decreases sickle reticulocyte adhesion to resting endothelium by inhibiting endothelial lutheran/basal cell adhesion molecule (Lu/BCAM) through phosphodiesterase 4A activation. J Biol Chem 289(16):11512–11521

Chantrathammachart P, Mackman N, Sparkenbaugh E et al (2012) Tissue factor promotes activation of coagulation and inflammation in a mouse model of sickle cell disease. Blood 120(3):636–646

Charache S, Terrin ML, Moore RD et al (1995) Effect of hydroxyurea on the frequency of painful crises in sickle cell anemia. Investigators of the Multicenter Study of Hydroxyurea in Sickle Cell Anemia. N Engl J Med 332(20):1317–1322

Charache S, Barton FB, Moore RD et al (1996) Hydroxyurea and sickle cell anemia. Clinical utility of a myelosuppressive "switching" agent. The Multicenter Study of Hydroxyurea in Sickle Cell Anemia. Medicine (Baltimore) 75(6):300–326

Chen GY, Nunez G (2010) Sterile inflammation: sensing and reacting to damage. Nat Rev Immunol 10(12):826–837

Chen G, Zhang D, Fuchs TA et al (2014) Heme-induced neutrophil extracellular traps contribute to the pathogenesis of sickle cell disease. Blood 123(24):3818–3827

Cheung ATW, Chan MS, Ramanujam S et al (2004) Effects of poloxamer 188 treatment on sickle cell vaso-occlusive crisis: computer-assisted intravital microscopy study. J Invest Med 52(6):402–406

Chistiakov DA, Orekhov AN, Sobenin IA, Bobryshev YV (2014) Plasmacytoid dendritic cells: development, functions, and role in atherosclerotic inflammation. Front Physiol 5:279

Colella MP, De Paula EV, Conran N et al (2012) Hydroxyurea is associated with reductions in hypercoagulability markers in sickle cell anemia. J Thromb Haemost 10(9):1967–1970

Colin Y, Le Van Kim C, El Nemer W (2014) Red cell adhesion in human diseases. Curr Opin Hematol 21(3):186–192

Conran N, Almeida CB, Lanaro C et al (2007a) Inhibition of caspase-dependent spontaneous apoptosis via a cAMP-protein kinase A dependent pathway in neutrophils from sickle cell disease patients. Br J Haematol 139(1):148–158

Conran N, Saad ST, Costa FF, Ikuta T (2007b) Leukocyte numbers correlate with plasma levels of granulocyte-macrophage colony-stimulating factor in sickle cell disease. Ann Hematol 86(4):255–261

Croizat H, Nagel RL (1999) Circulating cytokines response and the level of erythropoiesis in sickle cell anemia. Am J Hematol 60(2):105–115

Cruz PR, Lira RP, Pereira Filho SA et al (2015) Increased circulating PEDF and low sICAM-1 are associated with sickle cell retinopathy. Blood Cells Mol Dis 54(1):33–37 da Silva RR, Pereira MC, Melo Rego MJ et al (2014) Evaluation of Th17 related cytokines associated with clinical and laboratorial parameters in sickle cell anemia patients with leg ulcers. Cytokine 65(2):143–147

Davila J, Manwani D, Vasovic L et al (2015) A novel inflammatory role for platelets in sickle cell disease. Platelets 26(8):726–729

De Montalembert M, Wang W (2013) Cerebrovascular complications in children with sickle cell disease. Handb Clin Neurol 113:1937–1943

Diebold I, Kraicun D, Bonello S, Gorlach A (2008) The 'PAI-1 paradox' in vascular remodeling. Thromb Haemost 100(6):984–991

Dominical VM, Samsel L, Nichols JS et al (2014) Prominent role of platelets in the formation of circulating neutrophil-red cell heterocellular aggregates in sickle cell anemia. Haematologica 99(11):e214–e217

Dong JF, Moake JL, Nolasco L et al (2002) ADAMTS-13 rapidly cleaves newly secreted ultralarge von Willebrand factor multimers on the endothelial surface under flowing conditions. Blood 100(12):4033–4039

Driss A, Wilson NO, Mason K et al (2012) Elevated IL-1alpha and CXCL10 serum levels occur in patients with homozygous sickle cell disease and a history of acute splenic sequestration. Dis Markers 32(5):295–300

Duits AJ, Pieters RC, Saleh AW et al (1996) Enhanced levels of soluble VCAM-1 in sickle cell patients and their specific increment during vasoocclusive crisis. Clin Immunol Immunopathol 81(1):96–98

Duits AJ, Rodriguez T, Schnog JJ, CURAMA Study Group (2006) Serum levels of angiogenic factors indicate a pro-angiogenic state in adults with sickle cell disease. Br J Haematol 134(1):116–119

Dutra FF, Bozza MT (2014) Heme on innate immunity and inflammation. Front Pharmacol 5:115

Dutra FF, Alves LS, Rodrigues D et al (2014) Hemolysis-induced lethality involves inflammasome activation by heme. Proc Natl Acad Sci U S A 111(39):E4110–E4118

Dworkis DA, Klings ES, Solovieff N et al (2011) Severe sickle cell anemia is associated with increased plasma levels of TNF-R1 and VCAM-1. Am J Hematol 86(2):220–223

Elshazly SA, Heiba NM, Abdelmageed WM (2014) Plasma PTX3 levels in sickle cell disease patients, during vaso occlusion and acute chest syndrome (data from Saudi population). Hematology 19(1):52–59

Field JJ, Krings J, White NL et al (2009) Urinary cysteinyl leukotriene E(4) is associated with increased risk for pain and acute chest syndrome in adults with sickle cell disease. Am J Hematol 84(3):158–160

Field JJ, Nathan DG, Linden J (2011) Targeting iNKT cells for the treatment of sickle cell disease. Clin Immunol 140(2):177–183

Field JJ, Ataga KI, Majerus EM et al (2013) A phase I single ascending dose study of NKTT120 in stable adult sickle cell patients. Blood 122(21):977

Field JJ, Nathan DG, Linden J (2014) The role of adenosine signaling in sickle cell therapeutics. Hematol Oncol Clin North Am 28(2):287–299

Francis RB Jr (1989) Elevated fibrin D-dimer fragment in sickle cell anemia: evidence for activation of coagulation during the steady state as well as in painful crisis. Haemostasis 19(2):105–111

Francis RB Jr, Haywood LJ (1992) Elevated immunoreactive tumor necrosis factor and interleukin-1 in sickle cell disease. J Natl Med Assoc 84(7):611–615

Franck PF, Bevers EM, Lubin BH et al (1985) Uncoupling of the membrane skeleton from the lipid bilayer. The cause of accelerated phospholipid flip-flop leading to an enhanced procoagulant activity of sickled cells. J Clin Invest 75(1):183–190

Gambero S, Canalli AA, Traina F et al (2007) Therapy with hydroxyurea is associated with reduced adhesion molecule gene and protein expression in sickle red cells with a concomitant reduction in adhesive properties. Eur J Haematol 78(2):144–151

Garraud O, Cognasse F (2015) Are platelets cells? and if yes, are they immune cells? Front Immunol 6:70

Garrido VT, Proenca-Ferreira R, Dominical VM et al (2012) Elevated plasma levels and platelet-associated expression of the pro-thrombotic and pro-inflammatory protein, TNFSF14 (LIGHT), in sickle cell disease. Br J Haematol 158(6):788–797

Ghosh S, Adisa OA, Chappa P et al (2013) Extracellular hemin crisis triggers acute chest syndrome in sickle mice. J Clin Invest 123(11):4809–4820

Gladwin MT, Ofori-Acquah SF (2014) Erythroid DAMPs drive inflammation in SCD. Blood 123(24):3689–3690

Graido-Gonzalez E, Doherty JC, Bergreen EW et al (1998) Plasma endothelin-1, cytokine, and prostaglandin E2 levels in sickle cell disease and acute vaso-occlusive sickle crisis. Blood 92(7):2551–2555

Gros A, Ollivier V, Ho-Tin-Noe B (2015) Platelets in inflammation: regulation of leukocyte activities and vascular repair. Front Immunol 5:678

Hammerman SI, Kourembanas S, Conca TJ et al (1997) Endothelin-1 production during the acute chest syndrome in sickle cell disease. Am J Respir Crit Care Med 156(1):280–285

Hasan RN, Schafer AI (2008) Hemin upregulates Egr-1 expression in vascular smooth muscle cells via reactive oxygen species ERK-1/2-Elk-1 and NF-kappaB. Circ Res 102(1):42–50

Hebbel RP (2014) Ischemia-reperfusion injury in sickle cell anemia: relationship to acute chest syndrome, endothelial dysfunction, arterial vasculopathy, and inflammatory pain. Hematol Oncol Clin North Am 28(2):181–198

Hebbel RP, Eaton JW, Balasingam M, Steinberg MH (1982) Spontaneous oxygen radical generation by sickle erythrocytes. J Clin Invest 70(6):1253–1259

Heinrich PC, Castell JV, Andus T (1990) Interleukin-6 and the acute phase response. Biochem J 265(3):621–636

Hibbert JM, Hsu LL, Bhathena SJ et al (2005) Proinflammatory cytokines and the hypermetabolism of children with sickle cell disease. Exp Biol Med (Maywood) 230(1):68–74

Hofmann SR, Rösen-Wolff A, Tsokos GC, Hedrich CM (2012) Biological properties and regulation of IL-10 related cytokines and their contribution to autoimmune disease and tissue injury. Clin Immunol 143(2):116–127

Hoppe C, Kuypers F, Larkin S et al (2011) A pilot study of the short-term use of simvastatin in sickle cell disease: effects on markers of vascular dysfunction. Br J Haematol 153(5):655–663

Hossain M, Qadri SM, Liu L (2012) Inhibition of nitric oxide synthesis enhances leukocyte rolling and adhesion in human microvasculature. J Inflamm (Lond) 9(1):28

Huang AL, Vita JA (2006) Effects of systemic inflammation on endothelium-dependent vasodilation. Trends Cardiovasc Med 16(1):15–20

Hyacinth HI, Gee BE, Adamkiewicz TV et al (2012) Plasma BDNF and PDGF-AA levels are associated with high TCD velocity and stroke in children with sickle cell anemia. Cytokine 60(1):302–308

Ibe BO, Morris J, Kurantsin-Mills J, Raj JU (1997) Sickle erythrocytes induce prostacyclin and thromboxane synthesis by isolated perfused rat lungs. Am J Physiol 272(4 Pt 1):L597–L602

Idzko M, Ferrari D, Eltzschig HK (2014a) Nucleotide signalling during inflammation. Nature 509(7500):310–317

Idzko M, Ferrari D, Riegel AK, Eltzschig HK (2014b) Extracellular nucleotide and nucleoside signaling in vascular and blood disease. Blood 124(7):1029–1037

Ikuta T, Adekile AD, Gutsaeva DR et al (2011) The proinflammatory cytokine GM-CSF downregulates fetal hemoglobin expression by attenuating the cAMP-dependent pathway in sickle cell disease. Blood Cells Mol Dis 47(4):235–242

Iwasaki K, Mackenzie EL, Hailemariam K, Sakamoto K, Tsuji Y (2006) Hemin-mediated regulation of an antioxidant-responsive element of the human ferritin H gene and role of Ref-1 during erythroid differentiation of K562 cells. Mol Cell Biol 26(7):2845–2856

Jakubowski JA, Zhou C, Winters KJ et al (2014) The effect of prasugrel on ADP-stimulated markers of platelet activation in patients with sickle cell disease. Platelets 1–6

Jennings JE, Ramkumar T, Mao J et al (2008) Elevated urinary leukotriene E4 levels are associated with hospitalization for pain in children with sickle cell disease. Am J Hematol 83(8):640–643

Joneckis CC, Ackley RL, Orringer EP, Wayner EA, Parise LV (1993) Integrin alpha 4 beta 1 and glycoprotein IV (CD36) are expressed on circulating reticulocytes in sickle cell anemia. Blood 82(12):3548–3555

Kalogeris T, Baines CP, Krenz M, Korthuis RJ (2012) Cell biology of ischemia/reperfusion injury. Int Rev Cell Mol Biol 298:229–317

Kanavaki I, Makrythanasis P, Lazaropoulou C et al (2012) Adhesion molecules and high-sensitivity C-reactive protein levels in patients with sickle cell beta-thalassaemia. Eur J Clin Invest 42(1):27–33

Kato GJ, Gladwin MT, Steinberg MH (2007) Deconstructing sickle cell disease: reappraisal of the role of hemolysis in the development of clinical subphenotypes. Blood Rev 21(1):37–47

Kaul DK, Nagel RL, Chen D, Tsai HM (1993) Sickle erythrocyte-endothelial interactions in microcirculation: the role of von Willebrand factor and implications for vasoocclusion. Blood 81(9):2429–2438

Kaul DK, Finnegan E, Barabino GA (2009) Sickle red cell-endothelium interactions. Microcirculation 16(1):97–111

Keikhaei B, Mohseni AR, Norouzirad R et al (2013) Altered levels of pro-inflammatory cytokines in sickle cell disease patients during vaso-occlusive crises and the steady state condition. Eur Cytokine Netw 24(1):45–52

Key NS, Slungaard A, Dandelet L et al (1998) Whole blood tissue factor procoagulant activity is elevated in patients with sickle cell disease. Blood 91(11):4216–4223

King SB (2003) The nitric oxide producing reactions of hydroxyurea. Curr Med Chem 10(6):437–452

Koenen RR, Weber C (2011) Chemokines: established and novel targets in atherosclerosis. EMBO Mol Med 3(12):713–725

Kolaczkowska E, Kubes P (2013) Neutrophil recruitment and function in health and inflammation. Nat Rev Immunol 13(3):159–175

Kowalska MA, Rauova L, Poncz M (2010) Role of the platelet chemokine platelet factor 4 (PF4) in hemostasis and thrombosis. Thromb Res 125(4):292–296

Krishnan S, Setty Y, Betal SG et al (2010) Increased levels of the inflammatory biomarker C-reactive protein at baseline are associated with childhood sickle cell vasocclusive crises. Br J Haematol 148(5):797–804

Kuruppu S, Rajapakse NW, Dunstan RA, Smith AI (2014) Nitric oxide inhibits the production of soluble endothelin converting enzyme-1. Mol Cell Biochem 396(1–2):49–54

Lanaro C, Franco-Penteado CF, Albuqueque DM et al (2009) Altered levels of cytokines and inflammatory mediators in plasma and leukocytes of sickle cell anemia patients and effects of hydroxyurea therapy. J Leukoc Biol 85(2):235–242

Lance EI, Casella JF, Everett AD, Barron-Casella E (2014) Proteomic and biomarker studies and neurological complications of pediatric sickle cell disease. Proteomics Clin Appl 8(11–12):813–827

Landburg PP, Nur E, Maria N et al (2009) Elevated circulating stromal-derived factor-1 levels in sickle cell disease. Acta Haematol 122(1):64–69

Lapoumeroulie C, Benkerrou M, Odievre MH et al (2005) Decreased plasma endothelin-1 levels in children with sickle cell disease treated with hydroxyurea. Haematologica 90(3):401–403

Lee SP, Ataga KI, Orringer EP, Phillips DR, Parise LV (2006) Biologically active CD40 ligand is elevated in sickle cell anemia: potential role for platelet-mediated inflammation. Arterioscler Thromb Vasc Biol 26(7):1626–1631

Leick M, Azcutia V, Newton G, Luscinskas FW (2014) Leukocyte recruitment in inflammation: basic concepts and new mechanistic insights based on new models and microscopic imaging technologies. Cell Tissue Res 355(3):647–656

Lira SA, Furtado GC (2012) The biology of chemokines and their receptors. Immunol Res 54(1–3):111–120

Lister MF, Sharkey J, Sawatzky DA et al (2007) The role of the purinergic P2X7 receptor in inflammation. J Inflamm (Lond) 4:5

Lopes FC, Ferreira R, Albuquerque DM et al (2014) In vitro and in vivo anti-angiogenic effects of hydroxyurea. Microvasc Res 94:106–113

Lopes FC, Traina F, Almeida CB et al (2015) Key endothelial cell angiogenic mechanisms are stimulated by the circulating milieu in sickle cell disease and attenuated by hydroxyurea. Haematologica 100(6):730–739

Lubin B, Chiu D, Bastacky J, Roelofsen B, Van Deenen LL (1981) Abnormalities in membrane phospholipid organization in sickled erythrocytes. J Clin Invest 67(6):1643–1649

Manwani DM, Chen C, Carullo V et al (2014) Vaso-occlusion-promoting neutrophil mac-1 integrin activation in human sickle cell crises is stabilized by a single dose of intravenous gammaglobulin. Blood 124(21), ASH abstract:4089

McCracken JM, Allen LA (2014) Regulation of human neutrophil apoptosis and lifespan in health and disease. J Cell Death 7:15–23

McGann PT, Ware RE (2011) Hydroxyurea for sickle cell anemia: what have we learned and what questions still remain? Curr Opin Hematol 18(3):158–165

McGregor L, Martin J, McGregor JL (2006) Platelet-leukocyte aggregates and derived microparticles in inflammation, vascular remodelling and thrombosis. Front Biosci 11:830–837

Medzhitov R (2008) Origin and physiological roles of inflammation. Nature 454(7203):428–435

Mehta P, Albiol L (1982) Prostacyclin and platelet aggregation in sickle cell disease. Pediatrics 70(3):354–359

Michaels LA, Ohene-Frempong K, Zhao H, Douglas SD (1998) Serum levels of substance P are elevated in patients with sickle cell disease and increase further during vaso-occlusive crisis. Blood 92(9):3148–3151

Minniti CP, Delaney KM, Gorbach AM et al (2014) Vasculopathy, inflammation, and blood flow in leg ulcers of patients with sickle cell anemia. Am J Hematol 89(1):1–6

Mohammed FA, Mahdi N, Sater MA, Al-Ola K, Almawi WY (2010) The relation of C-reactive protein to vasoocclusive crisis in children with sickle cell disease. Blood Cells Mol Dis 45(4):293–296

Mohan JS, Lip PL, Blann AD, Bareford D, Lip GY (2005) The angiopoietin/Tie-2 system in proliferative sickle retinopathy: relation to vascular endothelial growth factor, its soluble receptor Flt-1 and von Willebrand factor, and to the effects of laser treatment. Br J Ophthalmol 89(7):815–819

Moreth K, Iozzo RV, Schaefer L (2012) Small leucine-rich proteoglycans orchestrate receptor crosstalk during inflammation. Cell Cycle 11(11):2084–2091

Morganroth ML, Stenmark KR, Zirrolli JA et al (1984) Leukotriene C4 production during hypoxic pulmonary vasoconstriction in isolated rat lungs. Prostaglandins 28(6):867–875

Mukaida N, Harada A, Matsushima K (1998) Interleukin-8 (IL-8) and monocyte chemotactic and activating factor (MCAF/MCP-1), chemokines essentially involved in inflammatory and immune reactions. Cytokine Growth Factor Rev 9(1):9–23

Nath KA, Hebbel RP (2015) Sickle cell disease: renal manifestations and mechanisms. Nat Rev Nephrol 11(3):161–171

Nath KA, Grande JP, Haggard JJ et al (2001) Oxidative stress and induction of heme oxygenase-1 in the kidney in sickle cell disease. Am J Pathol 158(3):893–903

Natta CL, Chen LC, Chow CK (1990) Selenium and glutathione peroxidase levels in sickle cell anemia. Acta Haematol 83(3):130–132

Niu X, Nouraie M, Campbell A et al (2009) Angiogenic and inflammatory markers of cardiopulmonary changes in children and adolescents with sickle cell disease. PLoS One 4(11), e7956

Nsiri B, Gritli N, Bayoudh F et al (1996) Abnormalities of coagulation and fibrinolysis in homozygous sickle cell disease. Hematol Cell Ther 38(3):279–284

Nur E, van Beers EJ, Martina S et al (2011) Plasma levels of pentraxin-3, an acute phase protein, are increased during sickle cell painful crisis. Blood Cells Mol Dis 46(3):189–194

O'Donnell A, Premawardhena A, Arambepola M et al (2009) Interaction of malaria with a common form of severe thalassemia in an Asian population. Proc Natl Acad Sci U S A 106(44):18716–18721

Okocha C, Manafa P, Ozomba J et al (2014) C-reactive protein and disease outcome in Nigerian sickle cell disease patients. Ann Med Health Sci Res 4(5):701–705

Okpala I (2015) Investigational selectin-targeted therapy of sickle cell disease. Expert Opin Investig Drugs 24(2):229–238

Opene M, Kurantsin-Mills J, Husain S, Ibe BO (2014) Sickle erythrocytes and platelets augment lung leukotriene synthesis with downregulation of anti-inflammatory proteins: relevance in the pathology of the acute chest syndrome. Pulm Circ 4(3):482–495

Ortega-Gomez A, Perretti M, Soehnlein O (2013) Resolution of inflammation: an integrated view. EMBO Mol Med 5(5):661–674

Ozaki E, Campbell M, Doyle SL (2015) Targeting the NLRP3 inflammasome in chronic inflammatory diseases: current perspectives. J Inflamm Res 8:15–27

Page C, Pitchford S (2013) Neutrophil and platelet complexes and their relevance to neutrophil recruitment and activation. Int Immunopharmacol 17(4):1176–1184

Pallis FR, Conran N, Fertrin KY et al (2014) Hydroxycarbamide reduces eosinophil adhesion and degranulation in sickle cell anaemia patients. Br J Haematol 164(2):286–295

Papadimitriou CA, Travlou A, Kalos A, Douratsos D, Lali P (1993) Study of platelet function in patients with sickle cell anemia during steady state and vaso-occlusive crisis. Acta Haematol 89(4):180–183

Patel N, Kalra VK (2010) Placenta growth factor-induced early growth response 1 (Egr-1) regulates hypoxia-inducible factor-1alpha (HIF-1alpha) in endothelial cells. J Biol Chem 285(27):20570–20579

Patel N, Gonsalves CS, Malik P, Kalra VK (2008) Placenta growth factor augments endothelin-1 and endothelin-B receptor expression via hypoxia-inducible factor-1 alpha. Blood 112(3): 856–865

Patel N, Gonsalves CS, Yang M, Malik P, Kalra VK (2009) Placenta growth factor induces 5-lipoxygenase-activating protein to increase leukotriene formation in sickle cell disease. Blood 113(5):1129–1138

Patel N, Sundaram N, Yang M et al (2010) Placenta growth factor (PlGF), a novel inducer of plasminogen activator inhibitor-1 (PAI-1) in sickle cell disease (SCD). J Biol Chem 285(22): 16713–16722

Pathare A, Al Kindi S, Alnaqdy AA et al (2004) Cytokine profile of sickle cell disease in Oman. Am J Hematol 77(4):323–328

Perelman N, Selvaraj SK, Batra S et al (2003) Placenta growth factor activates monocytes and correlates with sickle cell disease severity. Blood 102(4):1506–1514

Pernow J, Shemyakin A, Bohm F (2012) New perspectives on endothelin-1 in atherosclerosis and diabetes mellitus. Life Sci 91(13–14):507–516

Platt OS, Orkin SH, Dover G et al (1984) Hydroxyurea enhances fetal hemoglobin production in sickle cell anemia. J Clin Invest 74(2):652–656

Platt OS, Thorington BD, Brambilla DJ et al (1991) Pain in sickle cell disease. Rates and risk factors. N Engl J Med 325(1):11–16

Proenca-Ferreira R, Franco-Penteado CF, Traina F et al (2010) Increased adhesive properties of platelets in sickle cell disease: roles for alphaIIb beta3-mediated ligand binding, diminished cAMP signalling and increased phosphodiesterase 3A activity. Br J Haematol 149(2):280–288

Proenca-Ferreira R, Brugnerotto AF, Garrido VT et al (2014) Endothelial activation by platelets from sickle cell anemia patients. PLoS One 9(2), e89012

Qari MH, Dier U, Mousa SA (2012) Biomarkers of inflammation, growth factor, and coagulation activation in patients with sickle cell disease. Clin Appl Thromb Hemost 18(2):195–200

Reiter CD, Wang X, Tanus-Santos JE et al (2002) Cell-free hemoglobin limits nitric oxide bioavailability in sickle-cell disease. Nat Med 8(12):1383–1389

Ricciotti E, FitzGerald GA (2011) Prostaglandins and inflammation. Arterioscler Thromb Vasc Biol 31(5):986–1000

Rodrigues L, Costa FF, Saad ST, Grotto HZ (2006) High levels of neopterin and interleukin-3 in sickle cell disease patients. J Clin Lab Anal 20(3):75–79

Rowley CA, Ikeda AK, Seidel M et al (2014) Microvascular oxygen consumption during sickle cell pain crisis. Blood 123(20):3101–3104

Rubanyi GM, Ho EH, Cantor EH, Lumma WC, Botelho LH (1991) Cytoprotective function of nitric oxide: inactivation of superoxide radicals produced by human leukocytes. Biochem Biophys Res Commun 181(3):1392–1397

Safaya S, Steinberg MH, Klings ES (2012) Monocytes from sickle cell disease patients induce differential pulmonary endothelial gene expression via activation of NF-kappaB signaling pathway. Mol Immunol 50(1–2):117–123

Sakamoto TM, Lanaro C, Ozelo MC et al (2013) Increased adhesive and inflammatory properties in blood outgrowth endothelial cells from sickle cell anemia patients. Microvasc Res 90:173–179

Sarray S, Saleh LR, Lisa Saldanha F et al (2015) Serum IL-6, IL-10, and TNFalpha levels in pediatric sickle cell disease patients during vasoocclusive crisis and steady state condition. Cytokine 72(1):43–47

Schacter L, Warth JA, Gordon EM, Prasad A, Klein BL (1988) Altered amount and activity of superoxide dismutase in sickle cell anemia. FASEB J 2(3):237–243

Schaer DJ, Buehler PW, Alayash AI, Belcher JD, Vercellotti GM (2013) Hemolysis and free hemoglobin revisited: exploring hemoglobin and hemin scavengers as a novel class of therapeutic proteins. Blood 121(8):1276–1284

Sedger LM, McDermott MF (2014) TNF and TNF-receptors: from mediators of cell death and inflammation to therapeutic giants – past, present and future. Cytokine Growth Factor Rev 25(4):453–472

Serhan CN, Chiang N, Dalli J, Levy BD (2014) Lipid mediators in the resolution of inflammation. Cold Spring Harb Perspect Biol 7(2), a016311

Setty BN, Betal SG (2008) Microvascular endothelial cells express a phosphatidylserine receptor: a functionally active receptor for phosphatidylserine-positive erythrocytes. Blood 111(2):905–914

Setty BN, Stuart MJ (2002) Eicosanoids in sickle cell disease: potential relevance of neutrophil leukotriene B4 to disease pathophysiology. J Lab Clin Med 139(2):80–89

Setty BN, Key NS, Rao AK et al (2012) Tissue factor-positive monocytes in children with sickle cell disease: correlation with biomarkers of haemolysis. Br J Haematol 157(3):370–380

Shah N, Thornburg C, Telen MJ, Ortel TL (2012) Characterization of the hypercoagulable state in patients with sickle cell disease. Thromb Res 130(5):e241–e245

Shen H, Kreisel D, Goldstein DR (2013) Processes of sterile inflammation. J Immunol 191(6):2857–2863

Shet AS, Aras O, Gupta K et al (2003) Sickle blood contains tissue factor-positive microparticles derived from endothelial cells and monocytes. Blood 102(7):2678–2683

Shiu YT, Udden MM, McIntire LV (2000) Perfusion with sickle erythrocytes up-regulates ICAM-1 and VCAM-1 gene expression in cultured human endothelial cells. Blood 95(10):3232–3241

Sikora J, Orlov SN, Furuya K, Grygorczyk R (2014) Hemolysis is a primary ATP-release mechanism in human erythrocytes. Blood 124(13):2150–2157

Solovey A, Gui L, Key NS, Hebbel RP (1998) Tissue factor expression by endothelial cells in sickle cell anemia. J Clin Invest 101(9):1899–1904

Solovey A, Kollander R, Milbauer LC et al (2010) Endothelial nitric oxide synthase and nitric oxide regulate endothelial tissue factor expression in vivo in the sickle transgenic mouse. Am J Hematol 85(1):41–45

Sparkenbaugh E, Pawlinski R (2013) Interplay between coagulation and vascular inflammation in sickle cell disease. Br J Haematol 162(1):3–14

Sparkenbaugh EM, Chantrathammachart P, Wang S et al (2015) Excess of heme induces tissue factor-dependent activation of coagulation in mice. Haematologica 100(3):308–314

Steinberg MH, Barton F, Castro O et al (2003) Effect of hydroxyurea on mortality and morbidity in adult sickle cell anemia: risks and benefits up to 9 years of treatment. JAMA 289(13): 1645–1651

Sultana C, Shen Y, Rattan V, Johnson C, Kalra VK (1998) Interaction of sickle erythrocytes with endothelial cells in the presence of endothelial cell conditioned medium induces oxidant stress leading to transendothelial migration of monocytes. Blood 92(10):3924–3935
Sundaram N, Tailor A, Mendelsohn L et al (2010) High levels of placenta growth factor in sickle cell disease promote pulmonary hypertension. Blood 116(1):109–112
Tadie JM, Bae HB, Jiang S et al (2013) HMGB1 promotes neutrophil extracellular trap formation through interactions with Toll-like receptor 4. Am J Physiol Lung Cell Mol Physiol 304(5): L342–L349
Tantawy AA, Adly AA, Ismail EA, Darwish YW, Ali Zedan M (2014) Growth differentiation factor-15 in young sickle cell disease patients: relation to hemolysis, iron overload and vascular complications. Blood Cells Mol Dis 53(4):189–193
Tomer A, Kasey S, Connor WE et al (2001) Reduction of pain episodes and prothrombotic activity in sickle cell disease by dietary n-3 fatty acids. Thromb Haemost 85(6):966–974
Tsoumani ME, Kalantzi KI, Goudevenos IA, Tselepis AD (2012) Platelet-mediated inflammation in cardiovascular disease. Potential role of platelet-endothelium interactions. Curr Vasc Pharmacol 10(5):539–549
Turhan A, Weiss LA, Mohandas N, Coller BS, Frenette PS (2002) Primary role for adherent leukocytes in sickle cell vascular occlusion: a new paradigm. Proc Natl Acad Sci U S A 99(5): 3047–3051
Turhan A, Jenab P, Bruhns P et al (2004) Intravenous immune globulin prevents venular vasoocclusion in sickle cell mice by inhibiting leukocyte adhesion and the interactions between sickle erythrocytes and adherent leukocytes. Blood 103(6):2397–2400
Turner MD, Nedjai B, Hurst T, Pennington DJ (2014) Cytokines and chemokines: at the crossroads of cell signalling and inflammatory disease. Biochim Biophys Acta 1843(11):2563–2582
van Beers EJ, Yang Y, Raghavachari N et al (2015) Iron, inflammation, and early death in adults with sickle cell disease. Circ Res 116(2):298–306
van Golen RF, van Gulik TM, Heger M (2012) The sterile immune response during hepatic ischemia/reperfusion. Cytokine Growth Factor Rev 23(3):69–84
Van Kaer L, Parekh VV, Wu L (2013) Invariant natural killer T cells as sensors and managers of inflammation. Trends Immunol 34(2):50–58
Vincent L, Vang D, Nguyen J et al (2013) Mast cell activation contributes to sickle cell pathobiology and pain in mice. Blood 122(11):1853–1862
Wallace JL (2005) Nitric oxide as a regulator of inflammatory processes. Mem Inst Oswaldo Cruz 100(Suppl 1):5–9
Walley KR, McDonald TE, Higashimoto Y, Hayashi S (1999) Modulation of proinflammatory cytokines by nitric oxide in murine acute lung injury. Am J Respir Crit Care Med 160(2):698–704
Walter MR (2014) The molecular basis of IL-10 function: from receptor structure to the onset of signaling. Curr Top Microbiol Immunol 380:191–212
Weber DJ, Allette YM, Wilkes DS, White FA (2015) The HMGB1-RAGE inflammatory pathway: implications for brain injury induced pulmonary dysfunction. Antioxid Redox Signal
Werdehoff SG, Moore RB, Hoff CJ, Fillingim E, Hackman AM (1998) Elevated plasma endothelin-1 levels in sickle cell anemia: relationships to oxygen saturation and left ventricular hypertrophy. Am J Hematol 58(3):195–199
Westwick J, Watson-Williams EJ, Krishnamurthi S et al (1983) Platelet activation during steady state sickle cell disease. J Med 14(1):17–36
Wood KC, Granger DN (2007) Sickle cell disease: role of reactive oxygen and nitrogen metabolites. Clin Exp Pharmacol Physiol 34(9):926–932
Wood BL, Gibson DF, Tait JF (1996) Increased erythrocyte phosphatidylserine exposure in sickle cell disease: flow-cytometric measurement and clinical associations. Blood 88(5):1873–1880
Wood KC, Hebbel RP, Granger DN (2005) Endothelial cell NADPH oxidase mediates the cerebral microvascular dysfunction in sickle cell transgenic mice. FASEB J 19(8):989–991
Wun T, Cordoba M, Rangaswami A, Cheung AW, Paglieroni T (2002) Activated monocytes and platelet-monocyte aggregates in patients with sickle cell disease. Clin Lab Haematol 24(2):81–88

Wun T, Styles L, DeCastro L et al (2014) Phase 1 study of the E-selectin inhibitor GMI 1070 in patients with sickle cell anemia. PLoS One 9(7), e101301

Xia Y, Dawson VL, Dawson TM, Snyder SH, Zweier JL (1996) Nitric oxide synthase generates superoxide and nitric oxide in arginine-depleted cells leading to peroxynitrite-mediated cellular injury. Proc Natl Acad Sci U S A 93(13):6770–6774

Xu H, Wandersee NJ, Guo Y et al (2014) Sickle cell disease increases high mobility group box 1: a novel mechanism of inflammation. Blood 124(26):3978–3981

Yasin Z, Witting S, Palascak MB et al (2003) Phosphatidylserine externalization in sickle red blood cells: associations with cell age, density, and hemoglobin F. Blood 102(1):365–370

Zachlederova M, Jarolim P (2000) Gene expression in human lung microvascular cells interacting with sickle and calcium-loaded red cells and with inflammatory cytokines. Blood 96(11):598A

Zhang Y, Dai Y, Wen J et al (2011) Detrimental effects of adenosine signaling in sickle cell disease. Nat Med 17(1):79–86

Chapter 9
Clinical Manifestations of Sickle Cell Anemia: Infants and Children

Robert Sheppard Nickel and Lewis L. Hsu

Abstract Children with sickle cell disease (SCD) have varied clinical problems. The hallmark manifestation of SCD, the pain crisis, typically first occurs in early childhood presenting as dactylitis. Pain increases in frequency and severity as children age, especially during adolescence. Due to functional asplenia, children with SCD are at significantly increased risk for certain infections, most notably *Streptococcus pneumoniae.* Other infections like parvovirus B19 are also special threats and can trigger an aplastic crisis. Unique, potentially life-threatening acute complications like splenic sequestration and acute chest syndrome occur in these children. They are at risk for neurologic disease, the most serious being stroke. In addition, the chronic hemolysis of SCD causes gallstones, which can lead to biliary tract disease. Children with SCD also frequently face chronic issues that include nocturnal enuresis and decreased growth. Despite these many potential problems, with advances in care including antibiotic treatment, stroke screening, blood transfusions, and hydroxyurea therapy, children with SCD rarely die in childhood and can become productive adults.

Keywords Dactylitis • Aplastic crisis • Splenic sequestration • Acute chest syndrome

9.1 Introduction

Historically associated with mortality in childhood, the prognosis of sickle cell disease (SCD) has significantly improved over the last few decades so that, with modern supportive care, all children with SCD are expected to survive to adulthood.

R.S. Nickel, M.D., M.Sc. (✉)
Children's National Health System, George Washington University School of Medicine and Health Sciences, 111 Michigan Avenue NW, Washington, DC 20010, USA
e-mail: rnickel@childrensnational.org

L.L. Hsu, M.D., Ph.D.
University of Illinois at Chicago, 840 S. Wood St., Chicago, IL 60612, USA
e-mail: lewhsu@uic.edu

© Springer International Publishing Switzerland 2016

F.F. Costa, N. Conran (eds.), *Sickle Cell Anemia*,
DOI 10.1007/978-3-319-06713-1_9

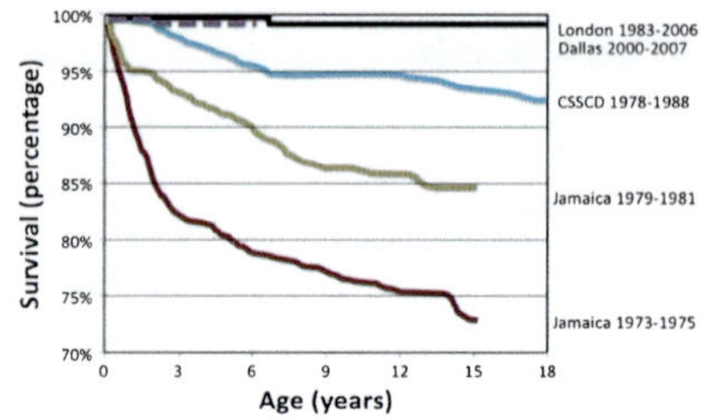

Fig. 9.1 Comparison of overall survival for children with HbSS and HbS-β^0 thalassemia from different cohorts during different time periods. Adapted from Quinn et al. (2010)

Analysis of death certificate data in the United States has demonstrated that death from SCD in childhood has decreased over time (Davis et al. 1997; Yanni et al. 2009). Multiple prospective cohort studies of newborns with SCD have similarly showed a trend of improved childhood survival (Fig. 9.1) (Lee et al. 1995; Telfer et al. 2007; Quinn et al. 2010). The largest such study, the Dallas Newborn Cohort, estimated overall survival at 18 years of age to be 93.9 % for HbSS and HbS-β^0 thalassemia patients, and 98.4 % for HbSC and HbS-β^+ thalassemia patients. Survival statistics for children with SCD today are likely even better as in the most recent analysis of this cohort from 2000 to 2007, no deaths occurred before the age of 18 (Quinn et al. 2010).

While death in childhood secondary to SCD is very rare in high-income nations, sadly children with SCD born in low-income nations (where the prevalence of SCD is greatest, particularly in Africa) still have a high risk of dying at a young age. Due to the lack of universal newborn screening in most low-income nations, young children may die from complications of SCD without ever being diagnosed. Accurate statistics on childhood mortality from SCD in low-income countries are thus not available, but it is clear that many children with SCD in these areas of the world die before age 5 (Makani et al. 2011).

With the proper supportive care that is routinely provided in high-income countries (and will hopefully become increasingly available in low-income countries) most children with SCD enjoy a fulfilling childhood with a good quality of life (Constantinou et al. 2014). Even with excellent supportive care, however, children with SCD may suffer from the complications summarized in this chapter. The clinical course of an individual child with SCD is highly variable; some may experience only minor issues, while others endure many of these serious complications.

9.2 Childhood Manifestations of SCD

9.2.1 Pain Crisis

The acute pain crisis, also referred to as vaso-occlusive crisis (VOC), is the most well-known clinical manifestation of SCD. Children with SCD have described this pain with various adjectives including: aching, pounding, sharp, and sore (Graumlich et al. 2001). The clinical presentation of VOC is variable. This pain can be steady or intermittent; it may come on suddenly or slowly (Dampier et al. 2002a), occur in a single body part, or affect many locations simultaneously with the extremities and lower back commonly affected. A pain crisis can be triggered by certain actions (swimming, overexertion), infection, or changes in the weather (colder temperatures, increased wind speed) (Rogovik et al. 2011), but may also occur without an inciting event.

Dactylitis (also termed "hand-foot syndrome") is a special manifestation of an acute pain crisis in young children in which the hands or feet are swollen, tender, and erythematous. It can occur before the age of 6 months but the highest incidence is between the ages of 6–12 months (Gill et al. 1995). The Cooperative Study of Sickle Cell Disease (CSSCD) estimated that, by age 2 years, ~25 % of all infants with HbSS sought medical care for this complication (Gill et al. 1995). Mild cases of dactylitis are likely more common. The BABY HUG study (discussed below) found that 36 % of infants (median age 13.6 months) had a history of dactylitis at the time of enrollment (Wang et al. 2011). Physical exam findings of VOC are much less common in older children and adolescents; however, VOC of any bone can cause accompanying swelling, tenderness, and erythema. These findings can be clinically indistinguishable from osteomyelitis (Almeida and Roberts 2005). If a joint is involved, VOC can cause effusions that appear similar to septic arthritis. VOC has been associated with a decreased hemoglobin and platelet count but an increased neutrophil count, lactate dehydrogenase (LDH), and C-reactive protein (CRP) (Najim and Hassan 2011). It is important to emphasize that, despite this association of laboratory values and VOC, the diagnosis of a pain crisis is based primarily on a patient's expression of pain.

The frequency and duration of pain crisis varies considerably. The CSSCD found that half of all children with HbSS required medical care for a pain crisis by age 4.9 years (7.1 years for HbSC) (Fig. 9.2) (Gill et al. 1995). In the United States, the average length of a pediatric hospitalization for a SCD pain crisis is ~4 days

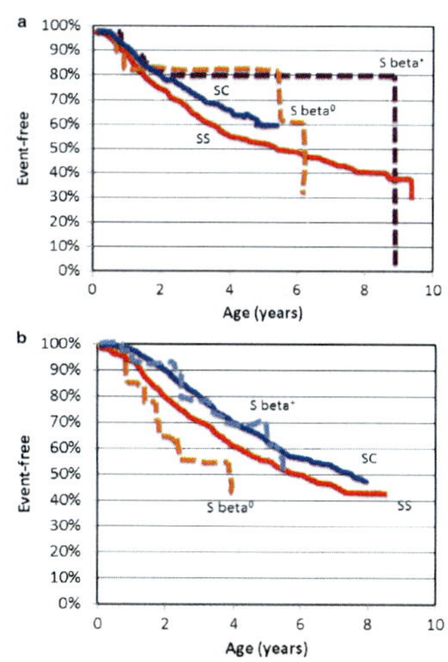

Fig. 9.2 Data from the cooperative study of sickle cell disease infant cohort (CSSCD), collected between 1978 and 1988; age at first clinical event in 694 infants with SCD from birth to 10 years of age for (**a**) painful event, (**b**) acute chest syndrome. Adapted from Gill et al. (1995)

(Panepinto et al. 2005; Raphael et al. 2012). Less severe pain episodes that are managed at home are more common. A study of infants with SCD not on hydroxyurea reported that the median age at first occurrence of any pain was 13.9 months for infants with HbSS (43.6 months for HbSC) (Dampier et al. 2014). A similar study documenting the daily pain of older children with SCD found that while 17 % of patients required admission for pain during the 6-month study period, 40 % experienced at least one episode of pain each month with most episodes lasting one day (Dampier et al. 2004). A striking range in the days of reported pain was also shown by this study group; a few children reported no days of pain versus a few who recorded pain on >90 % of days (Dampier et al. 2002b). These pain diary studies estimate that while young children (age < ~6 years) with SCD rarely experience pain (Dampier et al. 2014), older children and adolescents (age ~6–19 years) with SCD have pain more frequently, on one out of every six days (Dampier et al. 2002a). As children with SCD age into adolescence they also endure longer VOC hospitalizations (Panepinto et al. 2005; Raphael et al. 2012).

Hydroxyurea has the potential to decrease the burden of pain experienced by young children with SCD as demonstrated by the BABY HUG study. This multicenter clinical trial randomized infants (age 9–18 months) with HbSS or HbS-β^0 thalassemia, without regard to clinical severity, to receive daily hydroxyurea or placebo. With hydroxyurea treatment, the incidence of pain was significantly reduced from 203 to 94 events per 100 patient-years; the incidence of dactylitis was also significantly reduced from 66.5 to 12.7 events per 100 patient-years. With the increased use of hydroxyurea to treat young children with SCD, it is likely that VOC hospitalizations for children will decrease, as has already been demonstrated by one institution (Nottage et al. 2013).

9.2.2 *Infection*

Children with SCD are at increased risk for infection from encapsulated organisms due to functional asplenia. Damage to the spleen from sickle vaso-occlusion occurs early in life so that by 1 year of age the majority of infants with HbSS have evidence of splenic dysfunction (Rogers et al. 2011). With functional asplenia, invasive bacterial infections often progress rapidly. From the initial symptoms of fever and malaise, patients can develop potentially fatal septic shock in hours. Historically, bacterial infection was the major cause of death for children with SCD (Barrett-Connor 1971).

Today, deaths from bacteremia and meningitis among children with SCD have decreased due to various interventions such as urgent treatment of fever with antibiotics, penicillin prophylaxis, and vaccines. In the early 1980s the benefits of daily prophylactic penicillin was demonstrated in a landmark clinical trial in which young children (age 3–36 months) with HbSS were randomized to receive daily penicillin or placebo. This trial was stopped prematurely because significantly more children in the placebo arm had severe infections due to *Streptococcus pneumoniae* (placebo

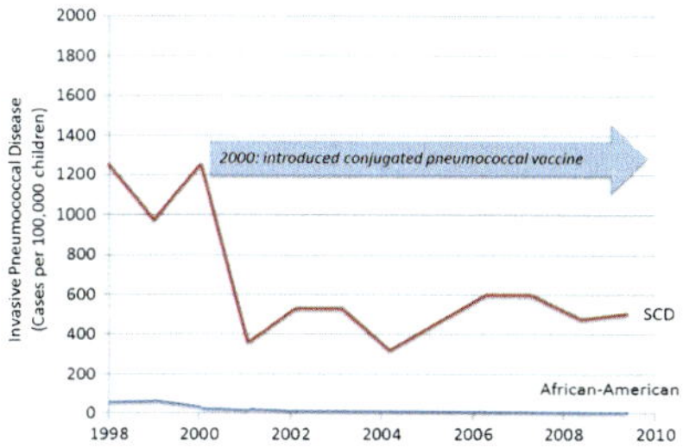

Fig. 9.3 Rates of invasive pneumococcal disease (IPD) in the United States: Rates of IPD in children under age 18 years with SCD, compared to overall rate of IPD in African-American children under age 18 in the Active Bacterial Core surveillance system. Adapted from Payne et al. (2013)

13/110 vs. penicillin 2/105; 84 % reduction) including three children receiving placebo who died from fulminant *S. pneumoniae* (Gaston et al. 1986). With the use of the 7-valent pneumococcal conjugate vaccine (PCV7) beginning in 2000, the incidence of invasive pneumococcal disease among young children with SCD has declined (Fig. 9.3) (Halasa et al. 2007; Payne et al. 2013). The 13-valent pneumococcal conjugate vaccine (PCV13) may further decrease the incidence of invasive pneumococcal disease, but it will not completely prevent this problem. The majority of recent cases of invasive pneumococcal disease in children with SCD were due to serotypes not included in PCV13 (Payne et al. 2013). Nonetheless, invasive bacterial infections are now rare with current vaccines and penicillin prophylaxis. Recent studies in Canada and the United States have shown that less than 1 % of febrile children with SCD have bacteremia (Rogovik et al. 2010; Baskin et al. 2013; Shihabuddin and Scarfi 2014).

Children with SCD are also at specifically increased risk of bacterial infections of the bone and joint. One study found that the prevalence of osteomyelitis in patients with HbSS was 12 % (Neonato et al. 2000). *Salmonella* is often the causative organism (Atkins et al. 1997; Burnett et al. 1998). It is hypothesized that sickle vaso-occlusion in the bowel may lead to increased mucosal barrier breakdown, resulting in transient bacteremia that can infect infarcted bone. Differentiating an acute bone infarct secondary to vaso-occlusion from osteomyelitis is difficult even with magnetic resonance imaging (MRI) (Lonergan et al. 2001). While VOC is much more common (Keeley and Buchanan 1982), osteomyelitis should be strongly considered in a child with SCD who has isolated bony pain and swelling with prolonged fever and pain (Berger et al. 2009).

Parvovirus B19 is another important infection in children with SCD. Children with SCD are not more prone to this common viral infection (Serjeant et al. 1993), but, in children with SCD, parvovirus can cause very severe anemia with reticulocytopenia termed an "aplastic crisis." While parvovirus infection is not the only cause of aplastic crisis in children with SCD, it is implicated in the vast majority of cases (Saarinen et al. 1986; Rao et al. 1992; Serjeant et al. 2001a). Children in aplastic crisis can present with increased pallor and lethargy. Delayed presentation with more profound anemia can include life-threatening complications like high-output heart failure, acute chest syndrome, ischemic stroke, or multiorgan failure. Most of these children have a history of fever but few have the characteristic "slapped cheek" rash (Goldstein et al. 1987; Kellermayer et al. 2003). Transfusion of red blood cells may be necessary while waiting for hematologic recovery. This recovery, defined as a rise in the reticulocyte count, can take up to 10 days (Saarinen et al. 1986; Goldstein et al. 1987). Fortunately, when individuals recover, immunity to parvovirus appears to prevent reoccurrence of aplastic crisis (Serjeant et al. 2001a). Many adolescents with SCD who had no history of an aplastic crisis have detectable IgG to parvovirus B19, demonstrating that parvovirus infection does not always cause clinical problems for children with SCD (Serjeant et al. 2001a; Zimmerman et al. 2003).

Other common childhood infections can also cause issues. Children with SCD are frequently hospitalized with viral infections, including influenza and respiratory syncytial virus (Bundy et al. 2010; Sadreameli et al. 2014). These infections may cause increased morbidity in some children with SCD as they are often implicated in triggering VOC or acute chest syndrome.

Malaria is a serious infection for children with SCD in areas of the world where it is endemic (Ambe et al. 2001). While children with sickle cell trait have a lower risk of complications and death from malaria (Aidoo et al. 2002; Williams et al. 2005), individuals with SCD do not appear to enjoy this same protection. It has been shown that children with SCD have lower rates of parasitemia (Komba et al. 2009; Makani et al. 2010), but it has also been demonstrated that children with SCD are *more* likely to die from malaria (McAuley et al. 2010).

9.2.3 Splenic Sequestration

A potentially critical manifestation of SCD is the acute trapping of blood in the spleen, termed splenic sequestration. Children with acute splenic sequestration present with an enlarging spleen, and may also have abdominal pain and symptoms of hypovolemia (pallor, lethargy, tachycardia). Nonspecific infectious symptoms, including fever, cough, diarrhea, and vomiting, are more commonly associated with splenic sequestration (Topley et al. 1981; Brousse et al. 2012). Severe episodes can progress to fatal shock in just a few hours. In addition to worsening anemia (traditionally defined as >2/dL drop in hemoglobin) with compensatory reticulocytosis, a decreased platelet count is often seen in children with splenic sequestration.

Splenic sequestration occurs primarily in young children with HbSS. In the Jamaican newborn cohort, 29 % of children with HbSS had an episode of splenic sequestration with the highest incidence occurring between 6 and 18 months and most episodes occurring before age 2 years (Emond et al. 1985). Similarly, a French study found that the median age at first splenic sequestration episode was 1.4 years (Brousse et al. 2012). Splenic sequestration may be the initial presenting clinical manifestation of SCD, and it has been reported in infants younger than 2 months (Pappo and Buchanan 1989; Airede 1992). The increased use of hydroxyurea therapy in infancy may change this natural history and possibly lead to more sequestration events occurring later in childhood.

Historically associated with significant mortality, death from splenic sequestration is rare today in settings with newborn diagnosis, parental education on spleen palpation, and accessible emergency medical care (Lee et al. 1995). While a study of children from the 1970s and early 1980s found a mortality rate of 12 % associated with acute splenic sequestration (Emond et al. 1985), a more recent study reported a 0.53 % risk of death (Brousse et al. 2012).

Children who have had acute splenic sequestration are at high risk for recurrent sequestration events in the future. The recurrence rate for children who recovered from their first episode of splenic sequestration has been reported to be 49–67 %, with most children experiencing another sequestration event within 6 months of the first episode (Emond et al. 1985; Brousse et al. 2012). Of note, even children with initially mild sequestration episodes have been shown to be at increased risk of future life-threatening sequestration events (Topley et al. 1981). In addition, after recovering from an episode of acute splenic sequestration, children are at increased risk of developing hypersplenism that is defined as a persistent reduction in steady state hemoglobin with increased reticulocyte count, reduced platelet count, and chronic splenic enlargement (Topley et al. 1981). Due to these future risks, surgical splenectomy is often recommended after a sequestration event.

9.2.4 Acute Chest Syndrome

Acute chest syndrome (ACS) is a term used to describe an acute pulmonary process that occurs exclusively in patients with SCD. ACS has been defined by the presence of a new pulmonary infiltrate that involves at least one complete lung segment on chest radiograph, and is accompanied by fever, chest pain, or respiratory symptoms (tachypnea, wheezing, cough). The most common presenting symptoms among children are fever and cough (Vichinsky et al. 1997). On physical exam, rales is the most common auscultory finding, yet many children may have a normal lung exam (Vichinsky et al. 1997). One study found that only 39 % of febrile children who presented to an emergency room (ER) and eventually diagnosed with ACS from an ER chest radiograph, were initially suspected by the provider to have ACS based on clinical findings (Morris et al. 1999). On chest radiograph, young children (age <2 years) have more upper lobe findings than older children, but all children most commonly have lower lobe involvement (Fig. 9.4) (Vichinsky et al. 1997). Moreover, on laboratory evaluation, patients typically have a decreased hemoglobin and increased white blood cell count compared to steady state values (Vichinsky et al. 1997).

Patients may not initially present with ACS but may instead develop it after a prodromal illness or a hospital admission for other indications (Creary and Krishnamurti 2014). In the CSSCD, 72 % of patients with ACS were admitted because of a VOC pain crisis, and among patients not admitted for ACS, ACS occurred a mean 2.5 days after admission (Vichinsky et al. 2000). ACS can also occur in the post-operative setting, particularly in younger children with greater blood and heat loss during surgery (Kokoska et al. 2004). The etiology of ACS

a b

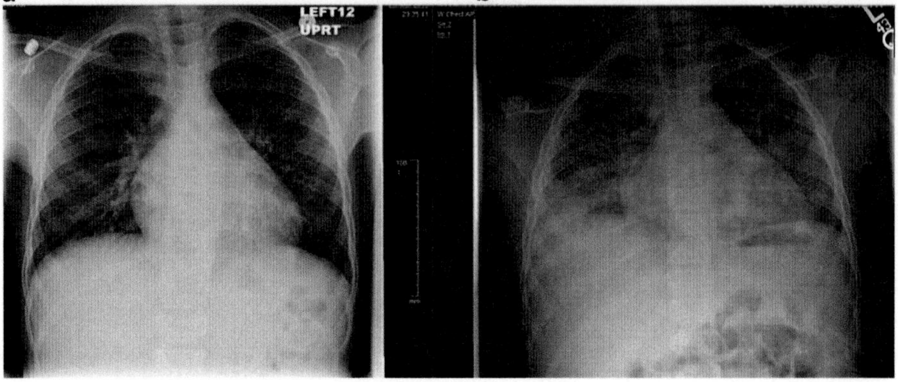

Fig. 9.4 Acute chest syndrome: chest radiographs of 10-year old with sickle cell anemia, hospitalized for pain and fever. Initial chest radiograph (**a**) was clear. Chest radiograph 36 h later (**b**) shows new infiltrates at the bases of both lungs

includes pulmonary infarction and fat embolism as well as infectious causes (specifically *Chlamydia pneumoniae, Mycoplasma pneumoniae*, and respiratory viruses) (Vichinsky et al. 2000). Likely due to respiratory infections, the incidence of ACS is highest during the winter months, especially for young children (Vichinsky et al. 1997).

Also of note, children with asthma appear to have an increased risk of developing ACS (Boyd et al. 2006; Sylvester et al. 2007). Most children with SCD will experience at least one episode of ACS. The CSSCD infant cohort found that 50 % of children with HbSS had ACS by 5.8 years of age (Fig. 9.2) (Gill et al. 1995). The increased use of hydroxyurea to treat SCD in childhood is expected to lead to less children suffering from ACS in the future. In the BABY HUG study, children in the hydroxyurea arm had significantly less ACS events than children in the placebo arm (4.2 vs. 14.6 events per 100 patient-years) (Thornburg et al. 2012).

The clinical course of ACS is variable (mild illness to respiratory failure/death) and likely highly influenced by supportive care practices and red blood cell transfusion. Evolving ACS often includes progression of pulmonary infiltrates, worsening hypoxia, and dropping hemoglobin. The CSSD found that the mean hospital stay for ACS among children was 5.4 days (Vichinsky et al. 1997). Adults generally have a more severe clinical course and higher risk of mortality associated with ACS (Vichinsky et al. 1997, 2000). Repeated episodes of ACS can lead to chronic lung disease (Powars et al. 1988).

9.2.5 Neurological Complications

Stroke is one of the most devastating complications of SCD. Children with SCD and stroke most commonly present with acute hemiparesis but may also have aphasia, cranial nerve abnormalities, seizures, or altered mental status (Powars et al. 1978;

Balkaran et al. 1992). Stroke can occur as an isolated clinical event, but also may occur in the setting of VOC pain crisis, ACS, splenic sequestration, or aplastic crisis (Balkaran et al. 1992; Powars et al. 1978). Children with SCD are more likely to have ischemic rather than hemorrhagic strokes and typically have partial or complete occlusion of large cerebral vessels (Ohene-Frempong et al. 1998; Powars et al. 1978; Stockman et al. 1972).

Stroke in SCD can occur throughout childhood, but children between the ages of 2 and 5 years have the highest rate (Ohene-Frempong et al. 1998). Before the implementation of stroke prevention with transcranial doppler (TCD) screening, the CSSCD estimated that 11 % of children with HbSS had a stroke by age 20 years (Ohene-Frempong et al. 1998). Similarly, a Jamaican newborn cohort study found that 7.8 % of children with HbSS had a stroke by age 14 years. Fortunately, since the landmark Stroke Prevention Trial in Sickle Cell Anemia (STOP), which established that chronic transfusion therapy could effectively prevent stroke in children with an elevated TCD velocity, the incidence of stroke in children with SCD has decreased (Adams et al. 1998; Fullerton et al. 2004; McCarville et al. 2008).

While most children with SCD who have had a stroke make substantial neurologic improvements, some children have severe, permanent disabilities and all appear to have some degree of intellectual impairment (Powars et al. 1978). Children who have suffered a stroke are also at very high risk for another stroke if they do not receive aggressive therapy (chronic red blood cell transfusion or stem cell transplant). One natural history study documented that 67 % of children with stroke had at least one recurrent stroke with most recurrent events occurring within 3 years of the first stroke (Powars et al. 1978).

"Silent strokes," defined as cerebral ischemia on MRI with no history of an acute neurologic event, are much more common than overt strokes in children with SCD (Fig. 9.5). In the CSSCD, 21.8 % of children, age 6–16 years, with HbSS had, on screening MRI, a silent stroke (Pegelow et al. 2002). These silent strokes can occur at a very young age; 13 % of infants (mean age 13.7 months) screened as part of the BABY HUG study had silent infarcts (Wang et al. 2008). Additionally, a more recent study found that 27.7 % of children with HbSS aged less than 6 years had silent infarcts (Kwiatkowski et al. 2009). Silent strokes are not benign findings; they are associated with neurocognitive deficits and school difficulties (Schatz et al. 2001; DeBaun et al. 2012; Armstrong et al. 1996). Additionally, children found to have silent strokes are at increased risk of both ischemia progression on MRI and new, overt strokes (Miller et al. 2001; Pegelow et al. 2002). Children with SCD also often develop cerebral vasculopathy before overt stroke (Fasano et al. 2015). In sum, neurologic abnormalities occur frequently in children with SCD. A recent study found that 49.9 % of children with SCD had either a stroke, abnormal TCD, cerebral stenosis, or silent stroke before age 14 (Bernaudin et al. 2011).

Headaches are a common complaint and are more prevalent in young (age <13 years) children with SCD compared to children without a chronic medical condition (Niebanck et al. 2007). Children with SCD who report frequent headaches are more likely to have frequent VOC pain crisis and also have cerebral vessel stenosis (Niebanck et al. 2007). Most children with SCD who present with acute headache do not have an acute central nervous system (CNS) event. Compared to children in

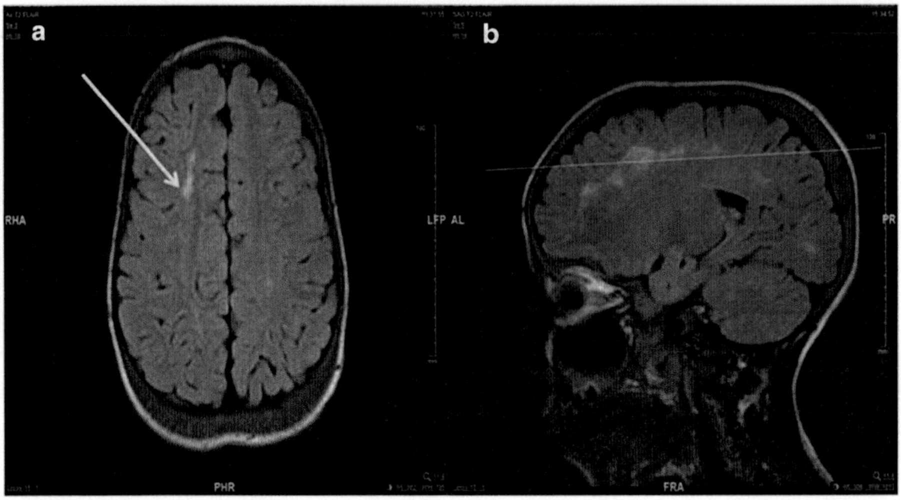

Fig. 9.5 MRI showing silent infarct of the deep white matter of the right cerebral hemisphere (*arrow*) in a 10-year old student on the honor roll. T2 FLAIR, axial view (**a**) and sagittal view (**b**)

the general population, however, children with SCD have an increased association of headaches with an acute CNS event. Children with SCD and headache who have a history of a previous CNS event or an abnormal neurologic exam are at increased risk for an acute CNS event like a cerebral sinovenous thrombosis or an intraventricular hemorrhage (Hines et al. 2011).

Sensorineural hearing loss can also occur in children with SCD, presumably from ischemic injury to the inner ear. Children with SCD very rarely develop deafness, but ~13 % have more mild hearing loss (Mgbor and Emodi 2004; Ajulo et al. 1993; Friedman et al. 1980). Spinal cord infarction causing lower extremity motor and sensory deficits has also been reported in children with SCD (Rothman and Nelson 1980; Edwards et al. 2013). Finally, while epilepsy is not typically associated with SCD, children with SCD have an increased risk of also developing this condition (Ali et al. 2010).

9.2.6 Hepatobiliary Complications

Bilirubin gallstones are common in children with SCD because of chronic, on-going sickle hemolysis. The prevalence of gallstones in children with SCD increases with age so that by age 20 years almost half of all individuals with HbSS have cholelithiasis (Walker et al. 2000; Bond et al. 1987). This biliary pathology, however, likely begins very early in childhood as 5 % of infants (mean age 12.9 months) in the BABY HUG study had biliary abnormalities (sludge, dilated common bile duct, thickened gallbladder wall, or cholelithiasis) (McCarville et al. 2011).

Cholelithiasis can cause a range of clinical problems including biliary colic, acute and chronic cholecystitis, cholangitis, and pancreatitis (see Chap. 12, Fig. 12.4 depicting a gallbladder with bilirubin stones). Biliary tract disease should be considered in patients with SCD who complain of right upper quadrant pain. However, cholelithiasis often does not cause symptoms and the risk of future clinical issues in asymptomatic children with cholelithiasis is unclear.

Children who have recovered from symptomatic biliary tract disease and do not undergo cholecystectomy are at high risk for continued clinical events secondary to their gallstones. One study found that 50 % of children had experienced recurrent cholelithiasis-related problems within 6 months after the initial event (Amoako et al. 2013). Cholecystectomy clearly decreases the risk of further problems but does not completely eliminate the risk of future biliary tract disease (Amoako et al. 2013).

Children with SCD also can rarely develop significant sickling in the hepatic sinusoids, which leads to a complication termed intrahepatic cholestasis. Individuals with intrahepatic cholestasis typically present with extreme conjugated hyperbilirubinemia, abdominal pain, hepatomegaly, coagulopathy, and elevated transaminases. The clinical course of intrahepatic cholestasis is variable. It may resolve in some with no treatment, but can cause liver failure and death in others even with aggressive support including exchange transfusion (Buchanan and Glader 1977) (Ahn et al. 2005).

9.2.7 Genitourinary Complications

Nocturnal enuresis, the persistence of urination in the bed at night, occurs more commonly in children with SCD. It has been estimated that almost 50 % of children with SCD age 5–10 years and approximately 15 % of adolescents with SCD age 16–20 years suffer from nocturnal enuresis (Wolf et al. 2014). The etiology of this increased prevalence of nocturnal enuresis is likely multifactorial. Due to sickle-related infarction to the renal medulla, children with SCD are unable to appropriately concentrate urine and thus produce dilute urine, termed hyposthenuria. This hyposthenuria results in polyuria, increased urinary frequency. In addition to hyposthenuria-induced nocturnal polyuria, disordered sleep breathing secondary to obstructive sleep apnea could contribute to nocturnal enuresis in SCD (Lehmann et al. 2012). Other potential reasons for SCD nocturnal enuresis include decreased bladder capacity and increased arousal thresholds (Readett et al. 1990).

Children with SCD can also present with painless hematuria due to renal papillary necrosis from sickling. This hematuria is usually benign and resolves with hydration (Scheinman 2009). Hematuria (red blood cells in the urine) should be distinguished from hemoglobinuria (hemoglobin in the urine), which can occur due to a hemolytic transfusion reaction.

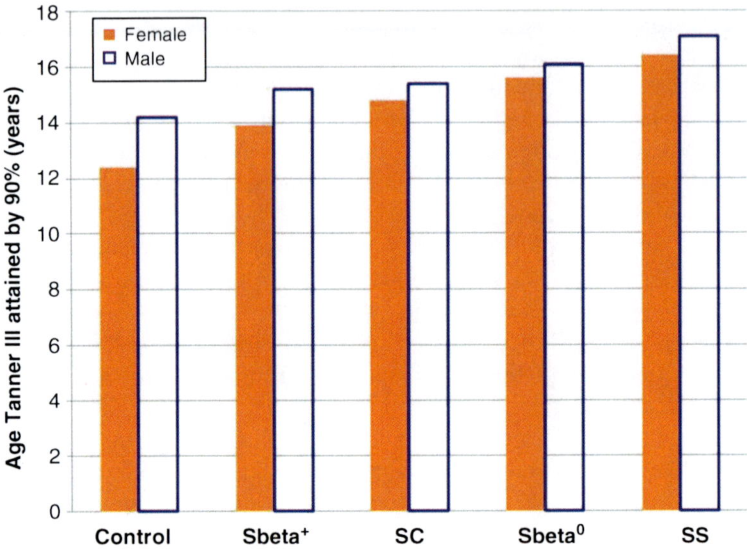

Fig. 9.6 Age by which 90 % of females and males with SCD had attained at least Tanner Stage III pubic hair. Data from the cooperative study of sickle cell disease infant cohort (CSSCD). Control data from the US Health Examination Survey of black females and white males are shown for reference, but have not been subjected to the same regression analysis. *SBeta*$^+$ HbS-β^+ thalassemia, *SC* HbSC, *SBeta*^{0} HbS-β^0 thalassemia, *SS* HbSS. Adapted from Platt et al. (1984)

9.2.8 Growth and Development

Children with SCD demonstrate a pattern of decreased growth consistent with constitutional delay. Low weight is more pronounced than short height (Platt et al. 1984). In a recent prospective study of children with HbSS, 38 % were below the 5th percentile for height, weight, or body mass index (BMI) at some point during the 4 years of observation (Zemel et al. 2007). By age 8 years, children with HbSS have been found to have significant delay in skeletal maturation on bone age testing (Stevens et al. 1986). Adolescents with HbSS begin pubertal development at older ages and also progress through puberty slower (Fig. 9.6) (Rhodes et al. 2009). Average age at menarche for girls with HbSS has been reported to range from 13.2 to 15.4 years, about 1–2 years later than matched controls (Zemel et al. 2007; Serjeant et al. 2001b).

Growth failure is not inherent to the genetics of SCD but likely a consequence of SCD chronic severe anemia, suboptimal nutrition, hypermetabolism, and possible endocrine dysfunction. Children with SCD on chronic transfusion therapy have been shown to have normalization of growth (Wang et al. 2005). Infants with HbSS treated with hydroxyurea for 2 years on the BABY HUG study had no significant differences in height and weight compared to both untreated infants with HbSS and World Health Organization standards (Rana et al. 2014). Long-term follow-up of a small number of individuals with HbSS treated with hydroxyurea since infancy suggests that hydroxyurea can normalize later growth and development in SCD (Hankins et al. 2014).

References

Adams RJ, McKie VC, Hsu L et al (1998) Prevention of a first stroke by transfusions in children with sickle cell anemia and abnormal results on transcranial Doppler ultrasonography. N Engl J Med 339(1):5–11

Ahn H, Li CS, Wang W (2005) Sickle cell hepatopathy: clinical presentation, treatment, and outcome in pediatric and adult patients. Pediatr Blood Cancer 45(2):184–190

Aidoo M, Terlouw DJ, Kolczak MS et al (2002) Protective effects of the sickle cell gene against malaria morbidity and mortality. Lancet 359(9314):1311–1312

Airede AI (1992) Acute splenic sequestration in a five-week-old infant with sickle cell disease. J Pediatr 120(1):160

Ajulo SO, Osiname AI, Myatt HM (1993) Sensorineural hearing loss in sickle cell anaemia – a United Kingdom study. J Laryngol Otol 107(9):790–794

Ali SB, Reid M, Fraser R, MooSang M, Ali A (2010) Seizures in the Jamaica cohort study of sickle cell disease. Br J Haematol 151(3):265–272

Almeida A, Roberts I (2005) Bone involvement in sickle cell disease. Br J Haematol 129(4): 482–490

Ambe JP, Fatunde JO, Sodeinde OO (2001) Associated morbidities in children with sickle-cell anaemia presenting with severe anaemia in a malarious area. Trop Doct 31(1):26–27

Amoako MO, Casella JF, Strouse JJ (2013) High rates of recurrent biliary tract obstruction in children with sickle cell disease. Pediatr Blood Cancer 60(4):650–652

Armstrong FD, Thompson RJ Jr, Wang W et al (1996) Cognitive functioning and brain magnetic resonance imaging in children with sickle cell disease. Neuropsychology Committee of the Cooperative Study of Sickle Cell Disease. Pediatrics 97(6 Pt 1):864–870

Atkins BL, Price EH, Tillyer L, Novelli V, Evans J (1997) Salmonella osteomyelitis in sickle cell disease children in the east end of London. J Infect 34(2):133–138

Balkaran B, Char G, Morris JS et al (1992) Stroke in a cohort of patients with homozygous sickle cell disease. J Pediatr 120(3):360–366

Barrett-Connor E (1971) Bacterial infection and sickle cell anemia. An analysis of 250 infections in 166 patients and a review of the literature. Medicine (Baltimore) 50(2):97–112

Baskin MN, Goh XL, Heeney MM, Harper MB (2013) Bacteremia risk and outpatient management of febrile patients with sickle cell disease. Pediatrics 131(6):1035–1041

Berger E, Saunders N, Wang L, Friedman JN (2009) Sickle cell disease in children: differentiating osteomyelitis from vaso-occlusive crisis. Arch Pediatr Adolesc Med 163(3):251–255

Bernaudin F, Verlhac S, Arnaud C et al (2011) Impact of early transcranial Doppler screening and intensive therapy on cerebral vasculopathy outcome in a newborn sickle cell anemia cohort. Blood 117(4):1130–1140, quiz 1436

Bond LR, Hatty SR, Horn ME et al (1987) Gall stones in sickle cell disease in the United Kingdom. Br Med J (Clin Res Ed) 295(6592):234–236

Boyd JH, Macklin EA, Strunk RC, DeBaun MR (2006) Asthma is associated with acute chest syndrome and pain in children with sickle cell anemia. Blood 108(9):2923–2927

Brousse V, Elie C, Benkerrou M et al (2012) Acute splenic sequestration crisis in sickle cell disease: cohort study of 190 paediatric patients. Br J Haematol 156(5):643–648

Buchanan GR, Glader BE (1977) Benign course of extreme hyperbilirubinemia in sickle cell anemia: analysis of six cases. J Pediatr 91(1):21–24

Bundy DG, Strouse JJ, Casella JF, Miller MR (2010) Burden of influenza-related hospitalizations among children with sickle cell disease. Pediatrics 125(2):234–243
Burnett MW, Bass JW, Cook BA (1998) Etiology of osteomyelitis complicating sickle cell disease. Pediatrics 101(2):296–297
Constantinou C, Payne N, Inusa B (2014) Assessing the quality of life of children with sickle cell anaemia using self-, parent-proxy, and health care professional-proxy reports. Br J Health Psychol 20:290–304
Creary SE, Krishnamurti L (2014) Prodromal illness before acute chest syndrome in pediatric patients with sickle cell disease. J Pediatr Hematol Oncol 36(6):480–483
Dampier C, Ely B, Brodecki D, O'Neal P (2002a) Characteristics of pain managed at home in children and adolescents with sickle cell disease by using diary self-reports. J Pain 3(6):461–470
Dampier C, Ely E, Brodecki D, O'Neal P (2002b) Home management of pain in sickle cell disease: a daily diary study in children and adolescents. J Pediatr Hematol Oncol 24(8):643–647
Dampier C, Setty BN, Eggleston B et al (2004) Vaso-occlusion in children with sickle cell disease: clinical characteristics and biologic correlates. J Pediatr Hematol Oncol 26(12):785–790
Dampier C, Ely B, Brodecki D et al (2014) Pain characteristics and age-related pain trajectories in infants and young children with sickle cell disease. Pediatr Blood Cancer 61(2):291–296
Davis H, Schoendorf KC, Gergen PJ, Moore RM Jr (1997) National trends in the mortality of children with sickle cell disease, 1968 through 1992. Am J Public Health 87(8):1317–1322
DeBaun MR, Armstrong FD, McKinstry RC et al (2012) Silent cerebral infarcts: a review on a prevalent and progressive cause of neurologic injury in sickle cell anemia. Blood 119(20): 4587–4596
Edwards A, Clay EL, Jewells V et al (2013) A 19-year-old man with sickle cell disease presenting with spinal infarction: a case report. J Med Case Rep 7:210
Emond AM, Collis R, Darvill D et al (1985) Acute splenic sequestration in homozygous sickle cell disease: natural history and management. J Pediatr 107(2):201–206
Fasano RM, Meier ER, Hulbert ML (2015) Cerebral vasculopathy in children with sickle cell anemia. Blood Cells Mol Dis 54(1):17–25
Friedman EM, Herer GR, Luban NL, Williams I (1980) Sickle cell anemia and hearing. Ann Otol Rhinol Laryngol 89(4 Pt 1):342–347
Fullerton HJ, Adams RJ, Zhao S, Johnston SC (2004) Declining stroke rates in Californian children with sickle cell disease. Blood 104(2):336–339
Gaston MH, Verter JI, Woods G et al (1986) Prophylaxis with oral penicillin in children with sickle cell anemia. A randomized trial. N Engl J Med 314(25):1593–1599
Gill FM, Sleeper LA, Weiner SJ et al (1995) Clinical events in the first decade in a cohort of infants with sickle cell disease. Cooperative Study of Sickle Cell Disease. Blood 86(2):776–783
Goldstein AR, Anderson MJ, Serjeant GR (1987) Parvovirus associated aplastic crisis in homozygous sickle cell disease. Arch Dis Child 62(6):585–588
Graumlich SE, Powers SW, Byars KC et al (2001) Multidimensional assessment of pain in pediatric sickle cell disease. J Pediatr Psychol 26(4):203–214
Halasa NB, Shankar SM, Talbot TR et al (2007) Incidence of invasive pneumococcal disease among individuals with sickle cell disease before and after the introduction of the pneumococcal conjugate vaccine. Clin Infect Dis 44(11):1428–1433
Hankins JS, Aygun B, Nottage K et al (2014) From infancy to adolescence: fifteen years of continuous treatment with hydroxyurea in sickle cell anemia. Medicine (Baltimore) 93(28), e215
Hines PC, McKnight TP, Seto W, Kwiatkowski JL (2011) Central nervous system events in children with sickle cell disease presenting acutely with headache. J Pediatr 159(3):472–478
Keeley K, Buchanan GR (1982) Acute infarction of long bones in children with sickle cell anemia. J Pediatr 101(2):170–175
Kellermayer R, Faden H, Grossi M (2003) Clinical presentation of parvovirus B19 infection in children with aplastic crisis. Pediatr Infect Dis J 22(12):1100–1101
Kokoska ER, West KW, Carney DE et al (2004) Risk factors for acute chest syndrome in children with sickle cell disease undergoing abdominal surgery. J Pediatr Surg 39(6):848–850

Komba AN, Makani J, Sadarangani M et al (2009) Malaria as a cause of morbidity and mortality in children with homozygous sickle cell disease on the coast of Kenya. Clin Infect Dis 49(2):216–222

Kwiatkowski JL, Zimmerman RA, Pollock AN et al (2009) Silent infarcts in young children with sickle cell disease. Br J Haematol 146(3):300–305

Lee A, Thomas P, Cupidore L, Serjeant B, Serjeant G (1995) Improved survival in homozygous sickle cell disease: lessons from a cohort study. BMJ 311(7020):1600–1602

Lehmann GC, Bell TR, Kirkham FJ et al (2012) Enuresis associated with sleep disordered breathing in children with sickle cell anemia. J Urol 188(4 Suppl):1572–1576

Lonergan GJ, Cline DB, Abbondanzo SL (2001) Sickle cell anemia. Radiographics 21(4):971–994

Makani J, Komba AN, Cox SE et al (2010) Malaria in patients with sickle cell anemia: burden, risk factors, and outcome at the outpatient clinic and during hospitalization. Blood 115(2):215–220

Makani J, Cox SE, Soka D et al (2011) Mortality in sickle cell anemia in Africa: a prospective cohort study in Tanzania. PLoS One 6(2), e14699

McAuley CF, Webb C, Makani J et al (2010) High mortality from Plasmodium falciparum malaria in children living with sickle cell anemia on the coast of Kenya. Blood 116(10):1663–1668

McCarville MB, Goodin GS, Fortner G et al (2008) Evaluation of a comprehensive transcranial doppler screening program for children with sickle cell anemia. Pediatr Blood Cancer 50(4):818–821

McCarville MB, Luo Z, Huang X et al (2011) Abdominal ultrasound with scintigraphic and clinical correlates in infants with sickle cell anemia: baseline data from the BABY HUG trial. AJR Am J Roentgenol 196(6):1399–1404

Mgbor N, Emodi I (2004) Sensorineural hearing loss in Nigerian children with sickle cell disease. Int J Pediatr Otorhinolaryngol 68(11):1413–1416

Miller ST, Macklin EA, Pegelow CH et al (2001) Silent infarction as a risk factor for overt stroke in children with sickle cell anemia: a report from the Cooperative Study of Sickle Cell Disease. J Pediatr 139(3):385–390

Morris C, Vichinsky E, Styles L (1999) Clinician assessment for acute chest syndrome in febrile patients with sickle cell disease: is it accurate enough? Ann Emerg Med 34(1):64–69

Najim OA, Hassan MK (2011) Lactate dehydrogenase and severity of pain in children with sickle cell disease. Acta Haematol 126(3):157–162

Neonato MG, Guilloud-Bataille M, Beauvais P et al (2000) Acute clinical events in 299 homozygous sickle cell patients living in France. French Study Group on Sickle Cell Disease. Eur J Haematol 65(3):155–164

Niebanck AE, Pollock AN, Smith-Whitley K et al (2007) Headache in children with sickle cell disease: prevalence and associated factors. J Pediatr 151(1):67–72, 72.e61

Nottage KA, Hankins JS, Smeltzer M et al (2013) Hydroxyurea use and hospitalization trends in a comprehensive pediatric sickle cell program. PLoS One 8(8), e72077

Ohene-Frempong K, Weiner SJ, Sleeper LA et al (1998) Cerebrovascular accidents in sickle cell disease: rates and risk factors. Blood 91(1):288–294

Panepinto JA, Brousseau DC, Hillery CA, Scott JP (2005) Variation in hospitalizations and hospital length of stay in children with vaso-occlusive crises in sickle cell disease. Pediatr Blood Cancer 44(2):182–186

Pappo A, Buchanan GR (1989) Acute splenic sequestration in a 2-month-old infant with sickle cell anemia. Pediatrics 84(3):578–579

Payne AB, Link-Gelles R, Azonobi I et al (2013) Invasive pneumococcal disease among children with and without sickle cell disease in the United States, 1998 to 2009. Pediatr Infect Dis J 32(12):1308–1312

Pegelow CH, Macklin EA, Moser FG et al (2002) Longitudinal changes in brain magnetic resonance imaging findings in children with sickle cell disease. Blood 99(8):3014–3018

Platt OS, Rosenstock W, Espeland MA (1984) Influence of sickle hemoglobinopathies on growth and development. N Engl J Med 311(1):7–12

Powars D, Wilson B, Imbus C, Pegelow C, Allen J (1978) The natural history of stroke in sickle cell disease. Am J Med 65(3):461–471

Powars D, Weidman JA, Odom-Maryon T, Niland JC, Johnson C (1988) Sickle cell chronic lung disease: prior morbidity and the risk of pulmonary failure. Medicine (Baltimore) 67(1):66–76

Quinn CT, Rogers ZR, McCavit TL, Buchanan GR (2010) Improved survival of children and adolescents with sickle cell disease. Blood 115(17):3447–3452

Rana S, Houston PE, Wang WC et al (2014) Hydroxyurea and growth in young children with sickle cell disease. Pediatrics 134(3):465–472

Rao SP, Miller ST, Cohen BJ (1992) Transient aplastic crisis in patients with sickle cell disease. B19 parvovirus studies during a 7-year period. Am J Dis Child 146(11):1328–1330

Raphael JL, Mueller BU, Kowalkowski MA, Oyeku SO (2012) Shorter hospitalization trends among children with sickle cell disease. Pediatr Blood Cancer 59(4):679–684

Readett DR, Morris J, Serjeant GR (1990) Determinants of nocturnal enuresis in homozygous sickle cell disease. Arch Dis Child 65(6):615–618

Rhodes M, Akohoue SA, Shankar SM et al (2009) Growth patterns in children with sickle cell anemia during puberty. Pediatr Blood Cancer 53(4):635–641

Rogers ZR, Wang WC, Luo Z et al (2011) Biomarkers of splenic function in infants with sickle cell anemia: baseline data from the BABY HUG Trial. Blood 117(9):2614–2617

Rogovik AL, Friedman JN, Persaud J, Goldman RD (2010) Bacterial blood cultures in children with sickle cell disease. Am J Emerg Med 28(4):511–514

Rogovik AL, Persaud J, Friedman JN, Kirby MA, Goldman RD (2011) Pediatric vasoocclusive crisis and weather conditions. J Emerg Med 41(5):559–565

Rothman SM, Nelson JS (1980) Spinal cord infarction in a patient with sickle cell anemia. Neurology 30(10):1072–1076

Saarinen UM, Chorba TL, Tattersall P et al (1986) Human parvovirus B19-induced epidemic acute red cell aplasia in patients with hereditary hemolytic anemia. Blood 67(5):1411–1417

Sadreameli SC, Reller ME, Bundy DG, Casella JF, Strouse JJ (2014) Respiratory syncytial virus and seasonal influenza cause similar illnesses in children with sickle cell disease. Pediatr Blood Cancer 61(5):875–878

Schatz J, Brown RT, Pascual JM, Hsu L, DeBaun MR (2001) Poor school and cognitive functioning with silent cerebral infarcts and sickle cell disease. Neurology 56(8):1109–1111

Scheinman JI (2009) Sickle cell disease and the kidney. Nat Clin Pract Nephrol 5(2):78–88

Serjeant GR, Serjeant BE, Thomas PW et al (1993) Human parvovirus infection in homozygous sickle cell disease. Lancet 341(8855):1237–1240

Serjeant BE, Hambleton IR, Kerr S, Kilty CG, Serjeant GR (2001a) Haematological response to parvovirus B19 infection in homozygous sickle-cell disease. Lancet 358(9295):1779–1780

Serjeant GR, Singhal A, Hambleton IR (2001b) Sickle cell disease and age at menarche in Jamaican girls: observations from a cohort study. Arch Dis Child 85(5):375–378

Shihabuddin BS, Scarfi CA (2014) Fever in children with sickle cell disease: are all fevers equal? J Emerg Med 47(4):395–400

Stevens MC, Maude GH, Cupidore L et al (1986) Prepubertal growth and skeletal maturation in children with sickle cell disease. Pediatrics 78(1):124–132

Stockman JA, Nigro MA, Mishkin MM, Oski FA (1972) Occlusion of large cerebral vessels in sickle-cell anemia. N Engl J Med 287(17):846–849

Sylvester KP, Patey RA, Broughton S et al (2007) Temporal relationship of asthma to acute chest syndrome in sickle cell disease. Pediatr Pulmonol 42(2):103–106

Telfer P, Coen P, Chakravorty S et al (2007) Clinical outcomes in children with sickle cell disease living in England: a neonatal cohort in East London. Haematologica 92(7):905–912

Thornburg CD, Files BA, Luo Z et al (2012) Impact of hydroxyurea on clinical events in the BABY HUG trial. Blood 120(22):4304–4310, quiz 4448

Topley JM, Rogers DW, Stevens MC, Serjeant GR (1981) Acute splenic sequestration and hypersplenism in the first five years in homozygous sickle cell disease. Arch Dis Child 56(10):765–769

Vichinsky EP, Styles LA, Colangelo LH et al (1997) Acute chest syndrome in sickle cell disease: clinical presentation and course. Cooperative Study of Sickle Cell Disease. Blood 89(5):1787–1792

Vichinsky EP, Neumayr LD, Earles AN et al (2000) Causes and outcomes of the acute chest syndrome in sickle cell disease. National Acute Chest Syndrome Study Group. N Engl J Med 342(25):1855–1865

Walker TM, Hambleton IR, Serjeant GR (2000) Gallstones in sickle cell disease: observations from The Jamaican Cohort study. J Pediatr 136(1):80–85

Wang WC, Morales KH, Scher CD et al (2005) Effect of long-term transfusion on growth in children with sickle cell anemia: results of the STOP trial. J Pediatr 147(2):244–247

Wang WC, Pavlakis SG, Helton KJ et al (2008) MRI abnormalities of the brain in one-year-old children with sickle cell anemia. Pediatr Blood Cancer 51(5):643–646

Wang WC, Ware RE, Miller ST et al (2011) Hydroxycarbamide in very young children with sickle-cell anaemia: a multicentre, randomised, controlled trial (BABY HUG). Lancet 377(9778):1663–1672

Williams TN, Mwangi TW, Wambua S et al (2005) Sickle cell trait and the risk of Plasmodium falciparum malaria and other childhood diseases. J Infect Dis 192(1):178–186

Wolf RB, Kassim AA, Goodpaster RL, DeBaun MR (2014) Nocturnal enuresis in sickle cell disease. Expert Rev Hematol 7(2):245–254

Yanni E, Grosse SD, Yang Q, Olney RS (2009) Trends in pediatric sickle cell disease-related mortality in the United States, 1983–2002. J Pediatr 154(4):541–545

Zemel BS, Kawchak DA, Ohene-Frempong K, Schall JI, Stallings VA (2007) Effects of delayed pubertal development, nutritional status, and disease severity on longitudinal patterns of growth failure in children with sickle cell disease. Pediatr Res 61(5 Pt 1):607–613

Zimmerman SA, Davis JS, Schultz WH, Ware RE (2003) Subclinical parvovirus B19 infection in children with sickle cell anemia. J Pediatr Hematol Oncol 25(5):387–389

Chapter 10
Treatment of Childhood Sickle Cell Disease

Rouba Abdennour and Miguel R. Abboud

Abstract With the advances in our understanding of the complex mechanisms that come into play in sickle cell disease (SCD), medical care improves and patients with SCD live longer. It is, thus, essential to have adequate knowledge of the available and potential treatment modalities for all SCD complications to reduce morbidity and mortality. As in all chronic illnesses, patient education is the most important aspect of treatment. Patients should be enrolled in a routine follow-up program with multidisciplinary care for better outcomes. Penicillin prophylaxis and adequate immunizations must be instated as soon as the diagnosis is made. Regular screening is warranted to predict the risk of central nervous system involvement, pulmonary hypertension, nephropathy and retinopathy. In this chapter, we also discuss the management of acute SCD complications including vaso-occlusive painful crises, fever, acute chest syndrome, acute splenic sequestration, cerebrovascular accidents, priapism, aplastic crisis, hepatobiliary complications and ophthalmologic complications. We also present approaches for chronic complications such as pulmonary hypertension, chronic kidney disease, chronic pain, sickle retinopathy, leg ulcers and avascular necrosis. The indications and risks of blood transfusions are discussed in addition to hematopoietic stem cell transplant, the only curative treatment for SCD.

Keywords Treatment • Acute complications • Chronic complications • Painful crisis • Hydroxyurea

Abbreviations

AAP	American Academy of Pediatrics
ACE	Angiotensin-converting enzyme
ACIP	Advisory Committee on Immunization Practices
ACS	Acute chest syndrome

R. Abdennour, M.D. • M.R. Abboud, M.D. (✉)
Department of Pediatrics and Adolescent Medicine, American University of Beirut Medical Center, Beirut, Lebanon
e-mail: ra190@aub.edu.lb; ma56@aub.edu.lb

© Springer International Publishing Switzerland 2016

F.F. Costa, N. Conran (eds.), *Sickle Cell Anemia*,
DOI 10.1007/978-3-319-06713-1_10

AHS	Acute hepatic sequestration
AIC	Acute intrahepatic cholestasis
ASS	Acute splenic sequestration
ATS	American Thoracic Society
AVN	Avascular necrosis
CBC	Complete blood count
CDC	Centers for Disease Control and Prevention
CKD	Chronic kidney disease
CRAO	Central retinal artery occlusion
CT	Computed tomography
ED	Emergency department
ESRD	End-stage renal disease
FDA	U.S. Food and Drug Administration
G6PD	Glucose-6-phosphate dehydrogenase
GvHD	Graft versus host disease
Hb	Hemoglobin
Hib	*Haemophilus influenzae* type B
Hib-MenCY-TT	*Haemophilus* b tetanus toxoid conjugate vaccine
HSCT	Hematopoietic stem cell transplantation
HU	Hydroxyurea
IOP	Intraocular pressure
IV	Intravenous
LIC	Liver iron content
MenACWY	Quadrivalent meningococcal conjugate vaccine
MRI	Magnetic resonance imaging
MTD	Maximum tolerated dose
NHLBI	US National Heart Lung and Blood Institute
NHS	UK National Health Service
NO	Nitric oxide
NSAID	Nonsteroidal anti-inflammatory drug
NT-Pro-BNP	N-terminal pro-brain natriuretic peptide
PCA	Patient-controlled analgesia
PCV13	13-valent pneumococcal vaccine
PCV7	7-valent pneumococcal vaccine
PH	Pulmonary hypertension
PPSV23	23-valent pneumococcal polysaccharide vaccine
PSR	Progressive sickle retinopathy
PT	Prothrombin time
PTT	Partial thromboplastin time
RBC	Red blood cell
SCD	Sickle cell disease
SNRI	Serotonin norepinephrine reuptake inhibitors
TCD	Transcranial doppler
TIA	Transient ischemic attack
TRV	Tricuspid regurgitant velocity
VOC	Vaso-occlusive crisis

10.1 Introduction

Sickle cell disease (SCD) is a chronic disease characterized by episodes of acute manifestations and progressive multi-organ damage (Rees et al. 2010). Therefore, health care professionals taking care or coming into contact with patients with SCD need to be knowledgeable about its acute and chronic complications and routine comprehensive multi-disciplinary medical care. This is essential to appropriately manage patients and reduce SCD morbidity and mortality. However, the relative rarity of the disease in most countries has resulted in practitioners not always having the knowledge required to manage the disease. It is our aim to provide a quick reference for practitioners who take care of patients either in comprehensive centers or in the setting of primary or emergency care.

10.2 Health Maintenance

10.2.1 Patient Education

As in all chronic illnesses, the patients and their families should be offered teaching, support and advice. Counseling sessions must be held as soon as the diagnosis is made. Patients should periodically followed-up by a pediatric hematologist and it is the physician's responsibility to educate the parents or caregivers regarding all aspects of the disease and the implications and importance of adherence to medications. Caregivers must be trained to recognize the symptoms of SCD complications, such as painful crises, dactylitis, fever, pallor, spleen enlargement by palpation, neurological manifestations and priapism among others, and when to contact the primary physician or seek immediate help at the emergency department. They should be taught how to manage pain at home and offered genetic counseling and advice on contraception.

10.2.2 Penicillin Prophylaxis

Due to the development of functional asplenia and the defective activation of the alternative complement pathway in patients with SCD (Johnston et al. 1973), children with any SCD subtype and particularly hemoglobin (Hb) SS are at an increased risk for invasive bacterial infections, most commonly those caused by Streptococcus pneumonia (Gill et al. 1989). Prophylactic penicillin significantly reduces the risk of pneumococcal infection in pediatric SCD patients, and is generally well tolerated with minimal adverse reactions (Hirst and Owusu-Ofori 2012). Prophylactic therapy with twice daily doses of oral penicillin should be promptly started as soon as the diagnosis is made and by 3 months of age to reduce the morbidity and risk of mortality of pneumococcal septicemia (Gaston et al. 1986). The American Academy of Pediatrics (AAP) recommends the use of penicillin for all children with SCD below 5 years of age. Erythromycin may be used as a substitute in patients with suspected or proven allergy to penicillin (AAP 2009). Penicillin prophylaxis may be discontinued in patients over 5 years of age provided they have not had a severe pneumococcal infection, they have not undergone splenectomy, and they are undergoing regular medical follow-up. If any of these three conditions are not met, the optimal duration of penicillin prophylaxis has not been studied, and most physicians continue prophylaxis into adulthood (AAP 2009; Falletta et al. 1995). Lifelong prophylaxis with penicillin has also been recommended (Davies et al. 2011). Children younger than 5 years of age should receive oral penicillin V at a dose of 125 mg twice daily, and children 5 years of age or older are given 250 mg twice daily (AAP 2009).

However, compliance with daily prophylaxis is not always achieved and resistance against penicillin is an increasing problem. Therefore, pneumococcal vaccination is of paramount importance (Davies et al. 2004). The use of the pneumococcal conjugate vaccine, in combination with penicillin prophylaxis and improved quality of care with prompt management of febrile episodes, has markedly decreased the incidence of fatal pneumococcal infections in children with SCD (Quinn et al. 2010).

10.2.3 Immunizations

In addition to following the regular Centers for Disease Control and Prevention (CDC) immunization schedule, special attention should be made to the following vaccinations in patients with SCD.

Pneumococcal Vaccine

The 13-valent pneumococcal vaccine (PCV13), which was approved by the U.S. Food and Drug Administration (FDA) in 2010, offers a broader coverage than the PCV7 vaccine and is more effective than the 23-valent pneumococcal polysaccharide vaccine (PPSV23) in children below 2 years of age. In addition, good antibody responses have been observed when PCV13 is administered to children previously vaccinated with PPSV23 (De Montalembert et al. 2015).

Infants with SCD should receive the primary 4-dose series of 13-valent pneumococcal conjugate vaccine (PCV13) at 2, 4, and 6 months of age and at 12 through 15 months as part of their routine immunization schedule.

In addition, for children with SCD of 2–5 years of age the Centers for Disease Control and Prevention (CDC) recommends the following:

- 1 dose of PCV13 should be given to those who previously received 3 PCV doses
- 2 doses of PCV13 should be given at least 8 weeks apart to those who previously received less than 3 PCV doses
- 1 supplemental dose of PCV13 should be given to those who completed their 4-dose series

- If there is no history of PPSV23 vaccination, PPSV23 should be given at least 8 weeks after the most recent dose of PCV13

For children 6–18 years of age:

- If there is no previous history of pneumococcal vaccination, 1 dose of PCV13 should be administered, followed by 1 dose of PPSV23 at least 8 weeks later
- If only PCV13 was previously received, 1 dose of PPSV23 should be administered at least 8 weeks after the most recent PCV13 dose
- If PPSV23 has been administered, but PCV13 has not, 1 dose of PCV13 should be given at least 8 weeks after the most recent dose of PPSV23.
- A single revaccination with PPSV23 should be administered 5 years after the first dose

For adults with SCD of 19–65 years of age, the Advisory Committee on Immunization Practices (ACIP) recommends the following:

- Pneumococcal vaccine-naïve patients should receive one dose of PCV13, followed by a dose of PPSV23 at least 8 weeks later. A second PPSV23 dose is recommended 5 years after the first PPSV23 dose.
- Patients with previous PPSV23 vaccination should be given a PCV13 dose at least 1 year after the last PPSV23 dose was received. For those who require additional doses of PPSV23, the first dose should be given at least 8 weeks after PCV13 and at least 5 years after the most recent dose of PPSV23 (CDC 2012).

For adults aged 65 years or older, the most recent ACIP guideline states that, if not previously vaccinated, patients should receive PCV13 first, then PPSV23, 6–12 months afterwards. If previously vaccinated with PPSV23, PCV13 should be administered at least 12 months after the PPSV 23 (CDC 2014a). The above recommendations are summarized in Table 10.1.

One major obstacle to immunization with the conjugated PCV 13 vaccine remains its cost and the fact that it is not part of routinely covered immunizations in many developing countries. In Lebanon, we have partially overcome this problem by partnering with parents and raising money through philanthropy to provide for care, including PCV 13 immunization, while discussing the possibilities of coverage with the Ministry of Public Health.

Haemophilus Influenzae Type B (Hib) Vaccine

One dose of Hib vaccine for SCD patients aged >5 years, if they have not previously received the Hib vaccine (CDC 2014b).

Meningococcal Vaccine

Infants with SCD should receive a 4-dose series at 2, 4, and 6 months of age, and again at 12 through 15 months with Meningococcal groups C and Y and *Haemophilus* b tetanus toxoid conjugate vaccine (Hib-MenCY-TT). Children aged 24 months and

Table 10.1 Pneumococcal immunization schedule in patients with SCD

Routine immunization schedule	Primary 4-dose series of PCV13: at 2, 4, 6 months and 12–15 months of age	
Age	Previous pneumococcal vaccination	Administer
2–5 years	3 PCV doses	1 dose of PCV13
	Less than 3 PCV doses	2 doses of PCV13 at least 8 weeks apart
	Completed 4-dose series	1 supplemental dose of PCV13
	No history of PPSV23	PPSV23 at least 8 weeks after the most recent dose of PCV13
6–18 years	Pneumococcal vaccine-naïve	1 dose of PCV13 followed by 1 dose of PPSV23 at least 8 weeks later
	Only PCV13	1 dose of PPSV23 at least 8 weeks after the most recent PCV13 dose
	PPSV23 but not PCV13	1 dose of PCV13 at least 8 weeks after the most recent dose of PPSV23
		Single revaccination with PPSV23 5 years after the first dose
19–65 years	Pneumococcal vaccine-naïve	1 dose of PCV13 followed by 1 dose of PPSV23 at least 8 weeks later. A second PPSV23 dose is recommended 5 years after the first PPSV23 dose
	PPSV23	PCV13 dose at least 1 year after the last PPSV23 dose
65 years or older	None	PCV13 followed by PPSV23 after 6–12 months
	PPSV23	PCV13 at least 12 months after PPSV23

PCV13 13-valent pneumococcal vaccine

PPSV23 23-valent pneumococcal polysaccharide vaccine

older, who have not received a complete meningococcal vaccination series, should receive two primary doses of quadrivalent meningococcal conjugate vaccine (MenACWY) at least 2 months apart. Children aged 2 months to 6 years should receive an additional dose of MenACWY 3 years after primary immunization; boosters should be repeated every 5 years thereafter. Patients above 7 years of age should receive an additional dose of MenACWY 5 years after primary immunization; boosters should be repeated every 5 years thereafter (CDC 2014b).

The above recommendations are periodically updated.

10.2.4 Clinic Visits

Survival and outcomes of patients with SCD have improved as a result of the combination of medical treatment, newborn screening, and integration of SCD patients into a routine follow-up program (Vichinsky et al. 1988). Therefore, specialized medical centers should be made available especially in endemic areas and patients should be routinely followed-up. The UK National Health Service (NHS) suggests scheduling a follow-up with the specialist every 3 months during the first 2 years, then every 6 months till the age of 5 years, and annually thereafter unless more frequent visits are needed (NHS 2010). There should also be regular communication between the primary care physician and the specialist.

Routine clinic visits should include the taking of a full medical history, interval history of painful crises, febrile illnesses and other SCD complications, frequency of emergency department visits and number of inpatient hospitalizations, school progress and attendance, compliance with medications and review of immunization record. A full physical exam should be performed with focus on vital signs, growth and development, pallor, jaundice, cardiac murmur and spleen size (NHS 2010). At the first consultation, laboratory studies should be performed with a complete blood count (CBC), reticulocyte count, hemoglobin electrophoresis and blood group. It may be worthwhile testing for glucose-6-phosphate dehydrogenase (G6PD) deficiency at the first newborn visit, if not done as part of the neonatal screening, as this condition is common in the same ethnic groups (Benkerrou et al. 2013). Blood tests including CBC and renal and liver function tests should be done as baseline and then at least once yearly and when needed.

10.2.5 Screening

Transcranial Doppler (TCD)

The value of TCD screening in predicting the risk of strokes in patients with SCD has been established since 1992 (Adams et al. 1992). TCD examination should be performed annually in children with sickle cell anemia between 2 and 16 years of age (Adams et al. 1998), and children with elevated TCD are candidates for chronic transfusion therapy for primary stroke prevention. The value of TCD in patients with genotypes other than hemoglobin SS or Sβ^0 has not been studied.

Pulmonary Hypertension

Both pulmonary arterial hypertension by cardiac catheterization and elevated tricuspid regurgitant velocity by echocardiogram have been shown to be independent risk factors for death in patients with SCD (Parent et al. 2011; Gladwin et al. 2004; Ataga et al. 2006; De Castro et al. 2008). While the latest US National Heart, Lung, and Blood Institute (NHLBI) expert panel report found insufficient evidence for screening in asymptomatic patients (NHLBI 2014), the American Thoracic Society (ATS) suggests performing echocardiography as a baseline in children with SCD to detect patients at high risk of morbidity and mortality, and every 1–3 years in adult SCD patients (Klings et al. 2014).

Renal Disease

Sickle cell nephropathy is one of the most common and severe manifestations of SCD. Renal dysfunction starts at an early age with evidence of hyperfiltration during infancy (Ware 2010). Microalbuminuria may start in late childhood and tends to increase with age as the kidney sustains more damage over time (Sharpe and Thein 2011). No definitive criteria exist for renal disease screening in SCD, but it is generally recommended to screen for albuminuria by standard dipstick urinalysis and to perform serum creatinine measurement at least once yearly. If urinalysis is positive for albuminuria, spot urine protein-to-creatinine ratio or 24-h urine collection should be performed (Ataga et al. 2014). Other non-invasive biomarkers such as urinary kidney injury molecule-1 (KIM-1) and N-acetyl-b-D-glucosaminidase (NAG) have shown associations with albuminuria in SCD patients and may be used in the future for further detection of patients with sickle nephropathy (Sundaram et al. 2011).

Retinopathy

Patients with SCD should undergo periodic dilated eye examination by an ophthalmologist starting at the age of 10 years, and every 1–2 years thereafter in individuals with a normal eye exam (NHLBI 2014).

Asthma

Signs and symptoms of asthma or hyperactive airway disease in pediatric and adult SCD patients should be assessed at every follow-up by history and physical exam. In patients with recurrent symptoms, pulmonary function tests should be performed. Patients with SCD and asthma are at higher risk of morbidity including VOC and ACS (Cohen et al. 2011) and mortality (more than twofold), compared to non-asthmatic SCD patients (Anim et al. 2011).

10.2.6 Transitioning into Adult Care

Despite the improvement in survival of young children with SCD, young adults who transition into adult medical care remain at high risk of death, especially in the 2-year period following their transition (Quinn et al. 2010). Several studies have looked into the possible causes, namely increasing complications with age, poor coordination between child-centered and adult-centered services during the transitioning (Callahan et al. 2001), non-adherence to follow-up appointments by adolescents or young adults due to personal, familial or hospital-related factors (Crosby et al. 2009), and health insurance issues (DeBaun and Telfair 2012). Perhaps one of the major factors is the fear of transitioning experienced by the adolescents when leaving the pediatric medical team and being transferred to a less familiar environment with less reliance on parents and more focus on self-management. Transition planning should be started as early as 13 years of age, and the process should involve the patient, parents, and pediatric and adult teams and it should occur over several years (de Montalembert et al. 2014).

10.3 Management of Acute Sickle Cell Disease Complications

Clinical manifestations and complications of SCD have been discussed in previous chapters. We now look into the treatment of each of these.

10.3.1 Vaso-Occlusive Painful Crisis

Vaso-occlusive crisis (VOC), also known as painful crisis, is the most common complication of SCD. It may present in infancy as dactylitis (Delicou and Maragkos 2013) and later in life manifest as pain most commonly involving the abdomen, back, femur and knees (Serjeant et al. 1994). Known triggers of VOC in patients with SCD include emotional stress, pain, hypoxic conditions, high altitude, dehydration (Wright and Ahmedzai 2010), extremes of temperature, alcohol and tobacco use and infections (Ahmed 2011). Patients should be instructed on how to avoid these triggers to prevent the development of VOC. Treatment of painful crisis starts at home and it is believed that most VOCs are entirely managed at home unless oral analgesia is not sufficient. Patients and their caregivers should be taught to identify alarming signs and should be instructed when to contact their caregiver and when to present to the hospital (Rees et al. 2003).

Most emergency department (ED) visits and hospitalizations in SCD patients are for treatment of VOCs (Yang et al. 1995). Suboptimal pain management increases morbidity and may contribute to mortality (Benjamin et al. 2000), therefore, it is essential to establish clinical pathways for the treatment of patients with acute VOC (Co et al. 2003). The initial step consists of assessing the intensity of the pain, using objective tools such as the Wong-Baker faces scale or the numerical scale for older children (Luffy and Grove 2003; Smith et al. 2008). Both rapid pain management and investigations to differentiate between VOC and other causes of pain or SCD complications should then be initiated. The three principles of management consist of analgesia, warmth and hydration, in addition to the treatment of the precipitating factor, if known.

Simple VOCs with mild pain can be managed with a trial of oral hydration and analgesics starting with standing dose of acetaminophen (paracetamol), unless contraindicated, every 6–8 h. If the pain is still uncontrolled, oral NSAIDs such as ibuprofen or ketoprofen every 8 h may be added in absence of any contraindications to NSAIDs treatment (e.g. renal insufficiency, peptic ulcers). This management can be started at home, in the clinic or the ED. Pain should be reassessed every 30 min.

Once pain is controlled, the treatment should be continued for 2 days and a follow-up with the treating physician should be ensured.

Hydration decreases sickling events. There are no established standards on the amount and duration of fluids required (Okomo and Meremikwu 2012), but the general trend is to give 1 to 1.5 times maintenance fluid requirement or 60 mL/kg/24 h (Delicou and Maragkos 2013), or 1.5 L/m^2/day (Okpala 2004b), care should be taken to avoid fluid overload. In patients who cannot tolerate oral hydration, intravenous (IV) fluids should be promptly initiated. In euvolemic patients it is safe to give maintenance IV fluids to avoid overhydration (NHLBI 2014). Normal saline infusion is avoided because it increases plasma osmolality leading to intracellular dehydration and ultimately RBC sickling (Okpala 2004b). Five percent dextrose in water is not used either as it may lead to hyponatremia (Miller 2011). Therefore, the maintenance intravenous solution of choice is 5 % dextrose in water with half-normal saline (D5% +0.45 % sodium chloride). Intravenous fluid boluses should be avoided in euvolemic patients.

Opioids are indicated in acute VOC in patients presenting with moderate-to-severe pain. After assessing the medication doses that have been taken prior to presentation and the patient's opiate intake history, opioids should be rapidly initiated. Morphine is the gold standard opiate used for VOC (Delicou and Maragkos 2013). There are no significant differences between oral sustained release morphine and parenteral morphine infusion with respect to mean pain scores, frequency of rescue analgesia, and adverse-effect profile (Jacobson et al. 1997). However, the general trend is to administer oral opioids for mild pain and IV or subcutaneous opioids for severe pain (Delicou and Maragkos 2013). Around-the-clock doses have been shown to be more effective than on-demand doses in reducing pain and decreasing hospital stay (Udezue and Herrera 2007). Morphine by patient-controlled analgesia (PCA) allows patients to titrate the doses based on pain intensity and was found to have fewer side-effects than continuous IV infusion of morphine (van Beers et al. 2007). Evidence supports the regular use of NSAIDs in acute VOCs in the absence of any contraindications, because of their efficacy in decreasing pain and their opioid-sparing effect (McQuay and Moore 1998).

Oxygen is administered if O_2 saturation falls below 95 % on room air or below the patient's steady-state levels. Laxatives are given to treat opioid-induced constipation and incentive spirometry to avoid acute chest syndrome. Adjunctive approaches such as applying heat to the painful area or distraction of children with games may be helpful (NHLBI 2014).

Indications for hospitalization of patients with acute VOC include:

- Failure to achieve adequate pain relief within 6–8 h at the ED or outpatient clinic
- Suspected infection
- Suspected organ involvement or other SCD complications
- Continued need for IV hydration and analgesia.

A suggested algorithm for management of acute severe VOC is outlined in Fig. 10.1.

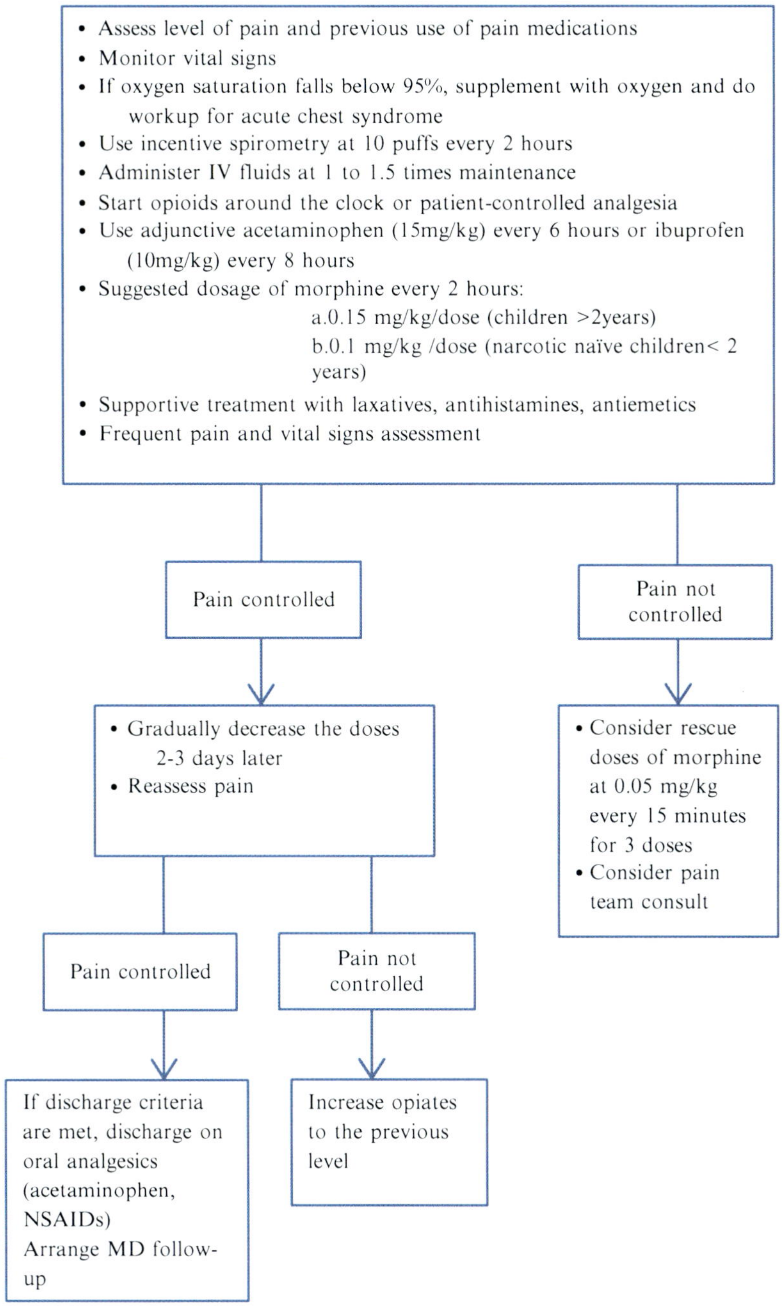

Fig. 10.1 Algorithm for inpatient management of acute severe VOC

Indications for hospital discharge include:

- Adequate pain relief on oral analgesics
- Tolerating oral hydration and medications
- Patient has been afebrile for more than 24 h with negative cultures (if applicable)
- Resolution of any pulmonary symptoms or documentation of adequate oxygenation on room air
- Stable hemoglobin or hematocrit
- Follow-up with MD is arranged.

10.3.2 Fever in a Patient with Sickle Cell Disease

Fever in patients with SCD is a medical emergency, especially with the emergence of penicillin-resistant organisms and possible non-compliance with the vaccination regimen. In addition, even in children who have been immunized with PCV 7, infections due to strains of pneumococcus that are not covered by the vaccine have been reported (McCavit et al. 2011). Patients and their caregivers should be instructed to present immediately to the emergency department (ED) or sickle cell clinic in any case of fever. In fact, fever is the second most common presenting symptom to the ED in patients with SCD (Yusuf et al. 2010).

The initial step in managing a febrile patient with SCD is to take an adequate history and physical exam to find a focus of infection and to search for signs of other SCD complications, such as acute chest syndrome and osteomyelitis. Laboratory workup should include complete blood count, reticulocyte count and blood culture. In patients with respiratory symptoms such as dyspnea, tachypnea, cough or abnormal breath sounds, a chest X-ray is warranted. Urinalysis and urine culture are performed in patients with no other focus or in patients with urinary symptoms. X-rays and/or magnetic resonance imaging (MRI) are done for patients with suspected osteomyelitis.

After cultures are taken, parenteral antibiotics should be administered to SCD patients with a temperature of 38.5 °C or greater to cover against *Streptococcus pneumoniae* and gram-negative enteric organisms (NHLBI 2014). Empiric ceftriaxone administration in febrile SCD patients has been linked to improved outcomes and decreased mortality (Wilimas et al. 1993). Subsequent management depends on the patient. Stable patients who are not ill-looking may be discharged on oral antibiotics with close follow-up, whereas toxic appearing patients need hospitalization and a course of parenteral antibiotics. Criteria for admission include fever above 39.5 °C, elevated white blood cell count, severe anemia, poor oral intake, surgical splenectomy, history of poor compliance and living far from a medical center.

Despite the low rate of true bacteremia shown in some studies (Shihabuddin and Scarfi 2014), fever must always be promptly managed in these patients. Some markers may be associated with a higher likelihood of bacteremia such as elevated absolute neutrophil count, high proportion of band cells, and the presence of vomiting (Savlov et al. 2014). In addition, patients should be closely evaluated for other complications such as the development of splenic sequestration, or aplastic crises. Newly detected splenomegaly and/or dropping platelet counts are, in our view, an indication for admission and close observation.

10.3.3 Acute Chest Syndrome

Acute chest syndrome (ACS) is a serious life-threatening condition that needs prompt management and hospitalization. Chest X-ray should be performed on any patient with SCD presenting with fever and respiratory symptoms. Management of ACS includes; oxygen saturation monitoring, supplemental oxygen, incentive spirometry, adequate antibiotic coverage, hydration, analgesia and transfusion. Antibiotics are always indicated in the treatment of ACS as the causative agent cannot always be determined. The regimen should combine a cephalosporin and a macrolide to treat both the common bacterial pathogens, in addition to atypical bacteria such as *Mycoplasma pneumonia* (Wright 2004).

Opiates are generally used to control the pain, but one must be cautious to achieve adequate analgesia without causing respiratory depression. They are usually supplemented with NSAIDs. Maintenance IV fluids are required but overhydration may worsen the symptoms and cause pulmonary edema. Incentive spirometry given at a regimen of 10 puffs every 2 h while the patient is awake has been shown to significantly reduce pulmonary complications (atelectasis or infiltrates) associated with ACS in patients hospitalized for acute chest or back pain (Bellet et al. 1995). The use of intermittent positive expiratory pressure has also been proposed (Hsu et al. 2005).

Transfusion is the cornerstone of ACS treatment as it improves oxygen delivery to the tissues by correcting severe anemia and decreasing HbS fraction (Emre et al. 1995). Exchange transfusion also decreases blood viscosity. Simple transfusion is effective and adequate in most patients with SS disease whose hemoglobin concentration is more than 1 g/dL below the baseline (NHLBI 2014). Exchange or partial exchange transfusion is preferred in patients with no acute drop in hemoglobin. The general target is to lower hemoglobin S below 30 %. Patients may require repetitive transfusions as hemoglobin concentrations may continue to drop in patients with ACS; therefore it is essential to follow hemoglobin and reticulocyte count (Miller 2011). Urgent exchange transfusion is indicated in rapidly deteriorating patients (oxygen saturation below 90 % despite oxygen supplementation, worsening respiratory distress, multilobar involvement, pleural effusions) (NHLBI 2014).

The use of bronchodilators such as inhaled salbutamol is encouraged in children with ACS even in the absence of wheezing (Vichinsky et al. 2000). Data on the use of corticosteroids for treatment of ACS has been conflicting (Miller 2011).

Dexamethasone use has been associated with higher readmission rates and VOCs after the resolution of ACS (Bernini et al. 1998; Sobota et al. 2010) and use of dexamethasone has been associated with hemorrhagic strokes in some series (Strouse et al. 2006). At this point, we do not recommend the routine use of steroids in patients with sickle cell disease who present with acute chest syndrome. Instead, we reserve steroids for the management of patients who also have asthma. One should thus be careful not to withhold steroids in these patients (Miller 2011). As mentioned earlier in this chapter, SCD patients with asthma are at a higher risk of developing ACS (Boyd et al. 2004). Therefore, adequate asthma control is essential. All practitioners taking care of individuals with SCD should familiarize themselves with the management of asthma.

The use of inhaled nitric oxide (NO) remains controversial. NO may be helpful in ACS because of its vasodilator and cytoprotective properties, which improve blood flow to hypoxic tissues. NO may also inhibit erythrocyte adhesion to the endothelium (Jia et al. 1996). Despite the fact that no adequate trials have been conducted to determine its efficacy in ACS treatment (Al Hajeri et al. 2008), some reports have shown positive results in critical cases that were treated with NO (Atz and Wessel 1997; Sullivan et al. 1999; Oppert et al. 2004), and NO may be considered in refractory cases of ACS (Miller 2011).

Recurrent ACS episodes are a risk factor for the development of chronic lung disease and ischemic strokes and are also associated with long-term increased mortality in patients with SCD (Vichinsky et al. 2000; Platt et al. 1994). Care should hence be taken to prevent the development of ACS in these patients. In the acute setting, the use of incentive spirometers for patients admitted with painful crises has been shown to effectively prevent the development of ACS. In a tertiary care center care setting, education of heath care providers and the implementation of guidelines to manage painful crises led to a 50 % decrease in the incidence of ACS in patients admitted for painful VOC (Reagan et al. 2011). ACS is a common post operative complication in patients with SCD and adequate care including preoperative transfusions, intra and post operative fluid management, incentive spirometry and post-operative pain management can decrease the incidence of this complication. Outside the acute setting, long-term hydroxyurea has been shown to decrease the incidence of ACS in infants, children and adults. Therefore, patients who have more than one episode of ACS should be started on hydroxyurea therapy. Chronic transfusions also effectively prevent the development of ACS (Miller et al. 2001), but should be recommended only for patients who fail hydroxyurea, given the cumbersome nature of the therapy and the risk of iron overload. As recurrent ACS is associated with increased mortality, patients who have suffered more than two episodes are considered candidates for bone marrow transplantation, which is very effective in preventing ACS. Some debate remains as to whether this modality of therapy should be offered only to patients who fail hydroxyurea. In our view, patients who have had two or more episodes of ACS and who have a matched sibling donor should be offered transplant regardless of the response to hydroxyurea.

10.3.4 Acute Splenic Sequestration

In patients with HbSS, acute splenic sequestration (ASS) usually occurs in infancy and early childhood. The risk decreases with age as they develop splenic fibrosis and autosplenectomy, which is usually complete by 5 years of age (Brousse et al. 2014). In patients with HbSC and HbSβ^{+}, ASS can occur later during childhood or even in adulthood. As mentioned earlier, parents must be taught to assess splenic size by palpation, especially when the patient has symptoms of severe anemia. The implementation of parental education programs has been shown to be associated with an increase in ASS incidence and a concomitant decrease in case fatality rate, probably reflecting increased awareness and earlier detection and management (Emond et al. 1985).

As ASS may lead to severe life-threatening anemia, immediate management consists of urgent blood transfusion to prevent hypovolemic shock. The target is to increase Hb to no greater than 8 g/dL in order to avoid the "overshoot" phenomenon, a process by which transfusion triggers the spleen to release the trapped erythrocytes into the circulation over the following days, leading to hyperviscosity.

Regular transfusion programs to prevent recurrence of splenic sequestration have shown limited benefits (Kinney et al. 1990). In addition, regular transfusions carry the risk of alloimmunization and iron overload (Rao and Gooden 1985) and have a high cost and poor availability of donor blood. Splenectomy is recommended for children with recurrent splenic sequestrations or a single life-threatening sequestration. It is also done in older children and adults with chronic splenic sequestration accompanied by local pain and hypersplenism. Patients should receive pneumococcal vaccine before splenectomy and every 3 years thereafter, in addition to Hib and meningococcal vaccines (Working Party of the British Committee for Standards in Haematology Clinical Haematology Task 1996). Partial splenectomy has been performed to retain some splenic function and immune competence, but the remaining splenic fragment might show recurrence of ASS (Owusu-Ofori and Hirst 2013). The efficacy of partial splenectomy, as compared to total splenectomy, remains unclear (Mouttalib et al. 2012). In our view, given the splenic dysfunction prevalent in patients with SCD, we see no role for partial splenectomy in this patient population.

10.3.5 Neurological Complications

As mentioned earlier in this chapter, children with a cerebral blood flow rate of 200 cm/s or more on TCD are at a high risk for cerebrovascular accidents (CVA). Chronic blood transfusion regimen is the mainstay of treatment for primary and secondary CVA prevention and it was reported as early as 1976 (Lusher et al. 1976). The Stroke Prevention in Sickle Cell (STOP 1) trial showed a 92 % reduction in stroke incidence in the study group receiving regular transfusion regimen (Adams et al. 1998). The STOP 2 trial showed normalization in TCD in patients receiving transfusions for a minimum of 30 months, and an increase in TCD and risk of stroke after discontinuing the transfusions (Adams et al. 2005). The Stroke With Transfusions Changing to Hydroxyurea (SWiTCH) trial revealed that transfusion and chelation are superior to hydroxyurea in the treatment of patients with SCD, stroke and iron overload (Ware et al. 2012). At this time, transfusions and chelation remain the mainstay of secondary stroke prevention in patients with SCD. For patients with elevated cerebral blood velocity, hydroxyurea may be effective in primary stroke prevention as suggested by the preliminary results of the TCD With Transfusions Changing to Hydroxyurea (TWiTCH) trial, but these have at this time not yet been published.

SCD patients who present with acute onset symptoms such as altered level of consciousness, paralysis, headache or slurred speech must undergo urgent computed tomography (CT) scan of the brain followed by MRI and magnetic resonance angiograpy (MRA) to evaluate for stroke (NHLBI 2014). A neurologist and a sickle cell specialist should be consulted. Exchange transfusion is preferred over simple transfusion as the first line treatment, as it is associated with a lower risk of recurrent stroke (Hulbert et al. 2006). These patients are then initiated on a monthly transfusion program for secondary stroke prevention. Management of SCD patient with acute stroke is outlined in Table 10.2.

The optimal duration of treatment is still unknown, and some patients remain at risk for recurrent strokes or transient ischemic attacks (TIAs) despite maintaining an HbS level below 30 % on transfusions (Scothorn et al. 2002; Pegelow et al. 1995). The risk of recurrence is highest within 2–3 years of the first stroke (Powars et al. 1978). In addition, regular transfusion regimens have not been shown to be effective in preventing progression of cerebral vasculopathy on MRI in children

Table 10.2 Management of sickle cell patients presenting with acute stroke

Primary assessment and management	History, physical exam and vital signs
	Stabilization, oxygenation, cautious IV hydration
Laboratory tests	CBC, reticulocytes, coagulation studies, BUN, creatinine, serum electrolytes
	Blood group and typing cross-match (extended RBC phenotyping if available)
	Lumbar puncture if meningitis is suspected
Imaging	Urgent CT scan of the brain
	Brain MRI and MRA
Transfusion	Exchange transfusion (manual or automated)
	Simple transfusion if exchange transfusion is not available
	Target Hb below 10 g/dL to avoid hyperviscosity

CBC complete blood count, *BUN* blood urea nitrogen

with SCD and stroke (Brousse et al. 2009).These patients will, as a result, require long-term follow up and we recommend that this includes yearly MRI and MRA.

10.3.6 Priapism

Priapism is a serious SCD complication that can lead to impotence if diagnosis and therapy are delayed. Recurrent priapism may lead to fibrosis. No controlled studies for prevention of recurrent priapism are available (Chinegwundoh and Anie 2004). Initial management of includes IV hydration, analgesia with morphine, oxygen and sedation if needed.

Several drugs have been used for the treatment of priapism. In the past, data have indicated benefits from stilboestrol (estrogen analogue) in preventing stuttering priapism, but possible side-effects include gynecomastia, loss of normal erections and gastrointestinal symptoms (Serjeant et al. 1985). Other hormonal agents have been used, as well such as finasteride (Rachid-Filho et al. 2009) and leuprolide (Maples and Hagemann 2004). The α-adrenergic agonist etilefrine is often used in the treatment and prevention of priapism, as various studies have shown its effectiveness in SCD patients with stuttering priapism or history of one major attack. Alpha-agonists act as vasoconstrictors and are thought to act on the penile arteries to force blood out of the corpora cavernosa (Powars and Johnson 1996). Blood pressure should be closely monitored in these patients. Contraindications to treating with etilefrine include hypertension, cerebral vascular disease, transient ischemic attacks, among others (Okpala et al. 2002; Gbadoe et al. 2001). Beta agonists have been used in some studies to induce smooth muscle relaxation and allow oxygenated blood to enter the corpora cavernosa and wash out the stagnant damaged sickle cells (Maples and Hagemann 2004). Combined alpha and beta agonists, such as pseudoephedrine, are also used. When these drugs do not achieve an immediate response, penile aspiration and irrigation with saline and alpha adrenergic agents is performed (Mantadakis et al. 2000). When a second irrigation is unsuccessful, surgical shunting of the blood away from the corpora cavernosa may be considered (Noe et al. 1981).

10.3.7 Aplastic Crisis

Parvovirus B19 infection in SCD patients causes acute severe anemia, characterized by low reticulocyte count, which differentiates it from acute splenic sequestration. Acute management consists of transfusing the patient to achieve a safe level of hemoglobin, not necessarily reaching the patient's baseline level. The patient's counts recover in 1–2 weeks. The patient should be isolated from vulnerable contacts such as siblings with SCD or pregnant women to prevent the spread of the infection (Okpala 2004a).

10.3.8 Hepatobiliary Complications

Liver Disease

Patients with SCD may develop acute hepatic sequestration (AHS), characterized by decreased Hb and increased reticulocyte count, in addition to increased liver size. Since about two-thirds of SCD patients have chronic mild hepatomegaly, change in size should be monitored. Some episodes of AHS self-resolve, while others might necessitate simple or exchange transfusion.

An uncommon complication of SCD is acute intrahepatic cholestasis (AIC) (Ahn et al. 2005). It may present with right upper quadrant pain and tenderness, fever, vomiting and leukocytosis. Laboratory findings include elevated total serum bilirubin (total 50 mg/dL or higher), hypoalbuminemia, thrombocytopenia, elevated alkaline phosphatase, variable levels of transaminases and increased prothrombin time (PT) and partial thromboplastin time (PTT). AIC can progress to liver failure (Issa and Al-Salem 2010). Treatment includes hydration, rest, close observation and exchange transfusion (Irizarry et al. 2006; Shao and Orringer 1995).

Gallbladder Disease

Despite the high prevalence of pigment gallstones in SCD patients due to hemolysis, acute cholecystitis occurs in less than 10 % of patients with SCD. Children and adults with asymptomatic cholelithiasis are treated with watchful waiting (NHLBI 2014). SCD patients presenting with acute cholecystitis are treated with antibiotics and supportive care, followed by elective cholecystectomy like in the general population (Johnson 2004). Symptomatic gallstones are also managed by cholecystectomy. Preoperative transfusion for patients undergoing cholecystectomy is warranted to decrease the risk of sickle cell events. The laparoscopic approach is preferred, when possible, as it incurs a shorter hospital stay, lower cost and fewer surgical complications than open cholecystectomy (Haberkern et al. 1997).

10.3.9 Ophthalmologic Complications

Acute ophthalmological complications of SCD include; hyphema secondary to blunt trauma, central retinal artery occlusion (CRAO), orbital and periorbital infections, orbital infarction, and orbital compression syndrome.

Hyphema can lead to elevated intraocular pressure (IOP) due to sickling in the anterior chamber of the eye and may cause permanent visual loss. Various agents including antifibrinolytics such as aminocaproic acid, corticosteroids and cycloplegics have been used, but data on management of SCD patients with hyphema is limited, and these approaches carry a risk of rebleed. Any elevation in IOP in SCD patients may cause vision loss, therefore, close monitoring of IOP is essential and any elevation might require paracentesis (Gharaibeh et al. 2013).

CRAO by sickled red cell sludge is an ocular emergency. It presents with acute painless loss of vision. Bilateral presentation is extremely rare. Pharmacological IOP reduction with carbonic anhydrase inhibitors, mechanical IOP reduction, ocular massage, direct thrombolysis and hyperbaric oxygen have been used without proven benefit. Most patients undergo exchange transfusion (Liem et al. 2008). The use of hyperbaric oxygen therapy combined with exchange transfusion has been successfully reported in a patient with SCD presenting with CRAO (Canan et al. 2014). Prognosis of CRAO in SCD is poor, and more studies are needed to establish guidelines for the management of this condition.

Orbital infarction is usually associated with VOC. Presentation may mimic periorbital cellulitis and the diagnosis is made with imaging studies. Surgical management may be required (NHLBI 2014). Orbital compression syndrome may be seen with orbital infarction. After an infectious cause is ruled-out, corticosteroids, like methylprednisolone, may be effective in decreasing orbital edema (Sokol et al. 2008). If optic nerve dysfunction or large hematomas are present, surgical evacuation is needed to prevent loss of vision and to speed recovery (Curran et al. 1997).

Any patient with SCD presenting with eye symptoms should be immediately referred to an ophthalmologist to prevent irreversible visual loss.

10.4 Management of Chronic Sickle Cell Disease Complications

As the life expectancy of people with SCD has increased, chronic complications are now a larger area of concern.

10.4.1 Pulmonary Hypertension

Pulmonary artery pressure can be assessed by echocardiography where the tricuspid regurgitant velocity (TRV) is used to calculate pulmonary artery pressure. Despite the unclear relationship between elevated TRV and true pulmonary hypertension (PH), the definite diagnosis of which is made by right heart catheterization (Pashankar et al. 2008), both parameters have been shown to be associated with higher mortality in adult SCD patients. The American Thoracic Society (ATS) defines patients with SCD who are at an increased risk of death as those who have elevated TRV, elevated serum N-terminal pro-brain natriuretic peptide (NT-pro-BNP) level, or PH confirmed by right heart catheterization (Klings et al. 2014).

Antihypertensive agents are no longer used in the treatment of PH in SCD, as SCD patients have lower systemic blood pressure compared to normal controls and are at risk of severe hypotension (Okpala 2004c). Hydroxyurea (HU) treatment decreases the frequency of ACS and VOC (Charache et al. 1995), both of which increase the risk of mortality in patients with SCD and PH (Mehari et al. 2013). In addition, the use of HU was shown to be associated with decreased mortality in SCD patients (Steinberg et al. 2003, 2010). Therefore, the ATS recommends the use of HU in patients with a high risk of mortality. Chronic transfusions are suggested as an alternative therapy, with no strong supportive evidence (Klings et al. 2014).

Other pharmacologic agents targeting PH have been studied. However, the presence of PH needs to be confirmed by right heart catheterization prior to considering therapy for PH. The phosophodiesterase type 5 inhibitor sildenafil is used for the treatment of pulmonary hypertension. However, its use in the setting of SCD has been controversial. While sildenafil was shown to improve PH and exercise capacity in a study performed on SCD patients with PH (Machado et al. 2005), a randomized double blind clinical trial evaluating the role of sildenafil in decreasing PH in SCD patients was closed early due to an increase in serious adverse events associated with sildenafil use (Machado et al. 2011). Therefore, the ATS strongly advises against the use of sildenafil in SCD patients with PH (Klings et al. 2014). The endothelin receptor antagonist, bosentan, has not been shown to significantly improve pulmonary vascular resistance or exercise tolerance in SCD patients with PH (Barst et al. 2010), but may be used in patients with confirmed PH, elevated pulmonary vascular resistance and normal pulmonary capillary wedge pressure (Hsu et al. 2005).

As mentioned earlier, NO has shown some benefit in patients with ACS and may benefit PH by the same mechanism. The use of NO requires special equipment and is cumbersome. Arginine is the nitrogen donor for synthesis of NO, and patients with SCD and PH who received L-arginine showed a 15.2 % mean reduction in estimated pulmonary artery systolic pressure, but these benefits were short-term (Morris et al. 2003). L-carnitine treatment may also decrease PH in SCD patients. The possible mechanisms include decreased production of tumor necrosis factor and improvement in endothelial dysfunction (El-Beshlawy et al. 2006).

At this point, the need for screening patients with echocardiography remains controversial and the management of patients with SCD and PH is also unclear. The high risk of mortality in patients with sickle cell disease and PH requires that these patients be managed in conjunction with pulmonary specialists who have experience in this domain. Optimizing HU therapy and chronic transfusions should be considered. Furthermore, a recent study utilizing reduced intensity conditioning and matched-sibling transplant was shown to effectively decrease TRV (Hsieh et al. 2014).

10.4.2 Chronic Kidney Disease

In infants with SCD, hydroxyurea may improve urine concentrating ability and decrease renal enlargement (Alvarez et al. 2012). Patients on HU are less likely to exhibit proteinuria, and the use of HU may prevent or slow the development of overt nephropathy or end-stage renal disease (ESRD) (Laurin et al. 2014). Therefore, HU should be considered in all patients with sickle cell nephropathy unless contraindicated (Sharpe and Thein 2014).

The benefits of angiotensin-converting enzyme (ACE) inhibitors in sickle cell nephropathy have been established since the early 1990s. Treatment with enalapril was shown to reduce the degree of proteinuria (Falk et al. 1992). Discontinuation of the drug may lead to increase in microalbuminuria to pre-treatment levels or higher (Aoki and Saad 1995). ACE inhibitors may slightly decrease blood pressure, so SCD patients on treatment need to be monitored to avoid hypotension (Foucan et al. 1998). Patients should also be monitored for hyperkalemia (McKie et al. 2007). ACE inhibitors are the current standard of care of pediatric and adult SCD patients with microalbuminuria or proteinuria (Ataga et al. 2014).

As individuals with SCD age, the risk of ESRD increases. Poor blood pressure control and use of nonsteroidal anti-inflammatory agents (NSAIDs) can increase the rate of renal disease progression. There are no clear guidelines on the treatment of hypertension in SCD patients, but diuretics should be used cautiously to avoid dehydration (Ataga et al. 2014). The risk of mortality in patients with SCD-ESRD is higher than for patients with ESRD due to other causes, especially when they reach the renal replacement therapy stage. This mortality rate, however, is lower in those who receive pre-dialysis nephrology care, highlighting the importance of follow-up with a nephrologist in SCD patients with chronic kidney disease (CKD) prior to reaching ESRD (McClellan et al. 2012). Erythropoietin-stimulating agents may be useful in CKD patients (Sharpe and Thein 2014). Hemodialysis and peritoneal dialysis are both performed, but renal transplant shows better outcomes (Ataga et al. 2014). Over the recent years, survival among SCD kidney transplant recipients has markedly improved (Huang et al. 2013). Candidates for kidney transplant should be carefully picked, as most SCD patients with ESRD have other SCD complications and poor prognosis.

10.4.3 Chronic Pain

Chronic pain in SCD is less frequent than acute VOCs. Its management, however, is more challenging and it involves analgesic medications, adjuvant therapy, physiotherapy, psychological support and possible surgery. This syndrome of chronic pain was originally described by Ballas and has gained increased recognition (Ballas et al. 2010). It is important in this context to trust patients and listen carefully to their complaints. In diagnosing chronic pain syndrome, it important to rule-out other types of chronic pain such as trauma or other comorbid conditions not related to SCD. Chronic SCD pain may also be due to an identifiable pathology such as leg ulcers or avascular necrosis, or may be due to chronic neuropathic pain or breakthrough pain in patients on opioids.

Oral opiates such as methadone, morphine, codeine, oxycodone, and hydroxycodone may be given (Delicou and Maragkos 2013). Combinations of long-acting opioid together with a short-acting opioid have been used (Shaiova and Wallenstein 2004). Morphine sulphate or hydromorphone tablets are given for breakthrough pain. When tolerance develops to one drug, the patient can be switched to another (Okpala 2004a). Methadone is effective for chronic pain, but is not widely used in SCD due to its side-effect profile. Patients should be referred for evaluation by a psychiatrist. Serotonin norepinephrine reuptake inhibitors (SNRIs) and tricyclic antidepressants may be helpful in altering the perception of pain, although their use has not been established in sickle cell pain (Co et al. 2003).

Psychotherapy, especially cognitive behavioral therapy, is effective for dealing with the emotional component of chronic pain and the psychological burden of SCD (Thomas 2000). Non-pharmacological methods have been suggested for the treatment of chronic SCD pain, such as meditation, progressive relaxation, dreaming, transcutaneous electrical nerve stimulation, hypnosis, music therapy and acupuncture, among others (Delicou and Maragkos 2013). Many patients report using complementary and alternative medicine as adjunctive therapy for pain management (Thompson and Eriator 2014). The values of these interventions need to be carefully evaluated and their benefits studied. It is, however, important to note that they may help individual patients and should be considered in this context.

10.4.4 Retinopathy

Progressive sickle retinopathy (PSR) may lead to vitreous hemorrhage and significant vision loss (Moriarty et al. 1988). Spontaneous regression may occur in up to 32 % of affected eyes (Downes et al. 2005). PSR is managed with laser photocoagulation. Photocoagulation helps decrease the rate of loss of visual acuity and reduces the incidence of vitreous hemorrhage (Farber et al. 1991). It can also help induce regression of pre-existing lesions (Kimmel et al. 1986). Surgical vitrectomy is used to treat severe vitreous hemorrhage and may show favorable outcomes (Williamson et al. 2009).

10.4.5 Leg Ulcers

Sickle cell ulcers are a debilitating, painful and often recurring complication of SCD. Initial treatment includes gentle debridement and wet to dry dressings, effective in most cases. A variety of topical agents have been used and studied.

Arginylglycylaspartic acid (RGD) peptide matrix acts as a topical synthetic substitute matrix at the ulcer site (Wethers et al. 1994). It was found to be the only intervention that significantly reduces ulcer size in a recent Cochrane review (Marti-Carvajal et al. 2014a). The administration of arginine butyrate combined with standard care (twice daily cleaning and wet-to-dry dressing changes) can promote healing of long-standing refractory ulcers. The mechanism is not well defined yet and may include a combination of the ability of butyrate to stimulate platelet-derived growth factor (PDGF) production, blockage of inflammatory cytokines and down-regulation of matrix metalloproteinases (McMahon et al. 2010).

One trial of topical preparation of neomycin, bacitracin, and polymyxin B resulted in a significant reduction in ulcer size (Baum et al. 1987). Solcoseryl has been shown to increase ulcer healing, but the effect was not statistically significant compared to controls (La Grenade et al. 1993). Oral zinc sulphate showed higher healing rates (Serjeant et al. 1970). A 6-week treatment regimen with subcutaneous heparin and human antithrombin concentrate showed improved healing (Cacciola et al. 1989).

Patients with chronic deep leg ulcers should be evaluated for osteomyelitis. Wound cultures should be taken and antibiotics should be started if infection is suspected (NHLBI 2014). Recently a nitrite cream has been used with encouraging results in this very frustrating condition (Minniti et al. 2014), this preparation is however only available on a research basis.

10.4.6 Avascular Necrosis

Avascular necrosis (AVN) of the femoral and humeral head is associated with reduced quality of life and chronic pain. It is a frequent and severe SCD complication and its treatment is not standardized (Marti-Carvajal et al. 2014b). The therapeutic approach depends on the radiographic staging of AVN. Initial treatment includes analgesia, physiotherapy and partial weight bearing on crutches and orthopedic assessment. A small study showed that physical therapy is as effective as hip core decompression, followed by physical therapy (Neumayr et al. 2006); however, other studies showed a significant benefit of surgical core decompression in improving pain and decreasing necrotic bone lesions (Mukisi-Mukaza et al. 2009). Conservative treatment has been shown to yield poor results (Ebong and Kolawole 1986). At this time, hip replacement seems to be the mainstay of therapy for patients with severe or very symptomatic disease. Despite the controversy, we recommend core decompression for patients with early symptomatic disease in a center with experience, as this may delay the need for hip replacement.

10.5 Blood Transfusions

Blood transfusions are a mainstay of treatment for patients with sickle cell disease. Chronic transfusions have the ability to prevent strokes and silent infarcts. Furthermore, in all the randomized studies of stroke prevention, i.e. STOP, SWiTCh and SIT (Miller et al. 2001; Alvarez et al. 2013; DeBaun et al. 2014; Beverung et al. 2015), patients in the transfusion arms had significantly fewer sickle cell related non-neurologic complications. In this section, we will briefly review the beneficial role of transfusions in SCD as well as the problems associated with this form of treatment.

10.5.1 Indications for Acute Transfusion

- *Acute exacerbation of anemia*: Seen in splenic sequestration, hepatic sequestration, aplastic crisis secondary to parvovirus B19 infection or any symptomatic anemia. The aim is to correct Hb to a level around 8 g/dL.
- *Acute chest syndrome*: Early simple transfusion is beneficial. Exchange transfusion is carried out if clinical deterioration occurs or if Hb levels are not low enough.
- *Multiorgan failure*
- *Preoperative management*: A conservative transfusion regimen to increase the hemoglobin level to 10 g per deciliter is effective in preventing perioperative complications in SCD patients (Vichinsky et al. 1995; Howard et al. 2013).
- *Stroke or acute neurological deficit:* Simple transfusion is given if exchange transfusion is not readily available.

10.5.2 Indications for Chronic Transfusion Regimen

- *Primary and secondary stroke prevention*: Regular transfusions to keep HbS less than 30 % (Wang and Dwan 2013).
- *Recurrent ACS:* In cases refractory to treatment with HU, chronic transfusion reduces the frequency of ACS (Miller et al. 2001).
- *Controversial indications*: Frequent VOCs (Miller et al. 2001), chronic pain, avascular joint necrosis, leg ulcers, priapism (Rees et al. 2010), recurrent splenic sequestration (limited data, splenectomy is the standard of care), pregnancy (Koshy et al. 1988; Mahomed 2000).

Chronic packed red blood cell (pRBC) transfusion reduces SCD complications by reducing the burden of sickled RBCs and decreasing hemolysis (Lezcano et al. 2006).

10.5.3 Exchange Transfusion

The benefits of exchange transfusion include increased HbA after transfusion, increased volume without increase in viscosity and reduced iron overload. Its risks are: higher potential rates of alloimmunization, high cost, need for specialized equipment and personnel and frequent need for permanent venous access.

Exchange transfusion is indicated in management of acute stroke and in severe worsening ACS.

10.5.4 Complications of Transfusions

Alloimmunization

Alloimmunization to minor RBC antigens is a significant complication of chronic transfusions that leads to increased risk of hemolytic transfusion reactions and limits the number of compatible RBC donors. Prevalence of alloimmunization can be as high as 35–40 % in the absence of minor RBC antigen phenotype matching (McPherson et al. 2010). Autoimmunization can also occur in this setting, and most autoantibodies are IgG and can fix complement. The risk of alloimmunization can be reduced by matching for the red cell antigens D, C, E, and Kell (Klings et al. 2014). SCD patients on chronic transfusions should undergo phenotype identification and RBC antigen matching (Godfrey et al. 2010).

Transfusional Iron Overload

Levels of serum ferritin correlate with volume of pRBCs transfused, but the rate of increase varies widely between different patients (Files et al. 2002). Data from the patients enrolled in the STOP 1 and 2 trials showed that ferritin levels of less than 1500 ng/mL are acceptable and levels of 3000 ng/mL or greater reflect significant iron overload and are associated with liver injury (Adamkiewicz et al. 2009).

Liver biopsy has been the gold standard in the diagnosis of iron overload as it allows a direct measure of iron stores and there is a poor correlation between serum ferritin levels and liver iron content (LIC) (Karam et al. 2008). New less invasive diagnostic tools using MRI have been developed to measure LIC and are being used in randomized controlled trials. Iron overload is treated with iron chelation to control LIC in order to reduce the risk of cirrhosis and hepatocellular carcinoma (Porter and Garbowski 2013). Cardiac overload may also occur in SCD patients on chronic transfusion regimens (Meloni et al. 2014), although the myocardium is relatively protected in SCD compared to thalassemia. Oral deferasirox and subcutaneous deferoxamine treatments have been compared in adults and children with SCD and transfusional iron overload and have yielded similar results (Vichinsky et al. 2007). High-dose intravenous desferrioxamine is a suitable option for poorly compliant patients (Kalpatthi et al. 2010).

Other risks of chronic transfusions include febrile reactions, allergic reactions, delayed hemolytic reactions, and volume overload. Taken together, these occur in 15 % of patients (Klings et al. 2014).

10.6 Pharmacotherapy in Sickle Cell Disease

10.6.1 Hydroxyurea

Hydroxyurea (HU), also known as hydroxycarbamide, is a ribonucleotide reductase inhibitor that was first synthesized in 1869 and has been used for several decades in the treatment of patients with myeloproliferative disorders. It was first shown to enhance HbF production in patients with SCD in a study published in 1984 (Platt et al. 1984). Increased HbF levels in the cells lead to a decrease in HbS concentration resulting in less polymerization, and less RBC sickling.

The exact mechanism by which HU increases HbF is not fully understood. One theory suggests that HU is cytotoxic to late erythroid precursors resulting in recruitment of early precursors with higher HbF production. Other hypotheses state that HU acts directly on late precursors to produce HbF or may alter transcription factors that act around the globin gene enhancer or promoter regions. HU may also act as a NO donor (Segal et al. 2008). Its rheological benefits include the ability to increase RBC water content and volume, to decrease the number of circulating leukocytes to limit the interaction of RBCs with the endothelium (Davies and Gilmore 2003).

A clinical trial published in 1995 showed that HU reduces the frequency of VOC and ACS, the need for transfusions and the frequency of hospitalization (Charache et al. 1995). A 9-year follow-up of the study showed significantly decreased mortality in patients whose HbF levels increased on HU treatment (Steinberg et al. 2003). The US FDA approved HU for the treatment of sickle cell anemia in adults in 1998.

The BABY HUG trial conducted on children 9–18 months of age showed significant benefit of HU use, including decreased VOC and dactylitis rates, and some evidence suggesting decreased ACS, hospitalization and transfusion rates (Wang et al. 2011). These effects are related to the increased Hb in patients on HU (Lebensburger et al. 2012). Currently, HU is the only approved disease-modifying drug for treatment of SCD in patients above 2 years of age.

Indications for initiation of HU include recurrent VOCs (3 or more severe episodes requiring admission in the last 12 months including dactylitis), 2 or more episodes of ACS, severe anemia, and as an alternative to transfusion to prevent new or recurrent stroke, in situations where transfusion therapy is not feasible (Ware et al. 2010). HU is also used in patients with evidence of sickle cell nephropathy to delay the onset of ESRD (Sharpe and Thein 2014). The efficacy of HU on chronic organ damage prevention or treatment has not yet been proven (McGann and Ware 2011). HU treatment should be discussed with and offered to all patients with SCD, starting from 9 months of age. Studies on HU have mostly included patients with

HbSS or HbSβ^0. However, treatment should also be considered for people with HbSβ+-thalassemia or HbSC who have recurrent sickle cell-associated pain.

HU is rapidly absorbed and has high bioavailability. Baseline investigations prior to initiation of HU therapy should include; complete blood count (CBC) with differential, reticulocyte count, quantitative measurement of HbF (e.g., hemoglobin electrophoresis, high-performance liquid chromatography), renal and liver function tests and pregnancy test for women (NHLBI 2014). HU can then be safely started at doses of 20 mg/kg/day in children and 15 mg/kg/day in adults given orally once daily. CBC is usually repeated weekly for the first 4 weeks then once every 4 weeks if the counts are stable (Ware 2010). HU dose may be escalated by 5 mg/kg/day at 8-week intervals if needed. Some patients only achieve a therapeutic effect at the maximum tolerated dose (MTD), of up to 35 mg/kg/day. MTD is usually well tolerated with sustained hematologic response (Zimmerman et al. 2004). If bone marrow suppression (thrombocytopenia or neutropenia) occurs, HU is withheld to allow for marrow recovery and CBC is monitored weekly. When counts recover, HU is restarted at a dose of 5 mg/kg/day less than the dose causing myelosuppression (Davies and Gilmore 2003). Clinical response usually occurs 3–6 months after initiation of adequate HU doses.

Short-term complications of HU include myelotoxicity, mouth ulceration, macrocytosis and megaloblastoid changes, gastrointestinal (GI) discomfort, skin toxicity-rashes and hyperpigmentation. GI complaints are not severe and may be reduced by changing the timing of the daily HU dose. Skin and nail complaints are mild and rarely significant (Ware 2010). Toxicity in children 9–18 months of age was found to be limited to mild-to-moderate neutropenia (Wang et al. 2011). HU toxicities are mild and similar for children, adolescents and adults with SCD (Kinney et al. 1999). Bone marrow suppression is common after dose escalation, but resolves within 2 weeks of temporary discontinuation of therapy (Steinberg et al. 2010).

To date, no significant long-term HU toxicities have been found in pediatric or adult SCD patients on chronic HU therapy. No adverse effects on growth, development, or number of acquired DNA mutations were found in pediatric patients (Zimmerman et al. 2004), and there have been no reported cases of myelodysplasia or leukemia in adults (Voskaridou et al. 2010).

10.6.2 Investigational Agents/Emerging Drugs

Besides HU, several HbF-inducing agents are under study in SCD patients, including the thalidomide analog pomalidomide, the short chain fatty acid derivative 2,3-sodium dimethyl butyrate (HQK-1001), and the hypomethylating agent decitabine and the histone deacetylase inhibitor vorinostat.

Other novel therapies targeting different disease mechanisms are being investigated (please see Chap. 16 for a full description of these therapies). Drugs targeting adhesion inhibit selectins and include rivipansel sodium, heparin and low molecular weight heparins, among others. Intravenous immunoglobulin (IVIg), propranolol, platelet aggregation inhibitors and factor Xa inhibitors are also being studied in clinical trials (Singh and Ballas 2015). Clinical trials on purified poloxamer 188 have also been conducted, as this molecule decreases blood viscosity, RBC aggregation and decreases friction between RBCs and the vascular endothelium (Gibbs and Hagemann 2004).

Anti-inflammatory drugs include regadenoson, carbon monoxide, statins, omega-3 fatty acids, zileton, prasugrel, NO and arginine. Prasugrel has reached Phase III trial. NO and arginine also function indirectly as fetal Hb induction agents. Arginine, a natural amino acid, is being evaluated in adults and children and has reached Phase III studies. Finally, drugs that prevent oxidative injury include glutamine, α-lipoic acid, acetyl-L-carnitine and Aes-103 (5-hydroxymethyl-2-furfural) are under study. The latter inhibits activation of the Gardos channel, leading to improved RBC hydration (Singh and Ballas 2015). A recent Cochrane review on phytomedicines highlights Niprisan(®) as a safe and effective intervention in reducing severe VOCs over a 6-month follow-up period (Oniyangi and Cohall 2013).

10.7 Stem Cell Transplant

Allogeneic hematopoietic stem cell transplantation (HSCT) is currently the only curative treatment for SCD. The objective of HSCT is to replace sickle erythropoiesis or to reduce its clinical impact by inducing the expression of β-globin chains (Walters 2005). HSCT is increasingly being used for young children with early SCD complications. Older adults are considered less favorable candidates for HSCT due to the higher risk for organ toxicities and greater susceptibility to severe graft versus host disease (GvHD) (Platt 2005). Several studies on HSCT in children showed good results with long-term disease-free survival ranging from 82 to 86 % (Bhatia and Walters 2008).

Indications for HSCT in SCD are weighed based on the risk-benefit ratio, depending on the patient's status and donor availability. When a matched sibling donor is available, indications for HSCT may include: stroke, elevated TCD velocity, ACS, recurrent VOCs (more than three episodes per year requiring hospitalization), pulmonary hypertension, TRV >2.5 m/s, AVN, alloimmunization, silent stroke especially with cognitive impairment, recurrent priapism and sickle nephropathy (Shenoy 2013). After the identification of a matched donor, the recipient undergoes extensive evaluation to check for organ dysfunction and health status. The recipient then receives the conditioning regimen, which usually provides both myeloablation and immunosuppression (Oringanje et al. 2013). The initial and most challenging step is to identify patients with severe disease requiring HSCT, but without conditions that would impede the use of intensive myeloablative regiments (Abboud 2009).

Myeloablative conditioning regimens have utilized a backbone consisting of busulfan and cyclophosphamide, with or without other immunosuppressive drugs such as anti-thymocyte globulin (ATG), anti-lymphocyte globulin (ALG) and total lymphoid irradiation (TLI) (Khoury and Abboud 2011). Most studies have used cyclosporine (CSP) and methotrexate (MTX) for post-transplant immunosuppression (Walters 2005).

The preparative regimen for myeloablative HSCT on children has severe adverse effects on growth and gonadal function. To reduce this toxicity, reduced intensity conditioning regimens have been used, including purine analogs (such as fludarabine, cladribine and pentostatin), alkylating agent or low-dose total body irradiation (TBI) (Oringanje et al. 2013). Adults with multiple comorbidities are not candidates for myeloblative transplant regimens. Recently, Hsieh and colleagues published a report on the successful transplant of adults using a non-myeloablative regimen (Hsieh et al. 2014). The applicability of transplants remains limited by the availability of donors and the willingness of parents and patients to undergo the procedure. Experimental approaches with haploidentical donors have shown some promise (Bolanos-Meade et al. 2012). The future will see more use of these techniques and the start of gene therapy protocols.

References

Abboud MR (2009) Hematopoietic stem-cell transplantation for adults with sickle cell disease. N Engl J Med 361(24):2380–2381

Adamkiewicz TV, Abboud MR, Paley C et al (2009) Serum ferritin level changes in children with sickle cell disease on chronic blood transfusion are nonlinear and are associated with iron load and liver injury. Blood 114(21):4632–4638

Adams R, McKie V, Nichols F et al (1992) The use of transcranial ultrasonography to predict stroke in sickle cell disease. N Engl J Med 326(9):605–610

Adams RJ, McKie VC, Hsu L et al (1998) Prevention of a first stroke by transfusions in children with sickle cell anemia and abnormal results on transcranial Doppler ultrasonography. N Engl J Med 339(1):5–11

Adams RJ, Brambilla D, Optimizing Primary Stroke Prevention in Sickle Cell Anemia Trial I (2005) Discontinuing prophylactic transfusions used to prevent stroke in sickle cell disease. N Engl J Med 353(26):2769–2778

Ahmed SG (2011) The role of infection in the pathogenesis of vaso-occlusive crisis in patients with sickle cell disease. Mediterr J Hematol Infect Dis 3(1):e2011028

Ahn H, Li CS, Wang W (2005) Sickle cell hepatopathy: clinical presentation, treatment, and outcome in pediatric and adult patients. Pediatr Blood Cancer 45(2):184–190

Al Hajeri A, Serjeant GR, Fedorowicz Z (2008) Inhaled nitric oxide for acute chest syndrome in people with sickle cell disease. Cochrane Database Syst Rev 1:CD006957

Alvarez O, Miller ST, Wang WC et al (2012) Effect of hydroxyurea treatment on renal function parameters: results from the multi-center placebo-controlled BABY HUG clinical trial for infants with sickle cell anemia. Pediatr Blood Cancer 59(4):668–674

Alvarez O, Yovetich NA, Scott JP et al (2013) Pain and other non-neurological adverse events in children with sickle cell anemia and previous stroke who received hydroxyurea and phlebotomy or chronic transfusions and chelation: results from the SWiTCH clinical trial. Am J Hematol 88(11):932–938

American Academy of Pediatrics (AAP) (2009) Immunization in special clinical circumstances. In: Pickering LK, Baker CJ, Long SS (eds) Red book: Report of the Committee on Infectious Diseases, 28th edn. American Academy of Pediatrics, Elk Grove Village

Anim SO, Strunk RC, DeBaun MR (2011) Asthma morbidity and treatment in children with sickle cell disease. Expert Rev Respir Med 5(5):635–645

Aoki RY, Saad ST (1995) Enalapril reduces the albuminuria of patients with sickle cell disease. Am J Med 98(5):432–435

Ataga KI, Moore CG, Jones S et al (2006) Pulmonary hypertension in patients with sickle cell disease: a longitudinal study. Br J Haematol 134(1):109–115

Ataga KI, Derebail VK, Archer DR (2014) The glomerulopathy of sickle cell disease. Am J Hematol 89(9):907–914

Atz AM, Wessel DL (1997) Inhaled nitric oxide in sickle cell disease with acute chest syndrome. Anesthesiology 87(4):988–990

Ballas SK, Lieff S, Benjamin LJ et al (2010) Definitions of the phenotypic manifestations of sickle cell disease. Am J Hematol 85(1):6–13

Barst RJ, Mubarak KK, Machado RF et al (2010) Exercise capacity and haemodynamics in patients with sickle cell disease with pulmonary hypertension treated with bosentan: results of the ASSET studies. Br J Haematol 149(3):426–435

Baum KF, MacFarlane DE, Maude GH, Serjeant GR (1987) Topical antibiotics in chronic sickle cell leg ulcers. Trans R Soc Trop Med Hyg 81(5):847–849

Bellet PS, Kalinyak KA, Shukla R, Gelfand MJ, Rucknagel DL (1995) Incentive spirometry to prevent acute pulmonary complications in sickle cell diseases. N Engl J Med 333(11): 699–703

Benjamin LJ, Swinson GI, Nagel RL (2000) Sickle cell anemia day hospital: an approach for the management of uncomplicated painful crises. Blood 95(4):1130–1136

Benkerrou M, Alberti C, Couque N et al (2013) Impact of glucose-6-phosphate dehydrogenase deficiency on sickle cell anaemia expression in infancy and early childhood: a prospective study. Br J Haematol 163(5):646–654

Bernini JC, Rogers ZR, Sandler ES et al (1998) Beneficial effect of intravenous dexamethasone in children with mild to moderately severe acute chest syndrome complicating sickle cell disease. Blood 92(9):3082–3089

Beverung LM, Strouse JJ, Hulbert ML et al (2015) Health-related quality of life in children with sickle cell anemia: impact of blood transfusion therapy. Am J Hematol 90(2):139–143

Bhatia M, Walters MC (2008) Hematopoietic cell transplantation for thalassemia and sickle cell disease: past, present, and future. Bone Marrow Transplant 41(2):109–117

Bolanos-Meade J, Fuchs EJ, Luznik L et al (2012) HLA-haploidentical bone marrow transplantation with posttransplant cyclophosphamide expands the donor pool for patients with sickle cell disease. Blood 120(22):4285–4291

Boyd JH, Moinuddin A, Strunk RC, DeBaun MR (2004) Asthma and acute chest in sickle-cell disease. Pediatr Pulmonol 38(3):229–232

Brousse V, Hertz-Pannier L, Consigny Y et al (2009) Does regular blood transfusion prevent progression of cerebrovascular lesions in children with sickle cell disease? Ann Hematol 88(8):785–788

Brousse V, Buffet P, Rees D (2014) The spleen and sickle cell disease: the sick(led) spleen. Br J Haematol 166(2):165–176

Cacciola E, Giustolisi R, Musso R, Longo A, Cacciola E (1989) Antithrombin III concentrate for treatment of chronic leg ulcers in sickle cell-beta thalassemia: a pilot study. Ann Intern Med 111(6):534–536

Callahan ST, Winitzer RF, Keenan P (2001) Transition from pediatric to adult-oriented health care: a challenge for patients with chronic disease. Curr Opin Pediatr 13(4):310–316

Canan H, Ulas B, Altan-Yaycioglu R (2014) Hyperbaric oxygen therapy in combination with systemic treatment of sickle cell disease presenting as central retinal artery occlusion: a case report. J Med Case Rep 8:370

Centers for Disease Control and Prevention (CDC) (2012) Use of 13-valent pneumococcal conjugate vaccine and 23-valent pneumococcal polysaccharide vaccine for adults with immunocom-

promising conditions: recommendations of the Advisory Committee on Immunization Practices (ACIP). MMWR Morb Mortal Wkly Rpt 61(40):816–819
Centers for Disease Control and Prevention (CDC) (2014a) Recommended adult immunization schedule, by vaccine and age group. http://www.cdc.gov/vaccines/schedules/hcp/imz/adult.html. Accessed 20 Nov 2014
Centers for Disease Control and Prevention (CDC) (2014b) Recommended immunization schedule for persons aged 0 through 18 years. http://www.cdc.gov/vaccines/schedules/hcp/imz/child-adolescent.html. Accessed 20 Nov 2014
Charache S, Terrin ML, Moore RD et al (1995) Effect of hydroxyurea on the frequency of painful crises in sickle cell anemia. Investigators of the Multicenter Study of Hydroxyurea in Sickle Cell Anemia. N Engl J Med 332(20):1317–1322
Chinegwundoh F, Anie KA (2004) Treatments for priapism in boys and men with sickle cell disease. Cochrane Database Syst Rev 4:CD004198
Co JP, Johnson KB, Duggan AK, Casella JF, Wilson M (2003) Does a clinical pathway improve the quality of care for sickle cell anemia? Jt Comm J Qual Saf 29(4):181–190
Cohen RT, Madadi A, Blinder MA et al (2011) Recurrent, severe wheezing is associated with morbidity and mortality in adults with sickle cell disease. Am J Hematol 86(9):756–761
Crosby LE, Modi AC, Lemanek KL et al (2009) Perceived barriers to clinic appointments for adolescents with sickle cell disease. J Pediatr Hematol Oncol 31(8):571–576
Curran EL, Fleming JC, Rice K, Wang WC (1997) Orbital compression syndrome in sickle cell disease. Ophthalmology 104(10):1610–1615
Davies SC, Gilmore A (2003) The role of hydroxyurea in the management of sickle cell disease. Blood Rev 17(2):99–109
Davies EG, Riddington C, Lottenberg R, Dower N (2004) Pneumococcal vaccines for sickle cell disease. Cochrane Database Syst Rev 1:CD003885
Davies JM, Lewis PN, Wimperis J et al (2011) Review of guidelines for the prevention and treatment of infection in patients with an absent or dysfunctional spleen: prepared on behalf of the British Committee for Standards in Haematology by a Working Party of the Haemato-Oncology Task Force. Br J Haematol 155:308–317
De Castro LM, Jonassaint JC, Graham FL, Ashley-Koch A, Telen MJ (2008) Pulmonary hypertension associated with sickle cell disease: clinical and laboratory endpoints and disease outcomes. Am J Hematol 83(1):19–25
de Montalembert M, Guitton C, French Reference Centre for Sickle Cell D (2014) Transition from paediatric to adult care for patients with sickle cell disease. Br J Haematol 164(5):630–635
De Montalembert M, Abboud MR, Fiquet A et al (2015) 13-valent pneumococcal conjugate vaccine (PCV13) is immunogenic and safe in children 6-17 years of age with sickle cell disease previously vaccinated with 23-valent pneumococcal polysaccharide vaccine (PPSV23): results of a phase 3 study. Pediatr Blood Cancer 62:1427–1436
DeBaun MR, Telfair J (2012) Transition and sickle cell disease. Pediatrics 130(5):926–935
DeBaun MR, Gordon M, McKinstry RC et al (2014) Controlled trial of transfusions for silent cerebral infarcts in sickle cell anemia. N Engl J Med 371(8):699–710
Delicou S, Maragkos K (2013) Pain management in patients with sickle cell disease – a review. EMJ Hema 1:30–36
Downes SM, Hambleton IR, Chuang EL et al (2005) Incidence and natural history of proliferative sickle cell retinopathy: observations from a cohort study. Ophthalmology 112(11):1869–1875
Ebong WW, Kolawole TM (1986) Aseptic necrosis of the femoral head in sickle-cell disease. Br J Rheumatol 25(1):34–39
El-Beshlawy A, Abd El Raouf E, Mostafa F et al (2006) Diastolic dysfunction and pulmonary hypertension in sickle cell anemia: is there a role for L-carnitine treatment? Acta Haematol 115(1-2):91–96
Emond AM, Collis R, Darvill D et al (1985) Acute splenic sequestration in homozygous sickle cell disease: natural history and management. J Pediatr 107(2):201–206

Emre U, Miller ST, Gutierez M et al (1995) Effect of transfusion in acute chest syndrome of sickle cell disease. J Pediatr 127(6):901–904
Falk RJ, Scheinman J, Phillips G et al (1992) Prevalence and pathologic features of sickle cell nephropathy and response to inhibition of angiotensin-converting enzyme. N Engl J Med 326(14):910–915
Falletta JM, Woods GM, Verter JI et al (1995) Discontinuing penicillin prophylaxis in children with sickle cell anemia. Prophylactic Penicillin Study II. J Pediatr 127(5):685–690
Farber MD, Jampol LM, Fox P et al (1991) A randomized clinical trial of scatter photocoagulation of proliferative sickle cell retinopathy. Arch Ophthalmol 109(3):363–367
Files B, Brambilla D, Kutlar A et al (2002) Longitudinal changes in ferritin during chronic transfusion: a report from the stroke prevention trial in sickle cell anemia (STOP). J Pediatr Hematol Oncol 24(4):284–290
Foucan L, Bourhis V, Bangou J et al (1998) A randomized trial of captopril for microalbuminuria in normotensive adults with sickle cell anemia. Am J Med 104(4):339–342
Gaston MH, Verter JI, Woods G et al (1986) Prophylaxis with oral penicillin in children with sickle cell anemia. A randomized trial. N Engl J Med 314(25):1593–1599
Gbadoe AD, Atakouma Y, Kusiaku K, Assimadi JK (2001) Management of sickle cell priapism with etilefrine. Arch Dis Child 85(1):52–53
Gharaibeh A, Savage HI, Scherer RW, Goldberg MF, Lindsley K (2013) Medical interventions for traumatic hyphema. Cochrane Database Syst Rev 12:CD005431
Gibbs WJ, Hagemann TM (2004) Purified poloxamer 188 for sickle cell vaso-occlusive crisis. Ann Pharmacother 38(2):320–324
Gill FM, Brown A, Gallagher D et al (1989) Newborn experience in the cooperative study of sickle cell disease. Pediatrics 83(5 Pt 2):827–829
Gladwin MT, Sachdev V, Jison ML et al (2004) Pulmonary hypertension as a risk factor for death in patients with sickle cell disease. N Engl J Med 350(9):886–895
Godfrey GJ, Lockwood W, Kong M, Bertolone S, Raj A (2010) Antibody development in pediatric sickle cell patients undergoing erythrocytapheresis. Pediatr Blood Cancer 55(6):1134–1137
Haberkern CM, Neumayr LD, Orringer EP et al (1997) Cholecystectomy in sickle cell anemia patients: perioperative outcome of 364 cases from the National Preoperative Transfusion Study. Preoperative Transfusion in Sickle Cell Disease Study Group. Blood 89(5):1533–1542
Hirst C, Owusu-Ofori S (2012) Prophylactic antibiotics for preventing pneumococcal infection in children with sickle cell disease. Cochrane Database Syst Rev 9:CD003427
Howard J, Malfroy M, Llewelyn C et al (2013) The Transfusion Alternatives Preoperatively in Sickle Cell Disease (TAPS) study: a randomised, controlled, multicentre clinical trial. Lancet 381(9870):930–938
Hsieh MM, Fitzhugh CD, Weitzel RP et al (2014) Nonmyeloablative HLA-matched sibling allogeneic hematopoietic stem cell transplantation for severe sickle cell phenotype. JAMA 312(1):48–56
Hsu LL, Batts BK, Rau JL (2005) Positive expiratory pressure device acceptance by hospitalized children with sickle cell disease is comparable to incentive spirometry. Respir Care 50(5):624–627
Huang E, Parke C, Mehrnia A et al (2013) Improved survival among sickle cell kidney transplant recipients in the recent era. Nephrol Dial Transplant 28(4):1039–1046
Hulbert ML, Scothorn DJ, Panepinto JA et al (2006) Exchange blood transfusion compared with simple transfusion for first overt stroke is associated with a lower risk of subsequent stroke: a retrospective cohort study of 137 children with sickle cell anemia. J Pediatr 149(5):710–712
Irizarry K, Rossbach HC, Ignacio JR et al (2006) Sickle cell intrahepatic cholestasis with cholelithiasis. Pediatr Hematol Oncol 23(2):95–102
Issa H, Al-Salem AH (2010) Hepatobiliary manifestations of sickle cell anemia. Gastroenterol Res 3(1):1–8
Jacobson SJ, Kopecky EA, Joshi P, Babul N (1997) Randomised trial of oral morphine for painful episodes of sickle-cell disease in children. Lancet 350(9088):1358–1361
Jia L, Bonaventura C, Bonaventura J, Stamler JS (1996) S-nitrosohaemoglobin: a dynamic activity of blood involved in vascular control. Nature 380(6571):221–226

Johnson CS (2004) The liver in sickle cell disease. In: Okpala IE (ed) Practical management of haemoglobinopathies. Blackwell Publishing, Oxford, pp 120–129

Johnston RB Jr, Newman SL, Struth AG (1973) An abnormality of the alternate pathway of complement activation in sickle-cell disease. N Engl J Med 288(16):803–808

Kalpatthi R, Peters B, Kane I et al (2010) Safety and efficacy of high dose intravenous desferrioxamine for reduction of iron overload in sickle cell disease. Pediatr Blood Cancer 55(7): 1338–1342

Karam LB, Disco D, Jackson SM et al (2008) Liver biopsy results in patients with sickle cell disease on chronic transfusions: poor correlation with ferritin levels. Pediatr Blood Cancer 50(1):62–65

Khoury R, Abboud MR (2011) Stem-cell transplantation in children and adults with sickle cell disease: an update. Expert Rev Hematol 4(3):343–351

Kimmel AS, Magargal LE, Stephens RF, Cruess AF (1986) Peripheral circumferential retinal scatter photocoagulation for the treatment of proliferative sickle retinopathy. An update. Ophthalmology 93(11):1429–1434

Kinney TR, Ware RE, Schultz WH, Filston HC (1990) Long-term management of splenic sequestration in children with sickle cell disease. J Pediatr 117(2 Pt 1):194–199

Kinney TR, Helms RW, O'Branski EE et al (1999) Safety of hydroxyurea in children with sickle cell anemia: results of the HUG-KIDS study, a phase I/II trial. Pediatric Hydroxyurea Group. Blood 94(5):1550–1554

Klings ES, Machado RF, Barst RJ et al (2014) An official American Thoracic Society clinical practice guideline: diagnosis, risk stratification, and management of pulmonary hypertension of sickle cell disease. Am J Respir Crit Care Med 189(6):727–740

Koshy M, Burd L, Wallace D, Moawad A, Baron J (1988) Prophylactic red-cell transfusions in pregnant patients with sickle cell disease. A randomized cooperative study. N Engl J Med 319(22):1447–1452

La Grenade L, Thomas PW, Serjeant GR (1993) A randomized controlled trial of solcoseryl and duoderm in chronic sickle-cell ulcers. West Indian Med J 42(3):121–123

Laurin LP, Nachman PH, Desai PC, Ataga KI, Derebail VK (2014) Hydroxyurea is associated with lower prevalence of albuminuria in adults with sickle cell disease. Nephrol Dial Transplant 29(6):1211–1218

Lebensburger JD, Miller ST, Howard TH et al (2012) Influence of severity of anemia on clinical findings in infants with sickle cell anemia: analyses from the BABY HUG study. Pediatr Blood Cancer 59(4):675–678

Lezcano NE, Odo N, Kutlar A, Brambilla D, Adams RJ (2006) Regular transfusion lowers plasma free hemoglobin in children with sickle-cell disease at risk for stroke. Stroke 37(6):1424–1426

Liem RI, Calamaras DM, Chhabra MS et al (2008) Sudden-onset blindness in sickle cell disease due to retinal artery occlusion. Pediatr Blood Cancer 50(3):624–627

Luffy R, Grove SK (2003) Examining the validity, reliability, and preference of three pediatric pain measurement tools in African-American children. Pediatr Nurs 29(1):54–59

Lusher JM, Haghighat H, Khalifa AS (1976) A prophylactic transfusion program for children with sickle cell anemia complicated by CNS infarction. Am J Hematol 1(2):265–273

Machado RF, Martyr S, Kato GJ et al (2005) Sildenafil therapy in patients with sickle cell disease and pulmonary hypertension. Br J Haematol 130(3):445–453

Machado RF, Barst RJ, Yovetich NA et al (2011) Hospitalization for pain in patients with sickle cell disease treated with sildenafil for elevated TRV and low exercise capacity. Blood 118(4):855–864

Mahomed K (2000) Prophylactic versus selective blood transfusion for sickle cell anaemia during pregnancy. Cochrane Database Syst Rev 2:CD000040

Mantadakis E, Ewalt DH, Cavender JD, Rogers ZR, Buchanan GR (2000) Outpatient penile aspiration and epinephrine irrigation for young patients with sickle cell anemia and prolonged priapism. Blood 95(1):78–82

Maples BL, Hagemann TM (2004) Treatment of priapism in pediatric patients with sickle cell disease. Am J Health Syst Pharm 61(4):355–363

Marti-Carvajal AJ, Knight-Madden JM, Martinez-Zapata MJ (2014a) Interventions for treating leg ulcers in people with sickle cell disease. Cochrane Database Syst Rev 12:CD008394

Marti-Carvajal AJ, Sola I, Agreda-Perez LH (2014b) Treatment for avascular necrosis of bone in people with sickle cell disease. Cochrane Database Syst Rev 7:CD004344

McCavit TL, Quinn CT, Techasaensiri C, Rogers ZR (2011) Increase in invasive Streptococcus pneumoniae infections in children with sickle cell disease since pneumococcal conjugate vaccine licensure. J Pediatr 158(3):505–507

McClellan AC, Luthi JC, Lynch JR et al (2012) High one year mortality in adults with sickle cell disease and end-stage renal disease. Br J Haematol 159(3):360–367

McGann PT, Ware RE (2011) Hydroxyurea for sickle cell anemia: what have we learned and what questions still remain? Curr Opin Hematol 18(3):158–165

McKie KT, Hanevold CD, Hernandez C et al (2007) Prevalence, prevention, and treatment of microalbuminuria and proteinuria in children with sickle cell disease. J Pediatr Hematol Oncol 29(3):140–144

McMahon L, Tamary H, Askin M et al (2010) A randomized phase II trial of Arginine Butyrate with standard local therapy in refractory sickle cell leg ulcers. Br J Haematol 151(5):516–524

McPherson ME, Anderson AR, Castillejo MI et al (2010) HLA alloimmunization is associated with RBC antibodies in multiply transfused patients with sickle cell disease. Pediatr Blood Cancer 54(4):552–558

McQuay H, Moore A (1998) An evidence-based resource for pain relief, 1st edn. Oxford University Press, Oxford

Mehari A, Alam S, Tian X et al (2013) Hemodynamic predictors of mortality in adults with sickle cell disease. Am J Respir Crit Care Med 187(8):840–847

Meloni A, Puliyel M, Pepe A et al (2014) Cardiac iron overload in sickle-cell disease. Am J Hematol 89(7):678–683

Miller ST (2011) How I treat acute chest syndrome in children with sickle cell disease. Blood 117(20):5297–5305

Miller ST, Wright E, Abboud M et al (2001) Impact of chronic transfusion on incidence of pain and acute chest syndrome during the Stroke Prevention Trial (STOP) in sickle-cell anemia. J Pediatr 139(6):785–789

Minniti CP, Gorbach AM, Xu D et al (2014) Topical sodium nitrite for chronic leg ulcers in patients with sickle cell anaemia: a phase 1 dose-finding safety and tolerability trial. The Lancet Haematol 1(3):e95–e103

Moriarty BJ, Acheson RW, Condon PI, Serjeant GR (1988) Patterns of visual loss in untreated sickle cell retinopathy. Eye (Lond) 2(Pt 3):330–335

Morris CR, Morris SM Jr, Hagar W et al (2003) Arginine therapy: a new treatment for pulmonary hypertension in sickle cell disease? Am J Respir Crit Care Med 168(1):63–69

Mouttalib S, Rice HE, Snyder D et al (2012) Evaluation of partial and total splenectomy in children with sickle cell disease using an Internet-based registry. Pediatr Blood Cancer 59(1):100–104

Mukisi-Mukaza M, Manicom O, Alexis C et al (2009) Treatment of sickle cell disease's hip necrosis by core decompression: a prospective case-control study. Orthop Traumatol Surg Res 95(7):498–504

NIH National Heart, Lung and Blood Institute (NHLBI) (2014). Evidence-based management of sickle cell disease. Expert panel report

Neumayr LD, Aguilar C, Earles AN et al (2006) Physical therapy alone compared with core decompression and physical therapy for femoral head osteonecrosis in sickle cell disease. Results of a multicenter study at a mean of three years after treatment. J Bone Joint Surg Am 88(12):2573–2582

Noe HN, Wilimas J, Jerkins GR (1981) Surgical management of priapism in children with sickle cell anemia. J Urol 126(6):770–771

Okomo U, Meremikwu MM (2012) Fluid replacement therapy for acute episodes of pain in people with sickle cell disease. Cochrane Database Syst Rev 6:CD005406

Okpala IE (2004a) Treatment modalities for pain in sickle cell disease. In: Okpala IE (ed) Practical management of haemoglobinopathies. Blackwell Publishing, Oxford, pp 72–75

Okpala IE (2004b) Sickle cell crisis. In: Okpala IE (ed) Practical management of haemoglobinopathies. Blackwell Publishing, Oxford, pp 63–71

Okpala IE (2004c) Pulmonary hypertension: a complication of haemolytic states. In: Okpala IE (ed) Practical management of haemoglobinopathies. Blackwell Publishing, Oxford, pp 130–133

Okpala I, Westerdale N, Jegede T, Cheung B (2002) Etilefrine for the prevention of priapism in adult sickle cell disease. Br J Haematol 118(3):918–921

Oniyangi O, Cohall DH (2013) Phytomedicines (medicines derived from plants) for sickle cell disease. Cochrane Database Syst Rev 1:CD004448

Oppert M, Jorres A, Barckow D et al (2004) Inhaled nitric oxide for ARDS due to sickle cell disease. Swiss Med Wkly 134(11-12):165–167

Oringanje C, Nemecek E, Oniyangi O (2013) Hematopoietic stem cell transplantation for people with sickle cell disease. Cochrane Database Syst Rev 5:CD007001

Owusu-Ofori S, Hirst C (2013) Splenectomy versus conservative management for acute sequestration crises in people with sickle cell disease. Cochrane Database Syst Rev 5:CD003425

Parent F, Bachir D, Inamo J et al (2011) A hemodynamic study of pulmonary hypertension in sickle cell disease. N Engl J Med 365(1):44–53

Pashankar FD, Carbonella J, Bazzy-Asaad A, Friedman A (2008) Prevalence and risk factors of elevated pulmonary artery pressures in children with sickle cell disease. Pediatrics 121(4):777–782

Pegelow CH, Adams RJ, McKie V et al (1995) Risk of recurrent stroke in patients with sickle cell disease treated with erythrocyte transfusions. J Pediatr 126(6):896–899

Platt OS (2005) Preventing stroke in sickle cell anemia. N Engl J Med 353(26):2743–2745

Platt OS, Orkin SH, Dover G et al (1984) Hydroxyurea enhances fetal hemoglobin production in sickle cell anemia. J Clin Invest 74(2):652–656

Platt OS, Brambilla DJ, Rosse WF et al (1994) Mortality in sickle cell disease. Life expectancy and risk factors for early death. N Engl J Med 330(23):1639–1644

Porter J, Garbowski M (2013) Consequences and management of iron overload in sickle cell disease. Hematology Am Soc Hematol Educ Program 2013:447–456

Powars DR, Johnson CS (1996) Priapism. Hematol Oncol Clin North Am 10(6):1363–1372

Powars D, Wilson B, Imbus C, Pegelow C, Allen J (1978) The natural history of stroke in sickle cell disease. Am J Med 65(3):461–471

Quinn CT, Rogers ZR, McCavit TL, Buchanan GR (2010) Improved survival of children and adolescents with sickle cell disease. Blood 115(17):3447–3452

Rachid-Filho D, Cavalcanti AG, Favorito LA, Costa WS, Sampaio FJ (2009) Treatment of recurrent priapism in sickle cell anemia with finasteride: a new approach. Urology 74(5):1054–1057

Rao S, Gooden S (1985) Splenic sequestration in sickle cell disease: role of transfusion therapy. Am J Pediatr Hematol Oncol 7(3):298–301

Reagan MM, DeBaun MR, Frei-Jones MJ (2011) Multi-modal intervention for the inpatient management of sickle cell pain significantly decreases the rate of acute chest syndrome. Pediatr Blood Cancer 56(2):262–266

Rees DC, Olujohungbe AD, Parker NE et al (2003) Guidelines for the management of the acute painful crisis in sickle cell disease. Br J Haematol 120(5):744–752

Rees DC, Williams TN, Gladwin MT (2010) Sickle-cell disease. Lancet 376(9757):2018–2031

Savlov D, Beck CE, DeGroot J, Odame I, Friedman JN (2014) Predictors of bacteremia among children with sickle cell disease presenting with fever. J Pediatr Hematol Oncol 36(5): 384–388

Scothorn DJ, Price C, Schwartz D et al (2002) Risk of recurrent stroke in children with sickle cell disease receiving blood transfusion therapy for at least five years after initial stroke. J Pediatr 140(3):348–354

Segal JB, Strouse JJ, Beach MC et al (2008) Hydroxyurea for the treatment of sickle cell disease. Evid Rep Technol Assess (Full Rep) 165:1–95

Serjeant GR, Galloway RE, Gueri MC (1970) Oral zinc sulphate in sickle-cell ulcers. Lancet 2(7679):891–892

Serjeant GR, de Ceulaer K, Maude GH (1985) Stilboestrol and stuttering priapism in homozygous sickle-cell disease. Lancet 2(8467):1274–1276

Serjeant GR, Ceulaer CD, Lethbridge R et al (1994) The painful crisis of homozygous sickle cell disease: clinical features. Br J Haematol 87(3):586–591

Shaiova L, Wallenstein D (2004) Outpatient management of sickle cell pain with chronic opioid pharmacotherapy. J Natl Med Assoc 96(7):984–986

Shao SH, Orringer EP (1995) Sickle cell intrahepatic cholestasis: approach to a difficult problem. Am J Gastroenterol 90(11):2048–2050

Sharpe CC, Thein SL (2011) Sickle cell nephropathy - a practical approach. Br J Haematol 155(3):287–297

Sharpe CC, Thein SL (2014) How I treat renal complications in sickle cell disease. Blood 123(24):3720–3726

Shenoy S (2013) Hematopoietic stem-cell transplantation for sickle cell disease: current evidence and opinions. Ther Adv Hematol 4(5):335–344

Shihabuddin BS, Scarfi CA (2014) Fever in children with sickle cell disease: are all fevers equal? J Emerg Med 47(4):395–400

Singh PC, Ballas SK (2015) Emerging drugs for sickle cell anemia. Expert Opin Emerg Drugs 20(1):47–61

Smith WR, Penberthy LT, Bovbjerg VE et al (2008) Daily assessment of pain in adults with sickle cell disease. Ann Intern Med 148(2):94–101

Sobota A, Graham DA, Heeney MM, Neufeld EJ (2010) Corticosteroids for acute chest syndrome in children with sickle cell disease: variation in use and association with length of stay and readmission. Am J Hematol 85(1):24–28

Sokol JA, Baron E, Lantos G, Kazim M (2008) Orbital compression syndrome in sickle cell disease. Ophthal Plast Reconstr Surg 24(3):181–184

Steinberg MH, Barton F, Castro O et al (2003) Effect of hydroxyurea on mortality and morbidity in adult sickle cell anemia: risks and benefits up to 9 years of treatment. JAMA 289(13):1645–1651

Steinberg MH, McCarthy WF, Castro O et al (2010) The risks and benefits of long-term use of hydroxyurea in sickle cell anemia: A 17.5 year follow-up. Am J Hematol 85(6):403–408

Strouse JJ, Hulbert ML, DeBaun MR, Jordan LC, Casella JF (2006) Primary hemorrhagic stroke in children with sickle cell disease is associated with recent transfusion and use of corticosteroids. Pediatrics 118(5):1916–1924

Sullivan KJ, Goodwin SR, Evangelist J, Moore RD, Mehta P (1999) Nitric oxide successfully used to treat acute chest syndrome of sickle cell disease in a young adolescent. Crit Care Med 27(11):2563–2568

Sundaram N, Bennett M, Wilhelm J et al (2011) Biomarkers for early detection of sickle nephropathy. Am J Hematol 86(7):559–566

Thomas V (2000) Cognitive behavioural therapy in pain management for sickle cell disease. Int J Palliat Nurs 6(9):434–442

Thompson WE, Eriator I (2014) Pain control in sickle cell disease patients: use of complementary and alternative medicine. Pain Med 15(2):241–246

Udezue E, Herrera E (2007) Pain management in adult acute sickle cell pain crisis: a viewpoint. West Afr J Med 26(3):179–182

UK National Health Service (NHS) (2010) Sickle cell disease in childhood. Standards and guidelines for clinical care, 2nd edn. London. ISBN:0-9554319-7-2

van Beers EJ, van Tuijn CF, Nieuwkerk PT et al (2007) Patient-controlled analgesia versus continuous infusion of morphine during vaso-occlusive crisis in sickle cell disease, a randomized controlled trial. Am J Hematol 82(11):955–960

Vichinsky E, Hurst D, Earles A, Kleman K, Lubin B (1988) Newborn screening for sickle cell disease: effect on mortality. Pediatrics 81(6):749–755

Vichinsky EP, Haberkern CM, Neumayr L et al (1995) A comparison of conservative and aggressive transfusion regimens in the perioperative management of sickle cell disease. The Preoperative Transfusion in Sickle Cell Disease Study Group. N Engl J Med 333(4):206–213

Vichinsky EP, Neumayr LD, Earles AN et al (2000) Causes and outcomes of the acute chest syndrome in sickle cell disease. National Acute Chest Syndrome Study Group. N Engl J Med 342(25):1855–1865

Vichinsky E, Onyekwere O, Porter J et al (2007) A randomised comparison of deferasirox versus deferoxamine for the treatment of transfusional iron overload in sickle cell disease. Br J Haematol 136(3):501–508

Voskaridou E, Christoulas D, Bilalis A et al (2010) The effect of prolonged administration of hydroxyurea on morbidity and mortality in adult patients with sickle cell syndromes: results of a 17-year, single-center trial (LaSHS). Blood 115(12):2354–2363

Walters MC (2005) Stem cell therapy for sickle cell disease: transplantation and gene therapy. Hematology Am Soc Hematol Educ Program 66–73

Wang WC, Dwan K (2013) Blood transfusion for preventing primary and secondary stroke in people with sickle cell disease. Cochrane Database Syst Rev 11:CD003146

Wang WC, Ware RE, Miller ST et al (2011) Hydroxycarbamide in very young children with sickle-cell anaemia: a multicentre, randomised, controlled trial (BABY HUG). Lancet 377(9778):1663–1672

Ware RE (2010) How I use hydroxyurea to treat young patients with sickle cell anemia. Blood 115(26):5300–5311

Ware RE, Rees RC, Sarnaik SA et al (2010) Renal function in infants with sickle cell anemia: baseline data from the BABY HUG trial. J Pediatr 156(1):66–70 e61

Ware RE, Helms RW, Investigators SW (2012) Stroke with transfusions changing to hydroxyurea (SWiTCH). Blood 119(17):3925–3932

Wethers DL, Ramirez GM, Koshy M et al (1994) Accelerated healing of chronic sickle-cell leg ulcers treated with RGD peptide matrix. RGD Study Group. Blood 84(6):1775–1779

Wilimas JA, Flynn PM, Harris S et al (1993) A randomized study of outpatient treatment with ceftriaxone for selected febrile children with sickle cell disease. N Engl J Med 329(7):472–476

Williamson TH, Rajput R, Laidlaw DA, Mokete B (2009) Vitreoretinal management of the complications of sickle cell retinopathy by observation or pars plana vitrectomy. Eye (Lond) 23(6):1314–1320

Working Party of the British Committee for Standards in Haematology Clinical Haematology Task F (1996) Guidelines for the prevention and treatment of infection in patients with an absent or dysfunctional spleen. BMJ 312(7028):430–434

Wright J (2004) Acute chest syndrome in sickle cell disease. In: Okpala IE (ed) Practical management of haemoglobinopathies. Blackwell Publishing, Oxford, pp 88–98

Wright J, Ahmedzai SH (2010) The management of painful crisis in sickle cell disease. Curr Opin Support Palliat Care 4(2):97–106

Yang YM, Shah AK, Watson M, Mankad VN (1995) Comparison of costs to the health sector of comprehensive and episodic health care for sickle cell disease patients. Public Health Rep 110(1):80–86

Yusuf HR, Atrash HK, Grosse SD, Parker CS, Grant AM (2010) Emergency department visits made by patients with sickle cell disease: a descriptive study, 1999-2007. Am J Prev Med 38(4 Suppl):S536–S541

Zimmerman SA, Schultz WH, Davis JS et al (2004) Sustained long-term hematologic efficacy of hydroxyurea at maximum tolerated dose in children with sickle cell disease. Blood 103(6): 2039–2045

Chapter 11
Priapism in Sickle Cell Disease: New Aspects of Pathophysiology

Mário A. Claudino, Carla F. Franco Penteado, and Kleber Yotsumoto Fertrin

Abstract Priapism is a prolonged, persistent, and painful penile erection unassociated with sexual interest or stimulation, which affects a large percentage of male sickle cell disease (SCD) patients. It manifests either as an acute, severe event, or as recurrent, stuttering priapism, with very limited therapeutic options. Untreated priapism can cause irreversible erectile dysfunction and surgical treatment remains the only option for severe cases. The mechanisms that contribute to the development of sickle cell disease-associated priapism are not fully understood, precluding efficacious pharmacological approaches. In this chapter, we review the physiology of penile erection, definitions of priapism, and summarize current knowledge of the pathophysiology underlying SCD-associated priapism. We discuss current and future possible therapeutic interventions, with emphasis on dysregulated signaling pathways that contribute to the development of this complication, such as the nitric oxide/cyclic guanosine monophosphate system and the RhoA/ROCK system, as well as the role of adenosine, opiorphins, and androgens in the pathogenesis of priapism.

Keywords Adenosine • Nitric oxide • Opiorphin • Priapism

M.A. Claudino, Ph.D. (✉)
Laboratory of Multidisciplinary Research, São Francisco University – USF,
Avenida São Francisco de Assis, 218, JD. São Jose, Braganca Paulista,
CEP 12916-900, São Paulo, Brazil
e-mail: mario.claudino@usf.edu.br

C.F. Franco Penteado, Ph.D. • K.Y. Fertrin, M.D., Ph.D.
Hematology Center, School of Medical Sciences, University of Campinas – UNICAMP,
Hemocentro, Rua Carlos Chagas 480, Campinas, São Paulo, CEP 13083-878, Brazil
e-mail: cffp@unicamp.br; fertrin@unicamp.br; kleberfertrin@gmail.com

© Springer International Publishing Switzerland 2016

F.F. Costa, N. Conran (eds.), *Sickle Cell Anemia*,
DOI 10.1007/978-3-319-06713-1_11

11.1 Introduction

Priapism is a pathologic condition consisting of a prolonged and persistent penile erection, unassociated with sexual interest or stimulation (Montague et al. 2003). This condition was first reported as being associated with sickle cell disease (SCD) in 1934 (Diggs and Ching 1934) and has been related by approximately 3.6–6.4 % of male children and adolescent patients (Tarry et al. 1987; Furtado et al. 2012) and by 20–89 % of adult male SCD patients (Adeyoju et al. 2002; Broderick et al. 2010; Lionnet et al. 2012). The rate of resulting erectile dysfunction (ED) may exceed 30 % (Bivalacqua and Burnett 2006; Claudino and Fertrin 2012). According to the American Urological Association Guidelines on the Management of Priapism and the European Association of Urology Guidelines on Priapism, priapism can be subdivided into three categories; ischemic (veno-occlusive, low flow), nonischemic (arterial, high flow) and stuttering (acute, intermittent).

Ischemic priapism is the most common forms of priapism, accounting for approximately 95 % of all priapic episodes, and is characterized by a painful and rigid penile erection. SCD is the primary cause of ischemic priapism in 23 % of adults, and 63 % of children (Salonia et al. 2014). Ischemic priapism beyond 4 h constitutes a compartment syndrome of the penis, resulting from a persistent erection, marked by rigidity of the corpora cavernosa (CC) and little or no cavernous arterial inflow. Penile sinusoids are regions prone to red blood cell sickling in men with SCD, due to blood stasis and slow flow rates; ischemic priapism is thought to result from the prolonged blockage of venous outflow by the vaso-occlusive process. This veno-occlusive episode requires emergency urological intervention to minimize potential irreversible consequences, such as corporal fibrosis and permanent erectile dysfunction (Spycher and Hauri 1986; El-Bahnasawy et al. 2002; Bivalacqua and Burnett 2006). In ischemic priapism, time-dependent changes occur in the corporal metabolic environment with progressive hypoxia, hypercapnia, and acidosis that typically generate penile pain (Muneer et al. 2008). The duration of priapism represents the most significant predictor of the maintenance of premorbid erectile function. Histologically, between 12 and 24 h after priapism ensues, corporal specimens show interstitial edema, progressive destruction of sinusoidal endothelium, exposure of the basal membrane, and platelet adhesion. After 48 h, thrombi are observed in the sinusoidal spaces, and fibroblast-like cell transformation takes place, along with smooth muscle necrosis. Thus, while interventions beyond 48–72 h after onset may eventually help relieve erection and pain, they have little benefit in preserving erectile function (El-Bahnasawy et al. 2002; Salonia et al. 2014). Studies show that 21–59 % of male SCD patients have experienced low-flow priapism for 24–48 h with impairment to erectile mechanisms, resulting in the development of erectile dysfunction (El-Bahnasawy et al. 2002; Adeyoju et al. 2002; Broderick 2012).

Non-ischemic priapism (arterial, high flow) is a persistent erection caused by unregulated cavernous arterial inflow. Typically, the corpora are tumescent but not fully rigid and not associated with pain (Broderick et al. 2010). High flow priapism is caused by trauma, and has not been associated with increased risk in SCD patients (Crane and Bennett 2011), or with the development of erectile dysfunction (Salonia et al. 2014).

Stuttering or recurrent ischemic priapism (acute, intermittent ischemic priapism) is a distinct condition characterized by recurrent painful penile erection, with complete detumescence between episodes (Salonia et al. 2014; Muneer et al. 2008). Stuttering priapic episodes are frequently self-limiting, but frequency and/or duration of these distressing priapic episodes may increase, and a single episode can sometimes develop into a major ischemic priapic event (Claudino and Fertrin 2012; Salonia et al. 2014). SCD is the most common cause of stuttering priapism and reaches a prevalence of 42–64 %. Of this group of patients, 89 % report their first priapic episode by the age of 20 years (Fowler et al. 1991; Mantadakis et al. 1999; Adeyoju et al. 2002). Recurrent episodes are usually nocturnal and may be triggered by sexual activities, which may suppress sexual desire for fear of episodes (Chow and Payne 2008). The underlying mechanism is similar to that of other types of ischemic priapism (Salonia et al. 2014), occurring due to a deficiency of endothelial nitric oxide in the penis, leading to downregulation of the phosphodiesterase type 5 (PDE5) enzyme (Champion et al. 2005), and causing alterations in the functioning of the control system of the corporal smooth muscle tone. Hence, responses to any sexual or nonsexual stimulus (such as that occurring during rapid eye movement sleep) can induce a prolonged erectile episode (Salonia et al. 2014). In addition, patients with short-lived intermittent priapic attacks are still at risk of erectile dysfunction (Adeyoju et al. 2002). Anele and Burnett (2015) showed that erectile dysfunction is associated with recurrent ischemic priapism, occurring in nearly 40 % of affected individuals overall. SCD patients with stuttering priapism are nearly five times more likely to develop erectile dysfunction, compared with those having stuttering priapism, when associated with non-SCD etiologies. Moreover, the frequency of episodes and minor episode durations (≤ 2 h) also seem to be associated with the development of erectile dysfunction in SCD patients (Anele and Burnett 2015).

Basic science investigations have focused on defining abnormalities in the penile tissue at the molecular level, which may reflect on the end-stage consequences of priapism. SCD-associated priapism involves dysfunction of the nitric oxide (NO) signaling pathway, increased oxidative stress, adenosine overproduction, alterations in the Rho A/Rho-kinase system, androgens and opiorphins.

11.2 Physiology of Normal Erectile Function

Penile erection is a hemodynamic biological phenomenon involving increased penile arterial inflow and reduced venous outflow from the penis. It is regulated by the smooth muscle tone of the CC and associated arterioles during sexual stimulation, along with afferences of neuronal, endocrine, and paracrine origin, determining the functional status of the penis (Giuliano 2011). Penile flaccidity (detumescent state) is mainly maintained by tonic release of norepinephrine through the sympathetic innervations of vascular and cavernosal smooth muscle cells. During penile erection (tumescent state), vascular smooth muscle relaxation decreases vascular resistance, thereby increasing blood flow through cavernous and helicine arteries and filling sinusoids, which are expanded due to the relaxation of smooth muscle cells in the CC (Andersson 2001b).

Physiological relaxation of penile smooth muscle is mainly, although not exclusively, mediated by the NO/cyclic guanosine monophosphate (cGMP) signaling pathway. NO is a gaseous molecule that is synthesized from its precursor amino acid, L-arginine, under the catalytic function of the NO synthases (NOSs). NOSs are subdivided into three isoforms, endothelial NOS (eNOS or NOS3), neuronal NOS (nNOS or NOS1), and inducible NOS (iNOS or NOS2) (Förstermann and Sessa 2012). In the penile smooth muscle, NO is released from both penile nitrergic nerves (nNOS enzyme) upon sexual stimulation, and the sinusoidal endothelium (eNOS enzyme) (Burnett 2004). Increased blood flow activates endothelial PI3-kinase to stimulate Akt, phosphorylate and activate eNOS, and provide persistent NO production for sustained penile erection (Hurt et al. 2002; Burnett 2004). Moreover, neuronal stimulation increases cAMP to activate PKA, which phosphorylates and stimulates nNOS catalytic activity, in turn increasing NO production (Hurt et al. 2012). NO release stimulates the soluble guanylyl cyclase (sGC) enzyme in the cavernosal smooth muscle, triggering increased synthesis of cGMP, which activates cGMP-specific protein kinase I (cGK I), providing the main signal for smooth muscle relaxation (Lucas et al. 2000). cGMP levels in the CC are regulated by the rate of cGMP synthesis by sGC and the rate of cGMP hydrolysis by phosphodiesterase type 5 (PDE5) (Gopal et al. 2001). In addition, PDE5 regulation (i.e., inhibition) then serves to control (i.e., promote) corporal smooth muscle relaxation (Corbin 2004).

Similarly to NO, adenosine is a potent vasodilator produced by adenine nucleotide degradation. Adenosine is predominantly generated by adenosine monophosphate (AMP) dephosphorylation, catalyzed by intracellular 5′-nucleotidase. Hydrolysis of s-adenosyl-homocysteine also contributes to the intracellular pool of adenosine (Phatarpekar et al. 2010). Extracellular adenosine may be generated by both adenine nucleotide degradation and dephosphorylation by ectonucleotidases (Colgan et al. 2006). Two enzymes then catabolize adenosine; adenosine kinase (ADK), which phosphorylates adenosine to AMP and is an important regulator of intracellular adenosine levels; and adenosine deaminase (ADA), which catalyzes the irreversible conversion of adenosine to inosine (Phatarpekar et al. 2010). Adenosine-induced vasodilation is mediated by increasing intracellular cyclic adenosine monophosphate (cAMP) levels in vascular smooth muscle cells via A2 receptor signaling (Olsson and Pearson 1990; Tager et al. 2008). cAMP activates protein kinase A (PKA), resulting in decreased calcium calmodulin-dependent MLC phosphorylation and enhanced smooth muscle relaxation (Lin et al. 2005). Its role in penile erection has been investigated in studies showing that intracavernous injection of adenosine results in tumescence and penile erection (Mi et al. 2008; Tostes et al. 2007; Prieto 2008). In addition, adenosine induces NO synthesis in endothelial cells through A2 receptor signaling, and adenosine-mediated CC relaxation is partially dependent on endothelium-derived NO (Faria et al. 2006; Mi et al. 2008; Wen et al. 2010; Sobrevia and Mann 1997).

Although the penile vascular endothelium and smooth muscle cells are sources of vasodilators such as NO and adenosine, vasoconstriction pathways are also important for penile hemodynamics. Penile vessels and cavernosal tissue receive rich adrenergic innervation that maintains the penis in the flaccid state, mainly via a tonic activity of these nerves. Hence, in the absence of an active NO/cGMP pathway, the cavernosal smooth muscle remains in the contracted state, possibly mediated by the effects of norepinephrine released from sympathetic nerves (Cellek 2000; Andersson 2001a). In addition to the well-established noradrenergic contraction mechanisms in the penis, the Rho A/Rho-kinase (ROCK) signal transduction pathway also controls erectile function by regulating smooth muscle tone through the modulation of the sensitivity of contractile proteins to Ca^{2+} (Linder et al. 2005; Musicki et al. 2009; Priviero et al. 2010). RhoA regulates smooth muscle contraction by cycling between a GDP-bound inactive form (coupled to a guanine dissociation inhibitor, RhoGDI) and a GTP-bound active form (Wettschureck and Offermanns 2002; Riento and Ridley 2003). Upstream activation of heterotrimeric G proteins leads to the exchange of GDP for GTP, an event carried out by the guanine exchange factors (GEFs) p115RhoGEF, PDZRhoGEF, and LARG (Leukemia-associated RhoGEF). These factors are able to transduce signals from G protein coupled receptors to RhoA (Riento and Ridley 2003). ROCK is activated by Rho A, which phosphorylates the regulatory subunit (MYPT1) of myosin light chain (MLC) phosphatase, causing inhibition of its phosphatase activity and enhancing the contractile response at a constant intracellular calcium concentration (Somlyo and Somlyo 2003; Webb 2003). The RhoA/ROCK Ca2+ sensitization pathway has been implicated in the regulation of penile smooth muscle contraction and tone both in animal models and in humans (Mills et al. 2003; Rees et al. 2002; Wang et al. 2002). ROCK is also involved in the modulation of calcium entry, induced by α1-adrenoceptor stimulation of the penile arteries (Villalba et al. 2007, 2008). Application of a vasoconstrictor agent combination of endothelin-1 and phenylephrine augments constrictor responses in CC tissue by a mechanism involving Rho A/ROCK (Filippi et al. 2003). Thus, several studies have shown that the RhoA/ROCK pathway is important for maintaining penile flaccidity (Mills et al. 2003; Bivalacqua et al. 2004; Linder et al. 2005; Priviero et al. 2010). The NO/cGMP system regulates the transcription of the gene encoding RhoA in corporal smooth muscle. In turn, cGK I inhibits the contractile system by phosphorylating RhoA and possibly other effectors of RhoA/ROCK signaling (Burnett and Musicki 2005; Priviero et al. 2010).

Penile erection regulation is also mediated by both pro-erectile and anti-erectile factors that are released locally or centrally by the brain and the spinal cord. Multiple regulatory systems/agents, such as purines (e.g., adenosine), peptides (e.g., opiorphins), and other gaseous molecules (e.g., carbon monoxide, hydrogen sulfide) are described as pro-erectile local factors (Srilatha et al. 2007; Liaw et al. 2011). Anti-erectile factors include norepinephrine, neuropeptide Y, and endothelin-1 (Bivalacqua et al. 2012). Androgens also serve a major modulatory role in the biology of penile erection and operate at both central and peripheral levels (Traish et al. 2011).

11.3 Nitric Oxide/cGMP and SCD Priapism

The NO/cGMP system is well-known to play a crucial role in the penile erection process and in the homeostasis of the penis; thus, it is paradoxical that chronically-impaired NO bioavailability accounts for priapism in SCD (Kato et al. 2007). Although the pathogenesis of SCD-associated priapism has not been completely elucidated, it has been suggested that hemolysis and oxidative stress in SCD contribute to a reduction in NO bioavailability in the erectile tissue, skewing the normal balance of smooth muscle tone towards vasoconstriction (Anele et al. 2015).

Due to the difficulty in exploring these mechanisms in patients, the use of animal models of priapism has become of extreme importance to decipher this devastating clinical challenge. In eNOS-deficient mice, electrical field stimulation promotes an increase in CC relaxation responses (mediated by a reduction in NO bioavailability). This suggests that the increased sensitivity of the cavernosal smooth muscle to nNOS-derived NO may be an important compensatory mechanism in eNOS-deficient mice, particularly since the cavernous nerves likely initiate the erectile process (Hurt et al. 2002). In addition, a study found similar results in CC for eNOS- or nNOS-deficient mice (both characterized by a reduction in NO bioavailability), where sodium nitroprusside (a NO donor) induced an enhanced relaxing response. These authors suggested a compensatory mechanism for eNOS-derived NO release in nNOS-deficient mice and nNOS-derived NO release in eNOS-deficient mice, inducing retained erectile function in these animals (Nangle et al. 2004). A subsequent study showed that the priapic phenotype exhibited by NOS-deficient mice and SCD transgenic mice is associated with downregulation of PDE5 expression and activity (Champion et al. 2005). SCD transgenic mice also present spontaneous priapism, an amplified CC relaxation response (mediated by the NO/cGMP signaling pathway), and increased intracavernosal pressure in vivo (Claudino et al. 2009; Bivalacqua et al. 2009), implying that the NO/cGMP pathway may indeed constitute a potential therapeutic target to treat priapism in SCD individuals.

11.4 Oxidative Stress and SCD Priapism

Oxidative stress is a major component of the pathophysiology of ischemic priapism as it affects the NO/cGMP system in the penis and reduces NO bioavailability. NO bioavailability is reduced by functional uncoupling of eNOS, characterized by the diversion of electron transfer within the enzyme from L-arginine oxidation.

This molecular event reduces molecular oxygen to superoxide, instead of producing NO (Kietadisorn et al. 2012). Thus, the uncoupled eNOS fails to produce NO and increases reactive oxygen species (ROS) formation, as can be observed in SCD-associated vasculopathy (Hsu et al. 2007; Kanika et al. 2010; Musicki et al. 2012).

The enzymes xanthine oxidase, NADPH oxidase, and uncoupled eNOS are all major sources of ROS (Wood et al. 2005, 2006). In the penises of SCD mice, oxidative stress increases due to eNOS uncoupling and upregulation of NADPH oxidase subunits $p67^{phox}$, $p47^{phox}$, and $gp91^{phox}$ (Musicki et al. 2012; Lagoda et al. 2013; Bivalacqua et al. 2013). Uncoupled eNOS and low NO bioavailability in both mice (Champion et al. 2005; Musicki et al. 2012, 2014; Bivalacqua et al. 2013) and humans with SCD (Lagoda et al. 2013) are associated with PDE5 downregulation. Resulting cGMP accumulation, upon neurostimulation, promotes an intense smooth muscle relaxation (Claudino et al. 2009) and priapism. More recently, long-term treatment with sildenafil was able to reverse both the nitrosative stress effect, oxidative stress generated by NADPH oxidase, and eNOS uncoupling in the penis of SCD mice, restoring endothelial NO synthesis, supporting the hypothesis that an "NO imbalance" in the penis is the molecular pathogenic basis for SCD-associated priapism (Bivalacqua et al. 2013; Musicki et al. 2014).

11.5 Rho A/ROCK and SCD Priapism

The Rho A/ROCK system exerts vasoconstriction of the penile vasculature via smooth muscle contraction effects due to the Ca^{2+}-independent promotion of myosin light chain (MLC) kinase or the attenuation of MLC phosphatase activity, and consequent reduction in endothelial-derived NO production (Linder et al. 2005; Musicki et al. 2009; Priviero et al. 2010). Two isoforms of ROCK are known, ROCK1 (ROK b) and ROCK2 (Rho-kinase or ROK a), and both are important for maintaining the penis in a flaccid state (Mills et al. 2003; Gratzke et al. 2010). Rho A activation, ROCK protein expression, and total ROCK activity, decline in the penile tissue of SCD transgenic mice, indicating that the molecular mechanism of priapism in SCD is associated with decreased vasoconstrictor activity in the penis (Bivalacqua et al. 2010). eNOS activity and endothelial NO levels directly influence ROCK activity to maintain the homeostasis of the penile vasculature, according to a feedback control mechanism. The eNOS-deleted mouse presents phenotypic in vivo evidence of priapism, similar to that seen in transgenic SCD mice. In this model, despite normal ROCK2 expression, its activity is reduced and can be rescued with eNOS gene transfer (Bivalacqua et al. 2007). ROCK2 protein expression is also reduced in the penis of the transgenic SCD mouse, along with reductions in RhoA GTPase and ROCK activities (Bivalacqua et al. 2010), which may contribute similarly to reduced NO bioavailability and the pathogenesis of priapism in SCD.

11.6 Adenosine and SCD Priapism

Adenosine is a potent vasodilator and is involved in normal and abnormal penile erection (Lue 2000; Andersson 2001a). The contribution of adenosine to the pathophysiology of priapism was first suggested after the observation that adenosine deaminase (ADA)-deficient mice display priapism. ADA is an enzyme of the purine metabolism that catalyses irreversible deamination of adenosine to inosine and its deficiency results in excess adenosine in the penile tissue (Mi et al. 2008). SCD transgenic mice also have higher levels of adenosine in whole blood and penile tissues (Mi et al. 2008; Zhang et al. 2011). Adenosine accumulation and PDE5 down-regulation were observed in cavernous smooth muscle cells under ischemic and hypoxic conditions (Lin et al. 2003). Adenosine mediated hypoxia-inducible factor 1 (HIF-1) induction and reduced PDE5 gene transcription via A2B receptor activation increases cGMP, leading to priapism in SCD mice (Ning et al. 2014). Moreover, both SCD transgenic mice and ADA-deficient mice present penile fibrosis, a late complication of priapism (Wen et al. 2010).

PEG-ADA enzyme therapy regulates adenosine levels, reduces increased cavernosal relaxation and prevents priapic events in both ADA-deficient and SCD transgenic mice. It also attenuates penile vascular damage and fibrosis and its effect is associated with reduced adenosine levels (Wen et al. 2010). Importantly, PEG-ADA therapy has long been used in humans as a life-saving therapy to treat ADA-deficient individuals (Hershfield 1995). Therefore, excess of adenosine contributes to the pathophysiology of priapism and this pathway is a potential therapeutic target for the treatment SCD priapism.

11.7 Opiorphins and SCD Priapism

Opiorphins are a class of peptides expressed in the penis that influence cavernosal tissue function (Davies 2009). This pentapeptide family has been described as a group of potent endogenous neutral endopeptidase (NEP) inhibitors, which act in the metabolism of multiple signaling peptides. Inhibition of NEP in the corporal smooth muscle leads to increased relaxation in response to peptide agonists (Wisner et al. 2006). In an experimental priapism model, opiorphins affect peptide signaling, mediated through the G protein-coupled receptor (GPCR) (Tong et al. 2008), whose activity affects intracellular levels of cAMP and cGMP, both involved in penile erection. Opiorphins also activate genes of mediators of the ornithine decarboxylase (ODC) pathway and the NOS/cGMP system, and can regulate HIF-1a and A2Br expression (Kanika et al. 2009). The administration of the ODC inhibitor, 1,3 diaminopropane, prevents the opiorphin-induced priapic state. Rats treated with plasmids encoding opiorphins display reduced cavernosal tissue PDE5 and eNOS expressions (Morrison and Burnett 2012). Additionally, transgenic SCD mice present up-regulation of mice opiorphin homologue genes in corporal tissue prior to any detectable indication of priapism (Kanika et al. 2009). Opiorphin up-regulation in response to SCD-associated hypoxia activates relaxant pathways in the smooth muscle and may increase blood flow, resulting in priapism. Interestingly, opiorphins can be measured in the bloodstream and saliva of patients and determining levels of this peptide in blood from SCD patients could be useful in the identification of patients at risk for priapism crisis (Fu et al. 2014).

11.8 Androgens and SCD Priapism

Androgens are involved in erectile physiology through the release of stimulatory neurotransmitters, such as dopamine, oxytocin, and nitric oxide (NO) in humans and animals (Traish and Kim 2005). These hormones control erectile function by affecting the release of pro-erectile and anti-erectile mediators (Isidori et al. 2014). The NO/cGMP system is controlled at different levels by androgens; NOS isoform expression in the CC is regulated by androgens in various animal species (Reilly et al. 1997; Morelli et al. 2004; Traish et al. 2007). In animal models of androgen deficiency, reduced PDE5 expression was restored by testosterone supplementation (Traish et al. 1999).

SCD patients present low levels of androgens (testosterone and dihydrotestosterone) (Osegbe and Akinyanju 1987; Parshad et al. 1994). Evidence suggests an association of priapism risk and testosterone levels. Clinical reports relate the development of priapism in two adolescents with SCD, about 1 week after receiving an intramuscular injection of testosterone enanthate (Slayton et al. 1995). However, testosterone replacement has been shown to improve sexual function without inducing priapism in hypogonadal men with SCD (Morrison et al. 2013). More recently, a study found no association between low testosterone levels and priapism risk in SCD patients, since only 25 % of SCD patients with a history of priapism had testosterone deficiency (Morrison et al. 2015).

Transgenic SCD mice have low systemic testosterone levels, and testosterone administration partially corrected the priapism phenotype (Morrison and Burnett 2012), suggesting that low testosterone levels could contribute to the development of priapism by affecting the NO/cGMP signaling pathway. Moreover, testosterone can also prevent priapism by regulating factors involved in the control of opiorphins (Chua et al. 2009). Furthermore, treatment with ketoconazole and prednisone prevented recurrent ischemic priapism by reducing testosterone levels, possibly through decreased opiorphin expression (Abern and Levine 2009). Further studies to clarify whether testosterone deficiency induces episodes of priapism and if testosterone replacement therapy may be indicated in SCD are needed.

11.9 Conclusions

Preventative and curative strategies for priapism must ideally address the pathophysiologic basis of this disorder. This may only be possible with a clear understanding of the pathogenesis of priapism in order to develop new therapeutic modalities targeting disease-specific molecular mechanisms. The NO-cGMP

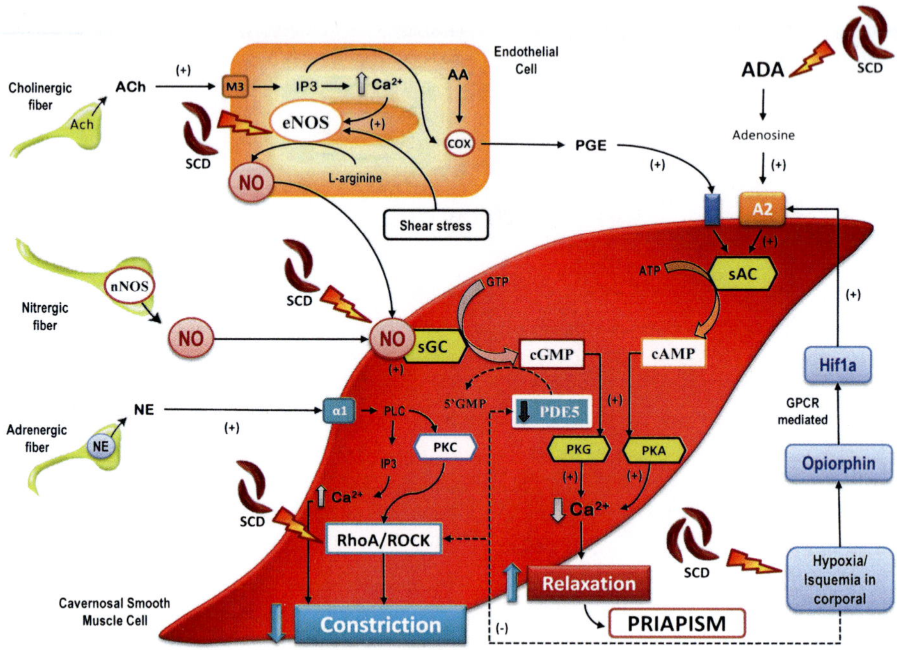

Fig. 11.1 Pathophysiological mechanisms involved in sickle cell disease (SCD)-associated priapism. The interaction of neuronal fibers, endothelial cells, and cavernosal smooth muscle cells in the penis is disturbed by SCD. Hemolysis causes uncoupling of nitric oxide synthase (eNOS), reducing endothelial NO production. Cholinergic stimulation contributes to the production of prostaglandin E2 (PGE2) by cyclo-oxygenase (COX). Hemolysis also releases ATP, which is converted to adenosine, a potent vasodilator. It activates its receptor A2B in smooth muscle cells linked to the soluble adenylate cyclase/cAMP/PKA pathway, resulting in decreased intracellular calcium and muscle relaxation. Vaso-occlusion and ischemia in corpora cavernosa stimulates the expression of adenosine A2B receptor via opiorphins, GPCR, and HIF1a. Free hemoglobin in SCD binds NO, and chronic low NO bioavailability causes PDE5 down-regulation, reducing cGMP hydrolysis and activating PKG, also lowering intracellular calcium. SCD affects the Rho A/ROCK system, interfering with norepinephrine-estimulated vasoconstrictor activity in penile tissue, favoring uncontrolled penile erection. These intracellular mechanisms may act alone or together to cause priapism associated with SCD

signaling pathway has been particularly explored as a means to target priapism treatment. While there are reports showing a potential role of hydroxyurea treatment in preventing recurrent priapism in SCD patients and in restoring erectile function loss subsequent to a very prolonged episode (Anele et al. 2015), most patients do not respond to this treatment modality. PDE5 inhibitors such as sildenafil and tadalafil have emerged as promising options, but results so far have not yet been convincing. Therefore, novel options are still needed, and there is potential for drugs interfering with other pathways involving adenosine, opiorphins, androgens and the RhoA/ROCK system (Fig. 11.1). Finally, it is also possible that priapism may be treatable with other therapeutic strategies, not specifically designed for priapism, which are currently under investigation, such as adhesion molecule adhesion inhibitors (rivipansel, formerly GMI-1070 and SelG21, an anti-P-selectin) and direct modulators of hemoglobin oxygen affinity, such as 5-hydroxymethylfurfural.

References

Abern MR, Levine LA (2009) Ketoconazole and prednisone to prevent recurrent ischemic priapism. J Urol 182(4):1401–1406

Adeyoju AB, Olujohungbe AB, Morris J et al (2002) Priapism in sickle-cell disease; incidence, risk factors and complications – an international multicentre study. BJU Int 90(9):898–902

Andersson KE (2001a) Pharmacology of erectile function and dysfunction. Urol Clin North Am 28(2):233–247

Andersson KE (2001b) Pharmacology of penile erection. Pharmacol Rev 53(3):417–450

Anele UA, Burnett AL (2015) Erectile dysfunction after sickle cell disease-associated recurrent ischemic priapism: profile and risk factors. J Sex Med 12(3):713–719

Anele UA, Morrison BF, Burnett AL (2015) Molecular pathophysiology of priapism: emerging targets. Curr Drug Targets 16:474–483

Bivalacqua TJ, Burnett AL (2006) Priapism: new concepts in the pathophysiology and new treatment strategies. Curr Urol Rep 7(6):497–502

Bivalacqua TJ, Champion HC, Usta MF et al (2004) RhoA/Rho-kinase suppresses endothelial nitric oxide synthase in the penis: a mechanism for diabetes-associated erectile dysfunction. Proc Natl Acad Sci U S A 101(24):9121–9126

Bivalacqua TJ, Liu T, Musicki B, Champion HC, Burnett AL (2007) Endothelial nitric oxide synthase keeps erection regulatory function balance in the penis. Eur Urol 51(6):1732–1740

Bivalacqua TJ, Musicki B, Hsu LL et al (2009) Establishment of a transgenic sickle-cell mouse model to study the pathophysiology of priapism. J Sex Med 6(9):2494–2504

Bivalacqua TJ, Ross AE, Strong TD et al (2010) Attenuated RhoA/Rho-kinase signaling in penis of transgenic sickle cell mice. Urology 76(2):510.e517–e512

Bivalacqua TJ, Musicki B, Kutlu O, Burnett AL (2012) New insights into the pathophysiology of sickle cell disease-associated priapism. J Sex Med 9(1):79–87

Bivalacqua TJ, Musicki B, Hsu LL et al (2013) Sildenafil citrate-restored eNOS and PDE5 regulation in sickle cell mouse penis prevents priapism via control of oxidative/nitrosative stress. PLoS One 8(7), e68028

Broderick GA (2012) Priapism and sickle-cell anemia: diagnosis and nonsurgical therapy. J Sex Med 9(1):88–103

Broderick GA, Kadioglu A, Bivalacqua TJ et al (2010) Priapism: pathogenesis, epidemiology, and management. J Sex Med 7(1 Pt 2):476–500

Burnett AL (2004) Novel nitric oxide signaling mechanisms regulate the erectile response. Int J Impot Res 16(Suppl 1):S15–S19

Burnett AL, Musicki B (2005) The nitric oxide signaling pathway in the penis. Curr Pharm Des 11(31):3987–3994

Cellek S (2000) Nitrergic-noradrenergic interaction in penile erection: a new insight into erectile dysfunction. Drugs Today (Barc) 36(2–3):135–146

Champion HC, Bivalacqua TJ, Takimoto E, Kass DA, Burnett AL (2005) Phosphodiesterase-5A dysregulation in penile erectile tissue is a mechanism of priapism. Proc Natl Acad Sci U S A 102(5):1661–1666

Chow K, Payne S (2008) The pharmacological management of intermittent priapismic states. BJU Int 102(11):1515–1521

Chua RG, Calenda G, Zhang X et al (2009) Testosterone regulates erectile function and Vcsa1 expression in the corpora of rats. Mol Cell Endocrinol 303(1-2):67–73

Claudino MA, Fertrin KY (2012) Sickling cells, cyclic nucleotides, and protein kinases: the pathophysiology of urogenital disorders in sickle cell anemia. Anemia 2012:723520

Claudino MA, Franco-Penteado CF, Corat MA et al (2009) Increased cavernosal relaxations in sickle cell mice priapism are associated with alterations in the NO-cGMP signaling pathway. J Sex Med 6(8):2187–2196

Colgan SP, Eltzschig HK, Eckle T, Thompson LF (2006) Physiological roles for ecto-5'-nucleotidase (CD73). Purinergic Signal 2(2):351–360

Corbin JD (2004) Mechanisms of action of PDE5 inhibition in erectile dysfunction. Int J Impot Res 16(Suppl 1):S4–S7

Crane GM, Bennett NE (2011) Priapism in sickle cell anemia: emerging mechanistic understanding and better preventative strategies. Anemia 2011, 297364

Davies KP (2009) The role of opiorphins (endogenous neutral endopeptidase inhibitors) in urogenital smooth muscle biology. J Sex Med 6(Suppl 3):286–291

Diggs LW, Ching RE (1934) Pathology of sickle cell anemia. Southern Med J 27:839–845

El-Bahnasawy MS, Dawood A, Farouk A (2002) Low-flow priapism: risk factors for erectile dysfunction. BJU Int 89(3):285–290

Faria M, Magalhães-Cardoso T, Lafuente-de-Carvalho JM, Correia-de-Sá P (2006) Corpus cavernosum from men with vasculogenic impotence is partially resistant to adenosine relaxation due to endothelial A(2B) receptor dysfunction. J Pharmacol Exp Ther 319(1):405–413

Filippi S, Marini M, Vannelli GB et al (2003) Effects of hypoxia on endothelin-1 sensitivity in the corpus cavernosum. Mol Hum Reprod 9(12):765–774

Förstermann U, Sessa WC (2012) Nitric oxide synthases: regulation and function. Eur Heart J 33(7):829–837, 837a–837d

Fowler JE, Koshy M, Strub M, Chinn SK (1991) Priapism associated with the sickle cell hemoglobinopathies: prevalence, natural history and sequelae. J Urol 145(1):65–68

Fu S, Tar MT, Melman A, Davies KP (2014) Opiorphin is a master regulator of the hypoxic response in corporal smooth muscle cells. FASEB J 28(8):3633–3644

Furtado PS, Costa MP, Ribeiro do Prado Valladares F et al (2012) The prevalence of priapism in children and adolescents with sickle cell disease in Brazil. Int J Hematol 95(6):648–651

Giuliano F (2011) Neurophysiology of erection and ejaculation. J Sex Med 8(Suppl 4):310–315

Gopal VK, Francis SH, Corbin JD (2001) Allosteric sites of phosphodiesterase-5 (PDE5). A potential role in negative feedback regulation of cGMP signaling in corpus cavernosum. Eur J Biochem 268(11):3304–3312

Gratzke C, Strong TD, Gebska MA et al (2010) Activated RhoA/Rho kinase impairs erectile function after cavernous nerve injury in rats. J Urol 184(5):2197–2204

Hershfield MS (1995) PEG-ADA replacement therapy for adenosine deaminase deficiency: an update after 8.5 years. Clin Immunol Immunopathol 76(3 Pt 2):S228–S232

Hsu LL, Champion HC, Campbell-Lee SA et al (2007) Hemolysis in sickle cell mice causes pulmonary hypertension due to global impairment in nitric oxide bioavailability. Blood 109(7): 3088–3098

Hurt KJ, Musicki B, Palese MA et al (2002) Akt-dependent phosphorylation of endothelial nitric-oxide synthase mediates penile erection. Proc Natl Acad Sci U S A 99(6):4061–4066

Hurt KJ, Sezen SF, Lagoda GF et al (2012) Cyclic AMP-dependent phosphorylation of neuronal nitric oxide synthase mediates penile erection. Proc Natl Acad Sci U S A 109(41):16624–16629

Isidori AM, Buvat J, Corona G et al (2014) A critical analysis of the role of testosterone in erectile function: from pathophysiology to treatment-a systematic review. Eur Urol 65(1):99–112

Kanika ND, Tar M, Tong Y et al (2009) The mechanism of opiorphin-induced experimental priapism in rats involves activation of the polyamine synthetic pathway. Am J Physiol Cell Physiol 297(4):C916–C927

Kanika ND, Melman A, Davies KP (2010) Experimental priapism is associated with increased oxidative stress and activation of protein degradation pathways in corporal tissue. Int J Impot Res 22(6):363–373

Kato GJ, Gladwin MT, Steinberg MH (2007) Deconstructing sickle cell disease: reappraisal of the role of hemolysis in the development of clinical subphenotypes. Blood Rev 21(1):37–47

Kietadisorn R, Juni RP, Moens AL (2012) Tackling endothelial dysfunction by modulating NOS uncoupling: new insights into its pathogenesis and therapeutic possibilities. Am J Physiol Endocrinol Metab 302(5):E481–E495

Lagoda G, Sezen SF, Cabrini MR, Musicki B, Burnett AL (2013) Molecular analysis of erection regulatory factors in sickle cell disease associated priapism in the human penis. J Urol 189(2):762–768

Liaw RL, Srilatha B, Adaikan PG (2011) Effects of hydrogen sulfide on erectile function and its possible mechanism(s) of action. J Sex Med 8(7):1853–1864

Lin G, Xin ZC, Lue TF, Lin CS (2003) Up and down-regulation of phosphodiesterase-5 as related to tachyphylaxis and priapism. J Urol 170(2 Pt 2):S15–S18; discussion S19

Lin CS, Lin G, Lue TF (2005) Cyclic nucleotide signaling in cavernous smooth muscle. J Sex Med 2(4):478–491

Linder AE, Webb RC, Mills TM et al (2005) Rho-kinase and RGS-containing RhoGEFs as molecular targets for the treatment of erectile dysfunction. Curr Pharm Des 11(31):4029–4040

Lionnet F, Hammoudi N, Stojanovic KS et al (2012) Hemoglobin sickle cell disease complications: a clinical study of 179 cases. Haematologica 97(8):1136–1141

Lucas KA, Pitari GM, Kazerounian S et al (2000) Guanylyl cyclases and signaling by cyclic GMP. Pharmacol Rev 52(3):375–414

Lue TF (2000) Erectile dysfunction. N Engl J Med 342(24):1802–1813

Mantadakis E, Cavender JD, Rogers ZR, Ewalt DH, Buchanan GR (1999) Prevalence of priapism in children and adolescents with sickle cell anemia. J Pediatr Hematol Oncol 21(6):518–522

Mi T, Abbasi S, Zhang H et al (2008) Excess adenosine in murine penile erectile tissues contributes to priapism via A2B adenosine receptor signaling. J Clin Invest 118(4):1491–1501

Mills TM, Lewis RW, Wingard CJ et al (2003) Vasoconstriction, RhoA/Rho-kinase and the erectile response. Int J Impot Res 15(Suppl 5):S20–S24

Montague DK, Jarow J, Broderick GA et al (2003) American Urological Association guideline on the management of priapism. J Urol 170(4 Pt 1):1318–1324

Morelli A, Filippi S, Mancina R et al (2004) Androgens regulate phosphodiesterase type 5 expression and functional activity in corpora cavernosa. Endocrinology 145(5):2253–2263

Morrison BF, Burnett AL (2012) Stuttering priapism: insights into pathogenesis and management. Curr Urol Rep 13(4):268–276

Morrison BF, Reid M, Madden W, Burnett AL (2013) Testosterone replacement therapy does not promote priapism in hypogonadal men with sickle cell disease: 12-month safety report. Andrology 1(4):576–582

Morrison BF, Anele UA, Reid ME et al (2015) Is testosterone deficiency a possible risk factor for priapism associated with sickle-cell disease? Int Urol Nephrol 47(1):47–52

Muneer A, Minhas S, Arya M, Ralph DJ (2008) Stuttering priapism – a review of the therapeutic options. Int J Clin Pract 62(8):1265–1270

Musicki B, Ross AE, Champion HC, Burnett AL, Bivalacqua TJ (2009) Posttranslational modification of constitutive nitric oxide synthase in the penis. J Androl 30(4):352–362

Musicki B, Liu T, Sezen SF, Burnett AL (2012) Targeting NADPH oxidase decreases oxidative stress in the transgenic sickle cell mouse penis. J Sex Med 9(8):1980–1987

Musicki B, Bivalacqua TJ, Champion HC, Burnett AL (2014) Sildenafil promotes eNOS activation and inhibits NADPH oxidase in the transgenic sickle cell mouse penis. J Sex Med 11(2): 424–430

Nangle MR, Cotter MA, Cameron NE (2004) An in vitro investigation of aorta and corpus cavernosum from eNOS and nNOS gene-deficient mice. Pflugers Arch 448(2):139–145

Ning C, Wen J, Zhang Y et al (2014) Excess adenosine A2B receptor signaling contributes to priapism through HIF-1α mediated reduction of PDE5 gene expression. FASEB J 28(6):2725–2735

Olsson RA, Pearson JD (1990) Cardiovascular purinoceptors. Physiol Rev 70(3):761–845

Osegbe DN, Akinyanju OO (1987) Testicular dysfunction in men with sickle cell disease. Postgrad Med J 63(736):95–98

Parshad O, Stevens MC, Preece MA, Thomas PW, Serjeant GR (1994) The mechanism of low testosterone levels in homozygous sickle-cell disease. West Indian Med J 43(1):12–14

Phatarpekar PV, Wen J, Xia Y (2010) Role of adenosine signaling in penile erection and erectile disorders. J Sex Med 7(11):3553–3564

Prieto D (2008) Physiological regulation of penile arteries and veins. Int J Impot Res 20(1):17–29

Priviero FB, Jin LM, Ying Z, Teixeira CE, Webb RC (2010) Up-regulation of the RhoA/Rho-kinase signaling pathway in corpus cavernosum from endothelial nitric-oxide synthase (NOS), but not neuronal NOS, null mice. J Pharmacol Exp Ther 333(1):184–192

Rees RW, Ziessen T, Ralph DJ et al (2002) Human and rabbit cavernosal smooth muscle cells express Rho-kinase. Int J Impot Res 14(1):1–7

Reilly CM, Lewis RW, Stopper VS, Mills TM (1997) Androgenic maintenance of the rat erectile response via a non-nitric-oxide-dependent pathway. J Androl 18(6):588–594

Riento K, Ridley AJ (2003) Rocks: multifunctional kinases in cell behaviour. Nat Rev Mol Cell Biol 4(6):446–456

Salonia A, Eardley I, Giuliano F et al (2014) European Association of Urology guidelines on priapism. Eur Urol 65(2):480–489

Slayton W, Kedar A, Schatz D (1995) Testosterone induced priapism in two adolescents with sickle cell disease. J Pediatr Endocrinol Metab 8(3):199–203

Sobrevia L, Mann GE (1997) Dysfunction of the endothelial nitric oxide signalling pathway in diabetes and hyperglycaemia. Exp Physiol 82(3):423–452

Somlyo AP, Somlyo AV (2003) Ca2+ sensitivity of smooth muscle and nonmuscle myosin II: modulated by G proteins, kinases, and myosin phosphatase. Physiol Rev 83(4):1325–1358

Spycher MA, Hauri D (1986) The ultrastructure of the erectile tissue in priapism. J Urol 135(1): 142–147

Srilatha B, Adaikan PG, Li L, Moore PK (2007) Hydrogen sulphide: a novel endogenous gasotransmitter facilitates erectile function. J Sex Med 4(5):1304–1311

Tager AM, LaCamera P, Shea BS et al (2008) The lysophosphatidic acid receptor LPA1 links pulmonary fibrosis to lung injury by mediating fibroblast recruitment and vascular leak. Nat Med 14(1):45–54

Tarry WF, Duckett JW, Snyder HM (1987) Urological complications of sickle cell disease in a pediatric population. J Urol 138(3):592–594

Tong Y, Tiplitsky SI, Tar M, Melman A, Davies KP (2008) Transcription of G-protein coupled receptors in corporeal smooth muscle is regulated by the endogenous neutral endopeptidase inhibitor sialorphin. J Urol 180(2):760–766

Tostes RC, Giachini FR, Carneiro FS et al (2007) Determination of adenosine effects and adenosine receptors in murine corpus cavernosum. J Pharmacol Exp Ther 322(2):678–685

Traish A, Kim N (2005) The physiological role of androgens in penile erection: regulation of corpus cavernosum structure and function. J Sex Med 2(6):759–770

Traish AM, Park K, Dhir V et al (1999) Effects of castration and androgen replacement on erectile function in a rabbit model. Endocrinology 140(4):1861–1868

Traish AM, Goldstein I, Kim NN (2007) Testosterone and erectile function: from basic research to a new clinical paradigm for managing men with androgen insufficiency and erectile dysfunction. Eur Urol 52(1):54–70

Traish AM, Miner MM, Morgentaler A, Zitzmann M (2011) Testosterone deficiency. Am J Med 124(7):578–587

Villalba N, Stankevicius E, Garcia-Sacristán A, Simonsen U, Prieto D (2007) Contribution of both Ca2+ entry and Ca2+ sensitization to the alpha1-adrenergic vasoconstriction of rat penile small arteries. Am J Physiol Heart Circ Physiol 292(2):H1157–H1169

Villalba N, Stankevicius E, Simonsen U, Prieto D (2008) Rho kinase is involved in Ca2+ entry of rat penile small arteries. Am J Physiol Heart Circ Physiol 294(4):H1923–H1932

Wang H, Eto M, Steers WD, Somlyo AP, Somlyo AV (2002) RhoA-mediated Ca2+ sensitization in erectile function. J Biol Chem 277(34):30614–30621

Webb RC (2003) Smooth muscle contraction and relaxation. Adv Physiol Educ 27(1-4):201–206

Wen J, Jiang X, Dai Y et al (2010) Increased adenosine contributes to penile fibrosis, a dangerous feature of priapism, via A2B adenosine receptor signaling. FASEB J 24(3):740–749

Wettschureck N, Offermanns S (2002) Rho/Rho-kinase mediated signaling in physiology and pathophysiology. J Mol Med (Berl) 80(10):629–638

Wisner A, Dufour E, Messaoudi M et al (2006) Human Opiorphin, a natural antinociceptive modulator of opioid-dependent pathways. Proc Natl Acad Sci U S A 103(47):17979–17984

Wood KC, Hebbel RP, Granger DN (2005) Endothelial cell NADPH oxidase mediates the cerebral microvascular dysfunction in sickle cell transgenic mice. FASEB J 19(8):989–991

Wood KC, Hebbel RP, Lefer DJ, Granger DN (2006) Critical role of endothelial cell-derived nitric oxide synthase in sickle cell disease-induced microvascular dysfunction. Free Radic Biol Med 40(8):1443–1453

Zhang Y, Dai Y, Wen J et al (2011) Detrimental effects of adenosine signaling in sickle cell disease. Nat Med 17(1):79–86

Chapter 12
Clinical Manifestations and Treatment of Adult Sickle Cell Disease

Fernando Ferreira Costa and Kleber Yotsumoto Fertrin

Abstract Despite being a disease that stems primarily from abnormalities in the erythrocytes, clinical manifestations and complications of sickle cell disease are known to affect virtually all organs and systems in the human body. Chronic hemolytic anemia and a systemic inflammatory state are the basic pathophysiological mechanisms that underlie the occurrence of both acute vaso-occlusive events (painful episodes, acute chest syndrome, priapism, stroke, etc.) and long-term end-organ damage (heart failure, chronic kidney disease, retinopathy, pulmonary hypertension, leg ulcers, osteoporosis, etc.). Adequate treatment for sickle cell disease in children with vaccination and prophylactic penicillin has allowed most of these patients to reach adulthood. Nevertheless, morbidity in the adult population is high, with many patients presenting with two or more vital organ complications by the age of 40. There is still room for improvement in the prevention, early diagnosis, and treatment of complications more frequently encountered by adult hematologists, and need for consultation with other subspecialties becomes a rule when caring for adult sickle cell patients. We review the clinical presentation, diagnosis, and management of the most relevant aspects of sickle cell disease in adults and summarize current treatment approaches, from supportive care with blood transfusions and hydroxyurea, to curative care with hematopoietic stem cell transplantation.

Keywords Vaso-occlusive event • End-organ damage • Hematopoietic stem cell transplantation • Blood transfusion • Hydroxyurea

---

F.F. Costa, MD, PhD (✉)
Hematology Center, School of Medical Sciences,
University of Campinas – UNICAMP, Campinas, São Paulo, Brazil
e-mail: ferreira@unicamp.br

K.Y. Fertrin, MD, PhD
Department of Clinical Pathology, School of Medical Sciences,
University of Campinas – UNICAMP, Campinas, São Paulo, Brazil
e-mail: fertrin@unicamp.br

© Springer International Publishing Switzerland 2016

F.F. Costa, N. Conran (eds.), *Sickle Cell Anemia*,
DOI 10.1007/978-3-319-06713-1_12

12.1 General Features and Major Manifestations of Adult Sickle Cell Disease

While the transition from childhood to adulthood in patients with sickle cell disease (SCD) is sometimes blurred by challenges in this process and can affect the achievement of adequate healthcare, some manifestations and complications of SCD remain unchanged, while others knowingly have a later onset, and are usually managed by adult hematologists and other specialists. Scheduled outpatient visits every 4–6 months may be the adequate follow-up for patients not presenting any complications, while the need for specific therapy will significantly shorten intervals between visits, e.g. patients starting hydroxyurea, or receiving chronic blood transfusions, iron chelation, etc.

Clinical features that characterize sickle cell disease at any age include pallor and jaundice secondary to chronic hemolytic anemia. Patients with SCD are usually of slender build, with normal to low body mass index. This may be the result of increased energetic expenditure due to bone marrow activity, in association with hypoxia and a chronic inflammatory state. Hemolysis results in a normocytic normochromic anemia in which levels of hemoglobin may vary between 6 and 10 g/dL, influencing the degree of pallor. Jaundice intensity varies widely across patients due to different levels of predominantly unconjugated hyperbilirubinemia. A typical complete blood count shows hyperproliferative anemia with reticulocyte counts ranging around 5–20%. Examination of peripheral blood smears shows red blood cells with evident polychromasia, a variable number of sickled or leaf-like cells, and occasional circulating erythroblasts can be observed. Hyposplenism (see Fig. 12.1) is usually present due to the splenic dysfunction that usually commences during early childhood (see Chap. 9), and explains the presence of erythrocytes containing Howell–Jolly bodies. Leukocytosis with neutrophilia and mild monocytosis is also a frequent feature, particularly in homozygous sickle cell anemia patients.

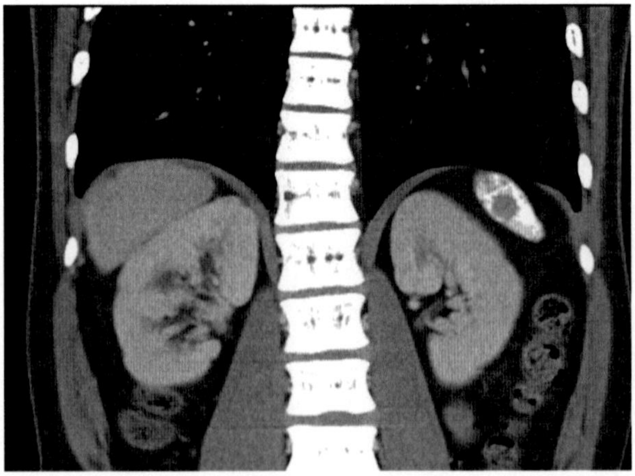

Fig. 12.1 Auto-splenectomy. Computerized tomography coronal section showing atrophic, calcified spleen in an adult male with sickle cell anemia

Thrombocytosis can be found and is probably caused both by hyposplenism and chronic inflammation.

There are distinct hematological features in other forms of SCD: HbSβ thalassemia presents with hypochromic microcytic anemia, which may range from mild to severe. While HbSC disease causes normochromic normocytic anemia, some patients may display mild microcytosis due to frequent co-inheritance of alpha thalassemia in some populations, and occasionally these patients are not even anemic, with only compensated hemolysis, which makes non-hematologists less likely to consider an inherited hemoglobin disorder as a diagnostic possibility in adults. Mild thrombocytopenia may occur in these milder phenotypes due to preserved splenic function resulting in hypersplenism; leukocytosis is a less frequent feature in complete blood counts.

Ensuing clinical complications of adult sickle cell disease vary from individual to individual and are extremely diverse. All complications stem, ultimately, from processes of vascular occlusion in organs or as a result of the hemolytic anemia that accompanies the disease. The variation in manifestations observed in a patients will depend on the type of sickle cell disease (HbSS, HbSβ^0 thalassemia, HbSβ^+ thalassemia, HbSC, etc.), on the many genetic modifiers of the disease (as covered in Chap. 15), in addition to some environmental factors. Complications of sickle cell disease can be divided into acute and chronic, as listed in Table 12.1.

While hematopoietic stem cell transplantation can be curative for SCD, most therapeutic options for adult patients are still palliative. Figure 12.2 represents schematically the basic pathophysiology of SCD and where in this process current treatment options intervene. Since the limited availability of matched sibling stem cell donors precludes most adult patients from being eligible for stem cell transplantation, treatment strategies for adult SCD aim at improving acute events and preventing chronic complications of the disease. Typical supportive care includes folic acid supplementation, pain management, fetal-hemoglobin induction with hydroxyurea, red blood cell transfusion, iron chelation, and specific screening and treatment of complications.

12.2 Folic Acid Supplementation

One of the cornerstones in the management of chronic hemolysis is folic acid supplementation. Red blood cells have a shortened lifespan in SCD and other chronic hemolytic anemias (Gillette et al. 1971), therefore it is generally accepted by physicians that these patients should receive prescription folic acid supplements to avoid megaloblastic anemia. Nevertheless, there is limited scientific evidence of either the benefits or potential harm of this approach. On one hand, the only double-blind controlled trial looking at folic acid supplementation in children failed to show hematologic improvement in the supplemented group, although an excess of cases of dactylitis was noticed in the control group (Rabb et al. 1983). Low serum zinc levels are known to occur in SCD patients and folate supplementation has been

Table 12.1 Manifestations and complications of adult sickle cell anemia

	Complication	Characteristics
Acute	Acute pain episodes (vaso-occlusive events)	Most common complication of SCD. Severity varies and may be manageable at home or require hospitalization
	Acute chest syndrome	Development of chest pain accompanied by fever, respiratory symptoms, and a chest X-ray with a new pulmonary opacity; associated with hypoxemia in severe cases
	Stroke	Both ischemic and hemorrhagic stokes may occur in adult SCD
	Thrombosis	Can occur in adult SCD, particularly during pregnancy and post-partum
	Liver complications	Acute pain in the right upper quadrant with jaundice requires workup to distinguish between acute cholecystitis, acute viral hepatitis, hepatic sequestration, and sickle cell intra-hepatic cholestasis
	Infections	Most frequently pneumonia, osteomyelitis, and urinary infections, may progress to or present primarily as sepsis
	Priapism	Compartment syndrome of the penis causing "stuttering" (short-lived, intermittent) or prolonged (lasting over 4 h) painful penile erections; can cause permanent erectile dysfunction
	Aplastic crisis	Exacerbated anemia accompanied by reticulocytopenia, usually caused by parvovirus B19 infection
Chronic	Hemolytic anemia	Normocytic, normochromic anemia; hemoglobin levels may vary between 6 and 10 g/dL, accompanied by reticulocytosis
	Functional asplenia	Splenic dysfunction and eventual autosplenectomy secondary to the splenic infarction that usually occurs during childhood
	Avascular necrosis	Can affect hip(s) or shoulder(s) causing early osteoarthritis and chronic pain
	Osteopenia and osteoporosis	Reduction of bone mass density occurs earlier than in the general population, is progressive and associated with hemolysis in SCD
	Pulmonary arterial hypertension	Exertional dyspnea or fatigue with chronic oxygen desaturation, caused by pulmonary artery lumen restriction and wall stiffening, linked to hemolysis, and associated with poor prognosis
	Gallstones/cholelithiasis	Caused by augmented heme breakdown due to hemolysis
	Retinopathy	Proliferative retinopathy is relatively frequent, especially in HbSC disease and may cause blindness
	Nephropathy	Hyperfiltration and hyposthenuria occur early, incidence of microalbuminuria increases with patient age and can result in end-stage kidney disease
	Heart disease	Includes diastolic dysfunction with increased mortality, overt heart failure, and underrecognized acute myocardial infarction
	Leg ulcers	Development of ulcers in the maleolar and distal leg skin can be a recurring complication. These ulcers are painful, disfiguring and are difficult to heal
	Neurological complications	Neurocognitive impairment is frequent, particularly in patients with previous stroke. Moyamoya syndrome may also occur, with proliferation of intracerebral blood vessels caused by stenosis or occlusion of cerebral arteries, increasing risk for acute cerebrovascular events

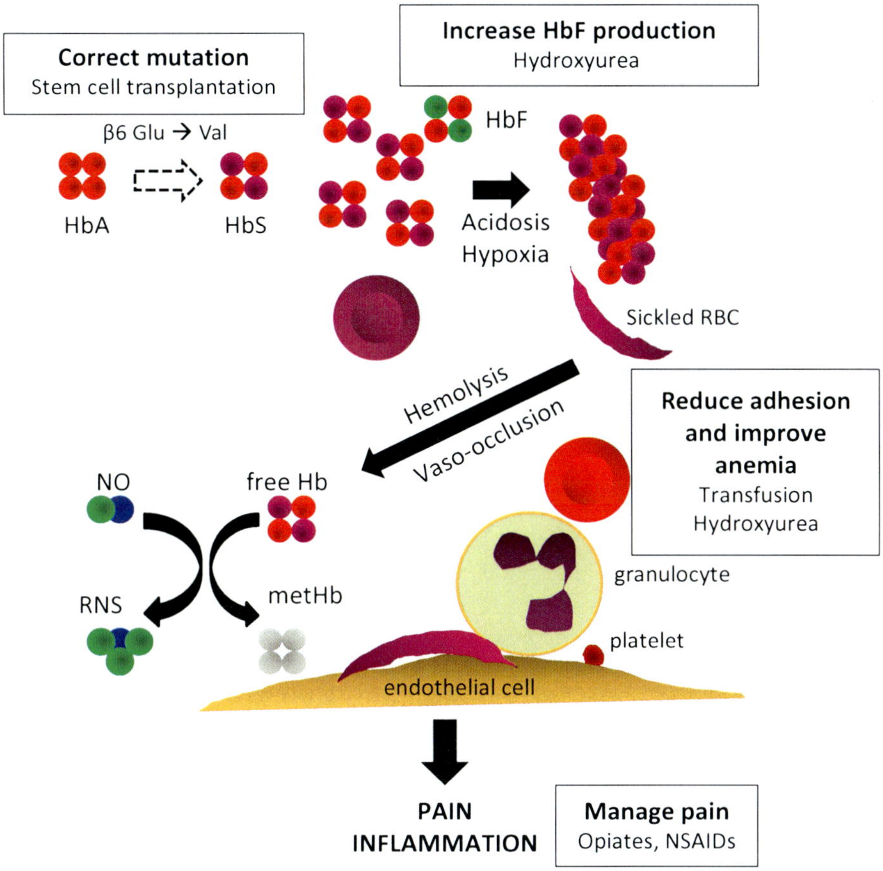

Fig. 12.2 Basic pathophysiology of sickle cell disease and currently available treatments

demonstrated to favor zinc deficiency (Simmer et al. 1987), while the chronic use of oral folate can mask cobalamin deficiency, and may allow SCD patients to develop neurological complications (Dhar et al. 2003). On the other hand, plasma homocysteine levels, known to correlate with endothelial dysfunction, are increased in children with SCD and decrease after folate supplementation, supporting a secondary beneficial role for folic acid supplements (Schnog et al. 2000). Epigenetic effects of folate on ovulation have also been considered as a possible explanation for an association between folate supplementation and increased incidence of twin pregnancies in SCD (Ballas et al. 2006). Besides the controversy over the indication of folic acid supplements, even less is known about the ideal dosage. One study studied homocysteine levels before and during progressive folic acid supplementation and proposed that 0.7 mg of daily folic acid may be an ideal dosage for children with SCD. Different formulations of folic acid supplement make the standard treatment schedule vary from 1 to 5 mg daily, depending on the country, and data from adult populations are still lacking.

12.3 Vaso-Occlusive Events and Pain Management

Of the serious acute presentations of the disease, the most frequent constitutes the acute pain crisis (or vaso-occlusive event, VOE), experienced as pain usually localized to bones and joints. The frequency of pain episodes requiring a clinic visit or hospitalization varies enormously from patient to patient, but was found by the Cooperative Study of Sickle Cell Disease (CSSCD) to average 1.0 pain episodes per patient year in male HbSS adults aged 20–39 years, with over 10 % of patients aged 20–29 years experiencing more than 3.0 pain episodes per patient year (Platt et al. 1991). The pain rate in patients over the age of 20 years was found to be indicative of clinical severity and to correlate with mortality.

Pain is a hallmark of SCD, so adequate pain management is of utmost importance in this population. While pain itself cannot be objectively measured, its presence should be evaluated by the clinician and care of pain will vary according to whether it occurs as an episodic event or as chronic pain. On average, painful episodes last for 4–5 days, but can sometimes last for weeks. A VOE is often the first diagnosis made for a SCD patient at the emergency department (ED) as almost any type of pain ensues. VOE should be only diagnosed once alternative diagnostic possibilities have been excluded, since there is no single exam that can confirm this diagnosis. Clinicians correctly seldom consider the diagnosis of VOE when pain is localized to the head. Pain localized elsewhere should also prompt consideration of other diseases, particularly during episodes of abdominal or chest pain, in which differential diagnosis for acute myocardial infarction, pulmonary embolism, acute cholecystitis, acute pancreatitis, or aortic aneurysm rupture can only be made with careful clinical evaluation, and sometimes demands appropriate laboratory and imaging exams. Figure 12.3 summarizes an example approach (described below) for an adult patient with SCD, arriving at the ED, whose complaint is, or includes, pain.

Example approach for an adult SCD patient, arriving at the ED, in pain

a. *Triage*: Nurses in EDs that treat SCD patients usually use triage scales. One of the most commonly used is the Emergency Severity Index (ESI), a simple five-level triage algorithm that helps to quickly classify patients according to acuity level. In the ESI algorithm, level 1 patients are the most severe and require immediate attention, while level 5 patients have the lowest priority and usually correspond to stable, mild cases. For example, ESI level for a typical SCD patient in pain will usually yield a minimum level 3 classification, since any such patient in this situation, will require more than one of the hospital "resources" (in this case, labs, imaging, IV fluids, and specialty consultation). Careful consideration should be taken as to whether the patient should be classified as more severe, since a pain score of 7 or higher on a scale from 0 to 10 due to intense ischemic pain is a possible level 2, and occasional patients will present with other level 2 criteria, such as low oxygen saturation, tachycardia, tachypnea, disorientation, or lethargy. Therefore, any SCD patient with pain should be considered a potential severe patient.

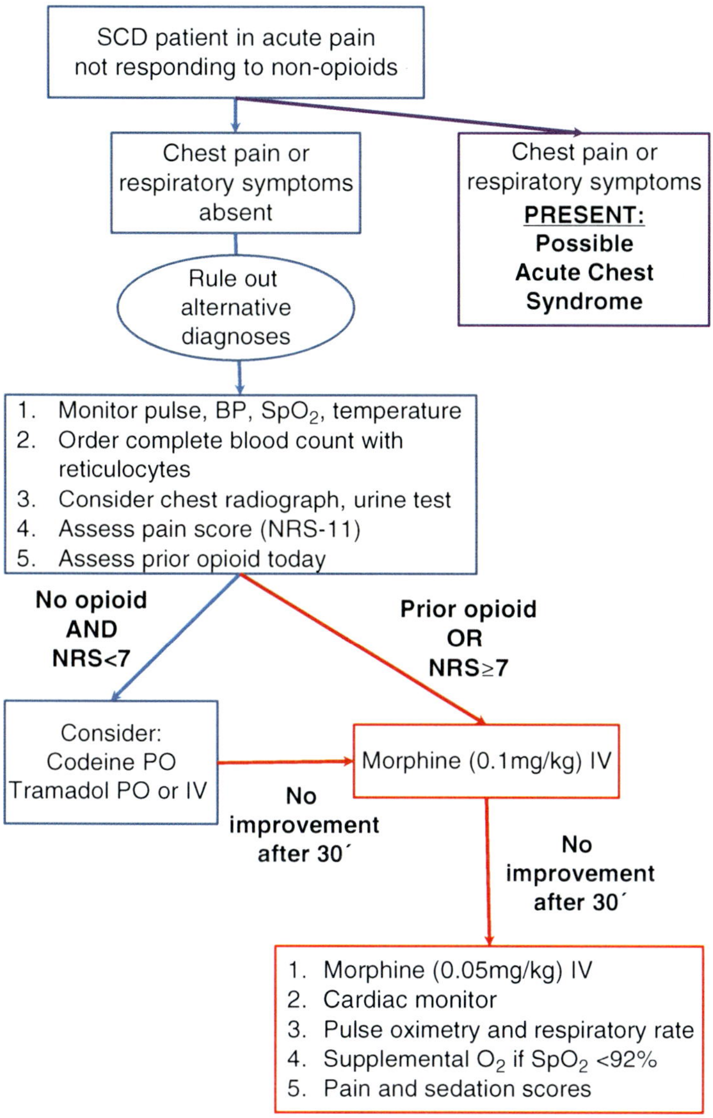

Fig. 12.3 Summarized example approach for an adult SCD patient, arriving at the emergency department, in pain

b. *Severity assessment*: After the initial assessment, VOE should be classified according to severity. Most clinicians are aware that pain scales, such as the Numeric Rating Scale (NRS-11, in which pain intensity is measured on a scale from 0 to 10) or the horizontal 100 mm Visual Analog Scale (Bijur et al. 2003) are useful and have been shown to be reasonably equivalent in pediatric SCD patients

(Myrvik et al. 2015), although data in the adult population are still lacking. Unfortunately, these scales are often misused as the only tool to decide whether to prescribe analgesic medication and which drug to choose. In the ED, NRS-11 is most beneficial if used to monitor pain improvement, not to decide treatment modality, since discrepancies between pain reported and visible distress frequently raise doubts about how urgently medication is needed (Patrick et al. 2015). A VOE should be classified as mild if pain subsides after common, over-the-counter (OTC) oral analgesic medications, such as acetaminophen (paracetamol), dipyrone (metamizole), or ibuprofen. Patients with mild VOEs may be treated as outpatients, and having mild VOEs come to the ED should be a sign of a possible loss of follow-up or that the primary caregiver failed to give proper orientation on how to handle mild pain before going to the ED. If the patient presents with pain that fails to respond to OTC medication, the event should be considered as at least moderate, and treated with lower potency opioids, such as tramadol or codeine. Patients may have used tramadol or codeine at home, or may be in chronic use of methadone and other potent opioids. Breakthrough pain or refractoriness to opioids in these cases already characterizes severe VOE.

c. *Acute pain treatment*: Parenteral opioids, such as IV morphine or hydromorphone, are the standard of care for situations of severe VOE in the ED. The usual initial dose of morphine is 0.1 mg/kg (maximum recommended single dose 10 mg, or one vial), and may range from 0.05 to 0.2 mg/kg depending on previous use of opioids, tolerance and comorbidities, such as chronic hepatic disease, advanced age, or pulmonary disease. Transdermal, transmucosal, intranasal or oral opioids have also been used in several reports and can be employed depending on previous experience of the staff and drug availability in a particular center. Patient controlled analgesia (PCA) is also encouraged if available, and has proven to be as successful in achieving pain control as continuous IV infusion with lower morphine doses. Undertreatment of severe pain with mild opiates or non-opiates only adds to the patient's degree of distress and actually contributes to increased unreliability of subjective assessment of pain (persistent "10 out of 10" pain score) and the development of apparent drug-seeking behavior. Clinicians, nurses, and all healthcare professionals involved in SCD patient care should be aware that opiate addiction is relatively uncommon, and at most as frequent in SCD patients as in oncologic patients, so denying opiates because of fear about addiction should be avoided, and concerns about drug addiction should be addressed in psychiatric consultation. Rescue doses of 25–50 % of the initial dose should be considered every 15–30 min until pain improves (typically a pain score below 7).
d. *Monitoring*: Reassessment of vital signs including pulse oximetry, respiratory rate, pain score, and level of consciousness (sedation score) every 15–30 min is mandatory for patients receiving IV opioids. Continuous cardiac and pulse oximetry monitoring is encouraged, particularly if several doses are required to improve pain.
e. *Supportive care*: Intravenous hydration should aim at normalizing the hydration status of clinically dehydrated patients. This means that so-called "hyperhydration"

should be avoided. About 3 L of fluids (PO and IV combined) should suffice for most cases, and clinicians should also consider insensible water loss due to fever, tachypnea, and elevated room temperature. There is no scientific evidence to suggest which type of fluid is more beneficial (Okomo and Meremikwu 2012), so the choice amongst a wide variety of crystalloid options (saline, NaCl 0.45 %, Ringer's solution, etc.) is often personal, although the idea of infusing hypotonic solutions is favored by many specialists as making pathophysiological sense, for promoting red blood cell rehydration and, probably, less sickling. Most adult SCD patients, particular those over 30, have either heart or kidney failure to some degree, so one should be cautious when prescribing bolus IV fluids to prevent iatrogenic pulmonary edema.

f. *Complementary evaluation*: Careful history and physical examination upfront can easily uncover precipitating factors such as cold exposure, dehydration or an obvious skin infection, for example. Additional exams for VOE assessment varies according to associated signs and symptoms, but typically should include a complete blood count with reticulocyte count, chest radiograph, and routine urine testing. Ordering blood or urine cultures and additional lab exams depend on the differential diagnoses considered.

g. *Admission*: Patients without pain improvement after two or more doses of IV opioids should be admitted and receive around-the-clock IV opioids every 4 h with rescue doses of 25–50 %. Association with non-steroidal anti-inflammatory drugs (NSAIDs), such as dipyrone, paracetamol or ibuprofen is also recommended. Hydroxyurea should not be withheld unless there are clear signs of toxicity due to hydroxyurea, such as reticulocytopenia or thrombocytopenia below 80,000/m^3, or neutrophil count below 2000/mm^3. Refractory pain is frequently an indication to consider exchange transfusion (or simple transfusion depending on Hb levels), and infections should be ruled out as cause for a refractory pain crisis. Patients presenting with generalized pain despite oral opioids before coming to the ED should be considered as particularly prone to admission, since the incidence of acute chest syndrome seems to be higher among such patients when compared to patients with more localized pain. Incentive spirometry is encouraged to reduce risk of acute chest syndrome in all patients admitted for VOE.

h. *Opioid tapering*: Once pain is controlled and no additional rescue doses are needed, daily morphine doses can be redistributed every 4 h, patients can be transitioned to oral medication, and slowly tapered.

i. *Discharge*: Patients can be discharged when they meet the following criteria: (1) pain improvement (either pain rate below 7 or at least 2 points lower than upon arrival); (2) pain controllable with oral medication; (3) tolerance to oral medication and hydration (adequate control of nausea/vomiting associated with opioid use, oral analgesics available); (4) absence of signs of infection; (5) no need for transfusion; (6) stable vital signs; (7) scheduled follow-up at the Hematology Clinic. These criteria also apply to patients at the ED within 4–6 h of arrival.

12.4 Acute Chest Syndrome in Adults

Acute chest syndrome (ACS) is classically defined by an acute event with the presence of: (1) acute onset of pain in the thoracic region; (2) respiratory symptoms, such as cough, dyspnea, or tachypnea; (3) a chest radiogram with a new pulmonary opacity; (4) fever; and (5) hypoxemia in severe cases. ACS may be triggered by events such as infection, fat embolism, or lung infarction and is still one of the most common causes of death in adults with sickle cell disease (Howard et al. 2015; Fitzhugh et al. 2010). It is noteworthy that only a few patients present with the full blown tetrad (or pentad if severe). Failing to promptly treat a patient lacking an abnormal chest X-ray (which is often the case), may result in rapidly evolving respiratory distress, need for mechanical ventilation, and even death. Therefore, it is safe to say that any physician encountering a SCD patient with acute chest pain should consider the possibility of ACS and, in our experience, early and aggressive treatment in cases presenting solely with chest pain and hypoxemia may prevent fatal outcomes.

Differential diagnoses of ACS include acute pulmonary thromboembolism (PE) and myocardial infarction (although rarely reported). PE incidence is increased in SCD, although one should remember that cases of ACS in adults result more frequently from fat embolism from the ischemic bone marrow, rather than blood clots formed in deep vein thromboses elsewhere. Patients undertreated for simple, localized pain crises tend to develop generalized pain, which increases the probability of bone marrow ischemia and subsequent ACS. Moreover, the presence of lower than usual platelet counts, under 200,000/mm^3, is non-specific, but may favor the diagnosis of fat embolism in homozygous sickle cell anemia patients, who normally have a much higher platelet count due to autosplenectomy and chronic inflammation.

Treatment of ACS is symptomatic, and includes both analgesia and adequate fluid management, as for VOEs, but also oxygen supplementation if oxygen saturation drops below 92 % in room air, and careful evaluation of the need for simple or exchange transfusion. Severe cases on mechanical ventilation or developing shock may benefit from erythrocytapheresis, if available. Large-spectrum parenteral antibiotics should be prescribed, aiming at the most common respiratory microbial agents in this population (*Streptococcus pneumoniae*, *Mycoplasma pneumoniae*, *Chlamydia pneumoniae*, and viruses), i.e. combination of third generation cephalosporin and macrolide (e.g. ceftriaxone and azithromycin), or so-called "respiratory" fluoroquinolones (e.g. levofloxacin) are frequent and adequate options, along with seasonal antivirals, such as oseltamivir for regions experiencing influenza virus outbreaks (e.g. H1N1). Patients with life-threatening ACS episodes or recurring ACS should be considered for long-term hydroxyurea therapy after discharge.

12.5 Vaso-Occlusive Episode Long-Term Management: Hydroxyurea

Hydroxyurea (HU), or hydroxycarbamide, is a chemotherapeutic agent that inhibits ribonucleotide reductase, an enzyme required for nucleotide and protein synthesis. The main beneficial effect of hydroxyurea in SCD is the induction of fetal hemoglobin (HbF) production (Charache et al. 1987). Ideally, HbF levels should reach 20 %, which corresponds to over 90 % of F-cells (erythrocytes that are rich in HbF), with decreased HbS polymerization, less sickling and reduced cell adhesion. Despite this primary effect on erythropoiesis, other beneficial effects of HU in SCD have been recognized. It also reduces the production of other cell types involved in vaso-occlusion, such as white blood cells and platelets, and is a nitric oxide donor. These effects are listed in Box 12.1.

The Multicenter Study of Hydroxyurea (MSH) was the largest study to prospectively address the clinical beneficial effects of chronic use of HU in SCD (Charache et al. 1995). Patients diagnosed with homozygous HbSS sickle cell anemia or sickle-beta zero thalassemia (HbSβ^0) that were treated with HU presented with decreased number of VOEs, decreased number of hospitalizations and a trend towards a lower transfusion requirement. There are several indications for chronic HU use, and while not all of them are evidence-based, particularly in the adult population, the absence of other therapeutic options often leads to a trial with HU in these patients. Common indications for initiation of HU therapy are listed in Box 12.2. Patients should provide informed consent, since HU therapy is associated with infertility with reversible azoospermia in men (Garozzo et al. 2000). Teratogenesis is still a concern in pregnant women, even though the contraindication of HU during pregnancy is based on animal studies using high doses of HU, and so far scientific

Box 12.1: Beneficial Effects of Hydroxyurea in SCA Patients

- Increases HbF production
- Decreases white blood cell count
- Decreases reticulocyte count
- Decreases hemolysis
- Decreases frequency of vaso-occlusive pain crisis and acute chest syndrome
- Decreases mortality
- Increases nitric oxide bioavailability
- Decreases red blood cell, white blood cell, and platelet adhesive properties
- Decreases endothelial dysfunction markers
- Decreases hypercoagulability

Box 12.2: Indications for Initiation of Hydroxyurea Therapy in Adults with SCD

Strongly recommended (Yawn et al. 2014)

1. Three or more hospitalizations for vaso-occlusive crisis in the past 12 months
2. Severe or recurrent acute chest syndrome
3. Sickle cell-associated pain that affects daily activities and quality of life
4. Symptomatic anemia that affects daily activities and quality of life (typically Hb < 6 g/dL)

Consider on case-by-case basis:

1. Adult onset stroke not eligible for chronic transfusion
2. Anemia (Hb < 8g/dL) in association with erythropoietin for end-stage renal disease to improve response
3. Anemia (Hb < 8g/dL) associated with structural cardiac disease
4. Pulmonary hypertension confirmed by right heart catheterization
5. Tricuspid regurgitant jet velocity above 2.5 m/s on echocardiography
6. Recurrent acute priapism
7. HbSC disease or HbS-β^+-thalassemia with complication affecting daily activities and quality of life

evidence fails to prove that HU increases the risk for human birth defects (Diav-Citrin et al. 1999). Nevertheless, we recommend women be screened for pregnancy with human chorionic gonadotrophin levels before treatment initiation and be advised to use contraceptives during the entire period of time they are on HU. In terms of toxicity, HU is a safe drug. A systematic review reported moderate level of causality with cytopenias, but there is insufficient evidence to associate HU with other cancers. Moreover, there is evidence to support HU does not increase the incidence of hematologic neoplasia in SCD patients (Lanzkron et al. 2008). A common concern amongst patients starting HU is the development or worsening of chronic leg ulcers. Hematologists should be aware that high-grade evidence of the association of HU with leg ulcer in other diseases does not apply to sickle cell disease patients, with good evidence that supports the absence of this association (Lanzkron et al. 2008). Similarly, association of HU in SCD patients has not been found with interstitial pneumonitis, hepatitis, corneal limbal stem cell deficiency, pruritus, or skin neoplasms, despite reports in other diseases (Lanzkron et al. 2008). Usual HU dosage, taken from the original MSH study (Charache et al. 1995, 1996), is 15–35 mg/kg/day, with monthly increments of 500 mg/day until a maximum tolerated dose (MTD) is reached (see Box 12.3 for recommendations for the use of hydroxyurea in adult sickle cell patients). MTD is defined as the maximum dose at which no significant toxicity occurs. Reticulocytopenia or thrombocytopenia below 80,000/μL or neutrophil count below 2000/μL are considered thresholds to define hematologic toxicity in SCD patients taking HU, since these patients primarily present with reticulocytosis, thrombocytosis and leukocytosis. HbF levels should be monitored at least every trimester and HU increased until HbF reaches 20 %, preferably with Hb levels above 9 g/dL, or MTD is reached. Although anecdotal, the occurrence of acute myocardial infarction was reported in association with an increase of Hb levels to over 10 g/dL (Fattori et al. 2005), so excessive increases in Hb levels with hyperviscosity should be avoided. Patients reaching MTD without HbF>20 % should be considered refractory, but suspension of HU therapy should be discussed on a case-to-case basis, since many patients report improvement of symptoms to their caregivers despite suboptimal HbF levels. Refractoriness to 35 mg/kg/day without any hematologic toxicity is very rare, and the possibility of low compliance should be investigated, particularly in the absence of a high MCV (usually above 120 fL). In the MSH study, patients were more likely to respond to HU if they were female, presented fewer VOEs at baseline, reticulocyte count over 300,000/μL, neutrophil count over 7500/μL, or a baseline fetal hemoglobin over 7.5 %. Patients bearing the Central African Republic haplotype were less likely to respond to HU, but this should not be grounds for not trying to reach MTD (Charache et al. 1996).

Box 12.3: Recommendations for the Use of Hydroxyurea in Adult Sickle Cell Patients

(modified from Yawn et al., JAMA 2014;312(10):1033–48)

Before initiating hydroxyurea:

1. **Explain** indication, aims, benefits that can be expected, and possible side effects of HU therapy to the patient—include possible supportive family members (spouse, children);
2. Order appropriate **laboratory exams**: CBC (including mean red blood cell corpuscular volume [MCV], neutrophil, platelet, and reticulocyte counts), renal function tests (BUN, creatinine), liver function tests (AST, ALT, total bilirubin and fractions), pregnancy test for women, baseline quantitative fetal hemoglobin (preferably HPLC);
3. Prescribe **contraceptive methods** and, if the patient intends to have children, stress the need for a planned pregnancy.

Starting dosage: 15 mg/kg/day, rounded up to the nearest 500 mg; 5–10 mg/kg/day if chronic kidney disease; pills can be taken as a single dose or multiple smaller doses.

Monitoring: CBC, renal and liver function tests every 4 weeks until MTD (see below); also measure fetal hemoglobin every 2–3 months afterwards.

(continued)

Box 12.3: (continued)

Maximum tolerated dose (MTD): Highest dose at which neutrophil count is above 2000/μL (may reach 1250/μL in young adults), with platelet and reticulocyte counts above 80,000/μL.

Dose escalation: Increase 5 mg/kg/day every 8 weeks until MTD is reached.

Toxicity: If neutrophils <2000/μL (depending on age), platelet <80,000/μL or reticulocytes <80,000/μL, stop hydroxyurea, monitor CBC weekly until recovery, and restart HU at dose 5 mg/kg/day lower than previously.

Maximum dose: 35 mg/kg/day or MTD.

Minimum duration of treatment: 6 months.

Do NOT:

1. Double up doses if patient misses dose;
2. Stop HU during hospitalization or acute illness;
3. Stop HU due to lack of increase in MCV or fetal hemoglobin.

CBC, complete blood count; HU, hydroxyurea; BUN, blood urea nitrogen; AST, aspartate aminotransferase; ALT, alanine aminotransferase; HPLC, high performance liquid chromatography

Compliance is one of the main challenges of HU therapy. With age and, depending on their weight, many patients will need to take four or more pills per day, which can prove to be cumbersome and lead to poor compliance for long periods of time. Another limitation is the fear of increasing the dose of HU to prevent hematologic toxicity. Physicians are encouraged to follow the blood count thresholds described and not be afraid to increase HU dosage before HbF levels rise to 20%, even if the patient reports improvement in the incidence of pain crises. In our experience, neutrophil counts of between 1500 and 2000 cells/μL are well tolerated and not associated with febrile neutropenia, and should not be considered an emergency. Hematologists should aim for the best compliance possible, since a minimum 80% of adherence to the treatment was associated with response to HU in the MSH study (Charache et al. 1996).

12.6 Aplastic Crisis

Aplastic crisis is a very particular type of acute complication that is not exclusive to SCD. It is typically caused by parvovirus B19 infection, and since this virus has tropism for erythroblastic precursors, it causes transient pure erythroid aplasia, resulting in acute onset of anemia with reticulocytopenia. This complication is most frequently seen in children, but may affect adults. Diagnostic confirmation depends on bone marrow aspirate showing typical viral inclusions in immature erythroblasts and serological tests. Since it is self-limited, management is based on blood transfusions, which should be only enough to reverse cardiac decompensation, such as congestive heart failure due to severe anemia (see comment under "Blood transfusion and iron chelation in SCD").

12.7 Heart Disease

Chronic hemolytic anemia causes a strain on the cardiovascular system, ultimately predisposing SCD patients to early development of high output heart failure, with left ventricle hypertrophy and dilation. Myocardial iron overload is a very rare occurrence in SCD, differently from what is found in thalassemia patients, and most probably SCD patients are protected from heart siderosis by a lower transfusional burden with exchange transfusion approaches, a later onset of transfusion programs, and chronic inflammation that may reduce the ability of iron to be transferred from the reticuloendothelial system to cardiomyocytes. Symptomatic patients with exertional dyspnea, cardiopulmonary abnormalities on physical examination, or peripheral edema should be evaluated with chest X-ray, electrocardiogram, and transthoracic Doppler echocardiography to screen for abnormalities. Asymptomatic patients may be screened annually in research centers dedicated to SCD. Since the severity of anemia impacts on the development of high cardiac output, hydroxyurea therapy can be recommended in some patients with very severe anemia (Hb under 6 g/dL) as an attempt to prevent heart disease, among other complications, but this indication should take into consideration the opinion of a SCD expert. Patients receiving blood transfusions had a lower left ventricle mass in one study, and this has been used as evidence to indicate chronic blood transfusion in more anemic patients (Hb under 7 g/dL) that do not respond to hydroxyurea (HU) and present with structural cardiac disease. Studies have also shown that diastolic dysfunction precedes overt cardiomyopathy and is a predictor of mortality (Sachdev et al. 2007; Caldas et al. 2008), reinforcing the idea that heart disease is a relative indication for more aggressive management. There are no specific guidelines for heart failure associated with SCD, but a small study reported a reduction in cardiac remodeling in SCD patients taking enalapril for microalbuminuria (Lima et al. 2008). Therefore, the use of angiotensin converting enzyme inhibitors (ACEi) or angiotensin receptor blockers (ARBs), as used for other causes of heart failure, is recommended in SCD-associated cardiomyopathy.

Myocardial infarction (MI) does occur in SCD patients, but it is probably underdiagnosed, and consequently underreported, in this patient population. Chest pain, epigastric pain, and dyspnea frequently guide physicians towards a diagnosis of vaso-occlusive crises, acute chest syndrome, or side effects secondary to non-steroidal anti-inflammatory drugs rather than MI, so physicians fail to order an electrocardiogram and appropriate serum cardiac enzymes (e.g. troponin I, which is less likely to be falsely elevated due to muscular ischemia or intramuscular analgesic administration). Coronary angiography is usually normal, but echocardiography may demonstrate segmental ventricular wall motion dysfunction. If MI is diagnosed, SCD patients should be treated with prompt analgesia, oxygenation, and hydration, along with exchange transfusions to ensure proper oxygen delivery, aiming at HbS below 30%, but with a hematocrit not exceeding 30%, as MI has been reported in a patient developing high hematocrit under hydroxyurea (HU) therapy (Fattori et al. 2005). Thrombolytic therapy or emergency coronary angioplasty are rarely indicated unless the patient has a high risk profile suggesting atherosclerotic etiology, rather than SCD-associated vascular occlusion. While hematologists may be unwilling to prescribe HU for fear of relative polycythemia and precipitation of a new MI, HU therapy has been shown to improve cardiac perfusion in some children evaluated with myocardial thallium-201 single photon emission computerized tomography (SPECT) (de Montalembert et al. 2004). Sudden cardiac death has become an increasing concern, not only in SCD patients, but also in sickle cell trait carriers, but efficient screening methods to determine which patients could be more susceptible to this complication are still unavailable. A review of heart complications in SCD has been published by Voskaridou et al. (2012).

12.8 Liver Complications

Hepatic disease can be challenging to diagnose and treat in SCD. Chronic liver disease or cirrhosis solely as a consequence of SCD is rare, so actively searching for alternative causes of liver disease, such as alcohol, medication, chronic viral hepatitis, autoimmune hepatitis, and even other genetic conditions, such as Wilson's disease, is mandatory. Iron overload is an expected complication in patients getting transfused throughout their lifetime which may result in chronic liver disease, and can be confirmed by magnetic resonance imaging with T2*. The use of liver transplantation in SCD patients has been reported, but worldwide experience does not exceed 30 cases (Gardner et al. 2014).

In the acute scenario, upper abdominal pain associated with jaundice, also known as "right upper quadrant syndrome", requires differential diagnosis among SCD-associated complications and other diseases, particularly when hyperbilirubinemia is severe (defined by some authors as a bilirubin level above 12–13 mg/dL) (Gardner et al. 2014; Ahn et al. 2005). Common conditions, such as acute cholecystitis (see Fig. 12.4 depicting gallstones), cholangitis, biliary pancreatitis, and viral hepatitis must be ruled out with the appropriate lab exams, i.e. liver and pancreatic enzymes, serology tests, and imaging exams, such as ultrasound, computerized tomography, or magnetic resonance cholangiopancreatography. Physicians at the ED should keep in mind that presentation of common liver diseases may be unusual in SCD patients, and careful history taking is crucial to reach a correct diagnosis in many cases. A SCD patient with acute pancreatitis may remember how the pain typically

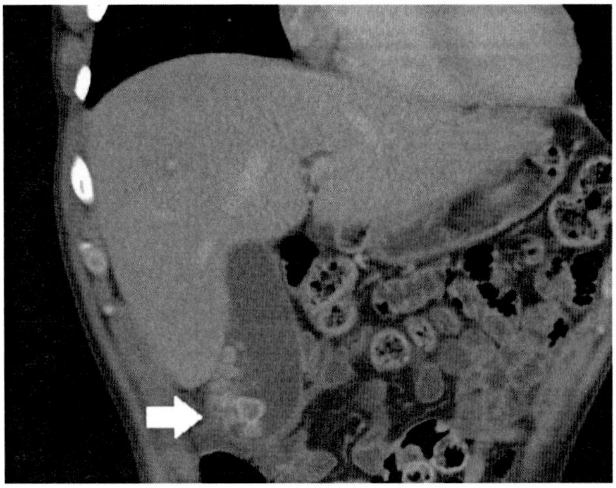

Fig. 12.4 Cholelithiasis. Computerized tomography coronal section showing multiple gallstones (*white arrow*) in an adult SCD patient

started in the abdomen and radiated to the back at first, but by the time he or she was brought to the ED, vaso-occlusive pain crisis had already ensued, precipitating secondary generalized pain and an acute chest syndrome that obscures the original cause of a severe VOE.

SCD-associated complications that should be considered in this setting are hepatic sequestration (HS) and sickle cell intrahepatic cholestasis (SCIC). HS is a life-threatening condition which usually presents with sudden onset of severe anemia associated with painful hepatomegaly and severe jaundice. Liver enzymes can increase by up to ten times normal, but median levels are between 100 and 200 UI/L and may be even only minimally elevated (Norris 2004). Bilirubin levels can reach 30 mg/dL and higher (Berry et al. 2007). Treatment requires emergent blood transfusion and erythrocytapheresis may eventually be considered, since HS has a high rate of mortality.

SCIC may present acutely, or as a chronic progressive complication. It is characterized by severe jaundice with predominantly conjugated bilirubin levels, similarly to those found in HS, with milder changes in liver enzymes than in HS. Absence of significant change in hemoglobin levels helps differentiate it from typical HS. Absence of liver enlargement makes HS less likely, but hepatomegaly may occur in SCIC. Liver failure with coagulopathy and encephalopathy may follow in adults, differently from the spontaneous improvement reported mostly in the pediatric population. Physicians should always consider keeping SCIC patients in hospital until it is certain that bilirubin levels are normalizing and hepatic function is preserved. Exchange blood transfusions to yield a HbS below 20 or 30% have been suggested (Gardner et al. 2014) and even chronic transfusion programs may be indicated for patients with recurrent SCIC, but no scientific evidence is available to determine the actual efficacy of this approach, and no specific treatment for SCIC exists.

12.9 Priapism

Priapism affects over 80% of men with SCD at least once in their lifetime (see Chap. 11). SCD-associated priapism is either acute ischemic or stuttering (Montague et al. 2003), and consists of a compartment syndrome of the penis, caused by sickling that blocks the venous drainage of the corpora cavernosa, resulting in prolonged painful penile erection. It may be bicorporal, affecting only the corpora cavernosa, a more common presentation in children, or tricorporal, also affecting the corpus spongiosum, which is more frequently the case in older SCD patients. Tricorporal priapism probably represents a later stage of bicorporal priapism developing a venous blockade by contiguous compression of the corpus spongiosum by the corpora cavernosa, so it would be reasonable for ED physicians to consider tricorporal priapism a more severe case upfront. Patients should be advised to seek medical attention if priapism does not subside after 4 hours, although, in our experience, a 2-hour long event typically prompts the patient to go to the ED, since 24/7 urology consultation is not widely available, and sometimes requires referencing the patient from a local ED to a tertiary care center, a process that may delay actual treatment. Patients should also be advised to try different strategies at home before coming to the ED (e.g. voiding the urinary bladder, exercise, warm or cold compresses, oral hydration, and even oral pseudoephedrine (Mantadakis et al. 2000) or etilefrine (Gbadoé et al. 2001), etc. Management in hospital should include oral and/or intravenous analgesics, hydration, and urological consultation. Urologists will both confirm ischemia and treat it by aspirating penile blood from the corpora cavernosa under dorsal nerve or penile shaft block. Irrigation of corpora cavernosa with saline or alpha-adrenergic agonists can be performed after aspiration. Phenylephrine injection can be associated to increase the efficacy of treatment, and can even be used as outpatient self-injection if the patient is trained to do so at home (Mantadakis et al. 2000). Other sympathomimetics agents, such as ephedrine, norepinephrine, or epinephrine may be used if phenylephrine is unavailable, but they carry a greater risk of cardiovascular side effects.

Refractoriness is a frequent possibility and can be managed with surgical shunts (e.g. Winter or Ebbehoj corporoglanular shunts, open proximal shunts, open distal shunts, etc.) with varying degrees of post-operative erectile dysfunction. Prosthetic surgery should also be considered for patients with permanent erectile dysfunction, but there still remains controversy on the best timing to perform this type of treatment. Recurrent acute priapism has been successfully managed with chronic low dose PDE5 inhibitors, such as sildenafil in a group of 13 patients (Burnett et al. 2014). Successful anti-androgen therapies with stilbestrol (Serjeant et al. 1985), flutamide (Costabile 1998), or ketoconazole (Hoeh and Levine 2014) have been reported in cases or series of cases, but side effects, such as diminished libido, gynecomastia, and oligo or azoospermia, prevent their use in boys and adolescents, or men wishing to conceive. Stuttering priapism can eventually also cause erectile dysfunction, so despite the lack of specific therapies, its impact should not be underestimated, and urological consultation is key in the search for adequate patient relief.

12.10 Osteopenia and Osteoporosis

Hemoglobin disorders, such as thalassemia and SCD, are recognized as causes of early onset of osteopenia and osteoporosis (Sarrai et al. 2007). Vitamin D deficiency seems to play a prominent role in the pathogenesis of bone mass reduction (Arlet et al. 2013), but other mechanisms involving hemolysis must be involved (Baldanzi et al. 2011). Bone density loss tends to be more severe to the spine than the femoral neck, and pathologic fractures may occur if osteoporosis is left unrecognized. Adults with SCD should be screened yearly with dual-energy X-ray absorptiometry (DXA) scans to measure bone mineral density, but frequency of scans may be reduced to once every other year if no bone density loss is detected. There are no randomized trials to guide treatment of SCD-associated osteopenia/ osteoporosis, so most hematologists rely on evidence obtained from the general population. It is not uncommon to encounter elevated T-scores when measuring bone mineral density in SCD patients, due to pathological fractures or bone infarcts that falsely elevate measurements, so an experienced specialist in scintigraphy should be consulted. Oral calcium carbonate (500 mg bid) and vitamin D (e.g. 50,000 UI of vitamin D2 daily) can be prescribed for osteopenic patients to improve bone marrow density (Adewoye et al. 2008), while full-blown osteoporosis should be additionally managed with oral bisphosphonates, such as sodium alendronate 70 mg weekly. Refractoriness to this approach may occur, and patients whose bone mineral density decreases despite adequate treatment should be considered for parenteral bisphosphonates, such as intravenous zoledronate or pamidronate. Newer therapeutic options, such as denosumab, have yet to be studied in the SCD setting. Patients should also be screened for hypomagnesemia, since low magnesium levels have been associated with lower absorption of vitamin D and may favor bone mass loss.

12.11 Avascular Necrosis

Avascular necrosis (AVN) or osteonecrosis is a well-recognized complication of SCD and prevalent in all genotypes (Mukisi-Mukaza et al. 2000; Mont et al. 2010; Milner et al. 1991). Bilateral involvement is frequent, and may affect femoral or humeral heads (Milner et al. 1993; Poignard et al. 2012). AVN of the femoral head (Fig. 12.5) has been reported more frequently in homozygous SCA, SCD with alpha thalassemia trait, lower HbF, and higher hemoglobin levels (Milner et al. 1991). Shoulder and hip girdle pain are most commonly reported before the range of motion is affected. While simple radiographs have long been used for evaluation when patients complain of pain, magnetic resonance imaging (MRI) should be preferred, since it can detect lesions in the contralateral hip or shoulder before the patient becomes symptomatic or develops femoral or humeral head collapse (Hernigou et al. 2006).

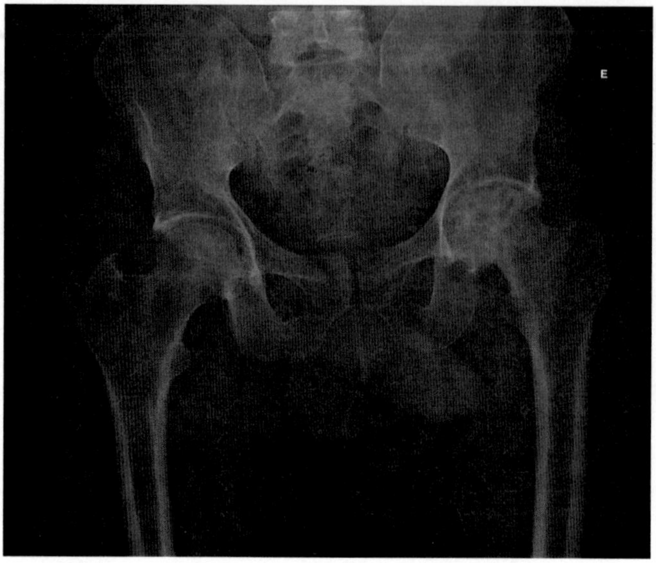

Fig. 12.5 Avascular necrosis of the femoral head. Plain radiograph showing left femoral head with severe collapse and deformation in a male adult sickle cell anemia patient

Compared with other causes of AVN of the femoral head, such as steroid use or alcohol, SCD-associated AVN has an earlier onset and more rapid progression (Hernigou et al. 2006). The natural history of femoral head AVN in SCD progresses from an asymptomatic stage without radiological abnormalities (Steinberg stage 0) to magnetic resonance imaging alterations (Steinberg stage I) (Steinberg et al. 1995), followed by radiographic alterations without (Steinberg stage II) or with a crescent sign (Steinberg stages III and IV); the crescent sign represents overt femoral head collapse, which occurs in 77% of patients. A positive MRI in an asymptomatic patient (stages I and II) represents 95% of chance of progression to pain in 3 years. The average time to progression between pain and collapse is about 35 months, but this can happen in a little as 3 months. Therefore, patients should be screened with MRI on a regular basis, and patients with pain should be evaluated as soon as possible, since pain always precedes collapse (Stoica et al. 2009). Total hip arthroplasty (THA) is the standard of care for end-stage femoral head AVN (Hernigou et al. 2008b; Clarke et al. 1989). Although the risk of post-operative infection and aseptic loosening have decreased with better perioperative care (transfusion, antibiotic prophylaxis), complication rates are still higher than in patients with other indications for THA. Acute chest syndrome is the main SCD-related complication, and patients should be also managed for ACS if fat embolism is considered. Joint preserving procedures, such as single coring or multiple drilling decompression (Al Omran 2013), and autologous stem cell grafting (Hernigou et al. 2008a, 2009) have been used in patients with less severe AVN and pain with improvement, although studies have not determined whether any of these approaches should be preferred. Physical therapy is also useful, and one study found no benefit in adding core decompression to physical therapy in pain management (Neumayr et al. 2006).

Humeral head AVN is more frequently observed in patients with hemoglobin SC disease and S-beta thalassemia than in homozygous SS (Poignard et al. 2012). Nevertheless, the SS genotype is a risk factor for more extensive lesion and more rapid progression to collapse. Patients that have already developed femoral head AVN are also more prone to humeral head AVN and hip involvement predicts earlier humeral collapse. Therefore, patients with isolated humeral head AVN should undergo bilateral hip MRI and be advised of their higher risk for hip AVN. Shoulder AVN also progresses more rapidly: the average time between pain and head collapse is 6 months, and differently from observations in steroid-related AVN, spontaneous regression does not occur. Shoulder arthroplasty is the mainstay of treatment, but as for AVN of any cause, core decompression, arthroscopic debridement, synovectomy, and capsular release may be used to improve pain and delay definitive surgery.

12.12 Ophthalmologic Complications

Retinopathy, particularly proliferative retinopathy (see Fig. 12.6a), is more common in HbSC than HbSS disease and probably caused by retinal ischemia and a proangiogenic component (Nagel et al. 2003; Lopes et al. 2015). SCD-associated retinopathy may also be non-proliferative, which is characterized by a variety of retinal lesions, such as black sunbursts (see Fig. 12.6b) and salmon patches, and while they indicate intraretinal hemorrhage, they do not need specific treatment.

Proliferative retinopathy is classified in five different Goldberg stages (Goldberg 1971):

Stage 1—Peripheral arteriolar occlusion;
Stage 2—Arteriolovenular anastomoses;
Stage 3—Neovascularization;
Stage 4—Vitreous hemorrhage;
Stage 5—Retinal detachment.

Stage 3 retinopathy can present with seafan formation (Fig. 12.6a), and indicates treatment (e.g. laser photocoagulation) to prevent progression and eventual visual loss. There is no preventative measure to avoid or slow the progression of SCD-associated proliferative retinopathy yet.

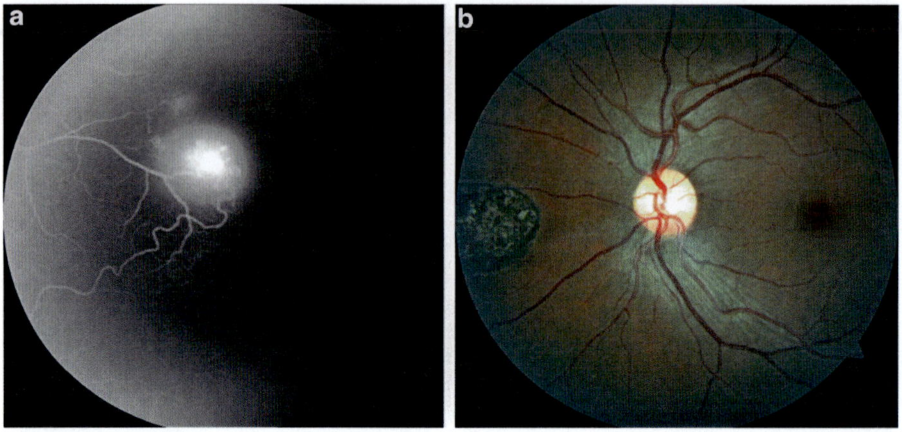

Fig. 12.6 Ophthalmologic complications. Proliferative retinopathy with neovascularization and seafan formation (**a**) in patient with hemoglobin SC disease. Non-proliferative retinopathy with black sunburst lesion (**b**). Courtesy of Dr. Monica Barbosa de Melo and Dr. José Paulo Cabral de Vasconcellos

12.13 Renal Disease

The most common renal manifestation of SCD is loss of concentrating capacity (hyposthenuria). Renal medullary infarctions can result from increased sickling inside the hypertonic milieu of the renal medulla, which is also known to occur in sickle cell trait individuals. This process also causes loss of urine acidification and decreased potassium excretion. Renal disease is one of the most severe chronic complications of SCD and its incidence increases with patients' age. Most patients over 40 years old will have some degree of microalbuminuria or overt proteinuria. Repeated cycles of ischemic injury in the inner medulla lead to sickle cell nephropathy, causing an increased cortical renal blood flow and glomerular filtration rate. Glomerular hyperfiltration leads to misleadingly low creatinine levels, frequently causing physicians to overlook proteinuria before glomerulosclerosis and tubulointerstitial fibrosis eventually result in chronic kidney disease (Sharpe and Thein 2014, 2011).

It is generally recommended to screen SCD adults for microalbuminuria at least once a year. Blood pressure (BP) is a major determinant of renal damage, so BP measurement every time the patients comes to the clinic is mandatory. Although solid scientific evidence in this regard is still lacking, it is safe to say that hypertension (systolic BP over 140 mmHg or diastolic BP over 90 mmHg) should be treated, and in our experience, anti-hypertensive treatment should be considered in patients with BP over 120/80 mmHg, similarly to recommendations for other high-risk populations, such as diabetics. The presence of microalbuminuria can be managed by using angiotensin converting enzyme (ACE) inhibitors, such as captopril and enalapril, although a Cochrane analysis searching for randomized trials addressing the efficacy of in SCD failed to find enough data to recommend ACE inhibitors in this setting. In the experience of our group and others, proteinuria levels may normalize with this strategy, and this approach is relatively safe, with only a mild risk of hypotension.

12.14 Leg Ulcers

Leg ulcers remain a challenge in SCD management. They are more prevalent among men and can affect 20% or more of patients, but are less common in SC disease and S-beta thalassemia. They are more commonly found around the maleolar regions, and frequently start with minor trauma or insect bites. Physicians should routinely examine the patients' ankles during outpatient visits, since small lesions may be overlooked before a full-blown ulcer appears. Leg ulcer may take years to heal or not heal at all, and sometimes can become large and mutilating (Fig. 12.7).

The use of a peptide gel containing a combination of arginine, glycine, and aspartate (RGD) was able to improve healing in a study with 55 patients, but its production has been discontinued (Wethers et al. 1994). Secondary infection should be treated with wide spectrum antibiotics that must be effective against *Salmonella* species. Bed rest and adequate pain management are often major factors for improvement in severe cases. There is no evidence that blood transfusions improve leg ulcers, and studies have failed to demonstrate an association between hydroxyurea and leg ulcer in SCD despite case reports in other populations taking hydroxyurea, such as myeloproliferative neoplasms. (Chaine et al. 2001). Although zinc deficiency has been associated with a higher incidence of leg ulcers, zinc supplementation did not improve leg ulcer healing in a study with 29 Jamaican patients (Serjeant et al. 1970). More recently, a phase I/II clinical trial showed improved leg ulcer

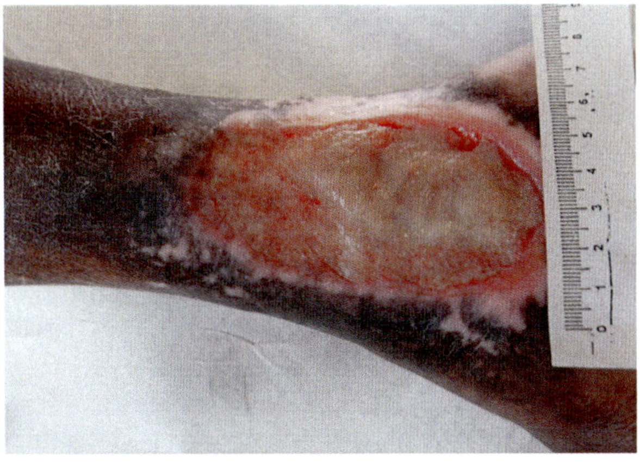

Fig. 12.7 Leg ulcer. Extensive perimaleolar skin ulceration in a 42-year old female sickle cell anemia patient

healing and reduced pain scores following the use of a topical sodium nitrite cream (Minniti et al. 2014). Underlying osteomyelitis should be considered in refractory infection of a leg ulcer, and can be evaluated with plain radiographs, computerized tomography, or magnetic resonance imaging, but sensitivity and specificity fall short from ideal to distinguish between osteomyelitis and bone infarct. Osteomyelitis is most often caused by *Salmonella*, *Staphylococcus aureus* or gram-negative bacilli, so treatment should include antibiotics with an adequate spectrum, but a definitive diagnosis of osteomyelitis should take clinical presentation and other exams into account before indicating sometimes extensive periods of treatment (e.g. treatment may exceed 6 weeks).

12.15 Pulmonary Arterial Hypertension

Pulmonary arterial hypertension (PAH) may represent a major cause of morbidity and mortality in adults with SCD and has been linked to hemolytic processes. PAH is defined as a resting mean pulmonary arterial pressure (mPAP) ≥25 mmHg by right heart catheterization (RHC) (Hoeper et al. 2013) and is caused by restriction in the lumen and wall stiffening of the pulmonary arteries, leading to exercise intolerance, fatigue, peripheral edema and chest pain (Gladwin et al. 2004; Yawn et al. 2014). Prevalence of PAH in SCD has not been accurately established, due to the practical difficulties of confirming the disease by RHC. A surrogate marker for the risk of PAH is increased echocardiography-derived regurgitant triscupid jet velocity (TRV), and TRV above 2.5 m/s has been associated with increased mortality in adults with SCD. A study carried out in 192 patients with SCD showed that 32% had a TRV greater than or equal to 2.5 m/s, while 9.2% presented a TRV of greater than or equal to 3 m/s (Gladwin et al. 2004). A more recent study reported that while 40 % of patients in an SCD cohort displayed a TRV of ≥ 2.5 m/s, right heart catheterization confirmed PH in 10% of the cohort and post-capillary and pre-capillary PH in 6.25% and 3.75%, respectively (Fonseca et al. 2012), although prevalence of PH in SCD, as confirmed by RHC, has been suggested to be approximately 6–11%, and therefore, not insignificant (Ataga and Klings 2014).

Patients should be screened every 1–3 years with transthoracic echocardiogram, or at shorter intervals if presenting with unexplained dyspnea or low oxygen saturation at rest or during exertion; patients with TRV over 3 m/s should be referred to RHC. Treatment options for PAH are still scarce. If PAH is confirmed by RHC, prostacyclin agonists and endothelin receptor antagonists, such as bosentan and ambrisentan, may be considered, although evidence supporting this recommendation is marginal, since no placebo-controlled randomized studies have been completed. A trial with sildenafil was interrupted due to an increase in the incidence of VOEs in the treatment arm. Hydroxyurea may be considered for patients with elevated TRV, since this by itself is a predictor of increased mortality, and red blood cell transfusions should be discussed on a case-by-case basis. Chronic definitive anticoagulation can also be employed in patients with a low risk of bleeding or with confirmed previous venous thromboembolism. There is no consensus as to whether PH constitutes a definitive indication for hematopoietic stem cell transplantation, but improvement in PAH after transplant has been reported (Colombatti et al. 2011).

12.16 Management of the Pregnant SCD Patient

Pregnancy is frequently a situation in which blood transfusions are considered, because of the general belief that HU should not be used in pregnant women, and that HU therapy should be stopped once pregnancy is confirmed. These recommendations are based on animal studies using doses of HU that are higher than those recommended for human use, and evidence that HU increases the risk for birth defects in pregnant women taking HU is lacking. Nevertheless, increased concern with such patients is justified, since SCD tends to be more severe during pregnancy. Even patients with milder forms of SCD, such as SC disease or S-β^+ thalassemia should discuss the risks and benefits of prophylactic transfusion. Only one randomized study has addressed prophylactic transfusion in pregnant SCD patients (Koshy et al. 1988) and failed to show any benefit to either the mothers or their offspring. Nevertheless, several case reports have leaned towards a more aggressive transfusional approach in pregnant women, since the risk of a fatal outcome to either the mother or the child does not seem to be negligible, and prophylactic erythrocytapheresis has emerged as one of the safest options in this setting. A recent systematic review based on the few studies available concluded that prophylactic transfusions may impact adverse maternal outcomes by reducing mortality, vaso-occlusive pain events, pyelonephritis, pulmonary complications including infection, infarction or embolism, and may improve neonatal outcomes by reducing perinatal mortality, neonatal death, and preterm birth (Malinowski et al 2015). The same review suggested that prophylactic transfusions did not affect the occurence of acute chest syndrome, lower urinary tract infection, endometritis, preeclampsia, intrauterine fetal demise or low-birth-weight infants, and highlighted the need for prospective, randomized trials. Combined follow-up with Ob/Gyn and Hematology experts is encouraged, since pregnant SCD women are at higher risk for eclampsia, preterm labor and delivery, deep venous thrombosis, intrauterine growth restriction, urinary tract infections, and sepsis.

In contrast to most pregnant women, SCD patients should not receive iron supplementation during pregnancy and lactation, except if iron deficiency is confirmed by low ferritin levels and transferrin saturation below 20 %.

12.17 Neurological Complications

Stroke, or cerebrovascular accident, while more common in children with SCD, can still occur during adulthood; in a retrospective cohort study of adult 2875 patients followed-up from 1970 through 2008 with SCD in France, 69 patients had experienced at least one stroke, where 27 ischemic strokes and 17 hemorrhagic strokes were recorded during adulthood (>20 years) (Gueguen et al. 2014), supporting suggestions that hemorrhagic strokes may be more common during young adulthood, while ischemic strokes become more frequent in later adulthood (Ohene-Frempong et al. 1998). A study showed that while ischemic stroke in childhood SCD is associated with vasculopathy in over 90% of the cases, the main cause of adult SCD stroke was sickle vaso-occlusion in only 41%, while cardioembolism contributed to 25% of cases (Calvet et al. 2015). Management of acute stroke in adults with SCD does not differ from children due to the lack of studies addressing this particular situation, so chronic blood transfusions are also recommended in ischemic stroke. Hemorrhagic stroke does not require specific treatment for SCD, and can be managed by neurosurgeons as in non-SCD patients. Nevertheless, patients with SCD will be more susceptible to other vaso-occlusive events and infections while hospitalized, so combined hematology and neurosurgery follow-up is recommended, and an SCD expert should recommend the appropriate pre-operative transfusion method for patients undergoing neurosurgical intervention.

Moyamoya syndrome, a chronic, occlusive cerebrovascular disease involving bilateral stenosis or occlusion of cerebral arteries, constitutes a relatively common manifestation of cerebral vasculopathy in SCD (Kassim and DeBaun 2013), more prominently seen in children. Moyamoya can be diagnosed in SCD by either cerebral angiography or magnetic resonance angiography and its development represents a grave prognostic finding in patients that may increase the risk of recurrence of cerebrovascular events, such as overt stroke or transient ischemic attack (Hulbert et al. 2011).

Neuroimaging abnormalities have been reported in adults with SCA and associated with altered cognition (Mackin et al. 2014). Neurocognitive impairment has been recognized to be common in SCD, particularly in those patients with a previous stroke, and probably accentuates with age due to continual hypoxia and chronic anemia even in neurologically intact SCD adults (Vichinsky et al. 2010). Silent cerebral infarcts (SCIs) have also been recognized in the adult SCD population (Vichinsky et al. 2010; Kugler et al. 1993; Silva et al. 2009), although most studies have focused in the pediatric population. There is still some discussion on the radiological definition of SCI in adults (DeBaun et al. 2012), which further complicates studies in this population. One study reported that almost 40% of the patients will reach the age of 18 with SCI (Bernaudin et al. 2015), but there still is no specific management for adults with SCD-associated SCI.

Finally, a high burden of, possibly pain-related, sleep disordered breathing and other sleep-related complaints have also been reported in the adult SCD population and may affect the quality of life of these individuals (Sharma et al. 2015).

12.18 Blood Transfusion and Iron Chelation in Adult SCD

The indication for blood transfusion in adults with SCD is less well studied than in children. Transfused blood should ideally always be matched for ABO, C, D, E, and K antigens, and donors must not carry sickle cell trait. Acute indication of blood transfusion should be considered in cases with symptomatic acute anemia, which usually only happens when hemoglobin levels drop more than 2 g/dL below basal hemoglobin levels. The amount of transfused blood should be just enough to improve symptoms, rather than aiming at specific hemoglobin values. Refractory pain crisis is a common indication for exchange transfusion in the acute setting, as well as acute chest syndrome. Emergent exchange transfusion or erythrocytapheresis is strongly recommended for acute stroke and acute chest syndrome that is developing the need for mechanical ventilation. Special care should be taken if transfusing patients with suspected aplastic crisis, because hemoglobin recovery can be more rapid than anticipated and result in overcorrection of anemia with severe complications, such as acute chest syndrome or stroke.

With regard to chronic blood transfusion, while the STOP study has clearly shown the benefits of transfusion in children with abnormal transcranial Dopplerfluxometry (TCD) for the prevention of stroke (Adams et al. 1998), there is no defined role for blood transfusion or TCD in the prevention of stroke in adults. Therefore, the use of chronic transfusion in SCD adults with stroke relies on the extrapolation of the results from the STOP 2 study, since no safe time interval for stopping blood transfusion could be determined. Other frequent indications of chronic use of blood transfusion include recurrent pain crisis with lack of response to HU, severe anemia not responsive to HU, end-stage renal disease, and heart failure. The aims of a transfusion program vary based on the indication; typically maintaining HbS levels below 30% for the first couple of years for stroke, HbS below 50% after the second year for stroke and for refractory pain crises, or an average Hb level of 9 g/dL for other indications. It is of utmost importance to refrain for overcorrecting anemia: Hb levels above 10 g/dL (or hematocrit above 30%) are associated with an increased risk of severe iatrogenic acute vaso-occlusive events, or even stroke. In spite of the improvements in the quality assurance of blood products, all patients should be immunized against hepatitis B, and patients that receive blood transfusions should be periodically screened (once a year) for hepatitis C and HIV.

Chronic blood transfusions will lead to a variable degree of iron overload. Severely anemic patients tend to receive "top-up" transfusion, with a higher iron balance than patients subjected to exchange transfusion, while erythrocytapheresis causes the least amount of iron load. High ferritin levels, combined with a transferrin saturation level above 45–50% and transfusional history, should be taken into account to determine the likelihood of iron overload, but more accurate assessment of iron overload in SCD patients should preferably be based on magnetic resonance imaging with T2* protocols (Porter and Garbowski 2013). In comparison with thalassemia patients, SCD patients present with a lower degree of iron overload, predominantly accumulated in the liver, with cardiac and pancreatic iron overload being extremely rare. Iron chelation can be prescribed with any of the three available agents (deferoxamine, deferiprone, and deferasirox). Studies have confirmed the efficacy of all chelators in removing excess liver iron in SCD, albeit with significant difference among the numbers of patients studied (Porter and Garbowski 2013). Deferasirox has been increasingly the drug of choice to chelate iron overloaded patients because of its oral route of administration (compared to parenteral use of deferoxamine) and convenient schedule of treatment (once daily dissolved in water, compared with thrice daily for deferiprone). Nevertheless, side effects of deferasirox include increases in creatinine levels and proteinuria. SCD patients are more prone to develop microalbuminuria and end stage renal disease than other patients treated with iron chelators, so it is still undetermined whether using this chelator in patients with renal disease is safe. Combination therapy with deferoxamine and deferiprone is preferred in the rare cases with documented cardiac iron overload.

12.19 Curative Treatment: Hematopoietic Stem Cell Transplantation

Similarly to the pediatric setting, the only curative treatment available for adults is hematopoietic stem cell transplantation (HSCT). As expected, published scientific reports show that, in contrast to younger children, patients over 16 years of age have only been offered cellular-based approaches for sickle cell disease from 2004 onwards.

Evidence in this group is much more scarce than in the pediatric population, and a retrospective search on PubMed yielded nine reports with a total not exceeding 60 cases of sickle cell anemia (SCA) patients over 21 years of age that have been transplanted, with only 21 patients aged over 30 years worldwide (Table 12.2). The Multicenter Pilot Investigation of Bone Marrow Transplantation in Adults with Sickle Cell Disease (STRIDE) has recently reported 22 SCD patients prepared for HSCT with busulfan 13.2mg/kg, fludarabine 150mg/m2 and anti-thymocyte globulin 6mg/kg (Krishnamurti et al. 2015, oral communication). Another oral communication from an international survey by Eurocord-Monacord/European Group for Blood and Marrow Transplantation (EBMT) and Center for International Blood and Marrow Transplant Research (CIBMTR) (Capelli et al. 2015), reported the outcomes after HLA-matched sibling HSCT of 154 SCD patients over 16 years of age prepared most frequently with myeloablative combination of busulfan and cyclophosphamide. There have been major concerns regarding the toxicity of myeloablative approaches, thus conditioning regimens used in these studies vary widely and employ different combinations of busulfan, cyclophosphamide, anti-thymocyte globulin (ATG), fludarabine, and total body irradiation. The type of ATG, the inclusion of other drugs, and radiation dose also vary. There is no consensus regarding the ideal stem cell source, which can range from matched sibling to haploidentical bone marrow, but encouraging results with

Table 12.2 Stem cell transplantation in adult SCD patients (over 16-21 years of age)

Year	Author	n	Age(s) or range reported (years)	Disease	Conditioning regimen	Reference
2004	Jacobsohn et al.	1	22.5	SCD	Busulfan 6.4 mg/kg Fludarabine 180 mg/m^2 hATG 40 mg/kg × 4 d	Jacobsohn et al. (2004)
2007	Bernaudin et al.	5	Over 15 (range 2.2–22.0)	SS, S-beta	Busulfan 485 mg/m^2 Cyclophosphamide 50 mg/kg × 4 d rATG 5 mg/kg × 4 d	Bernaudin et al. (2007)
2007	Panepinto et al.	3	Over 21 (range 2–27)	SS, S-beta, other	Busulfan 16 mg/kg Cyclophosphamide 50 mg/kg × 4 d ± other (fludarabine/TBI/ATG/bleomycin)	Panepinto et al. (2007)
2007	Horwitz et al.	2	21 and 27	2 SS	Fludarabine 24 or 30 mg/m^2 × 4 d Cyclophosphamide 50 mg/kg × 4 d TBI 200 cGy Alemtuzumab 100 mg × 5 d	Horwitz et al. (2007)
2008	Brodsky et al.	1	33	Combination of SC, PNH, and ITP	Fludarabine 30 mg/m^2 × 5 d Cyclophosphamide 14.5 mg/kg × 2 d TBI 200 cGy	Brodsky et al. (2008)
2010	Sauter et al.	1	22	Combination of SCD and Hodgkin's disease	"Reduced intensity regimen"	Sauter et al. (2010)
2012	Bolaños-Meade et al.	12	21–46	10 SS 2 SC	rATG 0.5 mg/kg × 1 d rATG 2 mg/kg × 2 d Fludarabine 30 mg/m^2 × 5 d Cyclophosphamide 14.5 mg/kg × 2 d TBI 2 Gy	Bolaños-Meade et al. (2012)
2013	Matthes-Martin et al.	1	24.8	SCD	Fludarabine 40 mg/m^2 × 4 d Thiotepa 5 mg/kg × 2 d Melphalan 140 mg/m^2 × 1 d ATG (not specified)	Matthes-Martin et al. (2013)
2014	Hsieh et al.	27	21–65	SS, SC, S-beta (1 beta thalassemia)	Alemtuzumab 0.03 mg/kg × 1 d Alemtuzumab 0.10 mg/kg × 1 d Alemtuzumab 0.30 mg/kg × 3 d TBI 300 cGy	Hsieh et al. (2014)

SCD sickle cell disease, *hATG* horse anti-thymocyte globulin, *SS* homozygous sickle cell anemia, *S-beta* S-beta thalassemia, *rATG* rabbit anti-thymocyte globulin, *TBI* total body irradiation, *PNH* paroxysmal nocturnal hemoglobinuria, *ITP* immune thrombocytopenic purpura, *SC* hemoglobin SC disease

the latter may mean that successful transplantation in sickle cell patients can become less dependent on the stem cell source than on the use of adequate conditioning regimens with optimized supportive care. Success rates have been largely similar to those found in children with very low mortality rates (under 10%) and a low incidence of graft-versus-host disease.

Other curative approaches to SCA are still under development—gene therapy targeting autologous stem cells for subsequent transplantation is one of the most promising options, and will be addressed in Chap. 16.

References

Adams RJ, McKie VC, Hsu L et al (1998) Prevention of a first stroke by transfusions in children with sickle cell anemia and abnormal results on transcranial Doppler ultrasonography. N Engl J Med 339(1):5–11

Adewoye AH, Chen TC, Ma Q et al (2008) Sickle cell bone disease: response to vitamin D and calcium. Am J Hematol 83(4):271–274

Ahn H, Li CS, Wang W (2005) Sickle cell hepatopathy: clinical presentation, treatment, and outcome in pediatric and adult patients. Pediatr Blood Cancer 45(2):184–190

Al Omran A (2013) Multiple drilling compared with standard core decompression for avascular necrosis of the femoral head in sickle cell disease patients. Arch Orthop Trauma Surg 133(5):609–613

Arlet JB, Courbebaisse M, Chatellier G et al (2013) Relationship between vitamin D deficiency and bone fragility in sickle cell disease: a cohort study of 56 adults. Bone 52(1):206–211

Ataga KI, Klings ES (2014) Pulmonary hypertension in sickle cell disease: diagnosis and management. Hematology Am Soc Hematol Educ Program 2014(1):425–431

Baldanzi G, Traina F, Neto JFM et al (2011) Low bone mass density is associated with hemolysis in Brazilian patients with sickle cell disease. Clinics 66(5):801–805

Ballas SK, Baxter JK, Riddick G (2006) Folate supplementation and twinning in patients with sickle cell disease. Am J Hematol 81(4):296–297

Bernaudin F, Socie G, Kuentz M et al (2007) Long-term results of related myeloablative stem-cell transplantation to cure sickle cell disease. Blood 110(7):2749–2756

Bernaudin F, Verlhac S, Arnaud C et al (2015) Chronic and acute anemia and extracranial internal carotid stenosis are risk factors for silent cerebral infarcts in sickle cell anemia. Blood 125(10):1653–1661

Berry PA, Cross TJ, Thein SL et al (2007) Hepatic dysfunction in sickle cell disease: a new system of classification based on global assessment. Clin Gastroenterol Hepatol 5(12):1469–1476

Bijur PE, Latimer CT, Gallagher EJ (2003) Validation of a verbally administered numerical rating scale of acute pain for use in the emergency department. Acad Emerg Med 10(4):390–392

Bolaños-Meade J, Fuchs EJ, Luznik L et al (2012) HLA-haploidentical bone marrow transplantation with posttransplant cyclophosphamide expands the donor pool for patients with sickle cell disease. Blood 120(22):4285–4291

Brodsky RA, Luznik L, Bolaños-Meade J et al (2008) Reduced intensity HLA-haploidentical BMT with post transplantation cyclophosphamide in nonmalignant hematologic diseases. Bone Marrow Transplant 42(8):523–527

Burnett AL, Anele UA, Trueheart IN, Strouse JJ, Casella JF (2014) Randomized controlled trial of sildenafil for preventing recurrent ischemic priapism in sickle cell disease. Am J Med 127(7):664–668

Caldas MC, Meira ZA, Barbosa MM (2008) Evaluation of 107 patients with sickle cell anemia through tissue Doppler and myocardial performance index. J Am Soc Echocardiogr 21(10):1163–1167

Calvet D, Bernaudin F, Gueguen A et al (2015) First ischemic stroke in sickle-cell disease: are there any adult specificities? Stroke 46(8):2315–2317

Cappelli B, Bernaudin F, Ruggeri A et al (2015) Hematopoietic stem cell transplantation from HLA identical sibling for sickle cell disease an international survey on behalf of eurocord-Monacord, EBMT paediatric disease working party and CIBMTR. Blood 126(23):541

Chaine B, Neonato MG, Girot R, Aractingi S (2001) Cutaneous adverse reactions to hydroxyurea in patients with sickle cell disease. Arch Dermatol 137(4):467–470

Charache S, Dover GJ, Moyer MA, Moore JW (1987) Hydroxyurea-induced augmentation of fetal hemoglobin production in patients with sickle cell anemia. Blood 69(1):109–116

Charache S, Terrin ML, Moore RD et al (1995) Effect of hydroxyurea on the frequency of painful crises in sickle cell anemia. Investigators of the Multicenter Study of Hydroxyurea in Sickle Cell Anemia. N Engl J Med 332(20):1317–1322

Charache S, Barton FB, Moore RD et al (1996) Hydroxyurea and sickle cell anemia. Clinical utility of a myelosuppressive "switching" agent. The Multicenter Study of Hydroxyurea in Sickle Cell Anemia. Medicine (Baltimore) 75(6):300–326

Clarke HJ, Jinnah RH, Brooker AF, Michaelson JD (1989) Total replacement of the hip for avascular necrosis in sickle cell disease. J Bone Joint Surg Br 71(3):465–470

Colombatti R, Varotto E, Ricato S et al (2011) Tricuspid regurgitant velocity elevation in a three-year old child with sickle cell anemia and recurrent acute chest syndromes reversed not by hydroxyurea but by bone marrow transplantation. Hematol Rep 3(2):e12

Costabile RA (1998) Successful treatment of stutter priapism with an antiandrogen. Tech Urol 4(3):167–168

de Montalembert M, Maunoury C, Acar P et al (2004) Myocardial ischaemia in children with sickle cell disease. Arch Dis Child 89(4):359–362

DeBaun MR, Armstrong FD, McKinstry RC et al (2012) Silent cerebral infarcts: a review on a prevalent and progressive cause of neurologic injury in sickle cell anemia. Blood 119(20):4587–4596

Dhar M, Bellevue R, Carmel R (2003) Pernicious anemia with neuropsychiatric dysfunction in a patient with sickle cell anemia treated with folate supplementation. N Engl J Med 348(22): 2204–2207

Diav-Citrin O, Hunnisett L, Sher GD, Koren G (1999) Hydroxyurea use during pregnancy: a case report in sickle cell disease and review of the literature. Am J Hematol 60(2):148–150

Fattori A, de Souza RA, Saad ST, Costa FF (2005) Acute myocardial infarction in sickle cell disease: a possible complication of hydroxyurea treatment. Hematol J 5(7):589–590

Fitzhugh CD, Lauder N, Jonassaint JC et al (2010) Cardiopulmonary complications leading to premature deaths in adult patients with sickle cell disease. Am J Hematol 85(1):36–40

Fonseca GH, Souza R, Salemi VM, Jardim CV, Gualandro SF (2012) Pulmonary hypertension diagnosed by right heart catheterisation in sickle cell disease. Eur Respir J 39(1):112–118

Gardner K, Suddle A, Kane P et al (2014) How we treat sickle hepatopathy and liver transplantation in adults. Blood 123(15):2302–2307

Garozzo G, Disca S, Fidone C, Bonomo P (2000) Azoospermia in a patient with sickle cell disease treated with hydroxyurea. Haematologica 85(11):1216–1218

Gbadoé AD, Atakouma Y, Kusiaku K, Assimadi JK (2001) Management of sickle cell priapism with etilefrine. Arch Dis Child 85(1):52–53

Gillette PN, Manning JM, Cerami A (1971) Increased survival of sickle-cell erythrocytes after treatment in vitro with sodium cyanate. Proc Natl Acad Sci U S A 68(11):2791–2793

Gladwin MT, Sachdev V, Jison ML et al (2004) Pulmonary hypertension as a risk factor for death in patients with sickle cell disease. N Engl J Med 350(9):886–895

Goldberg MF (1971) Classification and pathogenesis of proliferative sickle retinopathy. Am J Ophthalmol 71(3):649–665

Gueguen A, Mahevas M, Nzouakou R et al (2014) Sickle-cell disease stroke throughout life: a retrospective study in an adult referral center. Am J Hematol 89(3):267–272

Hernigou P, Habibi A, Bachir D, Galacteros F (2006) The natural history of asymptomatic osteonecrosis of the femoral head in adults with sickle cell disease. J Bone Joint Surg Am 88(12):2565–2572

Hernigou P, Daltro G, Filippini P, Mukasa MM, Manicom O (2008a) Percutaneous implantation of autologous bone marrow osteoprogenitor cells as treatment of bone avascular necrosis related to sickle cell disease. Open Orthop J 2:62–65

Hernigou P, Zilber S, Filippini P et al (2008b) Total THA in adult osteonecrosis related to sickle cell disease. Clin Orthop Relat Res 466(2):300–308

Hernigou P, Poignard A, Zilber S, Rouard H (2009) Cell therapy of hip osteonecrosis with autologous bone marrow grafting. Indian J Orthop 43(1):40–45

Hoeh MP, Levine LA (2014) Prevention of recurrent ischemic priapism with ketoconazole: evolution of a treatment protocol and patient outcomes. J Sex Med 11(1):197–204

Hoeper MM, Bogaard HJ, Condliffe R et al (2013) Definitions and diagnosis of pulmonary hypertension. J Am Coll Cardiol 62(25 Suppl):D42–D50

Horwitz ME, Spasojevic I, Morris A et al (2007) Fludarabine-based nonmyeloablative stem cell transplantation for sickle cell disease with and without renal failure: clinical outcome and pharmacokinetics. Biol Blood Marrow Transplant 13(12):1422–1426

Howard J, Hart N, Roberts-Harewood M et al (2015) Guideline on the management of acute chest syndrome in sickle cell disease. Br J Haematol 169(4):492–505

Hsieh MM, Fitzhugh CD, Weitzel RP et al (2014) Nonmyeloablative HLA-matched sibling allogeneic hematopoietic stem cell transplantation for severe sickle cell phenotype. JAMA 312(1):48–56

Hulbert ML, McKinstry RC, Lacey JL et al (2011) Silent cerebral infarcts occur despite regular blood transfusion therapy after first strokes in children with sickle cell disease. Blood 117(3):772–779

Jacobsohn DA, Duerst R, Tse W, Kletzel M (2004) Reduced intensity haemopoietic stem-cell transplantation for treatment of non-malignant diseases in children. Lancet 364(9429):156–162

Kassim AA, DeBaun MR (2013) Sickle cell disease, vasculopathy, and therapeutics. Annu Rev Med 64:451–466

Koshy M, Burd L, Wallace D, Moawad A, Baron J (1988) Prophylactic red-cell transfusions in pregnant patients with sickle cell disease. A randomized cooperative study. N Engl J Med 319(22):1447–1452

Krishnamurti L, Sullivan KM, Kamani NR et al (2015) Results of a multicenter pilot investigation of bone marrow transplantation in adults with sickle cell disease (STRIDE). Blood 126(23):543

Kugler S, Anderson B, Cross D et al (1993) Abnormal cranial magnetic resonance imaging scans in sickle-cell disease. Neurological correlates and clinical implications. Arch Neurol 50(6):629–635

Lanzkron S, Strouse JJ, Wilson R et al (2008) Systematic review: hydroxyurea for the treatment of adults with sickle cell disease. Ann Intern Med 148(12):939–955

Lima CS, Ueti OM, Ueti AA et al (2008) Enalapril therapy and cardiac remodelling in sickle cell disease patients. Acta Cardiol 63(5):599–602

Lopes FC, Traina F, Almeida CB et al (2015) Key endothelial cell angiogenic mechanisms are stimulated by the circulating milieu in sickle cell disease and attenuated by hydroxyurea. Haematologica 100(6):730–739

Mackin RS, Insel P, Truran D et al (2014) Neuroimaging abnormalities in adults with sickle cell anemia: associations with cognition. Neurology 82(10):835–841

Malinowski AK, Shehata N, D'Souza R et al (2015) Prophylactic transfusion for pregnant women with sickle cell disease: a systematic review and meta-analysis. Blood 126(21):2424-35

Mantadakis E, Ewalt DH, Cavender JD, Rogers ZR, Buchanan GR (2000) Outpatient penile aspiration and epinephrine irrigation for young patients with sickle cell anemia and prolonged priapism. Blood 95(1):78–82

Matthes-Martin S, Lawitschka A, Fritsch G et al (2013) Stem cell transplantation after reduced-intensity conditioning for sickle cell disease. Eur J Haematol 90(4):308–312

Milner PF, Kraus AP, Sebes JI et al (1991) Sickle cell disease as a cause of osteonecrosis of the femoral head. N Engl J Med 325(21):1476–1481

Milner PF, Kraus AP, Sebes JI et al (1993) Osteonecrosis of the humeral head in sickle cell disease. Clin Orthop Relat Res 289:136–143

Minniti CP, Gorbach AM, Xu D et al (2014) Topical sodium nitrite for chronic leg ulcers in patients with sickle cell anaemia: a phase 1 dose-finding safety and tolerability trial. Lancet Haematol 1(3):e95–e103

Mont MA, Zywiel MG, Marker DR, McGrath MS, Delanois RE (2010) The natural history of untreated asymptomatic osteonecrosis of the femoral head: a systematic literature review. J Bone Joint Surg Am 92(12):2165–2170

Montague DK, Jarow J, Broderick GA et al (2003) American Urological Association guideline on the management of priapism. J Urol 170(4 Pt 1):1318–1324

Mukisi-Mukaza M, Elbaz A, Samuel-Leborgne Y et al (2000) Prevalence, clinical features, and risk factors of osteonecrosis of the femoral head among adults with sickle cell disease. Orthopedics 23(4):357–363

Myrvik MP, Drendel AL, Brandow AM et al (2015) A comparison of pain assessment measures in pediatric sickle cell disease: visual analog scale versus numeric rating scale. J Pediatr Hematol Oncol 37:190–194

Nagel RL, Fabry ME, Steinberg MH (2003) The paradox of hemoglobin SC disease. Blood Rev 17(3):167–178

Neumayr LD, Aguilar C, Earles AN et al (2006) Physical therapy alone compared with core decompression and physical therapy for femoral head osteonecrosis in sickle cell disease. Results of a multicenter study at a mean of three years after treatment. J Bone Joint Surg Am 88(12):2573–2582

Norris WE (2004) Acute hepatic sequestration in sickle cell disease. J Natl Med Assoc 96(9):1235–1239

Ohene-Frempong K, Weiner SJ, Sleeper LA et al (1998) Cerebrovascular accidents in sickle cell disease: rates and risk factors. Blood 91(1):288–294

Okomo U, Meremikwu MM (2012) Fluid replacement therapy for acute episodes of pain in people with sickle cell disease. Cochrane Database Syst Rev 6, CD005406

Panepinto JA, Walters MC, Carreras J et al (2007) Matched-related donor transplantation for sickle cell disease: report from the Center for International Blood and Transplant Research. Br J Haematol 137(5):479–485

Patrick PA, Rosenthal BM, Iezzi CA, Brand DA (2015) Timely pain management in the emergency department. J Emerg Med 48(3):267–273

Platt OS, Thorington BD, Brambilla DJ et al (1991) Pain in sickle cell disease. Rates and risk factors. N Engl J Med 325(1):11–16

Poignard A, Flouzat-Lachaniette CH, Amzallag J, Galacteros F, Hernigou P (2012) The natural progression of symptomatic humeral head osteonecrosis in adults with sickle cell disease. J Bone Joint Surg Am 94(2):156–162

Porter J, Garbowski M (2013) Consequences and management of iron overload in sickle cell disease. Hematology Am Soc Hematol Educ Program 2013:447–456

Rabb LM, Grandison Y, Mason K et al (1983) A trial of folate supplementation in children with homozygous sickle cell disease. Br J Haematol 54(4):589–594

Sachdev V, Machado RF, Shizukuda Y et al (2007) Diastolic dysfunction is an independent risk factor for death in patients with sickle cell disease. J Am Coll Cardiol 49(4):472–479

Sarrai M, Duroseau H, D'Augustine J, Moktan S, Bellevue R (2007) Bone mass density in adults with sickle cell disease. Br J Haematol 136(4):666–672

Sauter C, Rausen AR, Barker JN (2010) Successful unrelated donor cord blood transplantation for adult sickle cell disease and Hodgkin lymphoma. Bone Marrow Transplant 45(7):1252

Schnog JB, van der Dijs FP, Brouwer DA et al (2000) Plasma homocysteine levels in sickle cell disease and the need for folate supplementation. J Pediatr Hematol Oncol 22(2):184–185, author reply 185–186

Serjeant GR, Galloway RE, Gueri MC (1970) Oral zinc sulphate in sickle-cell ulcers. Lancet 2(7679):891–892

Serjeant GR, de Ceulaer K, Maude GH (1985) Stilboestrol and stuttering priapism in homozygous sickle-cell disease. Lancet 2(8467):1274–1276

Sharma S, Efird JT, Knupp C et al (2015) Sleep disorders in adult sickle cell patients. J Clin Sleep Med 11(3):219–223

Sharpe CC, Thein SL (2011) Sickle cell nephropathy – a practical approach. Br J Haematol 155(3):287–297

Sharpe CC, Thein SL (2014) How I treat renal complications in sickle cell disease. Blood 123(24):3720–3726

Silva GS, Vicari P, Figueiredo MS et al (2009) Brain magnetic resonance imaging abnormalities in adult patients with sickle cell disease: correlation with transcranial Doppler findings. Stroke 40(7):2408–2412

Simmer K, Iles CA, James C, Thompson RP (1987) Are iron-folate supplements harmful? Am J Clin Nutr 45(1):122–125

Steinberg ME, Hayken GD, Steinberg DR (1995) A quantitative system for staging avascular necrosis. J Bone Joint Surg Br 77(1):34–41

Stoica Z, Dumitrescu D, Popescu M et al (2009) Imaging of avascular necrosis of femoral head: familiar methods and newer trends. Curr Health Sci J 35(1):23–28

Vichinsky EP, Neumayr LD, Gold JI et al (2010) Neuropsychological dysfunction and neuroimaging abnormalities in neurologically intact adults with sickle cell anemia. JAMA 303(18):1823–1831

Voskaridou E, Christoulas D, Terpos E (2012) Sickle-cell disease and the heart: review of the current literature. Br J Haematol 157(6):664–673

Wethers DL, Ramirez GM, Koshy M et al (1994) Accelerated healing of chronic sickle-cell leg ulcers treated with RGD peptide matrix. RGD Study Group. Blood 84(6):1775–1779

Yawn BP, Buchanan GR, Afenyi-Annan AN et al (2014) Management of sickle cell disease: summary of the 2014 evidence-based report by expert panel members. JAMA 312(10):1033–1048

Chapter 13
Hemoglobin Sβ Thalassemia, SC Disease and SD Disease: Clinical and Laboratorial Aspects

Sara T. Olalla Saad and Simone O. Gilli

Abstract Sickle cell disorders are inherited hemolytic anemias, associated with the presence of Hemoglobin S. This group of disorders comprises homozygotes (HbSS), compound heterozygotes for hemoglobin C (HbSC) or β-thalassemia (Sβ thalassemia) (the most frequent associations) and, uncommonly, hemoglobin D (HbSD) and hemoglobin E (HbSE). This abnormal phenotype is caused by mutations in the Beta globin genes of both chromosomes 11. Thus, these disorders are recessively inherited and abnormalities in both alleles lead to structural defects in the beta-globin chain (HbS, HbC, HbD, HbE), or a reduction in its expression (thalassemia and HbE). Consequently, normal HbA, which is an $\alpha_2\beta_2$ tetramer, is absent and substituted by the mutated hemoglobins, containing an $\alpha_2\beta_2^{\text{Mutated}}$ tetramer. Ultimately, the clinical phenotype is caused by the relatively high amounts of the $\alpha_2\beta_2^{\text{sickle}}$ tetramer, which allows hemoglobin polymerization and, in turn, leads to vasoocclusion, the hallmark of all sickle cell disorders. In this chapter, we will discuss clinical and laboratorial aspects of the compound sickle cell disorders SC, SD and Sβ thalassemia. In this book, sickle cell anemia is a synonymous for the homozygote state and it is approached elsewhere.

Keywords Genotype • Hemoglobinopathy SC • Hemoglobinopathy SD • Sβ thalassemia

---

S.T.O. Saad (✉) • S.O. Gilli
Hematology Center, School of Medical Sciences, University of Campinas/Hemocentro-Unicamp, Rua Carlos Chagas, 480, Cidade Universitaria Zeferino Vaz, 13083-878 Campinas, São Paulo, Brazil
e-mail: sara@unicamp.br; mona@unicamp.br

© Springer International Publishing Switzerland 2016

F.F. Costa, N. Conran (eds.), *Sickle Cell Anemia*,
DOI 10.1007/978-3-319-06713-1_13

13.1 Hemoglobinopathy SC

Despite the high prevalence of Hemoglobin SC disease, this hemoglobinopathy is often regarded as being clinically milder than homozygotic sickle cell anemia (HbSS) and very little is known specifically regarding this condition. After Hb SS disease, hemoglobinopathy SC is the most frequent sickle cell disorder worldwide. Hemoglobin C, as HbS, is also African-derived and is caused by a mutation in codon 6 of the Beta-globin chain; however this mutation changes glutamic acid to lysine, instead of to valine, as occurs in HbS. In HbSC disease, red cells contain approximately 50 % HbS and 50 % HbC; however, the presence of HbC is associated with increased K-Cl cotransport activity, which induces loss of K^+ and intracellular water, in turn facilitating the polymerization of HbS (Nagel et al. 2003), Thus, HbSC carriers suffer from acute episodes of vaso-occlusion and a number of complications that are secondary to chronic disease. While hemoglobinopathy SC is generally believed to be a clinically milder disease, compared to sickle cell anemia (homozygotes), it presents a higher frequency of proliferative retinopathy.

13.1.1 Epidemiology

Hemoglobin C is an African-derived mutation and reaches a frequency of 20 % in northern Ghana and Burkina Faso. Recently, genotypic data for sickle cell disease (Saraf et al. 2014) showed that the HbSC genotype ranges from 4 to 12 % of sickle cell diseases in Nigeria and Senegal, but reaches 49.6–92.2 % in Burkina Faso, located in northwestern Africa, bordering Benin. In the Americas and UK, the HbSC genotype ranges from 17.8 to 24.3 % of the total sickle cell disease patient population. Curiously, in Brazil, some regions in the North of the country and in the Northeast of the state of Minas Gerais present an equal incidence of HbSS and HbSC among newborns, reaching 0.1 % of neonates (Fernandes et al. 2010).

13.1.2 Clinical Data

Growth and Development In the Jamaica cohort, the height and weight of HbSC children was found not to differ from normal controls, from birth up to 5 years of age. Anthropometric measurements in 103 HbSC (47 male and 56 female) adult patients from our center (Hematology Center, University of Campinas, Brazil) show a median body mass index (BMI) of 25.9 (min–max; 18.8–46.6), median weight of 68 kg (39–109.2) and median height of 165 cm (143–183), which are similar those of the Brazilian population in general (http://www.ibge.gov.br/home/estatistica/populacao/censo2010/default.shtm). Data are presented in Table 13.1.

Painful Episodes In our cohort, at the time of writing, 8.7 % of HbSC patients had experienced at least two pain episodes per year requiring hospitalization. More than

Table 13.1 Clinical data for double heterozygotes for the sickle cell diseases

Diagnosis	HbSC	HbSβ^0	HbSβ$^+$
Number	103	31	15
Female:Male	56:47	19:12	6:9
Age (y)	38 (13–70)	35 (15:53)	37 (23:56)
Weight (kg)	68 (39.0–109.2)	51 (45:64)	69.4 (50–81)
Stature (m)	1.65 (1.43–1.83)	1.62 (1.57–1.69)	1.63 (1.52–1.82)
Body mass index (BMI)	25.9 (18.80–46.64)	19.7 (17.75–24.42)	25.1 (22.47–28.69)
Retinopathy	39.8 %	10.3 %	26.6 %
ACS	16.5 %	20.6 %	57.1 %
Priapism	2.9 %	10.0 %	0 %
Osteonecrosis	24.2 %	10.7 %	26.6 %
VTE	6.8 %	3.57 %	7.1 %
Stroke	3.9 %	6.9 %	6.6 %
Cholecystopathy	32.3 %	66.6 %	46.6 %
Splenic sequestration	2.9 %	0 %	6.6 %
Leg ulcer	2.9 %	7.1 %	0 %
Osteopenia	27.9 %	46 %	10 %
Osteoporosis	8.8 %	0 %	0 %
RBC transfusion	40.7 %	96.5 %	86.6 %
In hydroxyurea therapy	7.8 %	48 %	27 %

Clinical data were collected from cohorts of patients accompanied at the Hemoglobinopathies Clinic, Hematology Center, University of Campinas, at the time of writing. Percentages refer to the proportion of patients that had experienced the referred manifestation or were undergoing specified therapy

ACS acute chest syndrome, *VTE* venous thromboembolism, *RBC* red blood cell

50 % of patients were asymptomatic and had received an incidental diagnosis after routine blood counts, ophthalmological visits or family investigation of a proband with diagnosis of hemoglobinopathy, based on newborn screening. These data are in accordance with those of Platt et al. (1991) who reported an incidence of 0.4 painful episodes/HbSC patient-year, less than half the rate observed in homozygotes.

Complications Complications occur frequently in this population; in our cohort, 64.08 % of patients had experienced either an acute or a chronic clinical manifestation at least once. As shown in Table 13.1, retinopathy was the most frequent complication in the HbSC cohort with a prevalence of 39 %. Osteonecrosis occurred in 25 patients (24 %), whereas acute chest syndrome (ACS) had been experienced by 17 patients (16 %).

Additionally, cerebrovascular accidents had occurred in four patients (3.89 %); one patient had had a transient ischemic stroke with normal cerebral angiography and three patients had had an ischemic stroke. One patient in follow up and undergoing a transfusion program was uneventful. Other thromboembolic events occurred in 6.8 % of patients, including three patients with pulmonary thromboembolism, two of which occurred during labor or delivery. 32.3 % of patients presented cholecystopathy and only 2.9 % of patients developed other complications such as leg ulcers or priapism. Auto-splenectomy occurred in 45 % of our patients, corroborating data from Lane et al. (1995). Spleen enlargement had occurred in the remaining patients and, in three of them, at least one episode of splenic sequestration was noted. Osteopenia occurred in 27.9 % and osteoporosis in 8.8 % of the patients, where frequencies were lower than those in homozygotes (57 % with osteopenia and 24.5 % with osteoporosis) (Baldanzi et al. 2011). Our patients underwent at least one echocardiography every 2 years, which showed parameters suggestive of mild or moderate pulmonary hypertension in 5.8 % of the patients and left chamber diastolic dysfunction in 7 %. Hypertension was detected in 22 % of the patients, where two thirds of these individuals were older than 50 years old. In an important review published by Saraf et al. (2014), data regarding pulmonary and cardiac complications in HbSS, HbSC and HbSβ^+ thal patients are discussed (see Table 13.2).

In our HbSC cohort, liver complications were uncommon and appeared only in very severe cases. Two female patients developed chronic hepatopathy, as detected by ultrasound and liver biopsy. Both had a very severe phenotype, with basal hemoglobin levels of above 12 g/dL and were submitted to frequent phlebotomy due to pain. One of these patients (currently 58 years old) developed a cerebrovascular accident (CVA) and is on a red blood cell (RBC) transfusion program. We presume that the sickling process was the primary cause of liver disease in this patient, as we could not find any signs of hepatitis virus, cholelithiasis, clinical hemosiderosis, alcoholism or diabetes. The other patient had hepatitis C and died at 47 years due to G-bacteria infection. With regard to liver enzymes, only two female patients presented a mild increase in alanine aminotransferase (ALT; 69 U/L and 81 U/L respectively, normal < 33). Gamma-glutamyl transpeptidase (GGT) was higher than normal (normal female < 40 U/L and male < 60 U/L) in 25 % of the patients. Conjugated bilirubin was abnormal (above 0.4 mg/dL) in 54 % of the patients, but never reached values above 1.4 mg/dL. One patient had cirrhosis, as detected by ultrasound, and liver steatosis occurred in less than 30 % of the patients. A summary of the laboratorial data is presented in Table 13.3.

Kidney complications also seem to be uncommon in HbSC. In our cohort, the glomerular filtration rate (GFR), measured by clearance of ^{51}Cr-EDTA (Barros et al. 2006) and by serum creatinine values (Cockcroft and Gault 1976), was normal in most patients. Half of our patients older than 50 years old ($n=9$) showed a mild reduction in GFR (^{51}Cr-EDTA varying from 50 to 77 mL/min/1.73 m^2 and serum creatinine 0.94–1.47 mg/dL). Persistent microalbuminuria (20–200 μg/min) occurred in 15 % of the patients and two patients presented albuminuria (a 37 year old woman with albuminuria of 319 μg/min, serum creatinine of 0.61 mg/dL and GFR of 120 ml/min/1.73 m^2; and a 58 year old woman with albuminuria of 780 μg/min, serum creatinine of 0.94 mg/dL and GFR of 77 mL/min/1.73 m^2).

Pregnancy We evaluated the impact of prophylactic transfusion support in pregnant women diagnosed with HbSC disease. The patients were divided into two groups, according to the type of transfusion support received; 10 women received

Table 13.2 Sickle cell genotype and pulmonary and cardiac complications in the PUSH and Walk-PHaSST cohorts

General clinical manifestations

	>3 pain episodes PUSH	>3 pain episodes Walk-PHaSST	Leg ulcers PUSH	Leg ulcers Walk-PHaSST	Hb g/dL[a] PUSH	Hb g/dL[a] Walk-PHaSST	LDH U/L[b] PUSH	LDH U/L[a] Walk-PHaSST
Hb SS[c]	16.8 %	31.3 %	1.1 %	22.0 %	8.5 (0.1)	8.6 (0.1)	473 (459–488)	437 (428–446)
Hb SC[d]	10.1 %	27.9 %	0 %	9.0 %	11.5 (0.1)	11.6 (0.2)	279 (260–299)	245 (235–255)
Hb Sβ⁺-thal[e]	17.6 %	25.9 %	0 %	11.1 %	10.7 (0.3)	11.1 (0.4)	308 (276–344)	245 (213–268)
P	0.3	0.4	0.3	0.002	<0.001	<0.001	<0.001	<0.001

Pulmonary complications

	Acute chest syndrome PUSH	Acute chest syndrome Walk-PHaSST	O2 sat <95 % PUSH	O2 sat <95 % Walk-PHaSST	TRV ≥2.6 m/s PUSH	TRV ≥3.0 m/s Walk-PHaSST	BNP >160 ng/L PUSH	BNP >160 ng/L Walk-PHaSST
Hb SS[c]	51.3 %	65.3 %	11.1 %	21.6 %	11.7 %	15.0 %	27.7 %	25.8 %
Hb SC[d]	42.7 %	52.7 %	0 %	8.3 %	1.2 %	8.2 %	7.0 %	20.5 %
Hb Sβ⁺-thal[e]	44.4 %	64.0 %	0 %	0 %	7.1 %	0 %	16.7 %	8.3 %
P	0.17	0.09	<0.001	<0.001	0.013	0.007	<0.001	0.036

Table 13.2 (continued)

Left ventricular size and function								
	LV diastolic dimension Z score PUSH	LV diastolic area (cm^2) Walk-PHaSST	LV mass index (g/m^2) PUSH	LV mass index (g/m^2) Walk-pHaSST	Ejection fraction PUSH	Ejection fraction Walk-PHaSST	Mitral E/E_{tdi} PUSH	LV lateral E/Ea Walk-PHaSST
Hb SS[c]	1.6 (0.6–2.5)	35 (31–40)	94 (78–109)	113 (95–133)	64 (61–67)	61 (58–65)	6.5 (5.7–7.6)	6.4 (5.2–8.1)
Hb SC[d]	1.0 (−0.5–0.7)	29 (26–33)	67 (60–78)	87 (73–108)	64 (61–66)	61 (57–66)	6.1 (5.5–6.9)	6.4 (4.9–7.6)
Hb $S\beta^+$-thal[e]	0.4 (−0.4–1.4)	30 (28–33)	70 (64–90)	84 (69–97)	63 (59–66)	65 (60–68)	5.9 (4.9–6.5)	5.9 (4.8–8.2)
P	<0.001	<0.001	<0.001	<0.001	0.046	0.2	0.004	0.7

Table reproduced with permission from Saraf et al. (2014)

[a]In subjects without recent blood transfusion; adjusted for hydroxyurea

[b]In subjects without recent blood transfusion; adjusted for hydroxyurea, age and study site

[c]PUSH: N = 381 children; Walk-PHaSST: N = 505 predominantly adults

[d]PUSH: N = 90 children; Walk-PHaSST: N = 122 predominantly adults

[e]PUSH: N = 18 children: Walk-PHaSST: N = 27 predominantly adults

Table 13.3 Laboratorial data of double heterozygotes for sickle cell diseases

Parameters	HbSC mean (min–max)	HbSβ^0 mean (min–max)	HbSβ$^+$ mean (min–max)	Reference range
Number	103	31	15	
Hemoglobin, (g/dL)	11.9 (7.27–16.3)	8.7 (5.7–12.2)	9.9 (7.66–13.7)	11.8–16.7
Reticulocytes (×10^9/L)	244 (47.6–485.9)	231.3 (67.5–540)	187.5 (66.78–561.1)	22–139
MVC (fl)	80.8 (60.1–103.3)	77.4 (59.2–101.9)	72.1 (65.9–85.1)	82–98
MCHC (%)	34.3 (30.5–38.4)	33.2 (29.9–35.4)	31.5 (30.5–36.7)	31.6–34.9
Leukocytes (×10^9/L)	8.35 (1.52–16.01)	8.48 (3.99–15.07)	7.4 (3.01–16.01)	3.7–11.1
Neutrophils (×10^9/L)	4.55 (1.47–10.33)	4.0 (2.03–7.96)	3.73 (0.84–6.7)	1.5–7.5
Lymphocytes (×10^9/L)	2.75 (0.9–5.96)	2.86 (0.96–5.97)	2.0 (0.99–5.5)	1.0–3.5
Monocytes (×10^9/L)	0.45 (0.06–1.04)	0.45 (0.1–0.95)	0.32 (0.6–0.84)	0.2–0.92
Eosinophils (×10^9/L)	0.25 (0–0.67)	0.24 (0–1.02)	0.23 (0.01–0.6)	0.02–0.67
Platelets (×10^9/L)	319 (73–644)	418 (98–818)	174 (74–644)	130–400
HbF (%)	1.0 (0.2–5)	7.6 (1.3–24.9)	2.9 (0.3–6.6)	
Ferritin (ng/mL)	209.4 (8.97–1059)	415.7 (64.53–654.8)	316.1 (22.88–1955)	13–400
Serum iron (μg/dL)	81 (26–125)	114.5 (44–243)	70.5 (39.92)	30–160
TIBC (μg/dL)	277.5 (164–358)	230 (172–338)	273 (214–325)	228–428
Transferrin saturation (%)	29.4 (8.42–52.61)	47.52 (16.54–95.34)	27.03 (13.13–42.99)	
Lactate dehydrogenase (U/L)	471 (257–819)	612 (328–932)	469.5 (260–1050)	<480
Serum creatinin (mg/dL)	0.73 (0.39–1.16)	0.57 (0.32–0.96)	0.69 (0.48–1.1)	F<0.9; M<1.2
Clearance ^{51}Cr EDTA (ml/min)	98.5 (47–141)	105 (81–151)	106.6 (54.6–157)	<103.4 ± 15
Microalbumin (μg/min)	6.22 (0.78–25.7)	5.85 (1.99–41.8)	5.3 (1.99–9.3)	<30
AST (U/L)	25 (13–48)	33.5 (16–73)	27 (14–61)	<40
ALT (U/L)	19 (8–40)	22 (8–70)	23 (12–54)	<41
GGT (U/L)	27.5 (5–97)	27 (9–69)	42 (19–98)	5–61
Alkaline phosphatase (U/L)	67 (20–150)	83 (41–180)	86 (42–206)	35–129
Conjugated bilirubin (mg/dL)	0.5 (0.2–0.87)	0.6 (0.25–0.9)	0.66 (0.38–0.87)	<0.3
Unconjugated bilirubin (mg/dL)	1.0 (0.3–1.53)	1.2 (0.7–2.4)	0.9 (0.73–5.1)	<0.9

Clinical data were collected, at the time of writing, from cohorts of patients accompanied at the Hemoglobinopathies Clinic, Hematology Center, University of Campinas

AST aspartate aminotransferase, *ALT* alanine aminotransferase, *GGT* gamma glutamyl transpeptidase, *TIBC* total iron binding capacity

prophylactic erythrocytapheresis or manual exchange transfusion at 28 weeks of gestation, and 14 received transfusions only on demand, due to acute complications, or no transfusions at all. Our results indicate higher frequencies of SCD related complications in the group of women who had not received prophylactic transfusion support (35.7 % versus 10 % in the erythrocytapheresis group). The complications were also more severe in the latter group, including all cases of acute chest syndrome. Statistical difference was observed concerning gestational age at birth (38.7 weeks in the transfusion group versus 34.4 weeks, $p=0.037$), with a higher frequency of preterm births in the non-transfused group (69.23 % versus 30 % in the transfusion group). Thus, we observed a clear reduction in unfavorable outcomes in patients receiving prophylactic transfusions, probably reflecting better maternal and fetal conditions.

Survival Median survival of HbSC carriers is higher than that of HbSS individuals. Recently, Elmariah et al. (2014) reported that the median survival for HbSC is 66 years and 58 years for HbSS. Elevated white blood counts, lower estimated glomerular filtration rates, proteinuria, higher frequency of pain crises, pulmonary hypertension, cerebrovascular events, seizures, stroke, sVCAM-1, and short-acting narcotics use were significantly associated with decreased survival.

13.1.3 Laboratorial Data

Red Blood Cells HbSC blood smears show very few sickle cells, however many target cells are easily identified, as well as dense and microcytic cells. The low solubility of HbC induces intraerythrocytic crystal formation that may also be identified in the blood smear. Deformability of HbSC cells is lower than normal (Serjeant and Serjeant 2011a; Nagel and Steinberg 2009) and measurements by optical tweezer (Fontes et al. 2011; Brandão et al. 2003) demonstrate a huge heterogeneity; however, many cells show a very low elasticity, with elasticity being even lower than that of RBC of HbS homozygotes or patients with hereditary spherocytosis (Fig. 13.1). Recently, Mozar et al. (2015) reported increased activation of nitric oxide synthase in the RBC of HbSC patients, associated with increased RBC nitrite concentration, reflecting RBC-NOS dependent NO production.

Hematology Data Reticulocytes are usually mildly increased and leukocytes and platelets show normal values and distribution, except in patients with splenomegaly, who may have reduced neutrophil and platelet numbers due to sequestration. Hematological data are presented in Table 13.1.

Alpha thalassemia is common in African-derived populations, especially in populations from West African; therefore HbSC coexistence is expected. In our cohort, heterozygous alpha thalassemia occurred in 15.5 % of HbSC patients and three patients (2.91 %) were homozygotes. The effect of alpha thalassemia on clinical severity of HbSC is unknown; however, a mild clinical course in a 86 year old patient carrying both hemoglobinopathies has been reported (Rodgers et al. 1986).

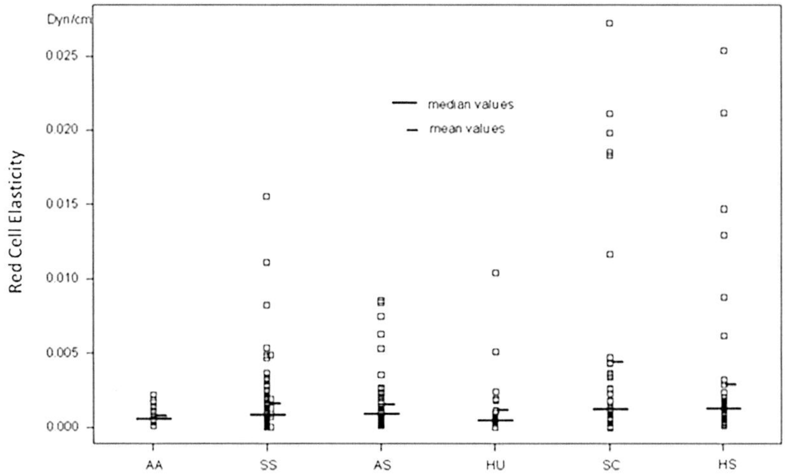

Fig. 13.1 Red cell elasticity (Dyn/cm), as measured by optical tweezers, in healthy controls (AA), and individuals with sickle cell anemia (SS), sickle cell trait (AS), sickle cell anemia on hydroxyurea therapy (HU), HbSC disease and hereditary spherocytosis (HS). Adapted from Brandão (2005)

In our cohort, disease was very severe in two of the alpha-thalassemia homozygotes, who presented CVA, pulmonary thromboembolism (PTE), ACS, pulmonary hypertension, osteonecrosis and retinopathy.

Haplotype Most HbC carriers present haplotype CI, nevertheless CII and CIII as well as atypical haplotypes can be found in a minority of patients. The association of these haplotypes with HbS haplotypes does not modify the hematological characteristics of the patients (Nagel and Steinberg 2009). In our cohort, Haplotypes CII, CIII and atypical, together, were found in less than 10 % of the HbSC patients.

Hemoglobin Distribution As mentioned above, red cells contain equal amounts of HbS and HbC, probably as a result of both abnormal chains competing similarly for alpha-globin chains. HbA2 and HbF are produced in normal amounts; however some patients exhibit a mild increase in HbF, probably related to the genetic background of HbS. In our cohort, HbF values were mostly normal and the median values in our sample were 1 %.

Hemolysis Hemolysis is known to be lower in HbSC, compared to HbSS homozygotes, and the severity of the disease is mainly attributed to high blood viscosity due to high hematocrit values. LDH has long been considered a clinical marker of intravascular hemolysis, which could contribute to complications associated with sickle cell disease (Kato et al. 2006). As such, we investigated associations between LDH and markers of hemolysis and organ dysfunction in our population of 103 patients with HbSC disease. LDH was positively correlated with markers of hemolysis and correlated significantly with reticulocyte counts, but was inversely correlated with haptoglobin levels (Table 13.4). Among patients who did not have complications,

Table 13.4 Correlations between LDH levels and hemolytic parameters in HbSC disease

	Number of patients	rho	*p*
Hemoglobin	85	–0.014	0.901
Reticulocyte count	80	0.471	<0.001
Haptoglobin	69	–0.323	0.007
Indirect bilirubin	57	0.059	0.661

Data collected, at the time of writing, from HbSC patients accompanied at the Hemoglobinopathies Clinic, Hematology Center, University of Campinas. Spearman's rank test

the median LDH concentration was 449 UI/L [257–603 UI/L]. This differed significantly from the median LDH concentration in patients with complications; 479 UI/L [322–2283 UI/L] ($p = 0.012$). Interestingly, an association was observed between LDH and platelet counts (*rho* 0.304, $p = 0.005$). These findings could be related to disease severity, as inflammation may induce thrombocytosis (Griesshammer et al. 1999); however, the high platelet count in our cohort was correlated with auto-splenectomy.

13.1.4 Association between LDH and Clinical Manifestations in HbSC

Although the intensity of hemolysis, as assessed by plasma LDH levels, is expected to be lower in HbSC than in HbSS patients, we investigated this specific parameter and analyzed its correlation with HbSC complications. We found a significant difference between median LDH levels in the subgroups with or without retinopathy and venous thromboembolism (VTE) (451.5 IU/L [257–1816] versus 537 IU/L [354–2283], $p = 0.03$ and 461 IU/L [257–1816] versus 664 IU/L [389–2283] $p = 0.018$, respectively). To further investigate the application of this marker, we determined the associations between LDH levels and complications. ROC curve analysis showed that for retinopathy, LDH>535 UI/L had a sensitivity of 51.3 % and a specificity of 76 % [95 % confidence interval: 51.8–75.5 %], $p = 0.013$ and OR: 3.3. For VTE, LDH>606.5 UI/L had a sensitivity of 71.4 % and a specificity of 84.6 % [95 % confidence interval: 55.3–99.2 %], $p = 0.003$ and OR = 13.1. For stroke, LDH>614.5 UI/L had a sensitivity of 75 % and a specificity of 85.2 % [95 % confidence interval: 38.7–100 %], $p = 0.016$ and OR = 16.3. Finally, for leg ulcer, LDH>668.5 UI/L had a sensitivity of 100 % and a specificity of 89 % [95 % confidence interval: 83.64–96.85 %], $p = 0.002$ and OR = 2.8 (Fig. 13.2). When these four complications were grouped together, LDH>535.5 UI/L had a sensitivity of 51.2 % and specificity of 78.6 % [95 % confidence interval: 52.09–75.96 %], $p = 0.007$ and OR = 3.78 (Fig. 13.3).

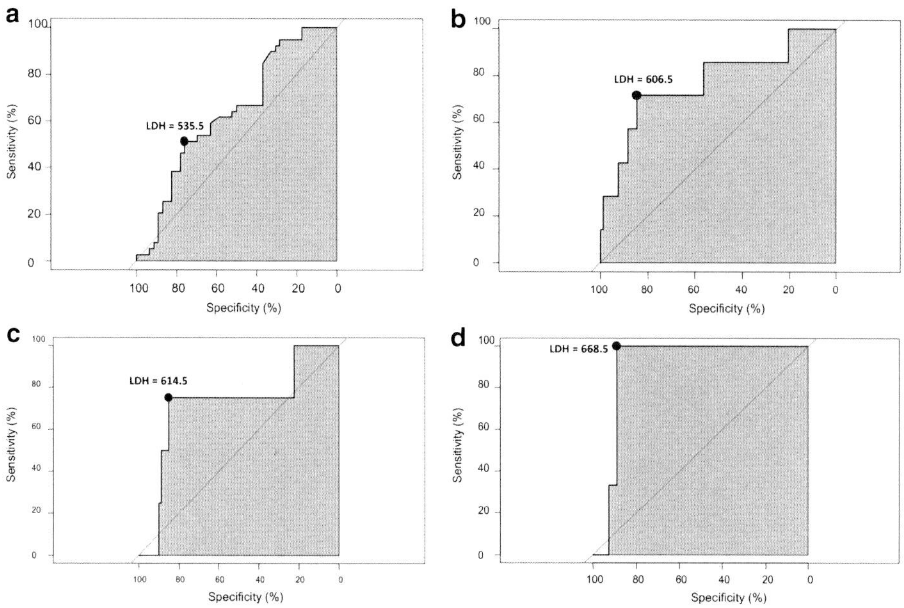

Fig. 13.2 Receiver operating characteristic (ROC) analysis using plasma lactate dehydrogenase levels as a parameter for the prediction of (**a**) stroke, (**b**) venous thromboembolism, (**c**) leg ulcer and (**d**) retinopathy in HbSC patients accompanied at the Hemoglobinopathies Clinic, Hematology Center, University of Campinas

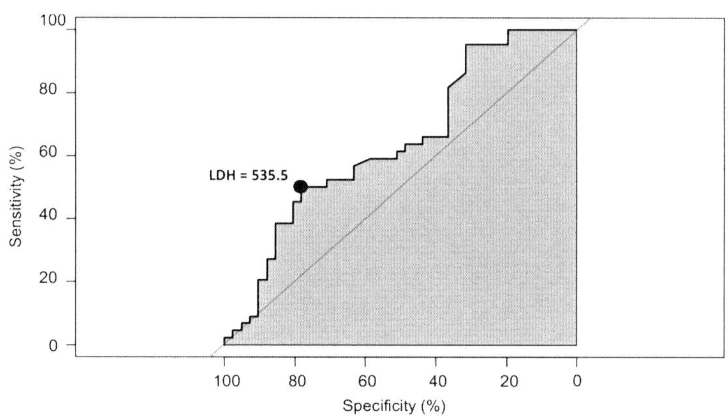

Fig. 13.3 Receiver operating characteristic (ROC) analysis using plasma lactate dehydrogenase levels as a parameter for the prediction of grouped complications (stroke, venous thromboembolism, leg ulcer and retinopathy) in HbSC patients accompanied at the Hemoglobinopathies Clinic, Hematology Center, University of Campinas

13.1.5 Elevated Hypercoagulability Markers in Hemoglobin SC Disease

While an increased risk for thromboembolic events in SC disease has been related (Stein et al. 2006; Novelli et al. 2012), there is a lack of studies evaluating hemostatic alterations in this population. We described a cross-sectional observational study to evaluate coagulation activation markers in adult SC patients, in comparison with SS patients and healthy controls. A total of 56 SC and 39 SS patients were included in the study, all in steady state, and 27 healthy controls. None of the patients were in use of hydroxyurea. HbSC patients presented a significantly upregulated relative expression of *tissue factor*, as well as elevations in thrombin-antithrombin complex and D-dimer, in comparison to controls ($p<0.01$). Furthermore, HbSC patients presented lower *tissue factor* expression, and thrombin-antithrombin complex and D-dimer levels, when compared to SS patients ($p<0.05$). Endothelial activation (soluble thrombomodulin and soluble vascular cell adhesion molecule-1), and inflammation (tumor necrosis factor-alpha) markers were both significantly elevated in HbSC patients when compared to controls, being as high as the levels seen in HbSS. Overall, in HbSC patients, higher hemolytic activity and inflammation were associated with a more intense activation of coagulation, and hemostatic activation was associated with two very prevalent chronic complications seen in HbSC disease; retinopathy and osteonecrosis. In summary, our results demonstrate that HbSC patients present a hypercoagulable state, although this manifestation was not as intense as that seen in sickle cell anemia (Colella et al. 2015).

13.1.6 Blood Cell Transfusion and Alloimmunization in HbSC Disease

Overall, patients with HbSC disease have a milder clinical course with a later onset of symptoms. Despite fewer episodes of acute chest syndrome (ACS) and vaso-occlusive crisis (VOC), the incidence of avascular necrosis, retinopathy, and pregnancy-related complications may be high in patients with HbSC. Furthermore, disease severity presents marked variability and some patients with HbSC disease have the same amount of complications as those patients with HbSS disease.

RBC transfusion remains an essential part of the management of patients with SC hemoglobinopathy. Despite the benefits, this procedure increases the risk of serious hazards related to transfusions such as delayed hemolytic transfusion reactions and alloimmunization. Alloantibody formation against RBC antigens is a major complication associated with RBC transfusions in patients with sickle cell disease (which comprises HbSC disease). The alloimmunization rate in this population ranges considerably; dependent primarily on the extent of minor RBC antigen matching and exposure frequency, and the development of multiple alloantibodies is not uncommon, often delaying the location of compatible RBCs.

There are few data in the literature reporting on alloimmunization rates in HbSC disease, specifically. Rosse et al. (1990) found no significant difference between the proportion of alloimmunized HbSS patients (13.1 %) and the proportion of alloimmunized non-HbSS patients (9.1 %) ($p=0.07$). Studies have reported that in the United Kingdom (UK), United States (US) and Kuwait, rates for alloimmunization in SCD patients are 18–76 % with ABO and D matching alone (Davies et al. 1986; Ambruso et al. 1987; Vichinsky et al. 1990; Olujohungbe et al. 2001; Aygun et al. 2002; Castro et al. 2002; Sakhalkar et al. 2005; Ameen et al. 2009), 5–11 % with additional limited phenotype matching for C, E, and K antigens (Sakhalkar et al. 2005; Vichinsky 2001), and 0–7 % for extended minor RBC antigen matching beyond C, E, and K (Tahhan et al. 1994; Lasalle-Williams et al. 2011). In Jamaica and Uganda, alloimmunization rates in SCD patients are even lower: 2.6–6.1 % with ABO and D matching alone (Olujohungbe et al. 2001; Natukunda et al. 2010). The lower incidence of RBC sensitization in these reports is probably influenced by low transfusion burdens as well as homogeneity between recipients and donors of African origin, compared to the UK and US, where donors of African descent represent a minority (Osby and Shulman 2005).

The rate of alloimmunization in our HbSC patients is 21.3 % which is apparently lower than the rate in HbSS patients (32.7 %); however with no statistical difference ($p=0.13$). Despite the current employment of extended phenotyping, we believe that several factors contribute to this result, including transfusions in other services that do not employ the use of the extended phenotype and the age of the patients who were alloimmunized during childhood when only ABO and RH typing were used. Finally, the high rates of Rh gene variants, which are not identified in conventional serological tests, may also have contributed to this index.

13.1.7 Diagnosis

The diagnosis of HbSC is based on the identification of hemoglobin S and hemoglobin C, in equal amounts, in the red cells. They are both easily identified by electrophoresis, isoeletric focusing or HPLC. However, since other hemoglobins may run in the position of HbC, it is important to differentiate them by acid citrate agar. Moreover, in alkaline electrophoresis, HbA2 and HbC migrate in the same region however, the amount of HbA2 is usually below 5 %, thus, when more than 40 % is observed in the HbA2 position, we presume that it is HbC.

13.2 Sβ Thalassemia

The occurrence of Sβ thalassemia is dependent on the distribution and prevalence of both alleles in a given region. Beta-thalassemia is very prevalent in individuals of Italian, Greek and Mediterranean region descent. As such, Sβ thalassemia is more frequent in areas where miscegenation of African descendants and descendants from these populations occur and can be more prevalent than HbSS in homozygosis in some parts of Greece; however in the Americas, beta thalassemia gene frequency is lower than 0.005 (Saraf et al. 2014; Christakis et al. 1990; Serjeant and Serjeant 2011b).

In patients with Sβ^0 thalassemia, the relative amount of HbS inside the RBCs is comparable to that observed in homozygotes and, as such, the phenotype of the disease is similar to that of HbSS. Conversely, the Sβ^+ phenotype may vary depending on the expression of HbA. Thus, the amount of HbS in RBCs may be similar to that observed in HbSC, with Hb levels of higher than 9 g/dL, splenomegaly and mild hemolysis. Additionally, the Sβ^+ phenotype may be even better if more than 20 % HbA is synthesized. This variation in hemoglobin synthesis is related to the mutational profile of the beta-thalassemic allele. Data from Sβ^0 and Sβ^+ patients seen in our clinic are shown in Tables 13.1 and 13.3. A comparison of hematological data for Sβ thalassemia individuals from the northeastern region of Brazil is shown in Table 13.5. In our cohort of S beta thalassemia patients (Table 13.1), Sβ^0 patients (compared to Sβ^+ patients) presented a significantly lower weight (median, 51 kg vs 69.4 kg; $p=0.002$), BMI (median 19.7 vs 25.1; $p<0.001$), lower densitometry values for lumbar spine (median –0.8 vs 0.95; $p=0.01$) and femoral neck (median –0.2 vs 1.2; $p=0.015$), hemoglobin levels (8.7 vs 9.9 g/dL, $p=0.005$), higher platelet number (418 vs 174×10^9/L; $p=0.021$), HbF (7.6 vs 2.9 %, $p=0.001$), serum iron (114 vs 70 μg/dL; $p=0.014$) and transferrin saturation (47.5 vs 27 %; $p=0.004$). These differences are easily understood, since the absence of HbA in the RBC may lead to greater anemia, lower growth, more hemolysis and consequently more osteoporosis/osteopenia and more iron absorption, which would increase transferrin saturation. Moreover, severity of sickle cell disorder is also related to early auto-splenectomy, which causes increased platelet number.

13.2.1 Diagnosis

The diagnosis of Sβ thalassemia is based on the presence of HbS and increased Hb A2 in a patient with low MCV and MCH. The amount of HbA varies according to the molecular defect of the βthal allele.

13.3 Hemoglobinopathy SD

SD disease is a rare sickle cell syndrome, characterized by compound heterozygosity for HbS and HbD. HbD Punjab or Los Angeles is the result of a mutation in codon 121 of the beta-globin chain, which substitutes glutamic acid for glutamine. The glutamine residue facilitates HbS polymerization and patients with both alleles exhibit vaso-occlusion and hemolytic anemia. Both hemoglobins have the same electrophoretic behavior at alkaline pH; however the solubility test, acid pH electrophoresis, HPLC and isoelectric focusing distinguish SD from homozygotes. Data from two patients with HbSD are shown in Table 13.6.

Table 13.5 Hematological data of patients with sickle cell disease

	SS n=20	SC n=20	S/β-IVS-I-6 n=18	S/β-IVS-I-5 n=16	S/β-Cd39 N=12	Reference range
Male:Female	10:10	8:12	9:9	7:9	6:6	
Age (y)	30 (23–39)	28 (18–55)	28 (20–28)	24 (18:35)	34.5 (24–59)	
RBC ($10^6/mm^3$)	2.46 (1.94–3.41)	4.05 (3.29–5.58)	5.10 (4.64–5.61)	3.64 (2.72–4.56)	3.55 (2.74–4.11)	3.9–6.0
Hb (g/dL)	7.4 (6.3–8.8)	10.9 (9.4–13.2)	11.6 (10.1–12.8)	7.4 (6.3–9.2)	7.8 (6.0–9.6)	11.8–16.7
VCM (fL)	94.3 (84.5–107.7)	85.4 (77.7–92.4)	73.3 (67.2–77.2)	68.7 (61.1–76.8)	73.0 (66.2–76.3)	82–98
Ret (%)	8.6 (4.3–15.6)	3.8 (1.5–7.0)	2.7 (1.0–4.4)	8.8 (4.1–20.0)	8.7 (2.6–13)	0.5–2.5
HbS (%)	89.9 (85.7–92.5)	49.5 (48.1–53.1)	67.4 (64.6–70.1)	72.9 (64.0–85.9)	84.5 (72.5–88.7)	
HbF (%)	6.9 (3.4–11)	1.3 (0.3–3.6)	1.8 (0.3–3.9)	17.6 (8.1–24.8)	11.0 (6.8–23.8)	
HbA (%)	–	–	26.3 (23.3–28.3)	5.2 (3.5–8.7)	–	

Data collected from cohorts of patients accompanied at the Hemoglobinopathies Clinic, Hematology Center of Pernambuco, Brazil (Hospital de Hematologia da Fundação do Estado de Pernambuco, HEMOPE). Values are expressed as means (minimum–maximum). Definitions of β thalassemia-causing mutations: IVS-I-6, single mutation in the sixth nucleotide of intron I (IVS-1); IVS-I-5, single mutation in the fifth nucleotide of intron I (IVS-1); Cd39, mutation in codon 39 of the β-globin gene. Adapted from Bezerra (2009)

Table 13.6 Clinical and laboratorial data for patients with double heterozygosity for HbS and HbD

Parameter	CASE 1	CASE 2	Reference range
Gender	M	F	
Age	39	38	
Hb (g/dL)	9.5	8.5	11.8–16.7
Reticulocytes (×10^9/L)	251.7	241.3	22–139
MCV (fL)	104.1	99.3	82–98
MCHC (%)	32.9	33.6	31.6–34.9
Leukocytes (×10^9/L)	7.5	6.86	3.7–11.1
Neutrophils (×10^9/L)	2.88	3.23	1.5–7.5
Lymphocytes (×10^9/L)	3.24	2.76	1.0–3.5
Monocytes (×10^9/L)	0.76	0.5	0.2–0.92
Eosinophils (×10^9/L)	0.26	0.24	0.02–0.67
Platelets (×10^9/L)	346	376	130–400
HbF %	7.5	8.5	
Microalbuminuria (μg/min)	15.4	3.09	<30
Serum creatinin (mg/dL)	0.8	0.52	F<0.9; M<1.2
Clearance ^{51}Cr EDTA (ml/min)	94	129	<103.4±15
Lactate dehydrogenase (U/L)	2038	1650	<480
AST (U/L)	57	45	<40
ALT (U/L)	19	17	<41
GGT (U/L)	61	12	5–61
Alkaline phosphatase	62	199	35–129
Conjugated bilirubin (mg/dL)	0.7	0.6	<0.3
Unconjugated bilirubin (mg/dL)	5.1	2.04	<0.9
Osteonecrosis	Yes	Yes	
Retinopathy	Yes	No	
ACS	No	No	
stroke	No	No	
VTE	No	No	
Priapism	No	No	
Leg ulcer	No	No	
Transfusion	Yes	Yes	
Alloimmunization	No	No	
Cholecystopathy	Yes	Yes	
Alpha thalassemia	No	No	
Hydroxyurea	No	No	

Data are from patients accompanied at the Hemoglobinopathies Clinic, Hematology Center, University of Campinas

AST aspartate amino transferase, *ALT* alanine amino transferase, *GGT* gamma glutamyl transpeptidase, *HbF* fetal hemoglobin, *VTE* venous thromboembolism

An epidemiological study carried out at the Federal University of Minas Gerais in Brazil (Orsini et al. 2014) showed an incidence of SD carriers of approximately 0.7 % of all sickle cell disease patients, comprising equally SD-Punjab and SD-Korle Bu. SD-Punjab patients have the same clinical phenotype as that of HbS homozygotes and SD-Korle Bu behaves as a sickle cell trait. The β73 residue mutated in HbD Korle Bu does not reduce HbS polymerization.

13.4 Conclusion

Sickle cell disorders are heterogeneous with regard to clinical and laboratorial data, depending mostly on the genotype. $S\beta^0$ thalassemia patients present similar parameters to those of HbSS homozygotes; while $S\beta^+$ thalassemia, hemoglobinopathy SC and hemoglobinopathy SD have similar phenotypes. However, adults from any of these groups can demonstrate severe complications and early death.

References

Ambruso DR, Githens JH, Alcorn R et al (1987) Experience with donors matched for minor blood group antigens in patients with sickle cell anemia who are receiving chronic transfusion therapy. Transfusion 27(1):94–98

Ameen R, Al Shemmari S, Al-Bashir A (2009) Red blood cell alloimmunization among sickle cell Kuwaiti Arab patients who received red blood cell transfusion. Transfusion 49(8):1649–1654

Aygun B, Padmanabhan S, Paley C, Chandrasekaran V (2002) Clinical significance of RBC alloantibodies and autoantibodies in sickle cell patients who received transfusions. Transfusion 42(1):37–43

Baldanzi G, Traina F, Marques Neto JF, Santos AO, Ramos CD, Saad ST (2011) Low bone mass density is associated with hemolysis in Brazilian patients with sickle cell disease. Clinics (Sao Paulo) 66(5):801–805

Barros FB, Lima CS, Santos AO et al (2006) 51Cr-EDTA measurements of the glomerular filtration rate in patients with sickle cell anaemia and minor renal damage. Nucl Med Commun 27(12):959–962

Bezerra MAC (2009) Adhesive and functional properties of red blood cells, neurotrophils and platelets in patients with Hemoglobinopathy SC, Hb S-Beta thalassemia and thalassemia intermedia. Dissertation, University of Campinas, Brazil

Brandão MM (2005) Aplicação da pinça óptica para o estudo da deformabilidade das hemácias. Dissertation, University of Campinas, Brazil

Brandão MM, Fontes A, Barjas-Castro ML et al (2003) Optical tweezers for measuring red blood cell elasticity: application to the study of drug response in sickle cell disease. Eur J Haematol 70(4):207–211

Castro O, Sandler SG, Houston-Yu P, Rana S (2002) Predicting the effect of transfusing only phenotype-matched RBCs to patients with sickle cell disease: theoretical and practical implications. Transfusion 42(6):684–690

Christakis J, Vavatsi N, Hassapopoulou H et al (1990) Comparison of homozygous sickle cell disease in northern Greece and Jamaica. Lancet 335(8690):637–640

Cockcroft DW, Gault MH (1976) Prediction of creatinine clearance from serum creatinine. Nephron 16(1):31–41

Colella MP, de Paula EV, Machado-Neto JA et al (2015) Elevated hypercoagulability markers in hemoglobin SC disease. Haematologica 100(4):466–471

Davies SC, McWilliam AC, Hewitt PE, Devenish A, Brozovic M (1986) Red cell alloimmunization in sickle cell disease. Br J Haematol 63(2):241–245

Elmariah H, Garrett ME, De Castro LM et al (2014) Factors associated with survival in a contemporary adult sickle cell disease cohort. Am J Hematol 89(5):530–535

Fernandes AP, Januário JN, Cangussu CB, Macedo DL, Viana MB (2010) Mortality of children with sickle cell disease: a population study. J Pediatr 86(4):279–284

Fontes A, Barjas C-ML, Brandão MM et al (2011) Mechanical and electrical properties of red blood cells using optical tweezers. J Opt 13(1):044012

Griesshammer M, Bangerter M, Sauer T, Wennauer R, Bergmann L, Heimpel H (1999) Aetiology and clinical significance of thrombocytosis: analysis of 732 patients with an elevated platelet count. J Intern Med 245(3):295–300

Kato GJ, Earles A, McGowan V, Machado RF et al (2006) Lactate dehydrogenase as a biomarker of hemolysis-associated nitric oxide resistance, priapism, leg ulceration, pulmonary hypertension, and death in patients with sickle cell disease. Blood 107(6):2279–2285

Lane PA, O'Connell JL, Lear JL et al (1995) Functional asplenia in hemoglobin SC disease. Blood 85(8):2238–2244

Lasalle-Williams M, Nuss R, Le T et al (2011) Extended red blood cell antigen matching for transfusions in sickle cell disease: a review of a 14-year experience from a single center (CME). Transfusion 51(8):1732–1739

Mozar A, Grau M, Lamarre Y et al (2015) Red blood cell nitric oxide synthase activation is increased in patients with sickle cell hemoglobin C disease. Am J Hematol 90(2):E30–E32

Nagel RL, Steinberg MH (2009) Hemoglobin SC disease and Hb C disorders. In: Steinberg MH, Forget BG, Higgs DR, Weatherall DJ (eds) Disorders of hemoglobin genetics, pathophysiology, and clinical management, 2nd edn. Cambridge University Press, Cambridge, pp 756–785

Nagel RL, Fabry ME, Steinberg MH (2003) The paradox of hemoglobin SC disease. Blood Rev 17(3):167–178

Natukunda B, Schonewille H, Ndugwa C, Brand A (2010) Red blood cell alloimmunization in sickle cell disease patients in Uganda. Transfusion 50(1):20–25

Novelli EM, Huynh C, Gladwin MT, Moore CG, Ragni MV (2012) Pulmonary embolism in sickle cell disease: a case–control study. J Thromb Haemost 10(5):760–766

Olujohungbe A, Hambleton I, Stephens L, Serjeant B, Serjeant G (2001) Red cell antibodies in patients with homozygous sickle cell disease: a comparison of patients in Jamaica and the United Kingdom. Br J Haematol 113(3):661–665

Orsini P, Rezende PV, Santos MV et al (2014) Estudo das Manifestações Clínicas e Hematológicas das Crianças com Hemoglobinopatia SD do Programa Estadual de Triagem Neonatal – PETN/NUPAD. In: XXIII Semana de Iniciação Científica da UFMG, 2014, Belo Horizonte. Anais eletrônicos da XXIII Semana de Iniciação Científica da UFMG

Osby M, Shulman IA (2005) Phenotype matching of donor red blood cell units for nonalloimmunized sickle cell disease patients: a survey of 1182 North American laboratories. Arch Pathol Lab Med 129(2):190–193

Platt OS, Thorington BD, Brambilla DJ, Milner PF, Rosse WF, Vichinsky E, Kinney TR (1991) Pain in sickle cell disease. Rates and risk factors. N Engl J Med 325(1):11–16

Rodgers GP, Sahovic EZ, Pierce LE, Anagnou NP, Noguchi CT, Schechter AN (1986) Hemoglobin SC disease and alpha-thalassaemia. Prolonged survival and mild clinical course. Am J Med 80(4):746–750

Rosse WF, Gallagher D, Kinney TR et al (1990) Cooperative study of sickle cell disease transfusion and alloimmunization in sickle cell disease. Blood 76(7):1431–1437

Sakhalkar VS, Roberts K, Hawthorne LM et al (2005) Allosensitization in patients receiving multiple blood transfusions. Ann N Y Acad Sci 1054:495–499

Saraf SL, Molokie RE, Nouraie M et al (2014) Differences in the clinical and genotypic presentation of sickle cell disease around the world. Paediatr Respir Rev 15(1):4–12

Serjeant GR, Serjeant BE (2011a) Sickle cell-haemoglobin C disease. In: Serjeant GR, Serjeant BE (eds) Sickle cell disease, 3rd edn. Oxford University Press, New York, pp 445–455

Serjeant GR, Serjeant BE (2011b) Other forms of sickle cell disease. In: Serjeant GR, Serjeant BE (eds) Sickle cell disease, 3rd edn. Oxford University Press, New York, pp 472–477

Stein PD, Beemath A, Meyers FA, Skaf E, Olson RE (2006) Deep venous thrombosis and pulmonary embolism in hospitalized patients with sickle cell disease. Am J Med 119(10):897.e7–e11

Tahhan HR, Holbrook CT, Braddy LR, Brewer LD, Christie JD (1994) Antigen-matched donor blood in the transfusion management of patients with sickle cell disease. Transfusion 34(7):562–569

Vichinsky E (2001) Consensus document for transfusion-related iron overload. Semin Hematol 38(1 Suppl 1):2–4

Vichinsky EP, Earles A, Johnson RA, Hoag MS, Williams A, Lubin B (1990) Alloimmunization in sickle cell anemia and transfusion of racially unmatched blood. N Engl J Med 322(23):1617–1621

Chapter 14
Sickle Cell Disease in Africa and the Arabian Peninsula: Current Management and Challenges

Adekunle Adekile and Julie Makani

Abstract Africa and the Arabian Peninsula are two regions of the world that are of particular interest in sickle cell disease. While the former has the highest burden of the disease in the world, the latter has the highest variety in terms of the genotypes, haplotypes and phenotypes that are encountered. The disease is usually severe in Africa because of complex interactions between genetic and environmental factors, but the Arabian Peninsula has a relatively mild expression because of the prevalence of the high-HbF phenotype, although the presentation is still quite heterogeneous, with some patients having a severe clinical course and developing complications. One major difference in the two regions is that the vast majority of African patients are homozygous, SS, while among Arabs, there is a high prevalence of other compound heterozygotes especially Sβ^0-thal. This chapter presents the contrasting pictures in terms of the epidemiology, clinical presentation, management practices and the prevailing challenges. It looks at the peculiar issues of resource limitation in Africa and outlines strategies that could surmount some of the challenges. While most of the countries in the Arabian Peninsula are endowed with the necessary resources, the wide variation in the phenotypic patterns poses challenges in adopting uniform control strategies.

Keywords Genotypes • Haplotypes • Phenotypes • Distribution • Peculiarities • Management • Challenges

---

A. Adekile (✉)
Faculty of Medicine, Department of Pediatrics, Kuwait University,
PO Box 24923, Safat 13110, Kuwait
e-mail: Adekile@hsc.edu.kw

J. Makani
Department of Hematology and Blood Transfusion, Muhimbili University of Health and Allied Sciences, PO Box 65001, Dar-es-Salaam, Tanzania

University of Oxford, Oxford, UK
e-mail: Julie.Makani@muhimbili-wellcome.org

© Springer International Publishing Switzerland 2016
F.F. Costa, N. Conran (eds.), *Sickle Cell Anemia*,
DOI 10.1007/978-3-319-06713-1_14

14.1 Sickle Cell Anemia in Africa

14.1.1 Introduction

The greatest burden of sickle cell anemia (SCA) in the world is in Africa, with the highest rates of prevalence and mortality. The occurrence of severe forms of SCA in Africa is the result of complex interactions between genetic and environmental factors. This is compounded by the limitations in many African countries that result in the failure to implement interventions that are known to be effective for improving survival. This section explores the epidemiology of SCA in Africa, focusing on the prevalence, morbidity and mortality, as well as clinical presentation and factors determining its severity. This is followed by a review of management of SCA in Africa, exploring current practice, challenges and outlining strategies that are being adopted to improve its management in Africa.

14.1.2 Epidemiology: Prevalence and Geographical Distribution

Birth Prevalence of SCA

One of the parameters used to determine the magnitude of SCA in a population is the birth prevalence of the disease, defined as the number of affected births per 1000 live births. In an ideal setting, this is determined by screening of all live births and identifying all newborns with confirmed SCA. Unfortunately, newborn screening (NBS) for SCA is not available in many African countries. Due to the absence of this information, the birth prevalence has been estimated from the available data on the prevalence of sickle cell trait and assuming that the sickle gene is in Hardy–Weinberg equilibrium. There are several limitations in the series of assumptions that are made with these estimates. However, in the absence of more accurate information, these figures are currently used to estimate the birth prevalence of SCA, and suggest that four out of five of the countries with the highest birth prevalence of the disease in the world are in Africa [Nigeria, Democratic Republic of Congo (DRC), India, Tanzania and Uganda]. With increasing population growth from increasing birth rates, it is estimated that, globally, 14 million babies will be born with SCA between 2010 and 2050, with 80 % of these births being in sub-Saharan Africa (Piel et al. 2013a) (Fig. 14.1).

Population Prevalence of SCA

African countries recognize the need to provide accurate estimates of population prevalence of SCA in order to plan health care for affected patients. The population prevalence of SCA refers to the number of people with SCA within a specified population, which is reported per 100 or per 1000 or 100,000, depending on the magnitude of the condition. For most conditions, this is determined during

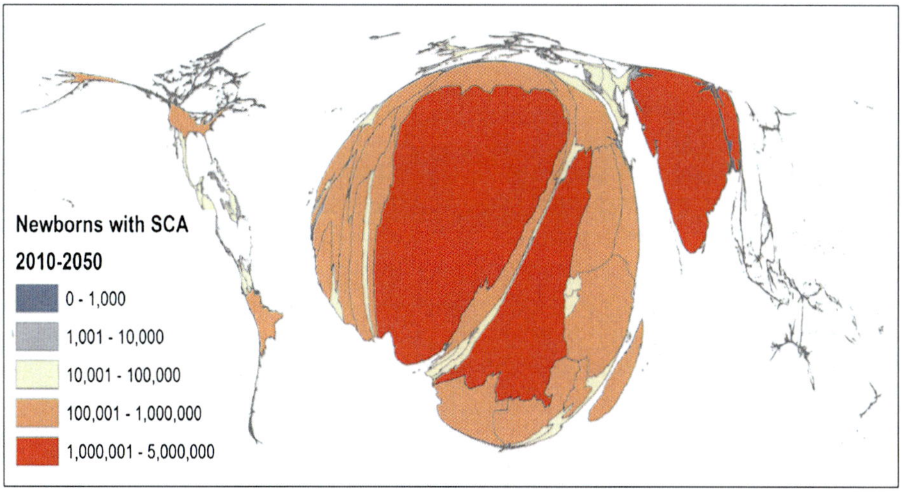

Fig. 14.1 Estimated number of newborns with sickle cell anemia, per country, between 2010 and 2050. Reproduced from Piel et al. (2013a)

population census or as part of demographic health surveillance programmes. However, most countries do not include the collection of information on SCA. Therefore, the estimate of population prevalence is determined by using the birth prevalence and mortality rate, as well as information from hospital records. In the United States of America (USA), it is estimated that there are 100,000 individuals with SCA (Hassell 2010). In sub-Saharan Africa, it is estimated that there could be over 6,000,000 individuals with SCA; assuming that life expectancy in individuals with SCA is 50 % that of the norm in Africa (Modell and Darlison 2008). Since the survival of individuals with SCA is bound to differ in different settings, depending on various genetic, environmental and social factors, definitive estimates of population prevalence are needed.

Geographical Distribution of SCA

The hypothesis proposed by Haldane suggested that individuals with the heterozygous state of thalassemia are protected from malaria, resulting in a high prevalence of thalassaemia in malaria-endemic areas (Haldane 1949). This hypothesis has been popularly referred to as the 'malaria hypothesis'. Allison, more specifically explored the relationship between sickle cell trait, SCA and malaria in Africa, which led to the description of lower prevalence of malaria in individuals with sickle cell trait and the geographical distribution of SCA in Eastern Africa (Allison 1954a, b). This led to further discussion on the natural selection of the sickle gene by malaria, which is balanced by the high mortality that occurs in individuals with the homozygous state. This state of balanced polymorphism is one of the factors that account for the occurrence of the high prevalence of the sickle gene in eastern Africa (Allison

1964). Allison further went on to discuss the occurrence of negative epistasis between two 'malaria-protective' genes within a population (Allison 1964), which may account for the geographical distribution of thalassaemia in Asia-India-Europe, and SCA in Africa (Penman et al. 2009). These hypotheses have led to maps that show the geographical distribution of the sickle gene, which matches the geographical distribution of malaria (Piel et al. 2010). However, there are two limitations to this approach. The first being that it uses information on prevalence of sickle cell trait from few data points to make assumptions on the prevalence within a country and continent. The second limitation is the assumption that malaria is the major factor that determines the prevalence of SCA. This simplified approach does not explain the maintenance of high prevalence of SCA in the Mediterranean (Penman et al. 2012) and there is a need to conduct micromapping studies to accurately determine the birth and population prevalence of the disease in different geographical areas within a country and continent (Weatherall et al. 2006).

Mortality

There is a high mortality rate in individuals with SCA in Africa. A study conducted in the Garki district in Nigeria reported that, within a population of individuals with SCA identified at birth, only 2 % were alive at the age of 5 years (Fleming et al. 1979). Recent literature suggests that childhood survival in SCA in Africa is likely to have improved, and is estimated to be 50 % in some settings (Weatherall et al. 2006). This however, does not approach the survival estimates that have been achieved in high-income countries, with childhood survival ranging between 94 and 95 % (Telfer et al. 2007; Quinn et al. 2004) (Fig. 14.2). There are limited reports of current mortality rates in SCA from African countries. Tanzania reported a sickle cell disease (SCD)-specific mortality rate of 1.9 [95 % confidence interval (CI): 1.5–2.9)] per hundred person-years of observation (100 PYO) (Makani et al. 2011a). This compares to 0.15 and 0.6 per 100 PYO in the United Kingdom (UK) and the United States of America (USA), respectively (Telfer et al. 2007; Quinn et al. 2010).

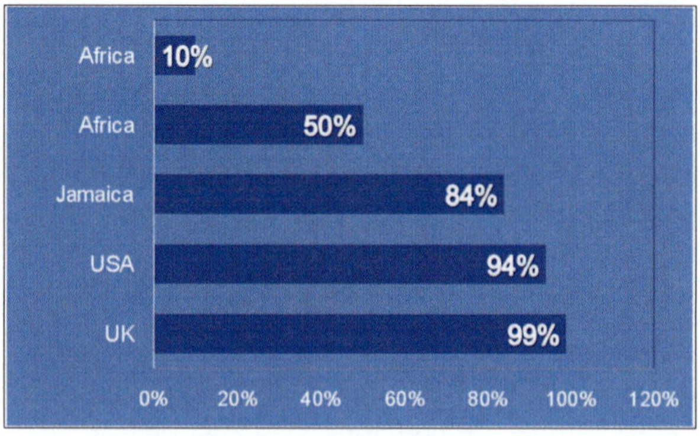

Fig. 14.2 Childhood survival for sickle cell anemia in different parts of the world

Globally, and within Africa, the period with the highest mortality in SCA is the first 5 years of life: 7.3 per 100 PYO in Tanzania, compared to 0.72 and 0.43 per 100 PYO for children ages 0–2 and 2–4 in the USA (Quinn et al. 2004). It is difficult to get accurate information on under-five mortality rates due to SCA in African countries, as there is no newborn screening and therefore most children with SCA will die before a diagnosis is made. Estimates by Modell et al. suggest that hemoglobin disorders contribute the equivalent of 3.4 % of mortality in children aged under 5 years worldwide or 6.4 % in Africa (Modell and Darlison 2008).

The causes of mortality, both in children and adults, in the USA, UK and Jamaica include infections, acute chest syndrome (ACS), acute splenic sequestration (ASS), and aplastic crisis (Thomas et al. 1982; Brozovic and Anionwu 1984; Leikin et al. 1989; Gill et al. 1995). Within Africa, it is likely that the most common causes of mortality are infections, anemia and acute episodes leading to stroke and acute chest syndrome (Makani et al. 2007). Other events such as pain, pulmonary hypertension, and hemolysis are associated with an increased risk of death. The absence of literature on SCA beyond childhood, as well as the limited number of adolescents and adults with SCA in hospital-based facilities, has resulted in the assumption that there is high childhood mortality in SCA in Africa. However, there is increasing evidence that the number of individuals with SCA is high (Rahimy et al. 2003; Tshilolo et al. 2008; Makani et al. 2011a). This suggests that there has either been a reduction in childhood mortality, or that the detection of individuals with SCA who have mild disease has increased.

14.1.3 Clinical Presentation: Different Phenotypes and Peculiarities

The heterogeneity of SCA that has been described in SCA populations in Europe and Americas is also seen in Africa. Its clinical presentation is heterogeneous in several ways. There is inter-individual variability with some individuals who are completely asymptomatic while others have extreme, debilitating illness. There is also variability within an individual, with changes in the type and frequency of clinical events with age. The general pattern of clinical disease is characterized by quiescent periods interspersed with episodes of acute illness, which were previously known as 'crises' that require emergency or urgent intervention. However, with improvement in healthcare and awareness about the natural history of SCA, there is increasing recognition of the chronic, life-long nature of the disease, which results in chronic complications involving end-organ dysfunction, as well as the effect of SCA on reducing the quality of life. As a result, there has been an increase in the number of health facilities that provide life-long care for SCA. Although there is limited information on clinical epidemiology of the illness in Africa, it is likely that there will be similarities with SCA populations in other parts of the world. However, it is important to explore and identify differences in the spectrum of disease in Africa due to the influence of various factors within genes, environment and society. Table 14.1 provides a summary of selected clinical phenotypes.

Table 14.1 Clinical features of sickle cell disease

Clinical event	Characteristics and comments	References
Pain	More than 60 % patients Most common cause of hospital admission Frequent pain is a risk factor for mortality	Platt et al. (1991), Gill et al. (1995), Ibidapo and Akinyanju (2000), Charles et al. (2006), Olabode and Shokunbi (2006), and Quinn et al. (2007)
Malaria	Risk factor for mortality. Chemoprophylaxis recommended in high transmission areas and children under 5 years	Fleming et al. (1979), Fleming (1989), Makani et al. (2010a), and Komba et al. (2009)
Bacterial infections	10 % of children under 5 years. Prophylaxis recommended against *Streptococcus pneumoniae*	Overturf et al. (1977), Ellison et al. (2013), Ramakrishnan et al. (2010), and Williams et al. (2009)
Anemia	Chronic. Acute episodes associated with mortality. Causes include infection, hemolysis, splenic sequestration	Hayes et al. (1985), El-Hazmi et al. (1987), Maude et al. (1987), Bayoumi et al. (1988), Christakis et al. (1990), Mohamed et al. (1992), and Akenzua et al. (1994)
Aplastic anemia	Associated with parvovirus B19 infection	Serjeant et al. (1981), Neonato et al. (2000), and Juwah et al. (2004)
Hyperhemolysis	Not common in Africa. Reduced with Hydroxyurea	Nolan et al. (2005), Kato et al. (2006), Ballas and Marcolina (2006), and Taylor et al. (2008)
Cholelithiasis	Prevalence is 40 % by adolescence	Childs (1995)
Acute splenic sequestration	Frequently occurs before the age of 3 years	Topley et al. (1981), Emond et al. (1985), and Gill et al. (1995)
Leg ulcers	Prevalence is 10–25 % in adults	Koshy et al. (1989) and Durosinmi et al. (1991)
Priapism	Prevalence is 10–40 % males. Occurs frequently in the 5–14 years age group	Gbadoe et al. (2007)
Stroke	Prevalence is 10 % in children. Risk factor for mortality. High rate of recurrence. Leads to poor quality of life	Ohene-Frempong et al. (1998)
Cognitive/silent stroke	Prevalence is 20 %. Risk factor for overt stroke Leads to impairment of executive function	DeBaun et al. (1998), Kinney et al. (1999), Miller et al. (2001), and Marouf et al. (2003a)
Retinopathy	Prevalence is >30 % in HbSC	Hayes et al. (1981) and Kent et al. (1994)
Acute chest syndrome (ACS)	Prevalence is 40 %. Occurs frequently in children, severe consequences in adults 12.8 per 100-patient years (Castro et al. 1994)	Vichinsky et al. (2000), Castro et al. (1994), and Platt et al. (1994)

(continued)

Table 14.1 (continued)

Clinical event	Characteristics and comments	References
Pulmonary hypertension	Prevalence of 30 % in adults Risk factor for mortality	Castro et al. (2003), Gladwin et al. (2004), Ataga et al. (2006), Nelson et al. (2007), and Onyekwere et al. (2008)
Avascular necrosis	Prevalence is 10–50 %	Griffiths (1968), Ebong (1977), and Lee et al. (1981)
Renal disease	Prevalence of chronic renal failure is 5–20 %	Abbott et al. (2002)

Adapted from Yardumian and Crawley (2001)

Genetic Determinants of Clinical Disease in Africa

There are four major β-globin haplotypes that have been described in Africa, each is associated with different levels of severity (see Fig. 14.3). In West Africa, the Senegal haplotype, which is associated with a high fetal hemoglobin level and a mild phenotype and the Benin haplotype, associated with a moderately severe phenotype, predominate. The Central African Republic (CAR), also known as the Bantu haplotype, occurs predominantly in East and Central Africa and carries a severe phenotype. The Arab/Indian haplotype, also associated with high fetal hemoglobin, is found predominantly in the Arabian Peninsula and the Indian subcontinent, but is also found in a few areas within Africa, such as Zanzibar, where there are populations of Arabs and Indians. The Cameroon haplotype, also found east of Nigeria in West Africa, is not widely distributed and is also associated with moderately severe disease. It should be noted that, in addition to SCA, West Africa has a high prevalence of hemoglobin C, resulting in occurrence of SC disease, which is another form of sickle cell disease (SCD) (Piel et al. 2013b).

One of the principal factors that determine severity in SCA, is the level of fetal hemoglobin (HbF). Following the genomic revolution and completion of the human genome project, efforts have been made to identify genetic loci that are associated with HbF production in SCA in Africa. Genetic variants at three principal loci have been shown to contribute to the inter-individual HbF variation in SCA (Thein et al. 2009; Lettre et al. 2008; Creary et al. 2009)—the region on chromosome 11p that contains the *HBB* and olfactory receptor gene clusters (Solovieff et al. 2010) and two hematopoietic regulator loci, on chromosome 6q (*HBS1L-MYB* intergenic polymorphism, *HMIP*) and on chromosome 2p (*BCL11A*). These loci are thought to account for less than 50 % of HbF variability in healthy European Caucasians (Thein and Menzel 2009). The genetic contribution to HbF in Africans is not clear; but is likely to be lower, with figures estimated at 2–20 % (unpublished observations). Initial work in Tanzania reported that of the three known genetic factors influencing HbF, only one is prevalent in Tanzanian patients, while the other two are rare in this population (Makani et al. 2011b). For this reason, there is a need to replicate genetic studies in African populations and conduct further studies to identify new loci.

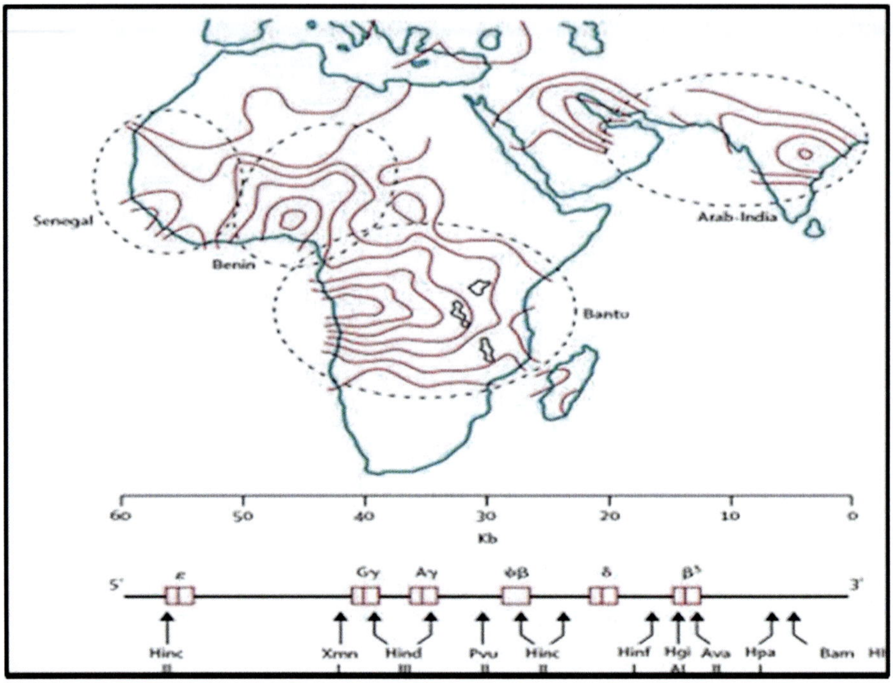

Fig. 14.3 Geographical distribution of the four haplotypes of the sickle gene. (**a**) Map identifies the three distinct areas in Africa and one in the Arab-India region where the sickle gene is present (*dotted lines*). Numbers of individuals with sickle-cell disease (*red lines*) in Senegal, Benin, and Bantu are higher near the coast, and falls concentrically inland. (**b**) The β-globin gene cluster haplotype is determined by DNA polymorphic sites (*boxes*) that are identified by endonuclease enzymes. Figure reproduced with permission from Stuart and Nagel (2004)

Environmental and Social Determinants of Clinical Disease in Africa

Infections, especially malaria and bacterial infections, due to *Streptococcus pneumoniae*, are the leading cause of mortality in SCA. In high-income countries, interventions to prevent infections with pneumococcal vaccination and penicillin prophylaxis are thought to be one of the major factors that have resulted in improved survival, particularly in the first 5 years of life. Unfortunately, few countries in Africa have implemented these interventions. The factors that have led to a delay in implementation of these interventions include debate about the burden of pneumococcal infection in SCA (Kizito et al. 2007; Obaro 2009). However, there is now unequivocal evidence that pneumococcal infection occurs with high prevalence in SCA in Africa (Reddy et al. 2010; Ramakrishnan et al. 2010; Campbell et al. 2004; Williams et al. 2009).

Within Africa, the prevalence of malaria is still high in some areas, although there is increasing evidence that there are changes in the transmission intensity with a decrease in prevalence, particularly in urban areas (O'Meara et al. 2008; Snow et al. 2005; Omumbo et al. 2005; Noor et al. 2014; Wang et al. 2006). However, malaria is still a cause of morbidity and mortality in some areas with the highest burden of disease in children under 5 years of age. The presence of sickle hemoglobin confers protection against malaria infection (Allison 1954b; Abdulhadi 2003; De Paz et al. 2006; Crompton et al. 2008; Rosenthal 2011; Aidoo et al. 2002). However, malaria is associated with increased mortality in SCA (McAuley et al. 2010; Makani et al. 2010; Komba et al. 2009). The issue of malaria chemoprophylaxis is complex due to the lack of evidence to guide the appropriate drug to be used. In the past, chloroquine was the chemoprophylactic agent of choice as it was cheap, effective, had minimal side effects and had a convenient dosing regime, being taken once a week. Current recommendations for chemoprophylaxis are limited because there is no agent that has a suitable profile that would be effective in the long-term for SCA in Africa (Kotila et al. 2007; Oniyangi and Omari 2006; Nwokolo et al. 2001; Mnyika et al. 2000). As a result, it is advisable to ensure malaria prevention with insecticide-treated nets as well as prompt diagnosis and treatment of malaria infection. This is of particular importance in areas with high malaria endemicity, as well as in children under 5 years of age.

The other factors that determine the natural history of SCA in Africa include access to healthcare, socioeconomic status, as well as cultural and religious beliefs (Wonkam et al. 2014; Fullwiley 2011; Brown et al. 2010; Addis et al. 2007; Ohaeri and Shokunbi 2002; Reese and Smith 1997). These factors have a significant role in determining the spectrum of disease, independently of its biological nature. There is a need for more research in Africa, as these factors will allow proper planning to ensure equitable access to health services.

14.1.4 Management (Healthcare)

Summary of Standard-of-Care Practice (Recommended Guidelines)

Management programmes for SCA should provide appropriate advice, counselling and support to parents and affected individuals. A key element of this is providing health education about SCA. This includes interventions such as drinking adequate quantities of fluid to avoid dehydration, recognition of acute events and triggers to seek medical care. Teaching mothers to recognise enlargement of the spleen and anemia was effective in diagnosing and treating anemia due to ASS (Emond et al. 1985; Al-Hawsawi and Ismail 2001). There are four options for SCA management that are recommended (Table 14.2). Most African countries are working towards option one, which involves providing the best possible patient care with the use of prophylactic penicillin following diagnosis, together with retrospective genetic counselling.

Current recommendations for management of SCA have been recently provided, following review of existing evidence (Yawn et al. 2014). These guidelines provide recommendations based on the level of strength of evidence available. Box 14.1

Table 14.2 Options for the management of sickle cell anemia

Option one: Best possible patient care with the use of prophylactic penicillin following diagnosis, together with retrospective genetic counseling
Option two: Best possible patient care, together with a neonatal screening program and the use of penicillin for all homozygous babies, together with retrospective screening and genetic counseling
Option three: Best possible patient care, together with a neonatal screening and the use of prophylactic penicillin from birth for homozygotes, together with population screening and prospective genetic counseling
Option four: As for option three, plus the availability of prenatal diagnosis, bone marrow transplantation, or both

Adapted from Weatherall et al. (2006)

Box 14.1: Selected Interventions for Sickle Cell Anemia That Can Be Implemented in Africa. Adapted from Yawn et al. (2014)

Preventive services

- Daily oral prophylactic penicillin up to the age of 5 years
- Annual transcranial Doppler examinations from the ages of 2 to 16 years in those with sickle cell anemia
- Long-term transfusion therapy to prevent stroke in those children with abnormal transcranial Doppler velocity (≥200 cm/s)

Management of acute complications

- Rapid initiation of opioids for treatment of severe pain associated with a vasoocclusive crisis
- Use of incentive spirometry in patients hospitalized for a vasoocclusive crisis

Management of chronic complications

- Use of analgesics and physical therapy for treatment of avascular necrosis
- Use of angiotensin-converting enzyme inhibitor therapy for microalbuminuria in adults with SCD
- Referral to expert specialists for consideration of laser photocoagulation for children and adults with proliferative sickle cell retinopathy
- Referral to expert specialists for consideration for echocardiography to evaluate signs of pulmonary hypertension

Indications for hydroxyurea therapy

- Adults with three or more severe vasoocclusive crises during any 12-month period
- Adults with SCD pain or chronic anemia interfering with daily activities
- Adults with severe or recurrent episodes of acute chest syndrome
- Consider offering treatment with hydroxyurea without regard to the presence of symptoms for infants, children, and adolescents

Blood transfusion for SCA

- Preoperative transfusion therapy to increase hemoglobin levels to 10 g/dl
- Maintain sickle hemoglobin levels of less than 30 % prior to the next transfusion during long-term transfusion therapy
- Assess iron overload, accompanied by a moderate strength recommendation to begin iron chelation therapy when indicated

outlines some of the recommendations based strong or moderate evidence. For most African counties, a limited diagnostic capacity exists; for example, many centers do not have access to transcranial Doppler ultrasonography. Furthermore, there are limitations in treatment capacity, for approaches such as long-term transfusion therapy, incentive spirometry and laser photocoagulation. However, most African countries should be able to provide at least the following: prophylactic penicillin, opioids for treatment of severe pain, hydroxyurea and blood transfusion for acute episodes of anemia, stroke and acute chest syndrome. Most centers are not in a position to provide long-term blood transfusion therapy for those with abnormal TCD (≥200 cms/s).

14.1.5 Current Practice, Challenges and Opportunities

Burden of Disease

Most African countries will have the challenge of dealing with large numbers of patients. As previously mentioned, estimates suggest that there will be 14,000,000 children born with SCA between 2010 and 2050 (Piel et al. 2013c). With increasing detection and survival, the number of individuals with SCA seeking healthcare will steadily increase (Modell and Darlison 2008). Furthermore, the SCA population in Africa will increasingly have individuals with the severe form of the disease, who will present with advanced complications in the acute and chronic form. This is within a background of limited diagnostic and treatment capacity, as well as within the context of complex ethical, social and cultural issues. As such, an approach that implements the best possible care within this setting is required, as well as the collection of evidence in the form of research in order to modify interventions based on locally appropriate evidence.

Health Systems

Health Facilities: Primary, Secondary and Tertiary Care Level Healthcare in Africa Healthcare in many African countries is administered at three levels. There has been an increase in the number of health facilities within African countries that provide care for SCA (Galadanci et al. 2014; Rahimy et al. 2003; Tshilolo et al. 2008; Makani et al. 2011a); most of these are in urban areas or centered in academic or research-oriented health facilities. In order to increase services beyond these few centers, there must be active strategies to ensure that appropriate management is built into services at all levels of healthcare with adequate support from these specialized centers. SCD stakeholders have been working with governments and international health agencies, such as the WHO, to ensure that there is appropriate management at different levels of healthcare with the development of referral centres for specialised diagnosis and treatment. This approach ensures a cost-effective way of effectively dealing with a highly prevalent condition in areas where resources are limited. However, to ensure adoption and sustainability of these strategies, there must be adequate political will on the part of national governments. Most African countries still do not have legislative policies for the control and management of sickle cell disease. It is doubtful whether much progress can be achieved until this is rectified.

Diagnostic Facilities: Laboratory Investigations for the Diagnosis of SCA There are three laboratory tests that are commonly used for diagnosis of SCA; hemoglobin electrophoresis (HbE), isoelectric focusing (IEF) and high performance liquid chromatography (HPLC). DNA-based tests can be done to precisely describe the genotype. However, for clinical purposes, diagnosis usually involves screening (sickling or solubility test), followed by confirmation of phenotype using one or two of these tests (HbE, IEF or HPLC). In most African hospitals, screening is done using the 'sickling test', which involves making a thin blood film, which is then put under hypoxic conditions by the addition of sodium metabisulphite, and the detection of 'sickled' red blood cells under a light microscope. A 'positive' sickling test identifies the presence of sickled RBCs, which occur in both homo- (SS) and heterozygous (AS) states. Confirmation of SCA is then usually carried out by hemoglobin electrophoresis, although for some hospitals in Africa there is capacity for IEF or HPLC. There is a rationale for centralizing the diagnostic services for confirmation of SCA in a few hospitals, which would receive samples in the form of dried blood spots. The screening could be done at point-of-care and there are currently efforts being made to develop rapid screening tests for SCA (Kumar et al. 2014; Yue et al. 2014).

The identification of individuals with SCA at birth by newborn screening (NBS) and the enrolment of these infants into care programs has been found to be associated with a 70 % decrease in mortality in the first 3 years of life (Yanni et al. 2009). Efforts are therefore being made to advocate the introduction of NBS for SCA within the health systems in Africa (Makani et al. 2015). There are challenges associated with the introduction of NBS such as financial costs, laboratory capacity, as well as logistical challenges associated with screening and feeding back results. However, there is increasing evidence that this is feasible (Tshilolo et al. 2009; Rahimy et al. 2009; Odunvbun et al. 2008; Mutesa et al. 2007). Furthermore, the survival benefits are evident as are the economic costs associated with the prevention of complications, as well as their prompt diagnosis and treatment.

Diagnostic Facilities: Laboratory Investigations for Acute and Chronic Complications In addition to developing capacity for diagnosis of SCA, most African countries need to strengthen their laboratories for the investigation of acute and chronic complications. The priority should be on tests that would identify conditions associated with increased risk of morbidity and mortality. This includes tests in hematology (blood counts, reticulocyte count, direct antiglobulin test for autoimmune hemolysis), chemistry (hemolysis, liver function tests) and infections (malaria, blood cultures). Most African countries have a health system that includes a referral process that will allow individuals to access these services.

Diagnostic Facilities: Imaging Important imaging tests that are needed for SCA management include ultrasound, X-Ray, neuroimaging (CT and MRI), as well as Transcranial Doppler ultrasonography (TCD). Most referral hospitals in African countries have ultrasound facilities, which are useful for the diagnosis of gall bladder disease as well as having capacity for X-ray services, which are needed for diagnosis of osteomyelitis (acute/chronic) and avascular osteonecrosis. With the increasing recognition of the prevalence of stroke, both overt and silent, the confirmation of cerebrovascular disease requires computerized tomography (CT) or magnetic resonance imaging (MRI) of the brain. Unfortunately, these services (including TCD) are limited to a few hospitals in most African countries, and the high cost associated with these tests means that they may not be accessible to everyone.

Medicines and Vaccines

There are a few hospitals in Africa that have a dedicated service for SCA or hematology. Therefore, most healthcare is provided by general practitioners or, where available, specialists in paediatrics and internal medicine. In areas where it is feasible, patients are seen on a regular basis and provided with folic acid supplements.

Prompt treatment of acute episodes, often caused by pain, fever or anemia, particularly at outpatient or in day-care facilities has been found to be effective and reduces the burden of hospitalization to the individual and the health system (Rahimy et al. 1999, 2003). This has been found to have a significant impact on, not only quality of life, but also mortality (Rahimy et al. 2003; Okpala et al. 2002).

Infection management is critical, as this is a major cause of morbidity and mortality. Although not widespread, many African countries are starting to provide penicillin prophylaxis in the under 5-year-old age group (Makani et al. 2015). Furthermore, where available, it is recommended that vaccination against pneumococcal infection should be done. However, there are areas with gaps in knowledge with regards to infection prevention in Africa, which would benefit from further research. The first uncertainty is whether oral penicillin is the best way of providing chemoprophylaxis, considering that this route requires daily administration, which may be associated with difficulties in compliance. The question is, therefore, whether intramuscular penicillin, administered on a monthly basis, would be a better alternative. This is the method used for the prevention of acute rheumatic fever in Africa for children with valvular and rheumatic heart disease. The second question is whether the pneumococcal vaccines that are available will provide coverage against the serotypes of *Streptococcus pneumoniae* that are prevalent in Africa. The third area is to determine the prevalence, pattern and antibiotic sensitivity of the bacterial organisms that cause infection in SCA. There is a surprising dearth of information in this area, which is compounded by the diagnostic capacity for blood stream infections.

It is recommended that the management of malaria in SCA should involve preventative measures, such as the use of insecticide-treated nets. There are challenges with regards to the agent that can be used for chemoprophylaxis, but mefloquine and malarone are recommended. Chloroquine is not recommended for treatment or prophylaxis because of the high prevalence of choloroquine-resistant malaria. Management should include prompt diagnosis and treatment of malaria.

Blood transfusion is used for the management of acute, life-threatening anemia in Africa, although the level of hemoglobin, which is used as a cut-off to make a clinical decision on whether to transfuse, is much lower. There has been an improvement in blood transfusion services in many African countries, with improvement in blood transfusion infection safety. This was triggered by strategies to address the HIV epidemic as part of the efforts to reduce transmission of HIV infections through transfusion. The current challenge is that the supply of blood is not adequate to meet the demand for acute interventions (acute stroke, acute chest syndrome, acute anemia). In addition, long-term transfusion programs, which have been found to be effective in reducing the incidence of stroke in high-risk individuals, are not an option for intervention in many African countries. The other challenge with blood transfusion in Africa is the risk of alloimmunization. Although the prevalence of alloimmunization may be lower than that in the West, due to similarities in ethnicity between the blood donor and SCA population, the risk is still present. Most hospitals and transfusion centers in Africa do not have the capacity to perform extended red blood cell phenotyping in order to provide appropriate blood for those known to have red blood cell antibodies. Finally, there is limited information on the prevalence of iron overload, particularly as a complication of blood transfusion. Despite these challenges, there is a need to increase efforts to improve blood transfusion practice for the management of SCA in Africa.

Hydroxyurea is used for SCA in some African countries (Akingbola et al. 2014; Makubi et al. 2012; Aloni and Nkee 2014; Galadanci et al. 2014). There has been discussion with regards to the potential risks within Africa, such as increased probability of bacterial infection due to myelosuppression, which is a recognized complication of hydroxyurea, as well as concern about an increase in the risk of malaria (Bakanay et al. 2005). However, the current thinking is that the benefits of hydroxyurea far outweigh the risks. It is, therefore, recommended that hydroxyurea should be used when indicated for SCA in Africa, whilst gathering evidence from clinical trials. However, even with encouraging use of hydroxyurea, there are challenges with regards to supply and access. Although it is a drug that has been used in many African countries for treatment of chronic myeloid leukaemia, its use for SCA is not widespread. As a consequence, it is not readily available in both public and private hospitals and pharmacies. Efforts are being made in African countries to increase drug accessibility, either by engaging pharmaceutical companies to support local production or improving local supply.

Hematopoietic stem cell transplantation (HSCT), which replaces the host's bone marrow with stem cells containing normal β-globin genotype, is a potential cure for SCA. Since the first successful transplant reported in 1984 (Johnson et al. 1984), there has been a significant reduction in risks due to SCT and increasing success, with the results, of up to 85 % event-free survival, occurring with HLA-matched sibling donors and transplantation early in the course of the disease before end-organ damage occurs (Walters et al. 1996, 2000; Bernaudin et al. 1993; Vermylen et al. 1998; Talano and Cairo 2015). In high-income countries, there are limitations regarding the availability of sibling donors (Krishnamurti et al. 2003) and therefore there have been attempts to improve survival for matched unrelated stem-cell donors (Woodard et al. 2002; Adamkiewicz et al. 2004). Within Africa, the issue of finding matched sibling donors may not be such a limiting factor, as families tend to be larger in size. Furthermore, although a huge proportion of individuals with SCA in Africa are from a background where HSCT is not an option, there is increasing demand for this intervention (Bazuaye et al. 2014). It is therefore critical that HSCT remains an option that is made available for some individuals with SCA in Africa (Pule and Wonkam 2014).

14.1.6 Conclusion

The course of SCA is heterogeneous, with a wider spectrum of disease-modifying factors in Africa. Despite the knowledge of the various genetic and environmental factors that alter disease severity, it is still difficult to accurately identify individuals with risk of severe disease before extensive damage has occurred, as well to target interventions.

In most African countries, SCA is a disorder of public health significance due to the high prevalence and considerable burden to individuals, communities and the health system. Therefore, there is an urgency to develop national policies and guidelines that will direct interventions that can be used in the short term, and start planning a more detailed management plan for the long term. In the medium to long term, with economic development in low resource countries in Africa, there will be a demographic transition, making chronic, non-communicable diseases such as SCA have increasing importance. Research has shown evidence of reductions in disease morbidity and mortality with the application of relatively simple interventional measures. Until such time that a low-risk, definitive cure is available, the cornerstone of management of SCA in many African countries, as is the case in other areas in the world, is the reduction of early childhood mortality, prevention of end-organ damage and improvement in the quality of life. Primary, community-based care, with facilities for referral to secondary and tertiary centers, would be the most cost-effective strategy to reach the large numbers of affected patients and their families.

14.2 Sickle Cell Disease in the Arabian Peninsula

14.2.1 Introduction

The Arabian Peninsula is home to some of the oldest civilizations in the world and it has witnessed massive migrations from time immemorial. While it contains extensive deserts, it also has fertile areas where agriculture thrived and malaria was endemic. Hemoglobinopathies, including thalassemias and sickle cell disease are quite prevalent. The region is noted for its variety of sickle genotypes, haplotypes, and phenotypes. The high prevalence rates of α- and β-thalassemia (thal) alleles lead to interesting interactions with HbS. The only known dominantly inherited sickle syndrome, in which heterozygotes present with severe phenotype, HbS Oman, is found in the region. Standard-of-care management practice is available in most countries, while newborn and premarital screening programs have also been instituted in many. However, the marked phenotypic heterogeneity is a challenge in formulating uniform management guidelines in the region. This section outlines the pattern of SCD found in the region and the lessons that can be learned from their study.

The Arabian Peninsula covers an area of ~3 million km^2, with an estimated population of ~52 million. It shares borders with Jordan and Iraq in the North, the Persian Gulf and the Gulf of Oman in the East, the Arabian Sea and the Gulf of Aden in the South and the Red Sea in the West. The countries of the Peninsula are Saudi Arabia, which is the largest and most populous with ~27 million people, Yemen, Oman, United Arab Emirates, Qatar, Bahrain and Kuwait. It is essentially a vast plateau, but there are mountain ranges in the Southeast and Southwest. The climate is extremely arid and there are extensive desert areas. However, there are oases and an outer ring of fertile tracts especially in Yemen, Oman and Eastern Saudi Arabia. These support agriculture and malaria was once endemic in parts of the Peninsula, but this has been relatively controlled with only sporadic and imported cases now occurring (Al-Hamidhi et al. 2014).

14.2.2 The Peoples of Arabia

Different peoples have continuously occupied the Peninsula since pre-historic times, with the earliest being Semites in the central region, Ubaidians on the Eastern coast, Hamites in the south and Negroids in the southern coast (Adekile 1997; Nayeem 1990). However, there were waves of migration out of the central part of the Peninsula with the Post-Pleistocene desertification, starting from the fourth millennium BC (Tixier 1986; Oates 1986). The initial centers of civilization were, therefore, established in the fertile area of Southwestern Arabia around Yemen from 1200 BC to 525 AD. The Mediterranean and Indian Seas also linked the great centers of civilization in Egypt, Mesopotamia, Southern Iran and the Indus Valley. An important link in the trade among these centers was the Dilmun civilization, which flourished between 3000 and 1200 BC and extended from present-day Kuwait to Eastern Saudi Arabia and Bahrain (Abu-Hakima 1988).

The greatest revolution in the region occurred with the flight of Prophet Mohammed to Medina in 622 AD, which was the onset of the Islamic Era that brought Arabian culture and influence to a large part of the Middle East, North Africa, Asia and Europe. More recent migrations followed inter-ethnic and recurrent drought in central Arabia. Significantly, members of the Utub tribe left Najd,

East–Central Saudi Arabia in the late seventeenth and early eighteenth centuries and founded settlements in present-day Qatar, Kuwait and the Bahrain Islands (Abu-Hakima 1988). However, both the United Arab Emirates (UAE) and Oman were never under Utub control, but were influenced by Southern Persia and Indus Valley civilizations and were favored by immigrants from Baluchistan over the last two millennia. Oman has maintained close contact with Yemen since the BC era, but by early nineteenth century, the country also controlled Mombasa, and the Island of Zanzibar in East Africa, establishing flourishing trade endeavors (Daar et al. 2000). These migrations and interactions have influenced the gene pool in the region and contributed significantly to the prevalent diversity and complexity of sickle cell and other genetic diseases.

14.2.3 Sickle Cell Disease in Arabia: Genotypes, Haplotypes and Phenotypes

The Arabian Peninsula presents the most variety, of any region of the world, in terms of the prevalent sickle genotypes, haplotypes and phenotypes, with all the known patterns being represented. Some variants are, indeed, peculiar to this part of the world and are not seen elsewhere. Socio-cultural factors also play a role in sustaining the prevalence of mutant genes in the Peninsula. Of importance is the high consanguinity rate, which is as high as 60 % in Saudi Arabia and about 54 % in Kuwait. The most common of these unions, is first-cousin, especially paternal, including double first-cousin marriages (El-Hazmi et al. 2011). The second factor is the large sibship size with averages of 6–7 children per family in many communities. The high prevalence of β- and α-thal alleles and glucose-6-phosphate dehydrogenase deficiency also accounts for different compound forms of SCD, much more than seen in other populations.

The prevalence of the β^S trait varies considerably in the different countries of the Peninsula, being highest in agricultural oases, where malaria was quite prevalent. In Saudi Arabia, prevalence of the trait varies from 2 to 27 %, with up to 1.4 % of the population having the disease in some areas (el-Hazmi and Warsy 1999; Jastaniah 2011; Lehmann et al. 1963). Patients in the Western provinces have a more severe phenotype compared to those in the Eastern provinces. Padmos et al. (1991) were the first to show that the former behave like West African patients and that the predominant β^S-globin haplotype is Benin, associated with low HbF levels, while patients in the Eastern provinces carry the Arab/Indian haplotype characterized by the *HBG2, −158 Xmn-1* (C→T) and have elevated Hb F levels. Patients in the Western province have a more severe phenotype compared to those in the East, although pain crisis and avascular necrosis of the femoral head occur in both. The incidence of overt stroke among hospitalized children with SCD in the former is about 9.4 % (Hawasawi et al. 1998), but is estimated to be lower in the latter (El Sayed et al. 1999).

White et al. (1986) reported a frequency of 0.95 % for sickle trait among Yemenis with a predominance of the Benin haplotype and high α-thal trait frequency (Al-Saqladi et al. 2010; el-Hazmi and Warsy 2000). The patients have a severe phenotype with the most common presenting symptom being dactylitis in 54 %, while the most common causes of hospitalization were pain crisis (36 %), anemic crisis (16 %) and acute chest syndrome in 11 % (Al-Saqladi et al. 2007).

Bahrain has the oldest and most comprehensive SCD prevention program in the Arabian Peninsula. The program was instituted in 1984, with newborn screening starting in 2007. The incidence of affected babies has reduced from 0.7 % in 2008 to 0.4 % in 2010 (Al Arrayed and Al Hajeri 2012). Screening of school children reported a prevalence of 1.2 % for SCD and 13.8 % for AS (Al-Arrayed et al. 2003), while among pregnant women, HbAS was found in 32.5 % (el-Shafei et al. 1992). The Arab/Indian haplotype predominates at about 90 % (Al-Arrayed 1995).

The first report of SCD from Kuwait was in 1970, of three siblings with a mild phenotype and high Hb F levels, who were asymptomatic until late childhood (Ali 1970). More recent reports have confirmed that the Arab/Indian haplotype is predominant with >85 % of the patients being either homozygous or compound heterozygous with the Benin haplotype (Adekile et al. 1994; Adekile and Haider 1996). The phenotype is, however, heterogeneous, but complications like dactylitis, leg ulcers and stroke are uncommon, while osteonecrosis is frequently seen. The commonest presentation is with pain crisis, with low incidence of hemolysis or severe infections.

The frequency of the sickle trait in the United Arab Emirates was reported at 1.9 % in a study of about 5000 Peninsular Arabs (White et al. 1986), while Miller reported a figure of 4.6 % in a survey of preschool children in the country (Miller et al. 2003). However, newborn screening showed a figure of 1.1 % incidence for both UAE nationals and expatriates (Al Hosani et al. 2005). The prevalence of the Arab/Indian haplotype has been put at about 52 %, with considerable phenotypic heterogeneity (Baysal 2001; el-Kalla and Baysal 1998).

According to a survey of ~1702 individuals, the frequency of HbAS in Qatar is about 7.5 % (Fawzi et al. 2003), with the predominant haplotype being Arab/India with a relatively mild, but variable phenotype. Oman presents the most variety in the distribution, haplotype and phenotypic patterns of SCD in the Peninsula. In an analysis of 7837 neonates, an incidence of 4.8 % was reported for HbAS and 0.3 % for SCD (Alkindi et al. 2010). This is similar to the figure of 5.8 % reported by Al-Riyami et al. who also showed a higher prevalence (>70 %) of the disease in areas of high malaria endemicity—Dharia, Dakhliya, North and South Shargiya (Al-Riyami et al. 2001). Because of the historical links to Yemen, Indian subcontinent and East Africa, the three main haplotypes are represented with Benin accounting for 48.7 %, Arab/India 25.8 % and Bantu 20.5 % (Daar et al. 2000). The phenotype of the disease therefore varies relative to the different haplotypes. Interestingly, the dominant sickle cell syndrome (HbS Oman), in which the heterozygote presents with a severe phenotype, has been described among some Omani families (Nagel et al. 1998).

14.2.4 *Peculiarities of SCD in the Arabian Peninsula*

More than any other region, the Arabian Peninsula presents a very interesting interplay of varieties of the disease that are either not encountered or are less prevalent in other populations. The region therefore presents natural models to study and understand these genetic variants. The presence of the Arab/Indian haplotype with high levels of HbF in many patients in the Peninsula, offers an opportunity to elucidate its role as a phenotype modifier. Secondly, the high prevalence of α- and β-thal alleles combines with HbS to produce SCD of variable phenotypes. Glucose-6-phosphate dehydrogenase is also quite prevalent and its influence on SCD has been reported in a number of studies in the region. Lastly, the region presents HbS Oman, which is the only known dominantly-expressed allele in which heterozygotes show a severe phenotype and homozygosity is not compatible with life.

Role of HbF as a Phenotype Modifier

The protective effects of HbF in SCD are evident from the absence of symptoms in affected newborns and young infants. Studies have shown that the heterotetramer, $\alpha_2\gamma\beta^S$, which is formed by the incorporation of γ chains into the HbS molecule is much more soluble than the homotetramer ($\alpha_2\beta^S{}_2$), thus polymerization is reduced in such patients (Poillon et al. 1993; Sunshine et al. 1979). SCD patients with HbF >8.6 % have a better survival and levels of ≥20 % have a milder phenotype and less end-organ pathology (Powars et al. 1984). Probably, the first publication alluding to the mild phenotype of some patients in the Arabian Peninsula was Ali's report of 1970 of older asymptomatic Kuwaiti SCD patients who happened to have elevated Hb F levels (Ali 1970). Padmos et al.'s study of 1991 compared Saudi patients in the Western province who had low Hb F levels to those in the Eastern province with high levels (Padmos et al. 1991). They showed the marked phenotypic differences in both, with the latter having a much more severe phenotype than the former. Western patients had more dactylitis and acute chest syndrome, while Eastern patients had more persistent splenomegaly, but painful crises and avascular necrosis of the femoral (AVN) head were common in both. More recently, Al-Sultan et al. have confirmed the severity of the SCD among Southwestern Saudi patients and reported prevalence figures of 22 %, 14 %, 11.5 % and 7.5 % for acute chest syndrome, osteonecrosis, serious infections and stroke, respectively (Alsultan et al. 2012). It must be stressed, however, that the genetics of HbF and its role as a phenotype modifier are not completely understood and there are still areas that need elucidation.

The distinguishing polymorphism that characterizes the Arab/Indian (AI) and Senegal haplotypes is the *HBG2 −158 Xmn-1*, (C→T) and this, to a large extent is responsible for the sustained elevated HbF levels seen in the patients, even as adults. Other QTLs especially the BCL11A on chromosome 2 and the HBS1L-MYB on chromosome 6 have been shown to be powerful inducers of HbF in the normal population and among patients with beta thalassemia in different ethnic backgrounds

(Akinsheye et al. 2011; Makani et al. 2011b; Thein and Menzel 2009). Indeed, polymorphisms in these two QTLs account for ~20 % of HbF expression in these groups. However, studies of SCD patients with the AI haplotype showed that they contribute only about 8 % to the HbF variance (Alsultan et al. 2013; Akinsheye et al. 2011). This raises the possibility that other yet-unknown, ethnocentric polymorphisms might be important in this group of patients.

It is intriguing, however, that among Arab patients with elevated HbF levels, there is still considerable phenotypic heterogeneity. Among patients in Kuwait, in whom the mean HbF is >20 % and, until the age of ~4 years, it is close to 30 % (Adekile et al. 2007), HbF levels do not significantly influence the frequency of vaso-occlusive crisis or AVN (Adekile and Haider 1996; Adekile et al. 2001). Indeed, AVN is particularly common in this population, being seen in ~26 % of children and 45 % of adults (Adekile et al. 2001; Gupta and Adekile 2004; Marouf et al. 2003b). However, there are some complications that are not encountered or are milder in Kuwaiti patients, including dactylitis, leg ulcers, priapism and acute chest syndrome.

Another distinguishing factor among children with the Arab/Indian haplotype is the absence of significant bacterial infections. This is also attributed to the high HbF levels, especially in the first 2 years of life when SCD patients are most vulnerable to sepsis with encapsulated organisms, especially pneumococcus. Several reports have alluded to the maintenance of spleen function to an older age among Arab patients. An early study (Al-Awamy et al. 1984) showed that a group of children with SCD from Eastern Saudi Arabia had low numbers of pocked RBCs in comparison to American patients who had high levels, indicating normal spleen function in the former. A study of 46 Kuwaiti patients with SCD, aged 2–16 years (Adekile et al. 2002a), using technetium splenic scintigraphy, showed that 39.1 % had normal function, 32.6 % had partial function and 28.3 % had no function. While there was no significant difference in HbF levels in the three groups, the prevalence of α-thal trait was significantly higher in the group with normal function. Similarly, another study from Eastern Saudi Arabia (Al-Jam'a et al. 2000) of 74 adults and children with SCD found that, among the children up to age 4 years, only 16.6 % had functional hyposplenism, which increased to 50 % by the age of 10 years. HbF also had no influence on spleen function and, while α-thal genotyping was not done, patients with low mean corpuscular volume (MCV) had better spleen function.

Of particular interest are central nervous system (CNS) manifestations, which are quite uncommon among Arab patients with the Arab/India haplotype. Stroke is seen in <1.0 % (Adekile 2001) and silent brain infarcts are rare in childhood (Adekile et al. 2002b). However, contrary to reports from the US (Kinney et al. 1999), where new silent infarcts are not seen in adult SCD patients, they are common in adult Kuwaiti patients in whom they are seen in ~20 % (Marouf et al. 2003a). It is, therefore, thought that the high HbF in these patients delays the onset and progression of cerebral small vessel vasculopathy such that brain infarcts are not seen in childhood. However, there is a cumulative, temporal effect, such that sequelae of the disease start to be expressed in adult patients in spite of the high HbF levels. Indeed, a recent study of 104 adult Saudi SCD patients, with elevated HbF levels (Alsultan et al. 2014), confirmed the non-benign nature of their disease. It reported that 47 % had at least one episode of acute chest syndrome; symptomatic osteonecrosis was reported in 18 %, priapism in 17 % and overt stroke in 6 %. Leg ulcers were not seen and there was a high prevalence of persistent splenomegaly. The findings from the Kuwait SCD registry also reflect this pattern of more complications in the adult patients compared to children (Adekile, unpublished data).

Influence of Co-existing α-Thal Trait

The Arabian Peninsula has some of the highest frequencies of α-thalassemia alleles in the world and this is reflected in the degree of its co-inheritance with SCD. The frequency of α-thal trait among Kuwait patients was found to be about 40.0 %, of whom ~30 % carried the α2 −3.7 kb deletion and ~10 % carried the T^{Saudi} non-deletional (AATAAA→AATAAG) allele (Adekile and Haider 1996; Adekile et al. 2007). Among 80 adult patients from Eastern Saudi Arabia with predominant Arab/India haplotype, as in Kuwait, 41 (51 %) had α-thalassemia trait of whom 16 (39 %) were homozygous for the −3.7 kb deletion, while 15 were heterozygous for the T^{Saudi} (Alsultan et al. 2014). While it is believed, in general, that α-thalassemia trait has an ameliorating effect in Arab SCD patients (el-Hazmi and Warsy 1993), studies from Saudi Arabia and Kuwait did not find an influence on the incidence of vaso-occlusive crisis, osteonecrosis or silent brain infarcts (Adekile et al. 2001, 2007; Alsultan et al. 2014; Adekile and Haider 1996). However, α-thalassemia trait significantly reduces the chance of developing gallstones or hyposplenia in Kuwaiti children with SCD (Haider et al. 1998; Adekile et al. 1996).

Influence of Glucose-6-Phosphate Dehydrogenase (G6PD) Deficiency

The frequency of G6PD deficiency varies from ~6 to ~40 % in the different countries of the Arabian Peninsula (Warsy and El-Hazmi 2001; White et al. 1986). There have been contradictory reports of its interaction with SCD with both ameliorating and enhancing effects on the phenotype described (El-Hazmi et al. 2011). G6PD deficiency was found in 47 % of SCD patients in Bahrain (Mohammad and Ardatl 1998), but there was no mention of how it influenced the phenotype. G6PD deficiency by itself did not alter the SCD phenotype among Saudi patients, but in addition to α-thal trait, there was an ameliorating effect (el-Hazmi et al. 1994).

HbSβThal

The high frequency of β-thalassemia in the Arabian Peninsula is reflected in the preponderance of Sβthal compound heterozygotes in the region. The phenotype is heterogeneous, determined to a large extent by the nature of the β-thal mutation (El-Hazmi et al. 2011). While $S\beta^{+}$thal carries a generally mild phenotype, $S\beta^{0}$thal is as severe, if not more so, than SS. Among SCD patients in Saudi Arabia, groups with the highest severity index were $S\beta^0$thal patients with one α-gene deletion and SS without α-thal (el-Hazmi et al. 1994). In Kuwait ~40 % of the patients in the SCD registry are $S\beta^0$thal and present more complications of the disease e.g. splenic sequestration, gallstone, osteopenia and osteonecrosis (Adekile, unpublished data).

HbSD-Punjab

HbD-Punjab or D-Los Angeles is a β-globin chain variant resulting from a Glu → Gln substitution at codon 121 (Itano 1951; Babin et al. 1964). It is most prevalent in the Indian sub-continent, but is seen sporadically in other ethnic groups. Both heterozygotes and homozygotes are clinically and hematologically normal. However, compound heterozygotes with HbS tend to present with a severe course, which may be indistinguishable from HbSS (Kelleher et al. 1984). HbSD is encountered in the Arabian Peninsula, where, indeed it is quite severe. Among Kuwaiti patients, in spite of elevated HbF levels of ~23 %, and HbD concentration of ~45 % and S of <30 %, the phenotype is, indeed, more severe than is generally seen in SS patients with similar Hb F levels (Adekile et al. 2010). It has been hypothesized that the Gluβ121 plays a vital role in gelation and that it weakens the α1/β2 contacts in HbS. When Glu is replaced by another residue (Gln in HbD and Lys in HbO-Arab), a pro-sickling molecule is created, thus explaining why HbSD and HbSO-Arab have such severe phenotypes (Adachi et al. 1988). When two pro-sickling mutations are inherited on the same chromosome, as happens in HbS Oman, a severe phenotype is seen, even in the heterozygote (see below).

HbS Oman

HbS Oman carries the β121 (Glu → Lys) and the β6 (Glu → Val) mutations (Langdown et al. 1989) on the same chromosome. The former is the mutation causing HbO_{Arab}, while the latter is the HbS mutation. The two, together, produce additive sickling effects such that heterozygotes for HbS Oman demonstrate a phenotype similar to HbSS. Nagel et al. (1998) described three individuals with 20–23 % HbS Oman and two others with levels of 13 % and 14 % respectively. The high HbS Oman group had co-existent silent α-thal (–α/αα), while the second group had α-thal trait (–α/-α). The latter had significantly lower MCV and MCH and higher Hb levels. The patients with high HbS Oman had frequent painful crises, acute chest syndrome and hypoxic encephalopathy. It is believed that the pathophysiology of the SCD syndrome in HbS Oman is due to the sickling propensity of both the β6 Val and β121 Lys mutations, but in addition, the latter also has an abnormal interaction with the RBC membrane, inducing hemolysis and RBC changes. Homozygosity for HbS Oman has not been described and it is thought to be incompatible with life.

14.2.5 Challenges to SCD Management in the Arabian Gulf

While many of the countries in the region have excellent facilities to provide adequate comprehensive care, this is not true of all. There is also a dearth of well-trained personnel in many centers, especially in the following cadres that are essential for a robust care program; nurses, social workers, counselors, psychologists, and technical staff. Newborn and obligatory premarital screening programs are available in some, but not all the countries. These programs have been quite successful in Bahrain, where they are starting to make an impact on the incidence of the disease.

Probably the greatest dilemma in producing uniform guidelines for the management of SCD in the region is the wide phenotypic variability encountered in the different affected populations. The β-globin haplotype, fetal hemoglobin level and co-inheritance of α-thalassemia trait have significant influences on the phenotype. Thus among those with the Arab/India haplotype, severe bacterial infections, stroke, leg ulcers and acute chest syndrome are relatively uncommon. Nonetheless, most patients receive penicillin prophylaxis in the first 5 years of life and pneumococcal vaccination is given. Folic acid is also administered on a routine basis. In Kuwait, where most patients have the Arab/India haplotype with elevated HbF, most patients do not present until the age of 4 or 5 years, penicillin prophylaxis is prescribed on an individual basis for those presenting in infancy and any patient <5 years of age with functional hyposplenism. In addition, folic acid is prescribed routinely for patients with Hb <10 g/dl.

Blood transfusion services are excellent in most of the countries with capability for extended phenotypic cross matching and screening for infective agents. Chronic transfusion therapy is available when indicated.

Transcranial Doppler (TCD) screening to identify patients at risk for stroke is advised in SCD patients with a severe phenotype and this is done in many of the centers. However, the two publications on TCD from Kuwait (Asbeutah et al. 2014) and Oman (Gujjar et al. 2013) did not find any abnormal values predictive of stroke using the STOP guidelines. It follows, therefore, that more studies are required to document the "normal" values for this region; otherwise, the current guidelines may not be applicable.

While most centers follow standard practice for the management of SCD acute events, the use of narcotic analgesics for pain control is not uniform. There is still reluctance on the part of some doctors and patients in using morphine especially among adult patients. There is therefore a need for more education in this area.

The use of hydroxyurea is widespread, following the usual indications of frequent, severe pain crisis, acute chest syndrome and severe anemia. Studies from Oman demonstrated the beneficial effects of the drug on hematological parameters, reduction in pain crisis and acute chest syndrome, even with low doses (Sharef et al. 2013; Wali and Moheeb 2011). Hydroxyurea is also effective in patients with high fetal hemoglobin, with no significant adverse effects. MRI hip studies have not shown any increase in avascular necrosis of the femoral head in patients on prolonged therapy (Adekile, unpublished data).

14.2.6 Conclusions

There is a wide variety of SCD genotypes, haplotypes and phenotypes in the countries of the Arabian Peninsula. While the Arabian/Indian haplotype is associated with generally mild disease, there is still considerable heterogeneity among the patients. Indeed, the adult patients may have significant morbidity. There is high level of care with excellent facilities for preventive services, immunization and penicillin prophylaxis and TCD screening in most centers. Blood transfusion services are excellent and hydroxyurea is readily available. However, newborn and premarital screening are still not available or mandatory in many of the countries. The main challenge to recommending uniform management guidelines is the marked phenotypic variability that exists across the region.

References

Abbott KC, Hypolite IO, Agodoa LY (2002) Sickle cell nephropathy at end-stage renal disease in the United States: patient characteristics and survival. Clin Nephrol 58(1):9–15

Abdulhadi NH (2003) Protection against severe clinical manifestations of Plasmodium falciparum malaria among sickle cell trait subjects is due to modification of the release of cytokines and/or cytoadherence of infected erythrocytes to the host vascular beds. Med Hypotheses 60(6):912–914

Abu-Hakima AM (1988) History of Eastern Arabia: the rise and development of Bahrain, Kuwait and Wahhabi Saudi Arabia. Probsthain, London

Adachi K, Kim J, Ballas S, Surrey S, Asakura T (1988) Facilitation of Hb S polymerization by the substitution of Glu for Gln at beta 121. J Biol Chem 263(12):5607–5610

Adamkiewicz TV, Mehta PS, Boyer MW et al (2004) Transplantation of unrelated placental blood cells in children with high-risk sickle cell disease. Bone Marrow Transplant 34:405–411

Addis G, Spector R, Shaw E, Musumadi L, Dhanda C (2007) The physical, social and psychological impact of priapism on adult males with sickle cell disorder. Chronic Illn 3(2):145–154

Adekile AD (1997) Historical and anthropological correlates of beta S haplotypes and alpha- and beta-thalassemia alleles in the Arabian Peninsula. Hemoglobin 21(3):281–296

Adekile AD (2001) Sickle cell disease in Kuwait. Hemoglobin 25(2):219–225

Adekile AD, Haider MZ (1996) Morbidity, beta S haplotype and alpha-globin gene patterns among sickle cell anemia patients in Kuwait. Acta Haematol 96(3):150–154

Adekile AD, Gu LH, Baysal E et al (1994) Molecular characterization of alpha-thalassemia determinants, beta-thalassemia alleles, and beta S haplotypes among Kuwaiti Arabs. Acta Haematol 92(4):176–181

Adekile AD, Tuli M, Haider MZ et al (1996) Influence of alpha-thalassemia trait on spleen function in sickle cell anemia patients with high HbF. Am J Hematol 53(1):1–5

Adekile AD, Gupta R, Yacoub F et al (2001) Avascular necrosis of the hip in children with sickle cell disease and high Hb F: magnetic resonance imaging findings and influence of alpha-thalassemia trait. Acta Haematol 105(1):27–31

Adekile AD, Owunwanne A, Al-Za'abi K et al (2002a) Temporal sequence of splenic dysfunction in sickle cell disease. Am J Hematol 69(1):23–27

Adekile AD, Yacoub F, Gupta R et al (2002b) Silent brain infarcts are rare in Kuwaiti children with sickle cell disease and high Hb F. Am J Hematol 70(3):228–231

Adekile A, Al-Kandari M, Haider M et al (2007) Hemoglobin F concentration as a function of age in Kuwaiti sickle cell disease patients. Med Princ Pract 16(4):286–290

Adekile A, Mullah-Ali A, Akar NA (2010) Does elevated hemoglobin F modulate the phenotype in Hb SD-Los Angeles? Acta Haematol 123(3):135–139
Aidoo M, Terlouw DJ, Kolczak M et al (2002) Protective effects of the sickle cell gene against malaria morbidity and mortality. Lancet 359(9314):1311–1312
Akenzua G, Akinyanju O, Kulozik A et al (1994) Sickle cell anaemia in Nigeria: a comparison between Benin and Lagos. Afr J Med Med Sci 23(2):101–107
Akingbola TS, Tayo BO, Salako B et al (2014) Comparison of patients from Nigeria and the USA highlights modifiable risk factors for sickle cell anemia complications. Hemoglobin 38(4): 236–243
Akinsheye I, Alsultan A, Solovieff N et al (2011) Fetal hemoglobin in sickle cell anemia. Blood 118(1):19–27
Al Arrayed S, Al Hajeri A (2012) Newborn screening services in Bahrain between 1985 and 2010. Adv Hematol 2012:903219
Al Hosani H, Salah M, Osman HM, Farag HM, Anvery SM (2005) Incidence of haemoglobinopathies detected through neonatal screening in the United Arab Emirates. East Mediterr Health J 11(3):300–307
Al-Arrayed SS (1995) Beta globin gene haplotypes in Bahraini patients with sickle cell anaemia. Bahrain Med Bull 17:15–20
Al-Arrayed S, Hafadh N, Amin S, Al-Mukhareq H, Sanad H (2003) Student screening for inherited blood disorders in Bahrain. East Mediterr Health J 9(3):344–352
Al-Awamy B, Wilson WA, Pearson HA (1984) Splenic function in sickle cell disease in the Eastern Province of Saudi Arabia. J Pediatr 104(5):714–717
Al-Hamidhi S, Mahdy MA, Idris MA et al (2014) The prospect of malaria elimination in the Arabian Peninsula: a population genetic approach. Infect Genet Evol 27:25–31
Al-Hawsawi ZM, Ismail GA (2001) Acute splenic sequestration crisis in children with sickle cell disease. Saudi Med J 22(12):1076–1079
Ali SA (1970) Milder variant of sickle-cell disease in Arabs in Kuwait associated with unusually high level of foetal haemoglobin. Br J Haematol 19(5):613–619
Al-Jam'a AH, Al-Dabbous IA, Chirala SK, Al-Majid H, Al-Ali J (2000) Splenic function in sickle cell anemia patients in Qatif, Saudi Arabia. Am J Hematol 63(2):68–73
Alkindi S, Al Zadjali S, Al Madhani A et al (2010) Forecasting hemoglobinopathy burden through neonatal screening in Omani neonates. Hemoglobin 34(2):135–144
Allison AC (1954a) Protection afforded by sickle-cell trait against subtertian malareal infection. Br Med J 4857:290–294
Allison AC (1954b) The distribution of the sickle-cell trait in East Africa and elsewhere, and its apparent relationship to the incidence of subtertian malaria. Trans R Soc Trop Med Hyg 48(4):312–318
Allison AC (1964) Polymorphism and natural selection in human populations. Cold Spring Harb Symp Quant Biol 29:137–149
Aloni MN, Nkee L (2014) Challenge of managing sickle cell disease in a pediatric population living in Kinshasa, Democratic Republic of Congo: a sickle cell center experience. Hemoglobin 38(3):196–200
Al-Riyami AA, Suleiman AJ, Afifi M, Al-Lamki ZM, Daar S (2001) A community-based study of common hereditary blood disorders in Oman. East Mediterr Health J 7(6):1004–1011
Al-Saqladi AW, Delpisheh A, Bin-Gadeem H, Brabin BJ (2007) Clinical profile of sickle cell disease in Yemeni children. Ann Trop Paediatr 27(4):253–259
Al-Saqladi AW, Brabin BJ, Bin-Gadeem HA et al (2010) Beta-globin gene cluster haplotypes in Yemeni children with sickle cell disease. Acta Haematol 123(3):182–185
Alsultan A, Aleem A, Ghabbour H et al (2012) Sickle cell disease subphenotypes in patients from Southwestern Province of Saudi Arabia. J Pediatr Hematol Oncol 34(2):79–84
Alsultan A, Alabdulaali MK, Griffin PJ et al (2014) Sickle cell disease in Saudi Arabia: the phenotype in adults with the Arab–Indian haplotype is not benign. Br J Haematol 164:597–604
Alsultan A, Ngo D, Bae H et al (2013) Genetic studies of fetal hemoglobin in the Arab–Indian haplotype sickle cell-beta(0) thalassemia. Am J Hematol 88(6):531–532

Asbeutah A, Gupta R, Al-Saeid O et al (2014) Transcranial Doppler and brain MRI in children with sickle cell disease and high hemoglobin F levels. Pediatr Blood Cancer 61(1):25–28

Ataga KI, Moore CG, Jones S et al (2006) Pulmonary hypertension in patients with sickle cell disease: a longitudinal study. Br J Haematol 134(1):109–115

Babin DR, Jones RT, Schroeder WA (1964) HEMOGLOBIN D-LOS ANGELES: ALPHA-2A BETA 2–121 GLUNH2. Biochim Biophys Acta 86:136–143

Bakanay SM, Dainer E, Clair B et al (2005) Mortality in sickle cell patients on hydroxyurea therapy. Blood 105:545–547

Ballas SK, Marcolina MJ (2006) Hyperhemolysis during the evolution of uncomplicated acute painful episodes in patients with sickle cell anemia. Transfusion 46(1):105–110

Bayoumi RA, Abu Zeid YA, Abdul Sadig A, Awad Elkarim O (1988) Sickle cell disease in Sudan. Trans R Soc Trop Med Hyg 82(1):164–168

Baysal E (2001) Hemoglobinopathies in the United Arab Emirates. Hemoglobin 25(2):247–253

Bazuaye N, Nwogoh B, Ikponmwen D et al (2014) First successful allogeneic hematopoietic stem cell transplantation for a sickle cell disease patient in a low resource country (Nigeria): a case report. Ann Transplant 19:210–213

Bernaudin F, Souillet G, Vannier JP et al (1993) Bone marrow transplantation (BMT) in 14 children with severe sickle cell disease (SCD): the French experience. GEGMO. Bone Marrow Transplant 12(Suppl 1):118–121

Brown BJ, Okereke JO, Lagunju A et al (2010) Burden of health-care of carers of children with sickle cell disease in Nigeria. Health Soc Care Community 18(3):289–295

Brozovic M, Anionwu E (1984) Sickle cell disease in Britain. J Clin Pathol 37(12):1321–1326

Campbell JD, Kotloff KL, Sow SO et al (2004) Invasive pneumococcal infections among hospitalized children in Bamako, Mali. Pediatr Infect Dis J 23(7):642–649

Castro O, Brambilla DJ, Thorington B et al (1994) The acute chest syndrome in sickle cell disease: incidence and risk factors. The Cooperative Study of Sickle Cell Disease. Blood 84(2):643–649

Castro O, Hoque M, Brown BD (2003) Pulmonary hypertension in sickle cell disease: cardiac catheterization results and survival. Blood 101(4):1257–1261

Charles KS, Osagie K, Battini RK (2006) Hospital admissions for acute painful crisis in Trinidad and Tobago. Are the British Committee for Standards in Haematology (BCSH) guidelines applicable? Clin Lab Haematol 28(5):299–302

Childs JW (1995) Sickle cell disease: the clinical manifestations. J Am Osteopath Assoc 95(10):593–598

Christakis J, Vavatsi N, Hassapopoulou H et al (1990) Comparison of homozygous sickle cell disease in northern Greece and Jamaica. Lancet 335(8690):637–640

Creary LE, Ulug P, Menzel S et al (2009) Genetic variation on chromosome 6 influences F cell levels in healthy individuals of African descent and HbF levels in sickle cell patients. PLoS One 4(1), e4218

Crompton PD, Traore B, Kayentao K et al (2008) Sickle cell trait is associated with a delayed onset of malaria: implications for time-to-event analysis in clinical studies of malaria. J Infect Dis 198:1265–1275

Daar S, Hussain H, Gravell D, Nagel R, Krishnamoorthy R (2000) Genetic epidemiology of HbS in Oman: multicentric origin for the betaS gene. Am J Hematol 64(1):39–46

De Paz FJ, Romero A, Diez D et al (2006) Malaria and sickle cell disease. Haematologica 91(12 Suppl):EIM03

DeBaun MR, Schatz J, Siegel MJ et al (1998) Cognitive screening examinations for silent cerebral infarcts in sickle cell disease. Neurology 50(6):1678–1682

Durosinmi MA, Gevao SM, Esan GJ (1991) Chronic leg ulcers in sickle cell disease: experience in Ibadan, Nigeria. Afr J Med Med Sci 20(1):11–14

Ebong WW (1977) Avascular necrosis of the femoral head associated with haemoglobinopathy. Trop Geogr Med 29(1):19–23

El Sayed MM, Adeuja AO, El-Nahrawy E, Olaish MA (1999) Characteristics of stroke in Hofuf, Saudi Arabia. Ann Saudi Med 19(1):27–31

el-Hazmi MA, Warsy AS (1993) On the molecular interactions between alpha-thalassaemia and sickle cell gene. J Trop Pediatr 39(4):209–213

el-Hazmi MA, Warsy AS (1999) Appraisal of sickle-cell and thalassaemia genes in Saudi Arabia. East Mediterr Health J 5:1147–1153

el-Hazmi MA, Warsy AS (2000) Xmn I polymorphic site in Yemeni sickle cell disease patients. J Trop Pediatr 46(1):25–29

El-Hazmi MA, Jabbar FA, Al-Faleh FZ, Al-Swailem AR, Warsy AS (1987) The haematological, biochemical and clinical – presentation of haemoglobin S in Saudi Arabia (i). Haematological & clinical expression. Trop Geogr Med 39(2):157–162

El-Hazmi MA, Warsy AS, al-Swailem AR, al-Faleh FZ, al-Jabbar FA (1994) Genetic compounds – Hb S, thalassaemias and enzymopathies: spectrum of interactions. J Trop Pediatr 40(3):149–156

el-Hazmi MA, Al-Hazmi AM, Warsy AS (2011) Sickle cell disease in Middle East Arab countries. Indian J Med Res 134(5):597–610

el-Kalla S, Baysal E (1998) Genotype-phenotype correlation of sickle cell disease in the United Arab Emirates. Pediatr Hematol Oncol 15(3):237–242

Ellison AM, Ota KV, McGowan KL, Smith-Whitley K (2013) Epidemiology of bloodstream infections in children with sickle cell disease. Pediatr Infect Dis J 32(5):560–563

el-Shafei AM, Dhaliwal JK, Sandhu AK (1992) Pregnancy in sickle cell disease in Bahrain. Br J Obstet Gynaecol 99(2):101–104

Emond AM, Collis R, Darvill D et al (1985) Acute splenic sequestration in homozygous sickle cell disease: natural history and management. J Pediatr 107(2):201–206

Fawzi Z, Al-Hilali A, Fakhroo N, Al-Bin-Ali A, Al-Mansour S (2003) Distribution of hemoglobinopathies and thalassaemias in Qatari nationals seen at Hamad Hospital in Qatar. Qatar Med J 12:20–24

Fleming AF (1989) The presentation, management and prevention of crisis in sickle cell disease in Africa. Blood Rev 3(1):18–28

Fleming AF, Storey J, Molineaux L, Iroko EA, Attai ED (1979) Abnormal haemoglobins in the Sudan savanna of Nigeria. I. Prevalence of haemoglobins and relationships between sickle cell trait, malaria and survival. Ann Trop Med Parasitol 73(2):161–172

Fullwiley D (2011) The enculturated gene: sickle cell health politics and biological difference in West Africa. Princeton University Press, Princeton

Galadanci N, Wudil BJ, Balogun TM et al (2014) Current sickle cell disease management practices in Nigeria. Int Health 6(1):23–28

Gbadoe AD, Geraldo A, Guedenon K et al (2007) Stuttering priapism in children with sickle cell anemia in Togo. Arch Pediatr 14(7):861–863

Gill FM, Sleeper LA, Weiner SJ et al (1995) Clinical events in the first decade in a cohort of infants with sickle cell disease. Cooperative Study of Sickle Cell Disease. Blood 86(2):776–783

Gladwin MT, Sachdev V, Jison ML et al (2004) Pulmonary hypertension as a risk factor for death in patients with sickle cell disease. N Engl J Med 350(9):886–895

Griffiths J (1968) Avascular necrosis of femoral head in Kenyan Africans. East Afr Med J 45(9):613–618

Gujjar AR, Zacharia M, Al-Kindi S et al (2013) Transcranial Doppler ultrasonography in sickle cell disease: a study in Omani patients. J Pediatr Hematol Oncol 35(1):18–23

Gupta R, Adekile AD (2004) MRI follow-up and natural history of avascular necrosis of the femoral head in Kuwaiti children with sickle cell disease. J Pediatr Hematol Oncol 26(6):351–353

Haider MZ, Ashebu S, Aduh P, Adekile AD (1998) Influence of alpha-thalassemia on cholelithiasis in SS patients with elevated Hb F. Acta Haematol 100(3):147–150

Haldane JBS (1949) The rate of mutation of human genes. Hereditas 35(Suppl):267–273

Hassell KL (2010) Population estimates of sickle cell disease in the U.S. Am J Prev Med 38(4 Suppl):S512–S521

Hawasawi ZM, Nabi G, Al Magamci MS, Awad KS (1998) Sickle cell disease in childhood in Madina. Ann Saudi Med 18(4):293–295

Hayes RJ, Condon PI, Serjeant GR (1981) Haematological factors associated with proliferative retinopathy in sickle cell-haemoglobin C disease. Br J Ophthalmol 65(10):712–717

Hayes RJ, Beckford M, Grandison Y et al (1985) The haematology of steady state homozygous sickle cell disease: frequency distributions, variation with age and sex, longitudinal observations. Br J Haematol 59(2):369–382

Ibidapo MO, Akinyanju OO (2000) Acute sickle cell syndromes in Nigerian adults. Clin Lab Haematol 22(3):151–155

Itano HA (1951) A third abnormal hemoglobin associated with hereditary hemolytic anemia. Proc Natl Acad Sci U S A 37(12):775–784

Jastaniah W (2011) Epidemiology of sickle cell disease in Saudi Arabia. Ann Saudi Med 31(3):289–293

Johnson FL, Look AT, Gockerman J et al (1984) Bone-marrow transplantation in a patient with sickle-cell anemia. N Engl J Med 311(12):780–783

Juwah AI, Nlemadim EU, Kaine W (2004) Types of anaemic crises in paediatric patients with sickle cell anaemia seen in Enugu, Nigeria. Arch Dis Child 89(6):572–576

Kato GJ, McGowan V, Machado RF et al (2006) Lactate dehydrogenase as a biomarker of hemolysis-associated nitric oxide resistance, priapism, leg ulceration, pulmonary hypertension, and death in patients with sickle cell disease. Blood 107(6):2279–2285

Kelleher JF Jr, Park JO, Kim HC, Schroeder WA (1984) Life-threatening complications in a child with hemoglobin SD-Los Angeles disease. Hemoglobin 8(3):203–213

Kent D, Arya R, Aclimandos WA, Bellingham AJ, Bird AC (1994) Screening for ophthalmic manifestations of sickle cell disease in the United Kingdom. Eye (Lond) 8(Pt 6):618–622

Kinney TR, Sleeper LA, Wang WC et al (1999) Silent cerebral infarcts in sickle cell anemia: a risk factor analysis. The Cooperative Study of Sickle Cell Disease. Pediatrics 103(3):640–645

Kizito ME, Mworozi E, Ndugwa C, Serjeant GR (2007) Bacteraemia in homozygous sickle cell disease in Africa: is pneumococcal prophylaxis justified? Arch Dis Child 92(1):21–23

Komba AN, Makani J, Sadarangani M et al (2009) Malaria as a cause of morbidity and mortality in children with homozygous sickle cell disease on the coast of Kenya. Clin Infect Dis 49(2):216–222

Koshy M, Entsuah R, Koranda A et al (1989) Leg ulcers in patients with sickle cell disease. Blood 74(4):1403–1408

Kotila R, Okesola A, Makanjuola O (2007) Asymptomatic malaria parasitaemia in sickle-cell disease patients: how effective is chemoprophylaxis? J Vector Borne Dis 44(1):52–55

Krishnamurti L, Abel S, Maiers M, Flesch S (2003) Availability of unrelated donors for hematopoietic stem cell transplantation for hemoglobinopathies. Bone Marrow Transplant 31(7):547–550

Kumar AA, Patton MR, Hennek JW et al (2014) Density-based separation in multiphase systems provides a simple method to identify sickle cell disease. Proc Natl Acad Sci U S A 111:14864–14869

Langdown JV, Williamson D, Knight CB, Rubenstein D, Carrell RW (1989) A new doubly substituted sickling haemoglobin: HbS-Oman. Br J Haematol 71(3):443–444

Lee RE, Golding JS, Serjeant GR (1981) The radiological features of avascular necrosis of the femoral head in homozygous sickle cell disease. Clin Radiol 32(2):205–214

Lehmann H, Maranjian G, Mourant A (1963) Distribution of sickle-cell hemoglobin in Saudi Arabia. Nature 198:492–493

Leikin SL, Gallagher D, Kinney TR et al (1989) Mortality in children and adolescents with sickle cell disease. Cooperative Study of Sickle Cell Disease. Pediatrics 84(3):500–508

Lettre G, Sankaran VG, Bezerra MA et al (2008) DNA polymorphisms at the BCL11A, HBS1L-MYB, and beta-globin loci associate with fetal hemoglobin levels and pain crises in sickle cell disease. Proc Natl Acad Sci U S A 105(33):11869–11874

Makani J, Williams TN, Marsh K (2007) Sickle cell disease in Africa: burden and research priorities. Ann Trop Med Parasitol 101(1):3–14

Makani J, Komba AN, Cox SE et al (2010) Malaria in patients with sickle cell anemia: burden, risk factors, and outcome at the outpatient clinic and during hospitalization. Blood 115(2):215–220

Makani J, Cox SE, Soka D et al (2011a) Mortality in sickle cell anemia in Africa: a prospective cohort study in Tanzania. PLoS One 6(2):e14699

Makani J, Menzel S, Nkya S et al (2011b) Genetics of fetal hemoglobin in Tanzanian and British patients with sickle cell anemia. Blood 117(4):1390–1392

Makani J, Soka D, Rwezaula S et al (2015) Health policy for sickle cell disease in Africa: experience from Tanzania on interventions to reduce under-five mortality. Trop Med Int Health 20:184–187

Makubi A, Soka D, Makani J (2012) Moyamoya disease, a rare cause of recurrent strokes in an African sickle cell child: does hydroxyurea have a role in this context? Int J Child Health Nutr 1(1):82–85

Marouf R, Gupta R, Haider MZ, Adekile AD (2003a) Silent brain infarcts in adult Kuwaiti sickle cell disease patients. Am J Hematol 73(4):240–243

Marouf R, Gupta R, Haider MZ, Al-Wazzan H, Adekile AD (2003b) Avascular necrosis of the femoral head in adult Kuwaiti sickle cell disease patients. Acta Haematol 110(1):11–15

Maude GH, Hayes RJ, Serjeant GR (1987) The haematology of steady state homozygous sickle cell disease: interrelationships between haematological indices. Br J Haematol 66(4):549–558

McAuley CF, Webb C, Makani J et al (2010) High mortality from Plasmodium falciparum malaria in children living with sickle cell anemia on the coast of Kenya. Blood 116(10):1663–1668

Miller ST, Macklin EA, Pegelow CH et al (2001) Silent infarction as a risk factor for overt stroke in children with sickle cell anemia: a report from the Cooperative Study of Sickle Cell Disease. J Pediatr 139(3):385–390

Miller CJ, Dunn EV, Berg B, Abdouni SF (2003) A hematological survey of preschool children of the United Arab Emirates. Saudi Med J 24(6):609–613

Mnyika SK, Kabalimu TK, Mbaruku G, Masisila R, Mpanju-Shumbusho W (2000) Randomised trial of alternative malaria chemoprophylaxis strategies among pregnant women in Kigoma, Tanzania: II. Results from baseline studies. East Afr Med J 77(2):105–110

Modell B, Darlison M (2008) Global epidemiology of haemoglobin disorders and derived service indicators. Bull World Health Organ 86(6):480–487

Mohamed AO, Bayoumi RA, Hofvander Y, Omer MI, Ronquist G (1992) Sickle cell anaemia in Sudan: clinical findings, haematological and serum variables. Ann Trop Paediatr 12(2):131–136

Mohammad AM, Ardatl KO (1998) Sickle cell disease in Bahrain: coexistence and interaction with glucose-6-phosphate dehydrogenase (G6PD) deficiency. J Trop Pediatr 44:70–72

Mutesa L, Boemer F, Ngendahayo L et al (2007) Neonatal screening for sickle cell disease in Central Africa: a study of 1825 newborns with a new enzyme-linked immunosorbent assay test. J Med Screen 14(3):113–116

Nagel RL, Daar S, Romero JR et al (1998) HbS-oman heterozygote: a new dominant sickle syndrome. Blood 92(11):4375–4382

Nayeem MA (1990) Prehistory and protohistory of the Arabian peninsula, vol 1. Hyderabad Publishers, Hyderabad, India

Nelson SC, Adade BB, McDonough EA, Moquist KL, Hennessy JM (2007) High prevalence of pulmonary hypertension in children with sickle cell disease. J Pediatr Hematol Oncol 29(5):334–337

Neonato MG, Guilloud-Bataille M, Beauvais P et al (2000) Acute clinical events in 299 homozygous sickle cell patients living in France. French Study Group on Sickle Cell Disease. Eur J Haematol 65(3):155–164

Nolan VG, Wyszynski DF, Farrer LA, Steinberg MH (2005) Hemolysis-associated priapism in sickle cell disease. Blood 106(9):3264–3267

Noor AM, Kinyoki DK, Mundia CW et al (2014) The changing risk of Plasmodium falciparum malaria infection in Africa: 2000–10: a spatial and temporal analysis of transmission intensity. Lancet 383(9930):1739–1747

Nwokolo C, Wambebe C, Akinyanju CO et al (2001) Mefloquine versus proguanil in short-term malaria chemoprophylaxis in sickle cell anaemia. Clin Drug Investig 21(8):537–544

Oates J (1986) The gulf in prehistory. In: H.A. Al Khalifa and M. Rice (eds) Bahrain through the ages: the archeology. London 79–86.

Obaro S (2009) Pneumococcal infections and sickle cell disease in Africa: does absence of evidence imply evidence of absence? Arch Dis Child 94(9):713–716

Odunvbun ME, Okolo AA, Rahimy CM (2008) Newborn screening for sickle cell disease in a Nigerian hospital. Public Health 122(10):1111–1116

Ohaeri JU, Shokunbi WA (2002) Psychosocial burden of sickle cell disease on caregivers in a Nigerian setting. J Natl Med Assoc 94(12):1058–1070

Ohene-Frempong K, Weiner SJ, Sleeper LA et al (1998) Cerebrovascular accidents in sickle cell disease: rates and risk factors. Blood 91(1):288–294

Okpala I, Thomas V, Westerdale N et al (2002) The comprehensiveness care of sickle cell disease. Eur J Haematol 68(3):157–162

Olabode JO, Shokunbi WA (2006) Types of crises in sickle cell disease patients presenting at the haematology day care unit (HDCU), University College Hospital (UCH), Ibadan. West Afr J Med 25(4):284–288

O'Meara WP, Bejon P, Mwangi TW et al (2008) Effect of a fall in malaria transmission on morbidity and mortality in Kilifi, Kenya. Lancet 372(9649):1555–1562

Omumbo JA, Guerra CA, Hay SI, Snow RW (2005) The influence of urbanisation on measures of Plasmodium falciparum infection prevalence in East Africa. Acta Trop 93(1):11–21

Oniyangi O, Omari AA (2006) Malaria chemoprophylaxis in sickle cell disease. Cochrane Database Syst Rev 4, CD003489

Onyekwere OC, Campbell A, Teshome M et al (2008) Pulmonary hypertension in children and adolescents with sickle cell disease. Pediatr Cardiol 29(2):309–312

Overturf GD, Powars D, Baraff LJ (1977) Bacterial meningitis and septicemia in sickle cell disease. Am J Dis Child 131(7):784–787

Padmos MA, Roberts GT, Sackey K et al (1991) Two different forms of homozygous sickle cell disease occur in Saudi Arabia. Br J Haematol 79(1):93–98

Penman BS, Pybus OG, Weatherall DJ, Gupta S (2009) Epistatic interactions between genetic disorders of hemoglobin can explain why the sickle-cell gene is uncommon in the Mediterranean. Proc Natl Acad Sci U S A 106(50):21242–21246

Penman BS, Gupta S, Buckee CO (2012) The emergence and maintenance of sickle cell hotspots in the Mediterranean. Infect Genet Evol 12(7):1543–1550

Piel FB, Patil AP, Howes RE et al (2010) Global distribution of the sickle cell gene and geographical confirmation of the malaria hypothesis. Nat Commun 1:104

Piel FB, Hay SI, Gupta S, Weatherall DJ, Williams TN (2013a) Global burden of sickle cell anaemia in children under five, 2010–2050: modelling based on demographics, excess mortality, and interventions. PLoS Med 10(7):e1001484

Piel FB, Howes RE, Patil AP et al (2013b) The distribution of haemoglobin C and its prevalence in newborns in Africa. Sci Rep 3:1671

Piel FB, Patil AP, Howes RE et al (2013c) Global epidemiology of sickle haemoglobin in neonates: a contemporary geostatistical model-based map and population estimates. Lancet 381(9861): 142–151

Platt OS, Thorington BD, Brambilla DJ et al (1991) Pain in sickle cell disease. Rates and risk factors. N Engl J Med 325(1):11–16

Platt OS, Brambilla DJ, Rosse WF et al (1994) Mortality in sickle cell disease. Life expectancy and risk factors for early death. N Engl J Med 330(23):1639–1644

Poillon WN, Kim BC, Rodgers GP, Noguchi CT, Schechter AN (1993) Sparing effect of hemoglobin F and hemoglobin A2 on the polymerization of hemoglobin S at physiologic ligand saturations. Proc Natl Acad Sci U S A 90(11):5039–5043

Powars DR, Weiss JN, Chan LS, Schroeder WA (1984) Is there a threshold level of fetal hemoglobin that ameliorates morbidity in sickle cell anemia? Blood 63(4):921–926

Pule G, Wonkam A (2014) Treatment for sickle cell disease in Africa: should we invest in haematopoietic stem cell transplantation? Pan Afr Med J 18:46

Quinn CT, Rogers ZR, Buchanan GR (2004) Survival of children with sickle cell disease. Blood 103(11):4023–4027
Quinn CT, Shull EP, Ahmad N et al (2007) Prognostic significance of early vaso-occlusive complications in children with sickle cell anemia. Blood 109(1):40–45
Quinn CT, Rogers ZR, McCavit TL, Buchanan GR (2010) Improved survival of children and adolescents with sickle cell disease. Blood 115(17):3447–3452
Rahimy MC, Gangbo A, Ahouignan G et al (1999) Outpatient management of fever in children with sickle cell disease (SCD) in an African setting. Am J Hematol 62(1):1–6
Rahimy MC, Gangbo A, Ahouignan G et al (2003) Effect of a comprehensive clinical care program on disease course in severely ill children with sickle cell anemia in a sub-Saharan African setting. Blood 102(3):834–838
Rahimy MC, Gangbo A, Ahouignan G, Alihonou E (2009) Newborn screening for sickle cell disease in the Republic of Benin. J Clin Pathol 62(1):46–48
Ramakrishnan M, Moisi JC, Klugman KP et al (2010) Increased risk of invasive bacterial infections in African people with sickle-cell disease: a systematic review and meta-analysis. Lancet Infect Dis 10(5):329–337
Reddy EA, Shaw AV, Crump JA (2010) Community-acquired bloodstream infections in Africa: a systematic review and meta-analysis. Lancet Infect Dis 10(6):417–432
Reese FL, Smith WR (1997) Psychosocial determinants of health care utilization in sickle cell disease patients. Ann Behav Med 19(2):171–178
Rosenthal PJ (2011) Lessons from sickle cell disease in the treatment and control of malaria. N Engl J Med 364(26):2549–2551
Serjeant GR, Topley JM, Mason K et al (1981) Outbreak of aplastic crises in sickle cell anaemia associated with parvovirus-like agent. Lancet 2(8247):595–597
Sharef SW, Al-Hajri M, Beshlawi I et al (2013) Optimizing Hydroxyurea use in children with sickle cell disease: low dose regimen is effective. Eur J Haematol 90(6):519–524
Snow RW, Guerra CA, Noor AM, Myint HY, Hay SI (2005) The global distribution of clinical episodes of Plasmodium falciparum malaria. Nature 434(7030):214–217
Solovieff N, Milton JN, Hartley SW et al (2010) Fetal hemoglobin in sickle cell anemia: genome-wide association studies suggest a regulatory region in the 5' olfactory receptor gene cluster. Blood 115(9):1815–1822
Stuart MJ, Nagel RL (2004) Sickle-cell disease. Lancet 364(9442):1343–1360
Sunshine HR, Hofrichter J, Eaton WA (1979) Gelation of sickle cell hemoglobin in mixtures with normal adult and fetal hemoglobins. J Mol Biol 133(4):435–467
Talano JA, Cairo MS (2015) Hematopoietic stem cell transplantation for sickle cell disease: state of the science. Eur J Haematol 94:391–399
Taylor JG, Nolan VG, Mendelsohn L et al (2008) Chronic hyper-hemolysis in sickle cell anemia: association of vascular complications and mortality with less frequent vasoocclusive pain. PLoS One 3(5):e2095
Telfer P, Coen P, Chakravorty S et al (2007) Clinical outcomes in children with sickle cell disease living in England: a neonatal cohort in East London. Haematologica 92(7):905–912
Thein SL, Menzel S (2009) Discovering the genetics underlying foetal haemoglobin production in adults. Br J Haematol 145(4):455–467
Thein SL, Menzel S, Lathrop M, Garner C (2009) Control of fetal hemoglobin: new insights emerging from genomics and clinical implications. Hum Mol Genet 18(R2):R216–R223
Thomas AN, Pattison C, Serjeant GR (1982) Causes of death in sickle-cell disease in Jamaica. Br Med J (Clin Res Ed) 285(6342):633–635
Tixier J (1986) The prehistory of the Gulf: recent findings. In: H.A. Al Khalifa and M. Rice (eds) Bahrain through the ages: the archeology. London 76–78.
Topley JM, Rogers DW, Stevens MC, Serjeant GR (1981) Acute splenic sequestration and hypersplenism in the first five years in homozygous sickle cell disease. Arch Dis Child 56(10):765–769

Tshilolo L, Kafando E, Sawadogo M et al (2008) Neonatal screening and clinical care programmes for sickle cell disorders in sub-Saharan Africa: lessons from pilot studies. Public Health 122(9):933–941

Tshilolo L, Aissi LM, Lukusa D et al (2009) Neonatal screening for sickle cell anaemia in the Democratic Republic of the Congo: experience from a pioneer project on 31 204 newborns. J Clin Pathol 62(1):35–38

Vermylen C, Cornu G, Ferster A et al (1998) Haematopoietic stem cell transplantation for sickle cell anaemia: the first 50 patients transplanted in Belgium. Bone Marrow Transplant 22(1):1–6

Vichinsky EP, Neumayr LD, Earles AN et al (2000) Causes and outcomes of the acute chest syndrome in sickle cell disease. National Acute Chest Syndrome Study Group. N Engl J Med 342(25):1855–1865

Wali YA, Moheeb H (2011) Effect of hydroxyurea on physical fitness indices in children with sickle cell anemia. Pediatr Hematol Oncol 28(1):43–50

Walters MC, Patience M, Leisenring W et al (1996) Bone marrow transplantation for sickle cell disease. N Engl J Med 335(6):369–376

Walters MC, Storb R, Patience M et al (2000) Impact of bone marrow transplantation for symptomatic sickle cell disease: an interim report. Multicenter investigation of bone marrow transplantation for sickle cell disease. Blood 95(6):1918–1924

Wang SJ, Lengeler C, Mtasiwa D et al (2006) Rapid Urban Malaria Appraisal (RUMA) II: epidemiology of urban malaria in Dar es Salaam (Tanzania). Malar J 5:28

Warsy AS, El-Hazmi MA (2001) G6PD deficiency, distribution and variants in Saudi Arabia: an overview. Ann Saudi Med 21(3–4):174–177

Weatherall D, Akinyanju O, Fucharoen S, Olivieri N, Musgrove P (2006) Inherited disorders of hemoglobin. In: Jamison D (ed) Disease control priorities in developing countries, 2nd edn. Oxford University Press, New York, pp 663–680

White JM, Byrne M, Richards R et al (1986) Red cell genetic abnormalities in Peninsular Arabs: sickle haemoglobin, G6PD deficiency, and alpha and beta thalassaemia. J Med Genet 23(3): 245–251

Williams TN, Uyoga S, Macharia A et al (2009) Bacteraemia in Kenyan children with sickle-cell anaemia: a retrospective cohort and case–control study. Lancet 374(9698):1364–1370

Wonkam A, Mba CZ, Mbanya D et al (2014) Psychosocial burden of sickle cell disease on parents with an affected child in Cameroon. J Genet Couns 23(2):192–201

Woodard P, Lubin B, Walters CM (2002) New approaches to hematopoietic cell transplantation for hematological diseases in children. Pediatr Clin North Am 49(5):989–1007

Yanni E, Grosse SD, Yang Q, Olney RS (2009) Trends in pediatric sickle cell disease-related mortality in the United States, 1983–2002. J Pediatr 154(4):541–545

Yardumian A, Crawley C (2001) Sickle cell disease. Clin Med 1(6):441–446

Yawn BP, Buchanan GR, Afenyi-Annan AN et al (2014) Management of sickle cell disease: summary of the 2014 evidence-based report by expert panel members. JAMA 312(10):1033–1048

Yue L, Lin M, Chen JT et al (2014) Rapid screening for sickle cell disease by polymerase chain reaction-high resolution melting analysis. Mol Med Rep 9(6):2479–2484

Chapter 15
Genetic Factors Modifying Sickle Cell Disease Severity

Kate Gardner and Swee Lay Thein

Abstract Sickle cell disease (SCD) is a monogenic disorder caused by a single base mutation but despite its apparent genetic simplicity, the clinical phenotype is hugely variable. In addition to environmental factors, family and epidemiological studies indicate that genetic variants co-inherited with the sickle mutation have a key role in modifying the disease course. This article provides an overview of the genetic modifiers of SCD known to date. Co-inheritance of α-thalassemia and persistent fetal hemoglobin (HbF) production are established major genetic modifiers but they do not explain the full spectrum of the phenotypic variability of SCD. While characterization of some of the key variants and pathways involved in HbF regulation have provided new therapeutic targets for HbF reactivation, generation of a personalized genetic risk score to inform prognosis and guide management requires a larger panel of genetic modifiers yet to be discovered. Elucidation of new genetic modifiers may also provide an insight into other "druggable" targets for therapeutic intervention.

Keywords Hemoglobin F • GWAS • Genotype/phenotype

K. Gardner
Molecular Haematology, Division of Cancer Studies, Faculty of Life Sciences & Medicine, King's College London, James Black Centre, 125 Coldharbour Lane, London SE5 9NU, UK

Department of Haematological Medicine, King's College Hospital NHS Foundation Trust, Denmark Hill, London SE5 9RS, UK
e-mail: kate.gardner@doctors.org.uk

S.L. Thein (✉)
Molecular Haematology, Division of Cancer Studies, Faculty of Life Sciences & Medicine, King's College London, James Black Centre, 125 Coldharbour Lane, London SE5 9NU, UK

Department of Haematological Medicine, King's College Hospital NHS Foundation Trust, Denmark Hill, London SE5 9RS, UK

Sickle Cell Branch, NIH/National Heart, Lung, and Blood Institute, Building 10-CRC/5E-5142, 10 Center Drive, Bethesda, MD 20892, USA
e-mail: sl.thein@kcl.ac.uk; sl.thein@nih.gov

© Springer International Publishing Switzerland 2016

F.F. Costa, N. Conran (eds.), *Sickle Cell Anemia*,
DOI 10.1007/978-3-319-06713-1_15

15.1 Introduction

Sickle cell disease (SCD) has been heralded as the first "molecular disease" when Pauling ascribed its basis to the presence of an abnormal hemoglobin in 1949 (Pauling et al. 1949). In 1957, Ingram (1957) described the abnormal hemoglobin as being caused by a single amino acid substitution (glutamic acid changed to valine) at position 6 of the β-globin chain of hemoglobin and in 1963, Goldstein et al. (1963) showed that this arose from a single base change of T>A at codon 6. Figure 15.1 summarizes a timeline of the significant events that have contributed to the understanding of the genetic basis, and management of SCD.

In addition to homozygosity for the β^S allele (HbSS, also referred to as sickle cell anemia, SCA), the syndrome of SCD includes HbSC disease (compound heterozygosity of HbS with HbC, Glu^6 to Lys^6), and HbSβ thalassemia (HbSβ^+ or HbSβ^0 thalassemia, depending on the type of the β-thalassemia mutation). Generally, the compound heterozygotes have a milder disease than HbSS, but even within each genotypic and ethnic group, a spectrum of clinical variability is the recurring theme. For example, within the HbSS group, at the mild end, patients can be asymptomatic while early mortality, frequent hospital admissions with acute pain episodes, childhood strokes and other end organ damage, typify the severe end of the clinical spectrum.

Both environmental and genetic factors contribute to this clinical variability. The importance of weather changes such as cold and rain as triggers of acute pain have been recognized and reported for many years but the conclusions were not consistent due to logistical difficulties in conducting such studies. Environmental factors also include nutritional state, access to social support, and medical care, all of which influence risk factors such as infections. The impact of environmental factors is demonstrated most graphically on the differences in the natural history and outcomes of SCD between the high- and low-income countries.

Twin studies, based on the concordance and discordance of disease complications and severity, have traditionally been used to assess the relative contributions of genetic and environmental factors in complex disorders such as diabetes and schizophrenia. Since monozygotic twins have identical DNA sequences, variation in their disease course can be attributed largely to the effects of the environment. There are three reports of this kind in SCD; two were limited to single pairs of identical twins, one with HbSS and α-thalassemia, and the other with HbSβ thalassemia (Amin et al. 1991; Joishy et al. 1976). The third study investigated nine pairs of identical twins, six with HbSS and three HbSC, from Jamaica (Weatherall et al. 2005). These twins have been followed for 15 years or more, and as a comparison group for examining degrees of concordance between laboratory parameters, 350 gender- and age-matched sibling pairs were also studied. These studies reported that while the twins showed similarities and concordance in laboratory parameters, and attained height and weight, there was discordance in frequency of acute painful episodes and other clinically critical complications. The conclusion was that environmental factors are of great importance in defining the clinical course of SCD.

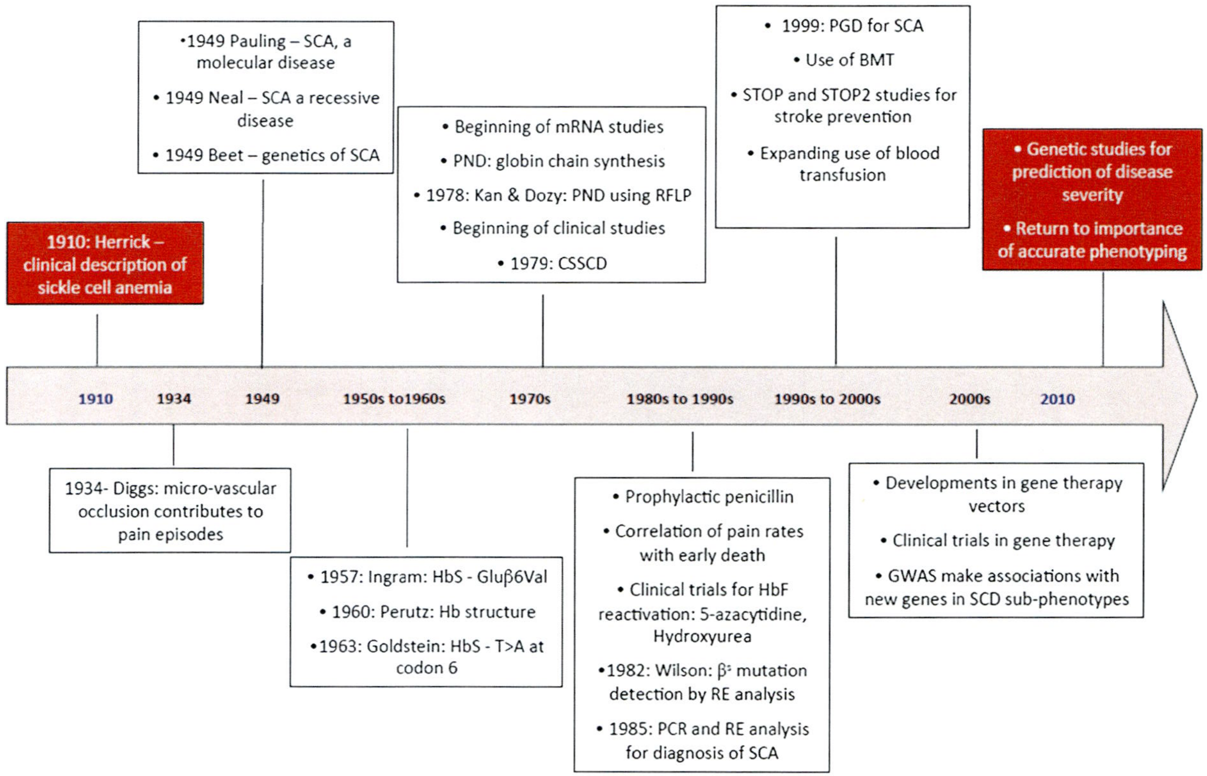

Fig. 15.1 A timeline of significant events that have contributed to the understanding of the genetic basis and management of SCD. *SCA* sickle cell anemia, *mRNA* messenger ribonucleic acid, *PND* prenatal diagnosis, *RFLP* restriction fragment length polymorphism, *CSSCD* co-operative study of sickle cell disease, *PGD* preimplantation genetic diagnosis, *BMT* bone marrow transplantation, *PCR* polymerase chain reaction, *RE* restriction enzyme, *GWAS* genome-wide association study

Family and epidemiological studies indicate that genes co-inherited with the sickle mutation have a key role in modifying the disease course, including higher incidence of stroke (Driscoll et al. 2003) and concordant response to hydroxycarbamide therapy in siblings (Steinberg et al. 1997). Co-inheritance of α-thalassemia and persistent fetal hemoglobin (HbF) production are established major genetic modifiers of SCD. Numerous candidate gene and genome-wide association studies (GWAS) have defined genetic differences in SCD patients and attempted to identify other genetic variants with particular disease complications. However, the disease complexity has presented immense challenges, and these studies have only provided a small amount of the variation in SCD severity observed in the clinic. Roles for other genetic modifiers of SCD severity have been proposed based on the pathophysiology downstream of the primary event (HbS polymerization), however, the majority of these putative markers have not been replicated.

The clinical diversity of SCD itself presents difficulties for genotype/phenotype correlation studies in terms of accurately defining clinical "sub-phenotypes" (Ballas et al. 2012; Smith-Whitley and Pace 2007; Rees et al. 2010). The clinical implications of a clearer understanding of the genetic variants and mechanisms responsible for the phenotypic variability of SCD are significant. First, the ability to predict disease severity based on a genetic SCD "panel" to facilitate risk stratification of patients: high risk patients might then be followed more intensively, and higher risk therapies (hematopoietic stem cell transplantation, hydroxycarbamide) could be targeted at these patients. Second, new modifying genetic variants might suggest new therapeutic targets for investigation.

We describe the current understanding in terms of determining this phenotypic diversity as well as provide an update of the genetic modifiers of severity in SCD.

15.2 Complications of SCD and Problems in Defining Severity of Phenotypes: Global vs Sub-phenotypes

While full genetic understanding of SCD remains incomplete, the emergence of genome-wide genotyping platforms, next generation sequencing, and rapid advances in genetic research has re-focused some attention back onto phenotyping. Clear and consistent definition of phenotypes is critical to the success of genetic association studies. This is particularly pertinent in SCD where there is profound variety in both the severity and nature of complications. Many of its complications are acute such as recurrent acute pain episodes, acute chest syndrome, priapism and stroke; some are intermittent, leading eventually to chronic complications and organ damage, such as chronic pain, pulmonary hypertension and sickle chronic lung disease, penile dysfunction and cognitive disability. The acute complications vary considerably not only between patients but also in the same patient with time.

Phenotypes can be clinical or laboratory parameters. While laboratory parameters are simple to measure, their values vary with the clinical state of the patient; for example, lactate dehydrogenase and white cell count which are normally elevated during steady-state, further increase during acute clinical events. Phenotypes are not always consistent or valid, e.g. pulmonary hypertension. Furthermore, some complications are uncommon (e.g. overt strokes) which makes related or "intermediate" traits a preferred endpoint (e.g. imaging results such as raised trans-cranial Doppler (TCD) velocities, or silent infarcts on magnetic resonance imaging).

Many studies focus on ***specific*** complications of SCD—sometimes described as "***sub-phenotypes***"—i.e. particular end organ damage/failure (e.g. stroke, proteinuria, osteonecrosis, pulmonary hypertension) as separate, individual phenotypic endpoints. ***Global*** markers of severity—for example mortality—offer the potential for a more cohesive endpoint that may be more informative overall. However, global severity scores have proved difficult to define. Accurate end-point definitions are crucial to enable differentiation of "cases" and "controls". Examples of proposed global severity scores include: (1) a "severity index" based on frequency of acute painful episodes, hospitalization, blood transfusion, infection and specific complications during the previous years starting from the birth of the child (el-Hazmi 1992); (2) the presence of dactylitis in infants, white cell count and hemoglobin (Hb) level to predict severe disease outcomes as defined by death, stroke, frequent pain and acute chest syndrome (Miller et al. 2000); and (3) a global severity score using a Bayesian network model (a "statistical" phenotype) (Sebastiani et al. 2007).

15.3 Genetic Methodologies

Generally, two approaches have been used to locate genetic variants in human disease: linkage analysis and association studies (Hirschhorn and Daly 2005). ***Linkage analysis studies*** aim to establish linkage between genes that co-segregate with a trait/disease within a family. This technique has been successful in highly penetrative single gene disorders, but has had limited success in many common diseases which comprise complex traits. ***Association studies*** look for differences in the frequencies of genetic variants between *cases* and *controls* to find genetic variants that are strongly associated with a trait/disease. If a variant is more common in cases than controls, an association is described. Such studies require large sample numbers and until recently have not been feasible due to genotyping cost. Crucially, SNPs identified in pilot studies ("***discovery cohort***") should always be replicated in additional independent populations ("***validation cohort***").

Prerequisites for any genetic association study include: (1) ***heritability*** (correlation of trait in sibling pairs, good r value); and (2) a clear distinction between ***cases*** and ***controls*** (or sufficient variability in a quantitative trait). These criteria present problems in many clinical manifestations of SCD. For example, hospital admissions and duration of stay have used for an objective definition of pain but these measures are influenced by cultural and social factors as well as intermittent illness, such as infections. For convenience, common or "pooled" controls have been used and this can compromize the analysis by contaminating cases in the controls. ***Adequate patient numbers*** are essential to allow robust statistical analysis and replication. Again, this presents problems in SCD genetic association studies; most institutions have small numbers of patients (in contrast to hypertensive or diabetic cohorts). Admixture of different ethnic groups is a confounder when different cohorts are pooled for analysis unless population stratification is accounted for prior to association analysis.

Two types of association studies have been utilized in SCD: candidate gene and genome wide association studies (GWAS). ***Candidate gene association studies*** look for differences in the frequencies of genetic variants in targeted genes between cases and controls, while ***GWAS*** involve an unbiased scan of the whole human genome (Manolio 2013). Many candidate gene association studies in SCD have been published, but often these associations have not been replicated/validated in independent cohorts. Furthermore, critics of candidate gene studies argue that our limited knowledge of SCD pathophysiology is inadequate to predict functional candidate genes (Manolio 2013). By design, GWAS are more likely to reveal unsuspected interactions as the GWAS approach delivers a "hypothesis free" method that could reveal new genes controlling SCD, and thereby exposing novel pathophysiological pathways.

GWAS will also confirm previous candidate genes if the association is robust (Menzel et al. 2007a; Milton et al. 2012). A case in point is the application of GWAS in the unexpected discovery of *BCL11A* (an oncogene that, hitherto, was not known to have a role in erythropoiesis) as a quantitative trait locus (QTL) controlling HbF (Menzel et al. 2007a; Uda et al. 2008). GWAS also confirmed association of the other two loci—*Xmn*1-*HBG2* (*rs782144*) on chromosome 11p and *HBS1L-MYB* (HMIP) on chromosome 6q—with HbF production, that were previously discovered through candidate gene (Labie et al. 1985) and genetic linkage studies (Craig et al. 1996). Similarly, GWAS confirmed the association between bilirubin level and *UGT1A1* polymorphism in SCD (Milton et al. 2012).

It has also become evident that simpler, "intermediate" phenotypes, such as HbF, that are reproducible and measurable, and disease-related, are much more successful in genetic association in SCD studies than clinical endpoints. Such intermediate endpoints or endo-phenotypes are often quantitative traits; they provide more power in genetic strategies. For example, blood flow velocity in the middle cerebral artery as detected by TCD screening is a biomarker of early cerebrovascular disease in SCD. Studies have shown that chronic blood transfusion therapy at this stage can prevent overt stroke (Adams et al. 1998). In this regard, TCD velocity would be an extremely attractive intermediate phenotype in studies for detecting genetic variants associated with sickle vasculopathy and stroke risk.

Whole genome or whole exome sequencing using next generation sequencing technology in combination with well-defined phenotypes offers the possibility of identifying new genetic variants (Bamshad et al. 2011). GWAS in combination with exome sequencing identified mutations in *GOLGB1* and *ENPP1* with stroke protection in sickle cell anemia (SCA) (Flanagan et al. 2013). In this study, overt stroke was the clinical marker but these variants have yet to be independently validated in a different population group.

15.4 Genetic Modifiers of SCD Severity

Global markers of SCD severity represent the "holy grail" of accurate clinical phenotyping. Multiple attempts at providing scoring systems, and using these for genetic associations have been made. Using the global severity index propounded by El-Hazmi (1992), Nishank identified three *eNOS* gene polymorphisms-*eNOS* 4a/b, *eNOS* 894G>T and *eNOS* -786 T>C associated with SCD severity (Nishank et al. 2013). A GWAS study (Sebastiani et al. 2010) utilized the global severity score devised by the same group (Sebastiani et al. 2007) in over 1200 SCD patients, and replicated in a validation set of samples. Validated SNPs included: *KCNK6* (potassium channel gene) and *TNKS* (telomere length regulator gene).

15.4.1 Modifiers of Global SCD Severity at the Primary Level

The central mechanism underlying the pathophysiology of SCD is the polymerization of deoxygenated HbS and formation of irreversibly sickled erythrocytes that lead to the two hallmarks of the disease—recurrent episodes of vaso-occlusion and pain, and chronic hemolytic anemia. Factors that impact the primary event of the disease process will thus have a global effect on the disease phenotype. They include the causative genotype, co-existing α-thalassemia and the innate ability to produce HbF.

Causative Sickle Genotype

In African-descended populations, HbSS typically accounts for 65–70 %, and HbSC 30–35 % of the cases of SCD, with most of the remainder having HbSβ thalassemia. Other genotypes of SCD have been described, including compound heterozygotes of HbS with HbD, HbO-Arab, but these are rare. While presence of HbS is fundamental to the pathobiology, the likelihood of HbS polymerization and sickling is also highly dependent on the concentration of intra-erythrocytic HbS, as well as the presence of non-HbS hemoglobin (Noguchi et al. 1983). Thus, individuals with HbSS or HbSβ^0 thalassemia, where the intra-cellular Hb is almost all HbS, tend to have the most severe disease, followed by HbSC and HbSβ^+ thalassemia. Most studies discussed below consider the homozygous SCD state of HbSS disease only.

HbA ($\alpha_2\beta_2$) or HbA$_2$ ($\alpha_2\delta_2$) do not participate in HbS polymerization. Since the β^+ thalassemia alleles in Africans are of the milder type with minimal deficit in β globin production, Africans with HbSβ^+ thalassemia have substantial proportions of intra-erythrocytic HbA and the SCD tends to be very mild. In contrast, individuals with HbSβ^+ thalassemia in the Mediterranean, have SCD almost as severe as that of HbSS (Serjeant and Serjeant 2001). Subjects with sickle cell trait (HbAS) with HbS of 35–40 %, rarely suffer from symptoms of SCD. Under exceptional circumstances, however, such as intense physical activity and dehydration, the consequent increased intracellular HbS concentration can induce vaso-occlusive pain (Bonham et al. 2010).

The HbS gene is found on a genetic background of four common β-globin haplotypes: Senegal, Benin, Central African Republic (or Bantu), and Arab-Indian. Clinical studies demonstrate variation in SCD severity between the β^S haplotypes, with decreasing severity from the Bantu>Benin>Senegal>Arab-Indian haplotypes. Disease severity correlates inversely with the HbF levels seen in these groups; lowest HbF seen in individuals with Bantu haplotype, and highest HbF in individuals with Arab-Indian haplotype (Nagel et al. 1985, 1987, 1991; Powars 1991; Figueiredo et al. 1996). The differences in clinical severity were ascribed to the difference in HbF levels implicating the *Xmn*1-*HBG2* site which is linked to the Senegal and Arab-Indian β^S haplotype but not to the Bantu haplotype (Labie et al. 1985) (see below for further discussion on modifying effects of HbF on SCD).

Other major genetic factors that influence the primary event of HbS polymerization include the co-inheritance of α-thalassemia and HbF ($\alpha_2\gamma_2$) levels.

Alpha Genotype

About one-third of African-descended patients with SCD have co-existing α-thalassemia (Steinberg and Embury 1986). Most commonly, this is due to the deletion variant ($-\alpha^{3.7}/$); the majority of patients are heterozygous ($\alpha\alpha/-\alpha^{3.7}$) with 3–5 % homozygous for the deletion ($-\alpha^{3.7}/-\alpha^{3.7}$) (Steinberg and Embury 1986; Vasavda et al. 2007). Co-inheritance of α-thalassemia affects SCD red cell phenotype; it reduces intracellular HbS concentration and the propensity of HbS polymerization, reducing the number of irreversibly sickled cells and decreasing hemolysis (Embury et al. 1982; Ballas 2001).

Clinically, co-inherited α-thalassemia protects against complications related to severe hemolysis including pulmonary hypertension, leg ulceration, priapism and albuminuria (Steinberg 2009; Buchanan et al. 2004). Conversely, the increased hematocrit and associated blood viscosity in α-thalassemia predispose to an increased likelihood of developing osteonecrosis, acute chest syndrome (ACS), retinopathy and acute painful vaso-occlusive episodes (Embury et al. 1994). Several studies have also demonstrated association of α-thalassemia with lower TCD measurements and, hence, reduced risk for stroke (Bernaudin et al. 2008; Rees et al. 2009; Flanagan et al. 2011; Cox et al. 2014) while another study could not demonstrate association between α-thalassemia and magnetic resonance angiography (MRA)-defined vasculopathy in paediatric patients with HbSS disease (Thangarajh et al. 2012). The lack of association in the latter study could be related to patient selection. Co-existing α-thalassemia also reduces bilirubin with a quantitative effect that is independent to that of the *UGT1A1* promoter polymorphism (Vasavda et al. 2007). Co-inheritance of α-thalassemia blunts the response to hydroxycarbamide therapy in SCD; this may be explained by its effect on HbF levels and MCV, two key parameters associated with hydroxycarbamide response (Vasavda et al. 2008).

In Jamaicans, the absence of α-thalassemia and higher HbF levels appeared to predict a more benign disease (Thomas et al. 1997), while a subsequent study reported that α-thalassemia did not promote survival in older Jamaicans with HbSS SCD (Serjeant et al. 2007).

Fetal Hemoglobin

Fetal hemoglobin (HbF, α2γ2) is a major ameliorating factor in SCD. Understanding fetal hemoglobin control and its therapeutic reactivation (pharmacological and genetic approaches) remains a top research priority. HbF reduces the propensity for HbS polymerization and its sequelae in two major ways: (1) the hybrid tetramers ($\alpha_2\gamma\beta^S$) do not partake in HbS polymerization, and (2) the presence of intra-erythocytic HbF dilutes the concentration of HbS (Noguchi et al. 1988). The clinical phenotype of SCD becomes evident within 6 months to 2 years of age as HbF levels decline.

HbF levels impact the "primary" level of disease pathology—HbS polymerization—thus HbF levels have a global beneficial effect. Indeed, in SCD, high HbF levels are a major predictor of survival (Platt et al. 1994), and reduced pain (Platt et al. 1991; Dampier et al. 2004); conversely, low levels of HbF have been associated with increased risk of brain infarcts in young children (Wang et al. 2008). At the sub-phenotype level, there appear to be disparities in its effects on complications such as renal impairment, retinopathy and priapism (Thein 2011; Steinberg and Sebastiani 2012). The failure of HbF to modulate all complications of SCD uniformly in the different reports may be related to the small sample sizes in genetic studies and even smaller numbers of end complications, and to ascertainment of phenotypes.

Update on the Genetic Control of Fetal Hemoglobin (HbF)

Developmental stage-specific expression of the β-like globin genes appears to be governed by two principles: competition for the upstream β-locus control region (LCR), and autonomous silencing of the embryonic and fetal globin genes involving various ubiquitous and erythroid-specific transcription factors (Wilber et al. 2011; Stamatoyannopoulos 2005). Although the fetal globin genes are autonomously silenced in adults, genetic variants lying both within and outside the *HBB* locus lead to natural variation in the level of expression of the fetal globin genes and HbF, of over 20-fold (Thein and Craig 1998). Some of these variants significantly ameliorate the clinical symptoms of the β-hemoglobinopathies. These variants account for 89 % of the quantitative variation but the genetic etiology is complex with no clear Mendelian inheritance patterns (Garner et al. 2000). Three known quantitative trait loci (QTLs) for the common HbF variation in adults include: *XmnI-HBG2* (*rs782144*) within the β-globin gene cluster on chromosome 11p, *HBS1L-MYB* intergenic region (HMIP) on chromosome 6q23, and *BCL11A* on chromosome 2p16 (Thein and Menzel 2009; Thein et al. 2009; Sankaran et al. 2010).

Variants in the *HBB*, *HMIP* and *BCL11A* loci account for 10–50 % of the variation in HbF levels in adults, healthy or with SCD or β-thalassemia, depending on the population studied (Menzel et al. 2007a; Lettre et al. 2008; Galanello et al. 2009; Bhatnagar et al. 2011; Makani et al. 2011; Badens et al. 2011; Bae et al. 2012; Mtatiro et al. 2014). The remaining variation ('missing heritability') is likely to be accounted for by many loci with relatively small effects, and/or rare variants with significant quantitative effects on γ-globin gene expression that are typically missed.

HBB Cluster on Chromosome 11p

Xmn1-HBG2 (rs782144) in the *HBB* cluster was the first known QTL for HbF and long-implicated by clinical genetic studies (Labie et al. 1985) (see section "Causative Sickle Genotype" above). The differences in clinical severity of SCD were ascribed to the difference in HbF levels implicating the *Xmn1-HBG2* site which is linked to the Senegal and Arab-Indian β^S haplotype but not to the Bantu haplotype (Labie et al. 1985). Recent high resolution genotyping, however, suggests that rs782144 is not likely to be the variant itself, but in tight linkage disequilibrium with causal element(s) that remain to be discovered in the β-globin cluster. In vitro reporter gene assays suggest that Gγ globin promoters isolated from Asian and Senegal chromosomes exert higher transcriptional activity than their counterparts from Benin and Bantu chromosomes (Ofori-Acquah et al. 2001). In particular, the Bantu Gγ promoter is 10 times weaker than the Asian promoter (Ofori-Acquah et al. 2001). However, the association between haplotypes, HbF levels and disease severity in SCD remains somewhat contentious due to the wide variation in HbF levels among individuals of the same haplotype.

BCL11A on Chromosome 2p16

Functional studies in primary human erythroid progenitor cells and transgenic mice demonstrated that BCL11A acts as a repressor of γ-globin gene expression that is effected by SNPs in intron 2 of this gene (Sankaran et al. 2008). Fine-mapping demonstrated that these HbF-associated variants, in particular rs1427407, localized to an enhancer that is erythroid-specific and not functional in lymphoid cells (Bauer et al. 2013). BCL11A does not interact with the γ-globin promoter but occupies discrete regions in the *HBB* complex (Jawaid et al. 2010). The silencing effect of BCL11A involves re-configuration of the *HBB* locus through interaction with GATA-1 and SOX6 that binds the proximal γ globin promoters (Xu et al. 2010, 2013). In a proof-of-principle, *bcl11a* knock-out in sickle mice increased HbF up to 30 %, reversing end-organ damage caused by the SCD (Xu et al. 2011).

HMIP on Chromosome 6q23

High resolution genetic mapping and resequencing refined the 6q QTL to a group of variants in tight linkage disequilibrium (LD) in a 24-kb block between the *HBS1L* and *MYB* gene, referred to as *HMIP-2* (Thein et al. 2007). The causal SNPs are likely to reside in two clusters within the block, at −84 and −71 kb respectively, upstream of *MYB* (Stadhouders et al. 2014; Menzel et al. 2014). Functional studies in transgenic mice and primary human erythroid cells provide overwhelming evidence that the SNPs at these two regions disrupt binding of key erythroid enhancers affecting long-range interactions with *MYB* and *MYB* expression, providing a functional explanation for the genetic association of the 6q *HBS1L-MYB* intergenic region with HbF and F cell levels (Stadhouders et al. 2012, 2014; Suzuki et al. 2013). A three-base pair (3-bp) deletion in *HMIP-2* -84 region is one functional element in the *MYB* enhancers accounting for increased HbF expression in individuals who have the sentinel SNP rs9399137 that was found to be common in European and Asian populations, although less frequently in African-derived populations (Farrell et al. 2011).

The *HBS1L-MYB* intergenic enhancers do not appear to affect expression of *HBS1L*, the other flanking gene (Stadhouders et al. 2014). *HBS1L* was excluded as having a role in the regulation of HbF and erythropoiesis in a recent report of rare uncharacterized disorders, where whole-exome sequencing revealed mutations in the *HBS1L* gene leading to a loss-of-function in the gene (Sankaran et al. 2013). The individual had normal blood counts and normal HbF levels. Thus, *HMIP-2* is likely to affect HbF and hematopoietic traits via regulation of *MYB*. *MYB* was also causally implicated by fine-mapping which identified rare missense *MYB* variants associated with HbF production (Galarneau et al. 2010).

MYB expression is also reduced by GATA-1 (Welch et al. 2004) and micro (mi) RNA-15a and -16-1 (Sankaran et al. 2011). Elevated levels of the latter have been proposed as the mechanism for the persistently elevated HbF levels, one of the unique features in infants with trisomy 13 (Huehns et al. 1964). These infants have increased expression of miRNAs 15a and 16-1 produced from an extra copy of the genes encoding miRNAs 15a and 16-1 on the triplicated chromosome 13. A recent study provided evidence that the increased HbF effect is mediated, at least in part, through down-modulation of *MYB* via targeting of its 3′ UTR by the miRNAs 15a and 16-1 (Sankaran et al. 2011).

The *MYB* transcription factor is a key regulator of erythropoiesis, and modulates HbF expression via two mechanisms: (1) indirectly through alteration of the kinetics of erythroid differentiation: low MYB levels accelerate erythroid differentiation leading to release of early erythroid progenitor cells that are still synthesizing predominantly HbF (Jiang et al. 2006), and (2) directly via activation of *KLF1* and other γ-globin repressors (e.g., nuclear receptors TR2/TR4) (Bianchi et al. 2010; Suzuki et al. 2013; Tallack and Perkins 2013).

Modulation of *MYB* expression also provides a functional explanation for the pleiotropic effect of the *HMIP-2* SNPs with other erythroid traits such as red cell count, MCV, MCH, HbA_2 levels, and also with platelet and monocyte counts (Menzel et al. 2007b, 2013; Soranzo et al. 2009; van der Harst et al. 2012).

KLF1 on Chromosome 19p13

KLF1 (previously termed *EKLF*), discovered by Jim Bieker in 1993 (Miller and Bieker 1993), re-emerged as a key transcription factor controlling HbF through genetic studies in a Maltese family with β-thalassemia and hereditary persistence of HbF (HPFH). Linkage studies identified a locus for the HPFH that segregated independently of the *HBB* locus on chromosome 19p13 which encompassed *KLF1* (Borg et al. 2010). Subsequent studies, which included expression profiling of erythroid progenitor cells, confirmed *KLF1* as the γ-globin gene modifier in this family. Family members with HPFH were heterozygous for the nonsense K288X mutation in *KLF1* that disrupted the DNA-binding domain of KLF1, a key erythroid gene regulator. Collective studies have now confirmed that *KLF1* is key in the switch from *HBG* to *HBB* expression; it not only activates *HBB* directly, providing a competitive edge, but also silences the γ-globin genes indirectly via activation of *BCL11A* (Siatecka and Bieker 2011; Zhou et al. 2010; Esteghamat et al. 2013). KLF1 may also play a role in the silencing of embryonic globin gene expression (Viprakasit et al. 2014; Magor et al. 2015).

Although there have been numerous reports of association of *KLF1* variants with increased HbF either as a primary phenotype, or in association with other red cell disorders (Borg et al. 2011), several GWASs of HbF (including ones in SCD patients of African descent) failed to identify common variants (Bhatnagar et al. 2011; Mtatiro et al. 2014).

The emerging network of HbF regulation also includes *SOX6*, chromatin-modeling factor *FOP* and the *NURD* complex, the orphan nuclear receptors TR2/TR4 (part of DRED) and the protein arginine methyltransferase PRMT5, involving DNA methylation and histone deacetylases 1 and 2 epigenetic modifiers. Regulators of the key transcription factors, such as miRNA-15a and 16-1 in *controlling MYB*, could also have a potential role in regulating HbF levels (Suzuki et al. 2014).

15.4.2 Glucose-6-Phosphate Dehydrogenase Deficiency

Glucose-6-phosphate dehydrogenase deficiency (G6PD) is common in patients with SCD of African ancestry (Bouanga et al. 1998). There is controversy about the effects of G6PD on TCD velocities, a biomarker for stroke risk in SCD; some studies report that G6PD increases the risk for high cerebral blood flow velocities (Bernaudin et al. 2008; Thangarajh et al. 2012) but others observed no effects (Rees et al. 2009; Cox et al. 2014; Flanagan et al. 2011). These conflicting reports could be related to the methodology used in the assay of the enzyme, or the panel of *G6PD* variants genotyped (Thangarajh et al. 2012; Flanagan et al. 2011). An earlier study showed that G6PD deficiency did *not* influence SCD clinical endpoints including survival, Hb levels, hemolysis, rate of acute pain or acute anemic episodes (Steinberg et al. 1988).

Genetic Modifiers of Organ-Specific Complications

The striking phenomenon in SCD is its clinical diversity. Multiple complications are common in SCD, both acute (frequent pain episodes, acute chest syndrome, strokes) and chronic (pulmonary hypertension, sickle nephropathy, gallstones, osteonecrosis). The variation in global severity of the disease, as well as the incidence of specific end-organ complications ("sub-phenotypes") in SCD, cannot be explained by these three major genetic modifiers—causative sickle genotype, HbF level and α-globin genotype—alone. While the primary etiology in SCD is HbS polymerization, multiple different (but inter-related) downstream pathological mechanisms contribute to SCD phenotype: hemolysis/heme damage, inflammation, oxidant injury, nitric oxide biology, vaso-regulation, cell adhesion and blood coagulation. These factors have modifying effects independent of HbS polymerization and are likely be multi-genic traits. All of these downstream pathways suggest candidate genes that could plausibly affect the different sickle-related complications. Based on this pathophysiology, researchers have identified candidate genes for ***gene association studies*** related to specific sickle complications or "sub-phenotypes".

Genetic association studies (both candidate gene studies and GWAS) have identified multiple possible genetic associations with SCD complications (Table 15.1).

Acute Pain Episodes

Acute pain episodes (APE) are the hallmark clinical feature in SCD. They are a measure of disease severity and a predictor of early mortality (Platt et al. 1991). Frequency of APE varies widely in SCD patients, with highest pain rates seen in those with high hematocrit and low HbF (Platt et al. 1991). Outwith these associations, there is no concrete further understanding of the genetic basis of APE frequency in SCD. It is probably the complication most affected by environmental factors. A compounding problem with pain studies is the clinical definitions of phenotypes. Nearly all patients with SCD have pain, and it is often difficult to quantitate objectively both frequency and severity of individual APE. Furthermore, the standard treatment for pain in APE is parenteral opioids, and individual response to opioid analgesia is itself related to genetic variability of their metabolism (Ballas 2007), making it harder still to dissect and measure APE accurately. As a result of these complicating features, many genetic studies on pain in SCD are poor, in particular because of lack of clear-cut definitions of *cases* versus *controls* required to make objective associations. Furthermore, some of the studies described are poorly conducted and not corrected for other key modifying factors including genotype and HbF levels. In African American patients and patients from Cameroon, association of HbF with the 3 loci (*BCL11A*, *HBS1L-MYB*, and *Xmn*I-*HBG2*) was accompanied by a corresponding reduction in APEs and hospitalization (Lettre et al. 2008; Wonkam et al. 2014).

Published studies have chosen candidate genes based on APE pathology, itself a complex event involving: red cell deformation, enhancement of white cell adhesion, inflammation, endothelial injury and activation of the coagulation and complement pathways. Examples of studies relating to APE in SCD include genes related to:

- *Oxidative stress*. SCD complications, and notably APE, are associated with oxidative stress. Glutathione S-transferases (GSTs) are a group of enzymes that

Table 15.1 Reported genetic associations with specific SCD sub-phenotypes

SCD sub-phenotype	Gene	References
Acute pain episodes	GSTM1 null genotype	Shiba et al. (2014)
Stroke	*VCAM1*/G1238C	Taylor et al. (2002)
	VCAM1/T1594C	Hoppe et al. (2004)
	IL4R/S503P	Hoppe et al. (2004)
	TNFA/G-308S	Hoppe et al. (2004)
	TNF-α/-308G>A allele	Belisario et al. (2015)
	LDLR/Ncol +/−	Hoppe et al. (2004)
	ADRB2/Q/27E	Hoppe et al. (2004)
	AGT/AG repeats	Tang et al. (2001)
	HLA genes	Styles et al. (2000) and Hoppe et al. (2003)
Osteonecrosis	*MTHFR*/C677T	Zimmerman and Ware (1998)
	IL-1β (-511C>T and +3954C>T)	Vicari et al. (2015)
	BMP6	Baldwin et al. (2005) and Ulug et al. (2009)
Acute chest syndrome	*NOS3*/T-786C	Sharan et al. (2004)
	NOS1/AAT repeats	Sullivan et al. (2001)
	COMMD7	Galarneau et al. (2013)
	HMOX1	Bean et al. (2012)
Gallstones	*UGT1A*/promoter repeats	Passon et al. (2001), Fertrin et al. (2003), and Vasavda et al. (2007)
Priapism	*KL*	Nolan et al. (2005) and Elliott et al. (2007)
Pulmonary hypertension	TGFβ/BMP pathway genes	Ashley-Koch et al. (2008)
	IL-1β (-511C>T and +3954C>T)	Vicari et al. (2015)
	MAPK8 A allele	Zhang et al. (2014)
	eNOS intron 4 VNTR polymorphism	Tantawy et al. (2015)
Leg ulcers	*KL*, *TEK*, TGFβ/BMP pathway genes	Nolan et al. (2006)
	IL-6 (-597G>A and -174G>C) genes	Vicari et al. (2015)
Bacteraemia	TGFβ/BMP pathway genes	Adewoye et al. (2006)
Renal disease	*APOL1*	Ashley-Koch et al. (2011)
Retinopathy	IL-6 (-597G>A and -174G>C) genes	Vicari et al. (2015)
Splenic sequestration	TNFA/-308G>A	Cajado et al. (2011)
	IL-8/-251A>T	Cajado et al. (2011)

Acute pain studies have not been included due to poor quality of the studies

protect against oxidative stress. Shiba found the *GSTM1* null genotype to be associated with increased risk of severe APE in Egyptian SCD patients (Shiba et al. 2014)

- *Vasculopathy*. Vascular endothelial growth factors (VEGF) are known to contribute to the pathogenesis of APE in SCD. A study in Bahrain associated multiple VEGF gene polymorphisms with the risk of APE (Al-Habboubi et al. 2012). Unfortunately, the differences between cases and controls was not clear cut (compared patients with SCD having had a recent APE or not).
- *Thrombosis*. Cystathionine beta-synthase (CBS) enzyme gene mutations are a risk factor for thromboembolic disorders. CBS 844ins68 was three times more frequent among SCD patients with APE (Alves Jacob et al. 2011). Again, there was poor clarification of the difference between "severe" and "mild" individuals with APE.
- *Infections*. *MBL2* codes for mannose-binding lectin (MBL), and is associated with modifications in the progression of infectious and inflammatory vascular diseases. Using better definitions of APE severity (using APE frequency), *MBL2* polymorphisms have been associated with APE in children with SCD (Oliveira et al. 2009; Mendonça et al. 2010). Unexpectedly, studies have observed no association of *MBL2* variants with susceptibility to infections (Oliveira et al. 2009) (Dossou-Yovo et al. 2009).

Gallstones

Jaundice and a predisposition to gallstones is associated with a variant in the promoter (TA repeats) of uridine diphosphate (UDP)-glucuronosyl-transferase 1A (*UGT1A1*), also referred to as Gilbert's syndrome. Co-inheritance of Gilbert's syndrome with SCD has been shown in multiple populations to increase the risk for developing gallstones (Passon et al. 2001; Fertrin et al. 2003; Vasavda et al. 2007). The influence of *UGT1A1* polymorphism became more evident in patients while on hydroxycarbamide therapy; children with 6/6 *UGT1A1* genotype achieved normal bilirubin levels while children with 6/7 or 7/7 *UGT1A1* genotypes did not (Heeney et al. 2003).

The association of Gilbert's syndrome with gallstones has also been validated in other populations with different hemolytic anemias e.g. hereditary spherocytosis (del Giudice et al. 1999), HbE/β-thalassemia (Premawardhena et al. 2001) and β-thalassemia (Galanello et al. 2001). Thus, the association of *UGT1A1* polymorphisms and gallstones in SCD is a well-replicated phenomenon. GWAS also confirmed the association between bilirubin level and *UGT1A1* polymorphism in SCD (Milton et al. 2012).

The triad of Gilbert's syndrome, SCD and gallstones presents a possible clinical context where genetic information may aid clinical decision-making. More widely in SCD, the role of elective cholecystectomy in asymptomatic gallstones remains controversial. While one study of SCD patients with asymptomatic gallstones showed significant increased morbidity in patients who were not electively cholecystectomized and subsequently had a symptomatic cholecystectomy (Curro et al. 2007), another study of SCD patients with gallstones demonstrated that the large majority remained asymptomatic over a 13-year follow up period (Attalla et al. 2013).

Thus, the addition of the (*UGT1A1*) genotype to the clinical phenotype of gallstones in SCD presents the question of whether these patients should have elective cholecystectomy.

Sickle Nephropathy

Renal impairment as measured by either proteinuria or glomerular filtration rate (GFR) are common complications of SCD (Sharpe and Thein 2014; Nath and Hebbel 2015), and in some cases sickle renal disease progresses to end-stage renal failure. Renal dysfunction is associated with severity of hemolysis (Becton et al. 2010; Maier-Redelsperger et al. 2010; Day et al. 2012). As a result of this, co-inheritance of α-thalassemia is protective against albuminuria (Nebor et al. 2010a).

The *MYH9-APOL1* locus, an important genetic risk factor for end-stage renal failure in non-SCD populations of African ancestry (Genovese et al. 2010), has also been shown to be associated with sickle cell nephropathy (Ashley-Koch et al. 2011). It is broadly considered that the true association is with *APOL1*, due both to the stronger statistical association with that gene and the lack of identification of causal functional variants in *MYH9*. The original association with *MYH9* has been attributed to the strong linkage disequilibrium between *MYH9* and *APOL1*.

Stroke

A familial predisposition to stroke in HbSS SCD was first identified by Driscoll et al. (2003). This has prompted numerous gene association studies where a variety of associations have been established between multiple genes and stroke—*VCAM1*/G1238C, *VCAM1*/T1594C, *IL4R*/S503P, *TNFA*/G-308S, TNF-α/-308G>A allele, *LDLR*/Ncol +/, *ADRB2*/Q/27E, *AGT*/AG repeats, HLA genes (Hoppe et al. 2004; Taylor et al. 2002; Belisario et al. 2015; Tang et al. 2001; Styles et al. 2000). In some studies, stroke was subdivided into large and small vessel disease based on imaging studies (Hoppe et al. 2004). Of the 38 published SNPs associated with stroke, the effects of α-thalassemia and SNPs in four genes (*ADYC9*, *ANXA2*, *TEK* and *TGFBR3*) could be replicated, although only nominally significant association results were obtained (Flanagan et al. 2011). More recently, GWAS in combination with whole exome sequencing have identified mutations in two genes—*GOLGB1* and *ENPP1*—associated with reduced stroke risk in pediatric patients but, again, this needs validation in independent studies (Flanagan et al. 2013).

Priapism

In males, priapism remains a common manifestation of SCD, found in about 35 % of men (Adeyoju et al. 2002). Independent association studies have identified KLOTHO (*KL*) with priapism in different populations (Nolan et al. 2005; Elliott et al. 2007). Separately, the *TGFβ/SMAD* pathway has also been implicated in priapism risk (Elliott et al. 2007).

Osteonecrosis

Osteonecrosis (avascular necrosis of the bone) occurs in about half of all adults in HbSS. Higher hematocrits are a predisposing factor, hence an increased incidence in HbSS patients with co-existing α-thalassemia, and patients with HbSC and HbSβ^{+} thalassemia genotypes. Association with bone morphogenic protein 6 (*BMP6*) have been replicated across populations (Baldwin et al. 2005; Ulug et al. 2009). This relates to TGF-β/SMAD/BMP pathway in bone metabolism. As for BMP6, regulating the activity of the TGF-β pathway to modulate its effects on bone may be possible (Callahan et al. 2002). Studies suggesting that factors in the coagulation pathway may be involved, such as *MTHFR* and platelet adhesion (*HPA-5B* allele), have been inconclusive (Castro et al. 2004; Zimmerman and Ware 1998; Galanello et al. 2001; Kutlar et al. 2001; Andrade et al. 1998).

Leg Ulcers

Leg ulceration varies widely in SCD with much higher prevalence in Jamaican patients than other cohorts (Alexander et al. 2004). This complication is closely associated with hemolysis severity, and therefore co-existing α-thalassemia is protective. Genetic association studies have implicated several genes in the TGF-β/SMAD/BMP pathway (Nolan et al. 2006). Duffy antigen receptor for chemokines (*DARC*) has also been shown to be associated with persistence of leg ulcers. It was suggested that the relatively higher white cell and neutrophil counts potentiate inflammation in the *Duffy* positive patients (Drasar et al. 2013).

Pulmonary Hypertension

Pulmonary hypertension has been defined in SCD studies using echocardiography, with tricuspid regurgitant jet velocity >2.5 m/s when right heart catheterization is unavailable (when it is defined as mean pulmonary artery pressure ≥25 mmHg and pulmonary capillary wedge pressure ≤15 mmHg). A tricuspid regurgitant jet (TRJ) velocity of >2.5 m/s occurs in about 30 % adults with SCD and is a risk factor for premature death (Gladwin et al. 2004). Pulmonary hypertension is associated with "hemolytic" sickle-complications—renal dysfunction, leg ulceration and priapism—which suggests a vasculopathy driven by chronic hemolysis underlies pulmonary hypertension, too (Taylor et al. 2008). Association studies have suggested multiple gene associations including: the *TGF-β/BMP* signalling pathway (*ACVRL1*, *BMPR2* and *BMP6*) (Ashley-Koch et al. 2008) and polymorphisms previously implicated in primary idiopathic pulmonary hypertension (Machado et al. 2001).

A more recent multi-center study (Zhang et al. 2014) considered the hypoxic response as contributory to pulmonary hypertension. To identify genes regulated by the hypoxic response and not other effects of chronic anemia, individuals with SCD were compared with patients with Chuvash polycythemia (constitutive upregulation of hypoxia-inducible factors in the absence of anemia or hypoxia). A SNP associated with reduced *MAPK8* expression (encoding a mitogen-activated protein kinase important for apoptosis, T-cell differentiation, and inflammatory responses), correlated with pulmonary hypertension. The association was further confirmed in an independent cohort (Walk-Treatment of Pulmonary Hypertension and Sickle Cell Disease With Sildenafil Therapy (walk-PHaSST) population). The homozygous AA genotype of *rs10857560* was present in all 14 patients with pulmonary hypertension.

Acute Chest Syndrome

Acute chest syndrome (ACS) represents a severe acute manifestation of SCD that is potentially life-threatening. One study showed increased susceptibility to ACS associated with a SNP in endothelial NO synthase gene (*eNOS* or *NOS3*) (Sharan et al. 2004), albeit in female patients only. Separately, low exhaled nitric oxide and a polymorphism in the *NOS1* gene has been implicated in ACS (Sullivan et al. 2001).

Galarneau et al. (2013) performed a gene-centric association study for ACS with individuals from the Cooperative Study of Sickle Cell Disease (CSSCD), with replication in independent cohorts. In the combined analysis, an association was found between ACS and *rs6141803*. This SNP is located 8.2 kb upstream of *COMMD7*, a gene highly expressed in the lung that interacts with nuclear factor-κB signalling.

Another candidate gene is Heme oxygenase-1 (*HMOX1*) which produces the protein HO-1, the rate-limiting enzyme in the catabolism of heme; *HMOX1* might attenuate the severity of APE and hemolysis. Bean et al. (2012) investigated a highly polymorphic (GT)n dinucleotide repeat in the promoter of *HMOX1* and showed that children with two shorter alleles had lower rates of ACS.

Splenic Sequestration

Cajado et al. (2011) identified an association between inflammatory markers TNF-α and IL-8 and splenic sequestration in children with SCD. Specifically, the A allele of the TNF-α -308G>A gene polymorphism was associated with an increased risk of splenic sequestration; and the T allele of the IL-8 -251A>T gene polymorphism was considered to be a protective factor for splenomegaly.

Infection

Infections are common events in SCD, especially in children. Studies have suggested that the incidence may be modulated by polymorphisms in the *HLA* locus, *MBL2* gene which encodes the mannose binding protein, *MPO* (gene encoding myeloperoxidase), Duffy antigen receptor for chemokines (*DARC*) and *TGF-β/BMP* pathway (*BMP6*, *TGFBR3*, *BMPR1A*, *SMAD6* and *SMAD3*) (Costa et al. 2005; Nebor et al. 2010b; Tamouza et al. 2002, 2007; Neonato et al. 1999; Cordero et al. 2009; Al-Ola et al. 2008; Adewoye et al. 2006).

Variable Response to Hydroxycarbamide Therapy

Hydroxycarbamide remains a major treatment option for SCD (Ware 2010; Yawn et al. 2014; National Institutes of Health: National Heart Lung and Blood Institute 2014). Clinical and laboratory response to hydroxycarbamide therapy however, is variable, a main determinant of response appears to be the baseline HbF level. Numerous association studies on HbF response to hydroxycarbamide have been reported, of which the association with baseline HbF levels and *Xmn*1-*HBG2* seems to be the most robust (Ware et al. 2002; Green et al. 2013).

15.5 Conclusion

Although environmental factors are important in determining the clinical outcome of SCD, it is evident that the genetic background of the affected individual imparts a substantial contribution to the clinical severity and response to medication. The attraction of being able to generate a personalized genetic risk score as prognostic marker, and to guide therapeutics, plus the relative ease of genotyping and reducing costs, has been a major driver underlying the recent output of genetic association studies in SCD. But the results are questionable in the majority of these genetic association studies because of lack of replication. Nonetheless, genetic studies have been successful in characterizing some of the key variants and pathways involved in HbF regulation, providing new therapeutic targets for HbF reactivation.

We must continue the quest to discover key modifier genes of SCD as a major research priority. This requires taking advantage of whole genome sequencing and the new genomic platforms, but much larger sample sizes (and therefore multicenter collaborations) are required to tease out small statistical differences. Care must be taken to consider, and appropriately classify, different ethnicities.

Additionally, we must focus on developing rigorous clinical phenotypes and the importance of identification of "cases" and "controls". Clinical researchers need to address the issue of defining and quantifying global sickle severity, as well as precise sub-phenotype definitions. As well as using clinical end points (stroke), it may be useful to use intermediate end points (trans-cranial Doppler velocities) with association studies. Many of the described association studies have highlighted the importance of identification of "cases" and "controls".

Finally, for those variants already identified, we must endeavour to: validate the variants in independent, large populations; identify the causal variants; support the genetic evidence by functional assays or relevant models to uncover the underlying pathogenesis. Understanding of the underlying mechanisms may guide translation of these genetic discoveries into clinical benefit as targeted, novel therapies.

References

Adams RJ, McKie VC, Hsu L et al (1998) Prevention of a first stroke by transfusions in children with sickle cell anemia and abnormal results on transcranial doppler ultrasonography. N Engl J Med 339(1):5–11

Adewoye AH, Nolan VG, Ma Q et al (2006) Association of polymorphisms of IGF1R and genes in the transforming growth factor- beta /bone morphogenetic protein pathway with bacteremia in sickle cell anemia. Clin Infect Dis 43(5):593–598

Adeyoju AB, Olujohungbe AB, Morris J et al (2002) Priapism in sickle-cell disease; incidence, risk factors and complications – an international multicentre study. BJU Int 90(9):898–902

Alexander N, Higgs D, Dover G, Serjeant GR (2004) Are there clinical phenotypes of homozygous sickle cell disease? Br J Haematol 126(4):606–611

Al-Habboubi HH, Mahdi N, Abu-Hijleh TM et al (2012) The relation of vascular endothelial growth factor (VEGF) gene polymorphisms on VEGF levels and the risk of vasoocclusive crisis in sickle cell disease. Eur J Haematol 89(5):403–409

Al-Ola K, Mahdi N, Al-Subaie AM et al (2008) Evidence for HLA class II susceptible and protective haplotypes for osteomyelitis in pediatric patients with sickle cell anemia. Tissue Antigens 71(5):453–457

Alves Jacob M, da Cunha Bastos C, Regina Bonini-Domingos C (2011) The 844ins68 cystathionine beta-synthase and C677T MTHFR gene polymorphism and the vaso-occlusive event risk in sickle cell disease. Arch Med Sci 7(1):97–101

Amin BR, Bauersachs RM, Meiselman HJ et al (1991) Monozygotic twins with sickle cell anemia and discordant clinical courses: clinical and laboratory studies. Hemoglobin 15(4): 247–256

Andrade FL, Annichino-Bizzacchi JM, Saad ST, Costa FF, Arruda VR (1998) Prothrombin mutant, factor V Leiden, and thermolabile variant of methylenetetrahydrofolate reductase among patients with sickle cell disease in Brazil. Am J Hematol 59(1):46–50

Ashley-Koch AE, Elliott L, Kail ME et al (2008) Identification of genetic polymorphisms associated with risk for pulmonary hypertension in sickle cell disease. Blood 111(12):5721–5726

Ashley-Koch AE, Okocha EC, Garrett ME et al (2011) MYH9 and APOL1 are both associated with sickle cell disease nephropathy. Br J Haematol 155(3):386–394

Attalla BA, Karrar ZA, Ibnouf G et al (2013) Outcome of cholelithiasis in Sudanese children with Sickle Cell Anaemia (SCA) after 13 years follow-up. Afr Health Sci 13(1):154–159

Badens C, Joly P, Agouti I et al (2011) Variants in genetic modifiers of beta-thalassemia can help to predict the major or intermedia type of the disease. Haematologica 96(11):1712–1714

Bae HT, Baldwin CT, Sebastiani P et al (2012) Meta-analysis of 2040 sickle cell anemia patients: BCL11A and HBS1L-MYB are the major modifiers of HbF in African Americans. Blood 120(9):1961–1962
Baldwin C, Nolan VG, Wyszynski DF et al (2005) Association of klotho, bone morphogenic protein 6, and annexin A2 polymorphisms with sickle cell osteonecrosis. Blood 106(1):372–375
Ballas SK (2001) Effect of alpha-globin genotype on the pathophysiology of sickle cell disease. Pediatr Pathol Mol Med 20(2):107–121
Ballas SK (2007) Current issues in sickle cell pain and its management. Hematology Am Soc Hematol Educ Program 97–105
Ballas SK, Kesen MR, Goldberg MF et al (2012) Beyond the definitions of the phenotypic complications of sickle cell disease: an update on management. ScientificWorldJournal 2012:949535
Bamshad MJ, Ng SB, Bigham AW et al (2011) Exome sequencing as a tool for Mendelian disease gene discovery. Nat Rev Genet 12(11):745–755
Bauer DE, Kamran SC, Lessard S et al (2013) An erythroid enhancer of BCL11A subject to genetic variation determines fetal hemoglobin level. Science 342(6155):253–257
Bean CJ, Boulet SL, Ellingsen D et al (2012) Heme oxygenase-1 gene promoter polymorphism is associated with reduced incidence of acute chest syndrome among children with sickle cell disease. Blood 120(18):3822–3828
Becton LJ, Kalpatthi RV, Rackoff E et al (2010) Prevalence and clinical correlates of microalbuminuria in children with sickle cell disease. Pediatr Nephrol 25(8):1505–1511
Belisario AR, Nogueira FL, Rodrigues RS et al (2015) Association of alpha-thalassemia, TNF-alpha (−308G>A) and VCAM-1 (c.1238G>C) gene polymorphisms with cerebrovascular disease in a newborn cohort of 411 children with sickle cell anemia. Blood Cells Mol Dis 54(1):44–50
Bernaudin F, Verlhac S, Chevret S et al (2008) G6PD deficiency, absence of alpha-thalassemia, and hemolytic rate at baseline are significant independent risk factors for abnormally high cerebral velocities in patients with sickle cell anemia. Blood 112(10):4314–4317
Bhatnagar P, Purvis S, Barron-Casella E et al (2011) Genome-wide association study identifies genetic variants influencing F-cell levels in sickle-cell patients. J Hum Genet 56(4):316–323
Bianchi E, Zini R, Salati S et al (2010) c-Myb supports erythropoiesis through the transactivation of KLF1 and LMO2 expression. Blood 116(22):e99–e110
Bonham VL, Dover GJ, Brody LC (2010) Screening student athletes for sickle cell trait--a social and clinical experiment. N Engl J Med 363(11):997–999
Borg J, Papadopoulos P, Georgitsi M et al (2010) Haploinsufficiency for the erythroid transcription factor KLF1 causes hereditary persistence of fetal hemoglobin. Nat Genet 42(9):801–805
Borg J, Patrinos GP, Felice AE, Philipsen S (2011) Erythroid phenotypes associated with KLF1 mutations. Haematologica 96(5):635–638
Bouanga JC, Mouele R, Prehu C et al (1998) Glucose-6-phosphate dehydrogenase deficiency and homozygous sickle cell disease in Congo. Hum Hered 48(4):192–197
Buchanan GR, DeBaun MR, Quinn CT, Steinberg MH (2004) Sickle cell disease. Hematology Am Soc Hematol Educ Program 35–47
Cajado C, Cerqueira BA, Couto FD et al (2011) TNF-alpha and IL-8: serum levels and gene polymorphisms (−308G>A and -251A>T) are associated with classical biomarkers and medical history in children with sickle cell anemia. Cytokine 56(2):312–317
Callahan JF, Burgess JL, Fornwald JA et al (2002) Identification of novel inhibitors of the transforming growth factor beta1 (TGF-beta1) type 1 receptor (ALK5). J Med Chem 45(5): 999–1001
Castro V, Alberto FL, Costa RN et al (2004) Polymorphism of the human platelet antigen-5 system is a risk factor for occlusive vascular complications in patients with sickle cell anemia. Vox Sang 87(2):118–123
Cordero EA, Veit TD, da Silva MA et al (2009) HLA-G polymorphism influences the susceptibility to HCV infection in sickle cell disease patients. Tissue Antigens 74(4):308–313

Costa RN, Conran N, Albuquerque DM et al (2005) Association of the G-463A myeloperoxidase polymorphism with infection in sickle cell anemia. Haematologica 90(7):977–979

Cox SE, Makani J, Soka D et al (2014) Haptoglobin, alpha-thalassaemia and glucose-6-phosphate dehydrogenase polymorphisms and risk of abnormal transcranial Doppler among patients with sickle cell anaemia in Tanzania. Br J Haematol 165(5):699–706

Craig JE, Rochette J, Fisher CA et al (1996) Dissecting the loci controlling fetal haemoglobin production on chromosomes 11p and 6q by the regressive approach. Nat Genet 12(1):58–64

Curro G, Meo A, Ippolito D, Pusiol A, Cucinotta E (2007) Asymptomatic cholelithiasis in children with sickle cell disease: early or delayed cholecystectomy? Ann Surg 245(1):126–129

Dampier C, Ely E, Eggleston B, Brodecki D, O'Neal P (2004) Physical and cognitive-behavioral activities used in the home management of sickle pain: a daily diary study in children and adolescents. Pediatr Blood Cancer 43(6):674–678

Day TG, Drašar ER, Fulford T, Sharpe CC, Thein SL (2012) Association between hemolysis and albuminuria in adults with sickle cell anemia. Haematologica 97(2):201–205

del Giudice EM, Perrotta S, Nobili B et al (1999) Coinheritance of Gilbert syndrome increases the risk for developing gallstones in patients with hereditary spherocytosis. Blood 94(7): 2259–2262

Dossou-Yovo OP, Zaccaria I, Benkerrou M et al (2009) Effects of RANTES and MBL2 gene polymorphisms in sickle cell disease clinical outcomes: association of the g.In1.1T>C RANTES variant with protection against infections. Am J Hematol 84(6):378–380

Drasar ER, Menzel S, Fulford T, Thein SL (2013) The effect of Duffy antigen receptor for chemokines on severity in sickle cell disease. Haematologica 98(8):e87–e89

Driscoll MC, Hurlet A, Styles L et al (2003) Stroke risk in siblings with sickle cell anemia. Blood 101(6):2401–2404

El-Hazmi MA (1992) Clinical and haematological diversity of sickle cell disease in Saudi children. J Trop Pediatr 38(3):106–112

Elliott L, Ashley-Koch AE, De Castro L et al (2007) Genetic polymorphisms associated with priapism in sickle cell disease. Br J Haematol 137(3):262–267

Embury SH, Dozy AM, Miller J et al (1982) Concurrent sickle-cell anemia and alpha-thalassemia: effect on severity of anemia. N Engl J Med 306(5):270–274

Embury SH, Hebbel RP, Mohandas N, Steinberg MH (eds) (1994) Sickle cell disease: basic principles and clinical practice. Raven, New York

Esteghamat F, Gillemans N, Bilic I et al (2013) Erythropoiesis and globin switching in compound Klf1::Bcl11a mutant mice. Blood 121(13):2553–2562

Farrell JJ, Sherva RM, Chen ZY et al (2011) A 3-bp deletion in the HBS1L-MYB intergenic region on chromosome 6q23 is associated with HbF expression. Blood 117(18):4935–4945

Fertrin KY, Melo MB, Assis AM, Saad ST, Costa FF (2003) UDP-glucuronosyltransferase 1 gene promoter polymorphism is associated with increased serum bilirubin levels and cholecystectomy in patients with sickle cell anemia. Clin Genet 64(2):160–162

Figueiredo MS, Kerbauy J, Goncalves MS et al (1996) Effect of alpha-thalassemia and beta-globin gene cluster haplotypes on the hematological and clinical features of sickle-cell anemia in Brazil. Am J Hematol 53(2):72–76

Flanagan JM, Frohlich DM, Howard TA et al (2011) Genetic predictors for stroke in children with sickle cell anemia. Blood 117(24):6681–6684

Flanagan JM, Sheehan V, Linder H et al (2013) Genetic mapping and exome sequencing identify 2 mutations associated with stroke protection in pediatric patients with sickle cell anemia. Blood 121(16):3237–3245

Galanello R, Piras S, Barella S et al (2001) Cholelithiasis and Gilbert's syndrome in homozygous beta-thalassaemia. Br J Haematol 115(4):926–928

Galanello R, Sanna S, Perseu L et al (2009) Amelioration of Sardinian beta-zero thalassemia by genetic modifiers. Blood 114(18):3935–3937

Galarneau G, Palmer CD, Sankaran VG et al (2010) Fine-mapping at three loci known to affect fetal hemoglobin levels explains additional genetic variation. Nat Genet 40(12):1049–1051

Galarneau G, Coady S, Garrett ME et al (2013) Gene-centric association study of acute chest syndrome and painful crisis in sickle cell disease patients. Blood 122(3):434–442
Garner C, Tatu T, Reittie JE et al (2000) Genetic influences on F cells and other hematologic variables: a twin heritability study. Blood 95(1):342–346
Genovese G, Friedman DJ, Ross MD et al (2010) Association of trypanolytic ApoL1 variants with kidney disease in African Americans. Science 329(5993):841–845
Gladwin MT, Sachdev V, Jison ML et al (2004) Pulmonary hypertension as a risk factor for death in patients with sickle cell disease. N Engl J Med 350(9):886–895
Goldstein J, Konigsberg W, Hill RJ (1963) The structure of human hemoglobin. VI. The sequence of amino acids in the tryptic peptides of the beta chain. J Biol Chem 238:2016–2027
Green NS, Ender KL, Pashankar F et al (2013) Candidate sequence variants and fetal hemoglobin in children with sickle cell disease treated with hydroxyurea. PLoS One 8(2):e55709
Heeney MM, Howard TA, Zimmerman SA, Ware RE (2003) UGT1A promoter polymorphisms influence bilirubin response to hydroxyurea therapy in sickle cell anemia. J Lab Clin Med 141(4):279–282
Hirschhorn JN, Daly MJ (2005) Genome-wide association studies for common diseases and complex traits. Nat Rev Genet 6(2):95–108
Hoppe C, Klitz W, Noble J et al (2003) Distinct HLA associations by stroke subtype in children with sickle cell anemia. Blood 101(7):2865–2869
Hoppe C, Klitz W, Cheng S et al (2004) Gene interactions and stroke risk in children with sickle cell anemia. Blood 103(6):2391–2396
Huehns ER, Hecht F, Keil JV, Motulsky AG (1964) Developmental hemoglobin anomalies in a chromosomal triplication: D_1 trisomy syndrome. Proc Natl Acad Sci U S A 51:89–97
Ingram VM (1957) Gene mutations in human haemoglobin: the chemical difference between normal and sickle cell haemoglobin. Nature 180(4581):326–328
Jawaid K, Wahlberg K, Thein SL, Best S (2010) Binding patterns of BCL11A in the globin and GATA1 loci and characterization of the BCL11A fetal hemoglobin locus. Blood Cells Mol Dis 45(2):140–146
Jiang J, Best S, Menzel S et al (2006) cMYB is involved in the regulation of fetal hemoglobin production in adults. Blood 108(3):1077–1083
Joishy SK, Griner PF, Rowley PT (1976) Sickle b-thalassemia: identical twins differing in severity implicate nongenetic factors influencing course. Am J Hematol 1(1):23–33
Kutlar A, Kutlar F, Turker I, Tural C (2001) The methylene tetrahydrofolate reductase (C677T) mutation as a potential risk factor for avascular necrosis in sickle cell disease. Hemoglobin 25(2):213–217
Labie D, Pagnier J, Lapoumeroulie C et al (1985) Common haplotype dependency of high G gamma-globin gene expression and high Hb F levels in beta-thalassemia and sickle cell anemia patients. Proc Natl Acad Sci U S A 82(7):2111–2114
Lettre G, Sankaran VG, Bezerra MA et al (2008) DNA polymorphisms at the BCL11A, HBS1L-MYB, and beta-globin loci associate with fetal hemoglobin levels and pain crises in sickle cell disease. Proc Natl Acad Sci U S A 105(33):11869–11874
Machado RD, Pauciulo MW, Thomson JR et al (2001) BMPR2 haploinsufficiency as the inherited molecular mechanism for primary pulmonary hypertension. Am J Hum Genet 68(1):92–102
Magor GW, Tallack MR, Gillinder KR et al (2015) KLF1 null neonates display hydrops fetalis and a deranged erythroid transcriptome. Blood 125:2405–2417
Maier-Redelsperger M, Levy P, Lionnet F et al (2010) Strong association between a new marker of hemolysis and glomerulopathy in sickle cell anemia. Blood Cells Mol Dis 45(4):289–292
Makani J, Menzel S, Nkya S et al (2011) Genetics of fetal hemoglobin in Tanzanian and British patients with sickle cell anemia. Blood 117(4):1390–1392
Manolio TA (2013) Bringing genome-wide association findings into clinical use. Nat Rev Genet 14(8):549–558
Mendonça TF, Oliveira MC, Vasconcelos LR et al (2010) Association of variant alleles of *MBL2* gene with vasoocclusive crisis in children with sickle cell anemia. Blood Cells Mol Dis 44(4): 224–228

Menzel S, Garner C, Gut I et al (2007a) A QTL influencing F cell production maps to a gene encoding a zinc-finger protein on chromosome 2p15. Nat Genet 39(10):1197–1199

Menzel S, Jiang J, Silver N et al (2007b) The HBS1L-MYB intergenic region on chromosome 6q23.3 influences erythrocyte, platelet, and monocyte counts in humans. Blood 110(10): 3624–3626

Menzel S, Garner C, Rooks H, Spector TD, Thein SL (2013) HbA2 levels in normal adults are influenced by two distinct genetic mechanisms. Br J Haematol 160(1):101–105

Menzel S, Rooks H, Zelenika D et al (2014) Global genetic architecture of an erythroid quantitative trait locus, HMIP-2. Ann Hum Genet 78:434–451

Miller IJ, Bieker JJ (1993) A novel, erythroid cell-specific murine transcription factor that binds to the CACCC element and is related to the *Krüppel* family of nuclear proteins. Mol Cell Biol 13(5):2776–2786

Miller ST, Sleeper LA, Pegelow CH et al (2000) Prediction of adverse outcomes in children with sickle cell disease. N Engl J Med 342(2):83–89

Milton JN, Sebastiani P, Solovieff N et al (2012) A genome-wide association study of total bilirubin and cholelithiasis risk in sickle cell anemia. PLoS One 7(4):e34741

Mtatiro SN, Singh T, Rooks H et al (2014) Genome wide association study of fetal hemoglobin in sickle cell anemia in Tanzania. PLoS One 9(11):e111464

Nagel RL, Fabry ME, Pagnier J et al (1985) Hematologically and genetically distinct forms of sickle cell anemia in Africa. The Senegal type and the Benin type. N Engl J Med 312(14):880–884

Nagel RL, Rao SK, Dunda-Belkhodja O et al (1987) The hematologic characteristics of sickle cell anemia bearing the Bantu haplotype: the relationship between ^{G}g and Hb F level. Blood 69:1026–1030

Nagel RL, Erlingsson S, Fabry ME et al (1991) The Senegal DNA haplotype is associated with the amelioration of anemia in African-American sickle cell anemia patients. Blood 77: 1371–1375

Nath KA, Hebbel RP (2015) Sickle cell disease: renal manifestations and mechanisms. Nat Rev Nephrol 11(3):161–171

National Institutes of Health: National Heart Lung and Blood Institute (2014) Evidence-based management of sickle cell disease NIH Expert Panel Report

Nebor D, Broquere C, Brudey K et al (2010a) Alpha-thalassemia is associated with a decreased occurrence and a delayed age-at-onset of albuminuria in sickle cell anemia patients. Blood Cells Mol Dis 45(2):154–158

Nebor D, Durpes MC, Mougenel D et al (2010b) Association between Duffy antigen receptor for chemokines expression and levels of inflammation markers in sickle cell anemia patients. Clin Immunol 136(1):116–122

Neonato MG, Lu CY, Guilloud-Bataille M et al (1999) Genetic polymorphism of the mannose-binding protein gene in children with sickle cell disease: identification of three new variant alleles and relationship to infections. Eur J Hum Genet 7(6):679–686

Nishank SS, Singh MP, Yadav R et al (2013) Endothelial nitric oxide synthase gene polymorphism is associated with sickle cell disease patients in India. J Hum Genet 58(12):775–779

Noguchi CT, Torchia DA, Schechter AN (1983) Intracellular polymerization of sickle hemoglobin. Effects of cell heterogeneity. J Clin Invest 72(3):846–852

Noguchi CT, Rodgers GP, Serjeant G, Schechter AN (1988) Levels of fetal hemoglobin necessary for treatment of sickle cell disease. N Engl J Med 318(2):96–99

Nolan VG, Baldwin C, Ma Q et al (2005) Association of single nucleotide polymorphisms in klotho with priapism in sickle cell anaemia. Br J Haematol 128(2):266–272

Nolan VG, Adewoye A, Baldwin C et al (2006) Sickle cell leg ulcers: associations with haemolysis and SNPs in Klotho, TEK and genes of the TGF-beta/BMP pathway. Br J Haematol 133(5):570–578

Ofori-Acquah SF, Lalloz MR, Layton DM (2001) Nucleotide variation regulates the level of enhancement by hypersensitive site 2 of the beta-globin locus control region. Blood Cells Mol Dis 27(5):803–811

Oliveira MC, Mendonca TF, Vasconcelos LR et al (2009) Association of the MBL2 gene EXON1 polymorphism and vasoocclusive crisis in patients with sickle cell anemia. Acta Haematol 121(4):212–215

Passon RG, Howard TA, Zimmerman SA, Schultz WH, Ware RE (2001) Influence of bilirubin uridine diphosphate-glucuronosyltransferase 1A promoter polymorphisms on serum bilirubin levels and cholelithiasis in children with sickle cell anemia. J Pediatr Hematol Oncol 23(7):448–451

Pauling L, Itano HA et al (1949) Sickle cell anemia, a molecular disease. Science 109(2835):443

Platt OS, Thorington BD, Brambilla DJ et al (1991) Pain in sickle cell disease: rates and risk factors. N Engl J Med 325(1):11–16

Platt OS, Brambilla DJ, Rosse WF et al (1994) Mortality in sickle cell disease: life expectancy and risk factors for early death. N Engl J Med 330(23):1639–1644

Powars DR (1991) Beta s-gene-cluster haplotypes in sickle cell anemia. Clinical and hematologic features. Hematol Oncol Clin North Am 5(3):475–493

Premawardhena A, Fisher CA, Fathiu F et al (2001) Genetic determinants of jaundice and gallstones in haemoglobin E beta thalassaemia. Lancet 357(9272):1945–1946

Rees DC, Lambert C, Cooper E et al (2009) Glucose 6 phosphate dehydrogenase deficiency is not associated with cerebrovascular disease in children with sickle cell anemia. Blood 114(3):742–743, author reply 743–744

Rees DC, Williams TN, Gladwin MT (2010) Sickle-cell disease. Lancet 376(9757):2018–2031

Sankaran VG, Menne TF, Xu J et al (2008) Human fetal hemoglobin expression is regulated by the developmental stage-specific repressor BCL11A. Science 322(5909):1839–1842

Sankaran VG, Xu J, Orkin SH (2010) Advances in the understanding of haemoglobin switching. Br J Haematol 149(2):181–194

Sankaran VG, Menne TF, Scepanovic D et al (2011) MicroRNA-15a and –16-1 act via MYB to elevate fetal hemoglobin expression in human trisomy 13. Proc Natl Acad Sci U S A 108(4):1519–1524

Sankaran VG, Joshi M, Agrawal A et al (2013) Rare complete loss of function provides insight into a pleiotropic genome-wide association study locus. Blood 122(23):3845–3847

Sebastiani P, Nolan VG, Baldwin CT et al (2007) A network model to predict the risk of death in sickle cell disease. Blood 110(7):2727–2735

Sebastiani P, Solovieff N, Hartley SW et al (2010) Genetic modifiers of the severity of sickle cell anemia identified through a genome-wide association study. Am J Hematol 85(1):29–35

Serjeant GR, Serjeant BE (2001) Sickle cell disease, 3rd edn. Oxford University Press, Oxford

Serjeant GR, Higgs DR, Hambleton IR (2007) Elderly survivors with homozygous sickle cell disease. N Engl J Med 356(6):642–643

Sharan K, Surrey S, Ballas S et al (2004) Association of T-786C eNOS gene polymorphism with increased susceptibility to acute chest syndrome in females with sickle cell disease. Br J Haematol 124(2):240–243

Sharpe CC, Thein SL (2014) How I treat renal complications in sickle cell disease. Blood 123(24):3720–3726

Shiba HF, El-Ghamrawy MK, Shaheen IA, Ali RA, Mousa SM (2014) Glutathione S-transferase gene polymorphisms (GSTM1, GSTT1, and GSTP1) in Egyptian pediatric patients with sickle cell disease. Pediatr Dev Pathol 17(4):265–270

Siatecka M, Bieker JJ (2011) The multifunctional role of EKLF/KLF1 during erythropoiesis. Blood 118(8):2044–2054

Smith-Whitley K, Pace BS (2007) Sickle cell disease: a phenotypic patchwork. In: Pace BS (ed) Renaissance of sickle cell disease research in the genome era, 1st edn. Imperial College Press, London, pp 45–67

Soranzo N, Spector TD, Mangino M et al (2009) A genome-wide meta-analysis identifies 22 loci associated with eight hematological parameters in the HaemGen consortium. Nat Genet 41(11):1182–1190

Stadhouders R, Thongjuea S, Andrieu-Soler C et al (2012) Dynamic long-range chromatin interactions control Myb proto-oncogene transcription during erythroid development. EMBO J 31(4): 986–999

Stadhouders R, Aktuna S, Thongjuea S et al (2014) HBS1L-MYB intergenic variants modulate fetal hemoglobin via long-range MYB enhancers. J Clin Invest 124(4):1699–1710
Stamatoyannopoulos G (2005) Control of globin gene expression during development and erythroid differentiation. Exp Hematol 33(3):259–271
Steinberg MH (2009) Genetic etiologies for phenotypic diversity in sickle cell anemia. ScientificWorldJournal 9:46–67
Steinberg MH, Embury SH (1986) Alpha-thalassemia in blacks: genetic and clinical aspects and interactions with the sickle hemoglobin gene. Blood 68(5):985–990
Steinberg MH, Sebastiani P (2012) Genetic modifiers of sickle cell disease. Am J Hematol 87(8):795–803
Steinberg MH, West MS, Gallagher D, Mentzer W (1988) Effects of glucose-6-phosphate dehydrogenase deficiency upon sickle cell anemia. Blood 71(3):748–752
Steinberg MH, Lu ZH, Barton FB et al (1997) Fetal hemoglobin in sickle cell anemia: determinants of response to hydroxyurea. Multicenter Study of Hydroxyurea. Blood 89(3):1078–1088
Styles LA, Hoppe C, Klitz W et al (2000) Evidence for HLA-related susceptibility for stroke in children with sickle cell disease. Blood 95(11):3562–3567
Sullivan KJ, Kissoon N, Duckworth LJ et al (2001) Low exhaled nitric oxide and a polymorphism in the NOS I gene is associated with acute chest syndrome. Am J Respir Crit Care Med 164(12):2186–2190
Suzuki M, Yamazaki H, Mukai HY et al (2013) Disruption of the Hbs1l-Myb locus causes hereditary persistence of fetal hemoglobin in a mouse model. Mol Cell Biol 33(8):1687–1695
Suzuki M, Yamamoto M, Engel JD (2014) Fetal globin gene repressors as drug targets for molecular therapies to treat the beta-globinopathies. Mol Cell Biol 34(19):3560–3569
Tallack MR, Perkins AC (2013) Three fingers on the switch: Kruppel-like factor 1 regulation of gamma-globin to beta-globin gene switching. Curr Opin Hematol 20(3):193–200
Tamouza R, Neonato MG, Busson M et al (2002) Infectious complications in sickle cell disease are influenced by HLA class II alleles. Hum Immunol 63(3):194–199
Tamouza R, Busson M, Fortier C et al (2007) HLA-E*0101 allele in homozygous state favors severe bacterial infections in sickle cell anemia. Hum Immunol 68(10):849–853
Tang DC, Prauner R, Liu W et al (2001) Polymorphisms within the angiotensinogen gene (GT-repeat) and the risk of stroke in pediatric patients with sickle cell disease: a case–control study. Am J Hematol 68(3):164–169
Tantawy AA, Adly AA, Ismail EA, Aly SH (2015) Endothelial nitric oxide synthase gene intron 4 VNTR polymorphism in sickle cell disease: relation to vasculopathy and disease severity. Pediatr Blood Cancer 62(3):389–394
Taylor JG, Tang DC, Savage SA et al (2002) Variants in the VCAM1 gene and risk for symptomatic stroke in sickle cell disease. Blood 100(13):4303–4309
Taylor JG, Nolan VG, Mendelsohn L et al (2008) Chronic hyper-hemolysis in sickle cell anemia: association of vascular complications and mortality with less frequent vasoocclusive pain. PLoS One 3(5):e2095
Thangarajh M, Yang G, Fuchs D et al (2012) Magnetic resonance angiography-defined intracranial vasculopathy is associated with silent cerebral infarcts and glucose-6-phosphate dehydrogenase mutation in children with sickle cell anaemia. Br J Haematol 159(3):352–359
Thein SL (2011) Genetic modifiers of sickle cell disease. Hemoglobin 35(5–6):589–606
Thein SL, Craig JE (1998) Genetics of Hb F/F cell variance in adults and heterocellular hereditary persistence of fetal hemoglobin. Hemoglobin 22:401–414
Thein SL, Menzel S (2009) Discovering the genetics underlying foetal haemoglobin production in adults. Br J Haematol 145(4):455–467
Thein SL, Menzel S, Peng X et al (2007) Intergenic variants of HBS1L-MYB are responsible for a major quantitative trait locus on chromosome 6q23 influencing fetal hemoglobin levels in adults. Proc Natl Acad Sci U S A 104(27):11346–11351
Thein SL, Menzel S, Lathrop M, Garner C (2009) Control of fetal hemoglobin: new insights emerging from genomics and clinical implications. Hum Mol Genet 18(R2):R216–R223

Thomas PW, Higgs DR, Serjeant GR (1997) Benign clinical course in homozygous sickle cell disease: a search for predictors. J Clin Epidemiol 50(2):121–126
Uda M, Galanello R, Sanna S et al (2008) Genome-wide association study shows BCL11A associated with persistent fetal hemoglobin and amelioration of the phenotype of beta-thalassemia. Proc Natl Acad Sci U S A 105(5):1620–1625
Ulug P, Vasavda N, Awogbade M et al (2009) Association of sickle avascular necrosis with bone morphogenic protein 6. Ann Hematol 88(8):803–805
van der Harst P, Zhang W, Mateo Leach I et al (2012) Seventy-five genetic loci influencing the human red blood cell. Nature 492(7429):369–375
Vasavda N, Menzel S, Kondaveeti S et al (2007) The linear effects of alpha-thalassaemia, the UGT1A1 and HMOX1 polymorphisms on cholelithiasis in sickle cell disease. Br J Haematol 138(2):263–270
Vasavda N, Badiger S, Rees D et al (2008) The presence of alpha-thalassaemia trait blunts the response to hydroxycarbamide in patients with sickle cell disease. Br J Haematol 143(4):589–592
Vicari P, Adegoke SA, Mazzotti DR et al (2015) Interleukin-1beta and interleukin-6 gene polymorphisms are associated with manifestations of sickle cell anemia. Blood Cells Mol Dis 54(3):244–249
Viprakasit V, Ekwattanakit S, Riolueang S et al (2014) Mutations in Kruppel-like factor 1 cause transfusion-dependent hemolytic anemia and persistence of embryonic globin gene expression. Blood 123:1586–1595
Wang WC, Pavlakis SG, Helton KJ et al (2008) MRI abnormalities of the brain in one-year-old children with sickle cell anemia. Pediatr Blood Cancer 51(5):643–646
Ware RE (2010) How I use hydroxyurea to treat young patients with sickle cell anemia. Blood 115(26):5300–5311
Ware RE, Eggleston B, Redding-Lallinger R et al (2002) Predictors of fetal hemoglobin response in children with sickle cell anemia receiving hydroxyurea therapy. Blood 99(1):10–14
Weatherall MW, Higgs DR, Weiss H, Weatherall DJ, Serjeant GR (2005) Phenotype/genotype relationships in sickle cell disease: a pilot twin study. Clin Lab Haematol 27(6): 384-390
Welch JJ, Watts JA, Vakoc CR et al (2004) Global regulation of erythroid gene expression by transcription factor GATA-1. Blood 104(10):3136–3147
Wilber A, Nienhuis AW, Persons DA (2011) Transcriptional regulation of fetal to adult hemoglobin switching: new therapeutic opportunities. Blood 117(15):3945–3953
Wonkam A, Ngo Bitoungui VJ, Vorster AA et al (2014) Association of variants at BCL11A and HBS1L-MYB with hemoglobin F and hospitalization rates among sickle cell patients in Cameroon. PLoS One 9(3):e92506
Xu J, Sankaran VG, Ni M et al (2010) Transcriptional silencing of {gamma}-globin by BCL11A involves long-range interactions and cooperation with SOX6. Genes Dev 24(8):783–798
Xu J, Peng C, Sankaran VG et al (2011) Correction of sickle cell disease in adult mice by interference with fetal hemoglobin silencing. Science 334(6058):993–996
Xu J, Bauer DE, Kerenyi MA et al (2013) Corepressor-dependent silencing of fetal hemoglobin expression by BCL11A. Proc Natl Acad Sci U S A 110(16):6518–6523
Yawn BP, Buchanan GR, Afenyi-Annan AN et al (2014) Management of sickle cell disease: summary of the 2014 evidence-based report by expert panel members. JAMA 312(10):1033–1048
Zhang X, Zhang W, Ma SF et al (2014) Hypoxic response contributes to altered gene expression and precapillary pulmonary hypertension in patients with sickle cell disease. Circulation 129(16):1650–1658
Zhou D, Liu K, Sun CW, Pawlik KM, Townes TM (2010) KLF1 regulates BCL11A expression and gamma- to beta-globin gene switching. Nat Genet 42(9):742–744
Zimmerman SA, Ware RE (1998) Inherited DNA mutations contributing to thrombotic complications in patients with sickle cell disease. Am J Hematol 59(4):267–272

Chapter 16
Future Perspectives for the Treatment of Sickle Cell Anemia

Kerri Nottage, Jeremie Estepp, and Jane Hankins

Abstract After decades with few treatment options for individuals with sickle cell disease (SCD), we have entered a treatment era of promising new therapeutic agents. These novel approaches target the diverse pathophysiology associated with SCD (e.g., increased blood cell adhesion, activated coagulation system, hyperinflammation, endothelial dysfunction). Potential therapies can be classified according to the "level" of the target intervention and related to the pathophysiology of SCD (upstream versus downstream events). In this chapter, "upstream therapies" refer to those that correct the genetic defect (correction of the sickle mutation in the beta globin gene via hematopoietic stem cell transplantation or gene therapy/gene editing), alter the natural hemoglobin switch phenomenon (enhancement of fetal hemoglobin production via gene therapy/gene editing), or prevent hemoglobin polymerization (e.g., drugs that alter the hemoglobin oxygen affinity or enhance fetal hemoglobin production). "Downstream therapies" are those aimed at quelling the downstream effects of hemolysis and vaso-occlusion (e.g., anti-adhesive, anti-inflammatory, or vaso-dilatory agents). This chapter discusses new therapies both in pre-clinical and clinical stages of investigation, and emphasizes those with the highest likelihood for impact on the disease and translation into clinical use over the next decade.

Keywords Intervention • Sickle cell disease • Gene therapy • Anti-adhesive • HbF inducer

16.1 Introduction

This chapter will cover current and future novel treatments for sickle cell disease (SCD), or those in pre-clinical development that appear promising in offering new avenues or in exploring new mechanisms or approaches to treat or cure SCD. The

K. Nottage, M.D., M.P.H. • J. Estepp, M.D. • J. Hankins, M.D., M.S. (✉)
Department of Hematology, St. Jude Children's Research Hospital,
262 Danny Thomas Place, MS # 800, Memphis, TN 38105-3678, USA
e-mail: kerri.nottage@stjude.org; jeremie.estepp@stjude.org; jane.hankins@stjude.org

© Springer International Publishing Switzerland 2016

F.F. Costa, N. Conran (eds.), *Sickle Cell Anemia*,
DOI 10.1007/978-3-319-06713-1_16

field is undergoing a true revolution in terms of development of new interventions for the disease, as exemplified by a current search within www.clinicaltrials.gov that resulted in 412 ongoing clinical trials for SCD (as of September 2014); thus, only a selection of the new therapies will be discussed here. Our criteria used for selecting an intervention to discuss in this chapter included (1) its potential for transforming the field, (2) the maturity of its associated clinical trials, or (3) new strategies for utilization of established therapies, the results of which could immediately alter current practice.

16.1.1 Single Mutation; Multi-System Disease

SCD is a genetic disorder caused by a single point mutation (adenine → thymine in the sixth codon of the β gene), resulting in valine being substituted for glutamic acid in the sixth position of the β chain. This mutation leads to polymerization of the hemoglobin (Hb) tetramer in deoxygenated conditions and gives rise to the classic "sickle-shaped" erythrocyte. The clinical consequences of this mutation are severe, wide-spread, and involve aberration of multiple downstream systems, including inflammatory, coagulation, and vaso-regulation (Fig. 16.1) (see Chaps. 3–8 for details). In this chapter, SCD refers to all disease genotypes (HbSS, HbSC, HbSβ^0thalassemia, HbSβ^+thalassemia, HbSD, HbSO, HbSE), whereas sickle cell anemia (SCA) refers to the two most severe ones: HbSS and HbSβ^0-thalassemia.

16.1.2 Therapeutic Classification

Many therapeutic agents will have multiple targets or overlapping mechanisms of action; however, for this chapter we have classified them based on their main mechanism of action, or target within the pathophysiology of SCD. We have divided therapies into two main groups: (1) those with "upstream" targets and (2) those with "downstream" targets (Table 16.1). Upstream therapeutic targets include therapies aimed at correcting the point mutation and those reversing the physiologic switch in hemoglobin production. These upstream strategies, such as genetic reprogramming of fetal hemoglobin (HbF) production, could profoundly alter all downstream events and provide significant clinical improvement or actually cure SCD (Sankaran and Nathan 2010). The downstream targets involve multiple systems (inflammation, coagulation, vaso-regulation, etc.) that can also be targeted to ameliorate symptoms of SCD, without a curative intent (Fig. 16.1). Selected therapies, some of which are listed in Table 16.1, will be discussed in the next two sections.

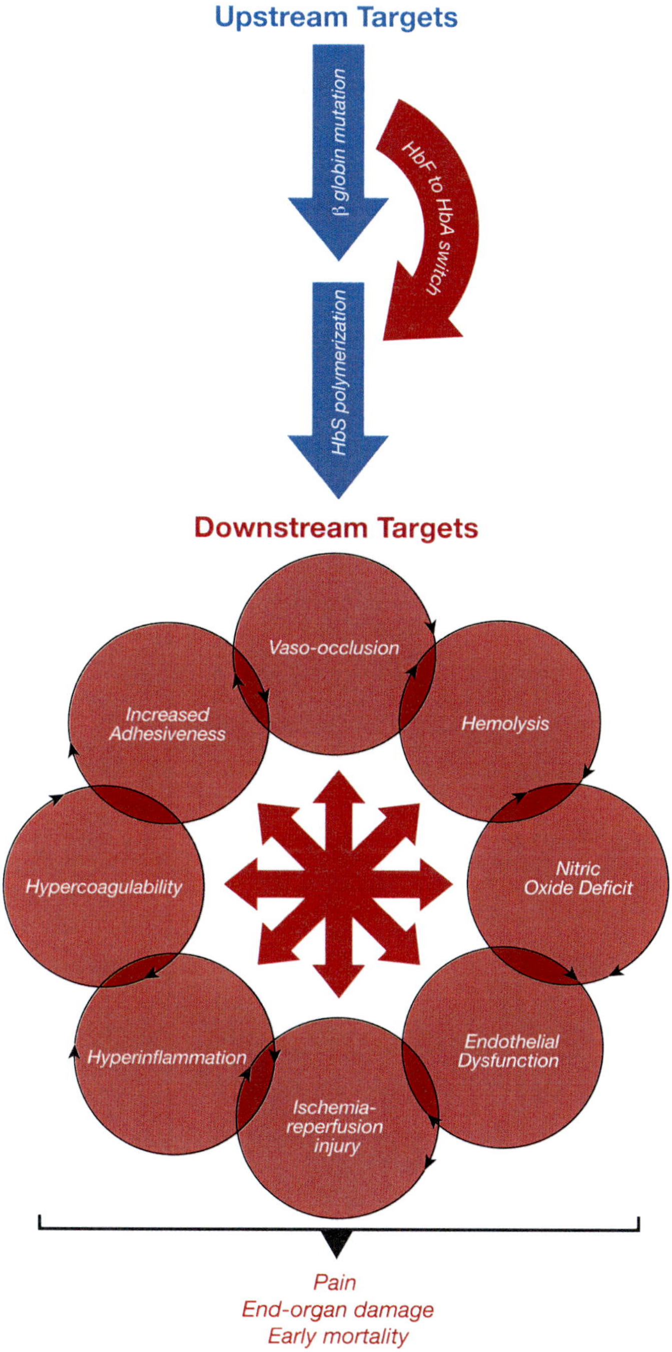

Fig. 16.1 Upstream and downstream targets in sickle cell disease. The pathophysiology of sickle cell disease is complex and involves a single point mutation in the beta globin gene that subsequently affects multiple systems downstream. An array of possible therapeutic targets are identified as upstream or downstream, according to the disease pathobiology

Table 16.1 New therapeutic approaches in SCD, grouped by physiologic target level

Upstream targets

HbF inducers	Modulator of HbO2 affinity	Bone marrow transplant using alternative sources of graft	Gene therapy
Suberoylanilide hydroxamic acid (SAHA)	AES103	Matched unrelated	Correction of beta globin gene
Hydroxyurea	GBT440 (formerly known as GTx011)	Haplo-identical related	Increased production of fetal hemoglobin (reversal of Hb switch phenomenon)
HQK-1001		Umbilical cord blood unrelated	
Lenalidomide and pomalidomide			
Decitabine			

Downstream targets

Anti-inflammatory agents	Vaso-dilators	Anti-thrombotic and anti-platelet agents	Anti-adhesives	Anti-RBC dehydration agent	Anti-oxidants
Regadenoson (adenosine 2A-receptor agonist)	Tadalafil	Rivaroxaban (anti Xa inhibitor)	GMI-1070 (E-selectin inhibitor)	ICA17043 (Senicapoc)	L-glutamine
NKTT120 (iNKT cell inhibitor)	Sildenafil	Heparin	SelG1 (monoclonal Ab anti-P-selectin)	Magnesium sulfate	Omega-3 fatty acid
Statins	Arginine	Aspirin	Poloxamer 188		N-acetyl cysteine
Vitamin D	Inhaled nitric oxide	Ticaglefor	Propanolol		Acetil L-carnitine
Zileuton	Sapropterin dihydrochloride (6R-BH4)	Prasugrel	Abciximab		Alpha lipoic acid
MP4CO (heme-oxygenase inhibitor)	Niacin		L-citruline		Broccoli sprouts homogenate
Phosphodiesterase 9 inhibitor			IVIG		

16.2 Therapies with Upstream Targets

16.2.1 Gene Therapy

Perhaps one of the most exciting prospects in the field is the potential for cure through gene transfer therapy. Therapeutic gene transfer for SCD is the process whereby a viral vector containing genetic information for normal β-globin production is administered to a patient; genetic material is inserted into the host genome to correct the underlying genetic defect. Gene therapy has proven successful in hemophilia B (Nathwani et al. 2011, 2014); however, this has not yet been tested in SCD, despite substantial effort over more than two decades. Early investigations using adeno-associated viruses failed because of the inability to maintain expression of the transferred genetic material (Nathwani et al. 2000). In addition, high levels of gene expression, estimated at 20 % of hematopoietic stem cells, are necessary to have therapeutic benefit (Nienhuis and Persons 2012). In the 1990s, a lentiviral vector was used to successfully transfer β- or γ-globin genetic material with resultant phenotypic expression in thalassemic mice (May et al. 2000; Rivella et al. 2003; Romero et al. 2013). Successful gene transfer was demonstrated in sickle murine models with improvement in the SCD phenotype (Levasseur et al. 2003; Pawliuk et al. 2001). Since this discovery, gene transfer therapy has continued to move forward with several clinical trials now open to evaluate safety and expression of gene transfer using γ-globin (NCT02186418) and β-globin lentivirus vectors (NCT02247843 and NCT02151526). As proof of principle, gene therapy has been used successfully in an adult with thalassemia (HbE/β^0-thalassemia), who has become transfusion-independent (Cavazzana-Calvo et al. 2010).

Most recently, a new modality of genetic engineering with theoretically greater precision and larger applicability is genome editing (or gene editing). This process involves a form of genetic engineering in which DNA is inserted into, replaced within, or removed from the genome using nucleases (Carroll 2011; Kim and Kim 2014; Sander and Joung 2014), which create double-stranded breaks at targeted locations, disrupting or repairing genetic defects. There are currently three nucleases in use: zinc finger nucleases, transcription activator-like effector nucleases, and clustered regularly interspaced short palindromic repeats (CRISPRs), such as the Cas9 system. Nuclease-induced double-stranded breaks are then repaired by different pathways, such as non-homologous end-joining and homology-directed repair; both repairing processes can allow the introduction of insertion or deletion mutations, or allow the introduction of specific desired coding sequences. The power of targeted genome editing is such that it can promote highly efficient alterations of the genome sequence and gene expression (e.g., enabling reverse genetics and assignment of function), and can be applied to several human diseases, such as SCD and thalassemia. Many different approaches are being investigated with application to different diseases, in which the mechanisms of certain genes are well understood. For example, gene editing might be applied in SCD through suppression of HbF controlling regions. KLF1 and BCL11A are genes whose natural role is suppression of γ-globin production during adulthood (Sankaran et al. 2008; Zhou et al. 2010). Inhibition of these genes in mice has led to increases in pancellular HbF (Xu et al. 2011). An alternative approach for HbF induction is activation of the γ-globin promoter in erythroblasts derived from human $CD34^+$ cells using an artificial zinc finger transcriptional activation factor (Hoban et al. 2015; Wilber et al. 2010). Given the fast pace at which this technique is being developed, it is conceivable that genome editing will be translated to the clinic in the next few years, providing a new generation of approaches to genetic correction of human disorders.

16.2.2 Bone Marrow (Hematopoietic Stem Cell) Transplantation (HSCT)

HSCT is currently the only curative therapy available for SCD. The first HSCT performed in a person with SCD occurred more than 30 years ago in a child with both SCD and acute myeloblastic leukemia; this patient was cured of both diseases (Johnson et al. 1984). Since then, over 1000 individuals with SCD (most selected for clinically severe disease) have been transplanted in the US and Europe using human leukocyte antigen (HLA)–identical sibling donors (Gluckman 2013). Overall survival (OS) and event-free survival (EFS) for HLA-identical sibling donor HSCT are very high today, ranging from 90–100 % to 80–100 %, respectively (Bernaudin et al. 2007; Bhatia et al. 2014; Gluckman 2013; Krishnamurti et al. 2008; Panepinto et al. 2007). The rate of graft versus host disease (GVHD) is progressively decreasing and is presently less than 10 %. Furthermore, the use of non-myeloablative HLA-identical conditioning regimens has allowed the extension of HSCT to adults with multiple co-morbidities and organ dysfunction, which would have been expected to increase their risk of HSCT-related complications (Hsieh et al. 2014). Non-myeloablative and reduced-intensity preparative regimens have also been successful in children and have provided excellent OS and EFS (Table 16.2) (Bhatia et al. 2014; Gluckman 2013; Krishnamurti et al. 2008).

Unfortunately, most individuals with SCD do not have an HLA-identical matched sibling bone marrow donor (Table 16.3). Therefore, it is imperative that future studies of HSCT in SCD explore the use of alternative sources of hematopoietic stem cells, which should include not only unrelated matched adult donors or partially-matched umbilical cord blood (UCB) grafts, but also related haplo-identical donors. Expanding the pool of donors could potentially increase the availability of HSCT to all eligible SCD individuals.

Results of HSCT using HLA-matched unrelated grafts (from both adult donors and UCB) in SCD are limited, but have been significantly inferior to HLA-identical or haplo-identical HSCT (Table 16.2) (Gluckman 2013; Kamani et al. 2012). Use of haplo-identical grafts could improve donor availability, but the risk of alloreactivity (GVHD) is higher. Reports of haplo-identical HSCT for hemoglobinopathies are scarce in the literature, but seem promising. In 31 children with thalassemia major, a T-cell depletion approach has been used to reduce the risk of GVHD in haplo-

Table 16.2 Outcome comparison of novel HSCT approaches in hemoglobinopathies

Disease	Group	# patients	Median age (range) (years)	Graft type	%OS	Graft failure (%)	DFS (%)	aGVHD (all types) (%)	aGVHD grade III/IV (%)	TRM (%)	BMT intensity	Reference
Matched sibling												
TM and SCD	Eurocord and EBMTR	BM: 389 UCB: 96	BM: 8.1 (0.2–24) UCB: 5.9 (2–20)	Match-sib marrow or UCB	BM: 97 UCB: 95	BM: 7.4 UCB: 10.4	BM: 88 UCB: 83	BM: 21 UCB: 11	BM: 2 (G-IV) UCB: 0	BM: 4 UCB: 3	Myeloablative	Locatelli et al. (2013)
SCD	Columbia, NY, USA	18	8.9 (2.3–20.2)	Match-sib marrow or UCB	100	0	100	17	11	0	Myeloablative with reduced toxicity	Bhatia et al. (2014)
SCD	Atlanta, GA, USA	7	(1.5–8)	Match-sib marrow	100	14	86	14	0	0	Reduced intensity	Krishnamurti et al. (2008)
SCD	NIH, USA	30	(16–65)	Match-sib marrow	97	13	87	0	0	0 (1 death after graft failure—ICH)	Non-myeloablative	Hsieh et al. (2014)
Matched unrelated												
SCD	BMT—CTN	8	(7–16)	UCB only (≥5/6 matched)	100	63	37	25	0	0	Reduced intensity	Kamani et al. (2012)
Haplo-identical related												
TM	Rome, Italy	31	Children (age?)	Parents or sibling	93	23	93	0	0	6	Myeloablative	Sodani et al. (2011)
SCD	Baltimore, MD, USA	14	30 (15–46)	Parents or sibling	100	43	78	0	0	0	Non-myeloablative	Bolanos-Meade et al. (2012)

TM beta thalassemia major, *SCD* sickle cell disease, *OS* overall survival, *EFS* event-free survival, *TRM* transplant-related mortality, *BM* bone marrow, *UCB* umbilical cord blood, *aGVHD* acute graft versus host disease, *ICH* intra-cranial hemorrhage, *CTN* Clinical Trials Network, *EBMTR* European Bone Marrow Transplantation Registry, *NIH* National Institutes of Health

Table 16.3 Probability of available graft for SCD, according to source of graft and degree of HLA matching (if considering the majority of SCD African American) (Gragert et al. 2014)

Type of graft	Likelihood of finding available donor
HLA-matched sibling (marrow or UCB)	14 %
Unrelated HLA-matched (adult donor marrow (8/8 alleles))	19 %
Unrelated 6/6 HLA-matched cord blood[a]	6 % for recipient < 20 years of age 2 % for recipient > 20 years of age
Unrelated 5/6 HLA-matched cord blood[a]	58 % for recipient < 20 years of age 24 % for recipient > 20 years of age

UCB umbilical cord blood

[a]With adequate cell dose

identical HSCT, and demonstrated both OS and EFS of 93 % (Table 16.2) (Sodani et al. 2011). A study with adults with SCD who received non-myeloablative haplo-identical non-manipulated grafts, with additional cyclophosphamide dosing post-graft infusion (to reduce GVHD risk), showed high OS (100 %), albeit with high graft rejection (43 %) (Table 16.2) (Bolanos-Meade et al. 2012). The non-myeloablative haplo-identical approach is now being tested in children with SCD (NCT00977691 and NCT01850108). Currently, T-cell depleted grafts (using CD34+ selection) are being tested in children and adults (NCT01966367) using HLA-identical sibling or unrelated donors and in children with haplo-identical donors (NCT01461837 and NCT02165007).

UCB is a valuable source of stem cells, which promote early engraftment and lower rates of acute GVHD even with one allele mismatch (5/6 HLA match). However, due to insufficient cell number (in relationship to the size of the recipient), the engraftment rate and sustainability of the graft may be reduced. An interesting study is investigating the use of UCB along with a new product, NiCord® (nicotinamide and noncultured T-cell fraction), a stem-cell based product composed of ex vivo expanded allogeneic cord blood cells (NCT01590628) (Horwitz et al. 2014). If successful, this approach could improve efficacy of HSCT using UCB grafts.

Finally, although the overwhelming majority of HSCT for SCD have occurred in patients with severe disease complications (stroke, recurrent episodes of acute chest syndrome [ACS] and pain), there has been recent discussion about considering individuals with less severe disease for HSCT (Nickel et al. 2014). This argument finds support from previously transplanted milder cases (e.g., children of African immigrants to Europe who returned to their home countries where the care for SCD was suboptimal) and went on to have excellent outcome post procedure. Unfortunately, in early life, there are no reliable predictors of those who eventually will develop severe complications, which might justify early lower risk transplants in patients who are in better overall health. This discussion will likely continue as a result of improved successes with HSCT and greater availability due to the use of alternative sources of graft.

16.2.3 HbF Inducers

HbF is one of the most powerful determinants of clinical severity (Platt et al. 1991; Serjeant 1995; Steinberg et al. 1995). Fetal hemoglobin ($\alpha_2\gamma_2$) inhibits the deoxygenation-induced polymerization of mutant sickle hemoglobin (HbS, $\alpha_2\beta^S{}_2$). This inhibition occurs mainly due to two factors: (1) neither HbF homotetramers ($\alpha_2\gamma_2$) nor heterotetramers ($\alpha_2\gamma\beta^s$) participate in the polymerization process; and (2) the intracellular concentration of HbS, which is the prime determinant of polymerization, is lessened by dilution with increased HbF (Eaton and Hofrichter 1987). In natural history studies, higher HbF levels are associated with reduced morbidity and mortality (Leikin et al. 1989; Platt et al. 1991, 1994; Stevens et al. 1981). These clinical observations provided strong evidence that pharmacologically induced HbF would be beneficial to individuals with SCD.

Several medications, with different mechanism of action, have the ability to induce HbF production. Any drug that substantially increases intracellular HbF in a homogenous distribution (pancellular HbF distribution) has the potential to improve clinical outcomes dramatically in patients with SCD.

Hydroxyurea

Hydroxyurea is an antimetabolite chemotherapeutic agent known to stimulate HbF production and is the only FDA-approved therapy for use in adult patients with SCD. Hydroxyurea has predictable laboratory benefits: it raises Hb concentrations and HbF levels, as well as promotes a parallel increase in red cell mean corpuscular volume (MCV) (Ferster et al. 2001; Kinney et al. 1999). The myelosuppressive and cytotoxic effects of hydroxyurea induce erythroid regeneration and the recruitment of earlier progenitors programmed to produce higher levels of HbF (Dover et al. 1986). The exact mechanism by which hydroxyurea increases HbF levels is unknown, but it seems to be mediated through a nitric oxide (NO)-dependent activation of soluble guanylyl cyclase within erythroid progenitor cells (Cokic et al. 2003, 2008). Hydroxyurea has additional beneficial laboratory effects in individuals with SCA, including lowering white blood cell count (WBC), reticulocytes, and platelets, increasing NO production (Nahavandi et al. 2002), improving RBC hydration (Orringer et al. 1991), and decreasing RBC adhesiveness to endothelium (Hillery et al. 2000).

The usual starting dose of hydroxyurea is 20 mg/kg/day given once daily orally (Heeney and Ware 2010; Platt et al. 1991), and therapy reduces the incidence of pain, ACS, hospitalization, and transfusions in adults and children (Charache et al. 1995; Ferster et al. 2001; Jayabose et al. 1996; Wang et al. 2011), but more importantly, hydroxyurea reduces mortality in individuals with SCD (Lobo et al. 2013; Steinberg et al. 2003). Additionally, when hydroxyurea is included in preconditioning regimens prior to bone marrow transplantation of patients with SCD, a lower incidence of rejection and engraftment failure is frequently seen (Brachet

Table 16.4 Qualitative evaluation of organ function in hydroxyurea versus placebo in the BABY HUG (Wang et al. 2011)

	Hydroxyurea				Placebo				Difference[b]	
	n	Entry	Exit	%Δ[a]	*n*	Entry	Exit	%Δ[a]	(95 % CI)	*p*-value
HJB (per 10^6 RBC)	76	663	1360	106 %	82	495	1470	197 %	−274 (−538 to −10)	0.04
Pitted cells (%)	85	4.3	5.7	32 %	82	4.6	8.4	84 %	−2.5 (−4.7 to −0.2)	0.04
Urine osmolality (mOsm/kg H_2O)	81	384	494	29 %	84	400	454	13 %	57 (3–110)	0.04
Urine-specific gravity	86	1.010	1.012	0 %	82	1.012	1.011	0 %	0.002 (0.0004–0.004)	0.02

HJB Howell-Jolly body, *RBC* red blood cell
[a]Percent difference from entry to exit
[b]*p*-value calculated with Student's t test comparing the exit versus entry differences between mean values in hydroxyurea and placebo groups

et al. 2004). When hydroxyurea is initiated early in life, there is evidence of protection for some end organs. In young children with SCA, splenic function was preserved and, in some cases, regained when hydroxyurea was escalated to the maximum tolerated dose (approximately 30 mg/kg/day) (Hankins et al. 2005, 2008a; Heeney and Ware 2010; Nottage et al. 2014). Similar beneficial findings in other organs have also been reported, such as improvement of renal function, proteinuria, retinopathy, resolution of hypoxemia, and protection against recurrent stroke (Aygun et al. 2013; Estepp et al. 2013; Fitzhugh et al. 2005; Singh et al. 2008; Ware et al. 2004). The BABY HUG study (Wang et al. 2011) (www.clinicaltrials.gov NCT00006400) was a landmark randomized multicenter trial investigating the role of hydroxyurea in organ preservation in very young (9–18 months) clinically asymptomatic children with SCA. Although the trial's primary endpoints, assessing organ preservation (spleen assessment by ^{99}Tc spleen scan and glomerular filtration rate by ^{99}Tc-DTPA clearance), were not met, other quantitative measures of splenic function (Howell-Jolly bodies and pit counts) and renal function (urine osmolality and specific gravity) suggested improvement with hydroxyurea therapy (Table 16.4).

Recently, several clinical trials evaluating the use of hydroxyurea for secondary protection in children with previous stroke, and primary prophylaxis for those with abnormal transcranial Doppler (TCD) velocities have been concluded. The SWiTCH trial (Ware et al. 2012) (NCT00122980) was a Phase 3 randomized trial comparing chronic erythrocyte transfusion and chelation versus hydroxyurea and phlebotomy in children with SCA who had a previous stroke and iron overload. This trial failed to demonstrate noninferiority of hydroxyurea in comparison with transfusions and, currently, transfusions and chelation therapy remain the preferred way to manage children with SCA, stroke, and iron overload. Recently, the TWiTCH trial (NCT01425307) compared erythrocyte transfusions to hydroxyurea therapy for the reduction of primary stroke risk in children with abnormal TCD velocities who did not have cerebral vasculopathy or history of stroke and had received at least 12 months of chronic transfusion. This trial was closed early since its primary endpoint was met. If results of the TWiTCH trial indicate that hydroxyurea is not inferior to chronic transfusion, hydroxyurea can be considered as an alternative therapy for children with SCA and abnormal TCD without significant vasculopathy.

Given the collective accumulated evidence of benefit of hydroxyurea, in 2014, the National Heart, Lung, and Blood Institute (NHLBI) issued evidence-based guidelines recommending that hydroxyurea therapy be offered to all children with SCA (≥9 months of age), independent of disease severity, and that it should be prescribed for all adults with clinically severe disease (Yawn et al. 2014).

Interestingly, limited information about the pharmacokinetics (PK) of hydroxyurea is available. In a small cohort of SCD patients, no significant differences in PK parameters occurred between adult and pediatric individuals (De Montalembert et al. 2006); however, in children receiving hydroxyurea for the first time, significant interparticipant variability has been reported, both in PK parameters and systemic drug exposure (Ware et al. 2011). Given the increasing use of hydroxyurea in the pediatric population and a paucity of PK information, the FDA offered a written request under the Best Pharmaceuticals for Children Act (BPCA) to specifically address the PK of hydroxyurea in children, specifically highlighting the need for data comparing liquid and capsule formulations. In response to this written request, the "Pharmacokinetics and Relative Bioavailability of a Liquid Formulation of Hydroxyurea in Pediatric Patients with Sickle Cell Anemia" (NCT01506544) trial was designed to characterize the disposition of a liquid hydroxyurea formulation in a cohort of toddlers (≥2 to ≤5 years) with SCA and to evaluate the relative bioavailability of a liquid formulation compared to a proprietary capsular formulation in older (>5 to ≤17 years) children. The results of this trial are forthcoming. Because hydroxyurea undergoes renal clearance, its dose must be adjusted in individuals with renal impairment. A reduced initial dose of hydroxyurea (7.5 mg/kg/day) is recommended in individuals with a creatinine clearance <60 mL/min (Yan et al. 2005), and close monitoring of myelotoxicity is essential in these patients.

The long-term safety of hydroxyurea continues to be of concern. The risk of cancer development no longer seems prominent, as no evidence suggests an increased rate of malignancy associated with hydroxyurea therapy (Brawley et al. 2008), and, in children treated with hydroxyurea therapy, no genotoxicity or chromosomal damage has been identified (McGann et al. 2011, 2012). Some effect on sperm production has been reported in men being treated with hydroxyurea, and this is a significant concern for both practitioners and patients (Berthaut et al. 2008; DeBaun 2014; Smith-Whitley 2014). However, data suggesting that there are issues with male fertility related to hydroxyurea therapy are limited and of poor quality. A prospective study was recently completed to evaluate this risk (NCT01609192) and results should be forthcoming.

Significant clinical questions still remain regarding hydroxyurea therapy that need to be addressed. For example: What is the optimal age of initiation? What is the optimal dosage, low fixed-dose or escalated to a level of moderate myelosuppression (i.e., maximum tolerated dose)? Are there laboratory benchmarks that should be targeted, such as HbF or Hb levels? Can hydroxyurea therapy be utilized safely in resource-poor countries, where the burden of SCA is the highest and co-morbidities (e.g., malaria, malnutrition) are common? What are its effects on quality of life? How do we maximize adherence to a daily medication to optimize long-term outcomes? How do we study novel therapeutic agents in SCD in combination with hydroxyurea in future clinical trials?

To address the issue of optimal dosing of hydroxyurea, a prospective cohort of children treated with hydroxyurea (NCT00305175) was evaluated for the effect of higher HbF levels. In this study, during intervals when children had HbF levels of 20 % or less, they were twice as likely to be hospitalized, both for SCD-related causes or any cause (Estepp et al. 2014). This suggests that the clinical threshold for achieving maximum clinical benefits of the drug is when HbF values are ≥20 %. These data suggest that hydroxyurea therapy (dose and adherence) should be tailored to achieve this HbF level, which could be used as a benchmark for future clinical trials using hydroxyurea (or other HbF inducers) alone or in combination.

Decitabine

Decitabine and its analogue, 5-azacytidine, are cytidine surrogates. Once incorporated into the DNA, they form covalent bonds with DNA methyltrasferase (DNMT), leading to depletion of this enzyme, and resulting in DNA hypomethylation (Creusot et al. 1982). Hypomethylation of the γ-globin gene promoter triggers its expression and induces γ-globin synthesis, resulting in the so called "γ-globin reverse switch," the postulated mechanism of action for increased HbF production (Charache et al. 1983; DeSimone et al. 1983). In addition, these compounds induce selective degradation of DNMT1, also resulting in re-expression of γ-globin genes (Ghoshal et al. 2005).

Following early reports of success in baboons, a remarkable increase in F-cell and HbF production was observed in patients with SCD and thalassaemia with 5-azacytidine use, in addition to a reduction in the proportion of dense RBCs in patients with SCD (DeSimone et al. 1982; Dover et al. 1985; Ley et al. 1983a, b). These initial reports were very encouraging; however, concerns related to malignant transformation in rats, presumed to be related to 5-azacytidine, halted future investigation (Carr et al. 1984). The 5-azacytidine analogue, decitabine (2-deoxy 5-azacytidine), was shown to promote similar molecular and cellular effects to its counterpart, with no apparent tumorigenic risks (DeSimone et al. 2002; Koshy et al. 2000). Prompted by the fact that some patients treated with hydroxyurea will have a poor response, even in the setting of good adherence (i.e., hydroxyurea low responders), more effort has been recently placed into the development of decitabine as an alternative or adjunct therapy in SCD. Low dose subcutaneous use of decitabine (0.2 mg/kg 1–3 times/week) was tested in a small group of adult patients who had responded poorly to hydroxyurea; decitabine promoted a marked increase in HbF, F cell proportion, and Hb concentration, and decreased reticulocyte and absolute neutrophil counts (Saunthararajah et al. 2003). In this study, however, the platelet count increased with decitabine therapy, an incompletely understood effect that may trigger undesirable clotting activation and will require close monitoring in subsequent studies. A report of four adult patients with multiple complications of SCD described clinical benefit of decitabine in reducing vaso-occlusive events and improved symptoms of heart dysfunction (Saunthararajah et al. 2008).

Decitabine has only been tested parenterally (IV or SQ) in human subjects. An oral form of decitabine, which was tested in baboons and seemed to offer the same benefits as the parenteral formulations (Lavelle et al. 2007), would improve the likelihood of this drug becoming an acceptable therapy for SCD. The long-term clinical effects (e.g., reduction in vaso-occlusive events and protection against end organ damage) and long-term side effects of decitabine (e.g., malignancy and male infertility) have not yet been investigated. Clinical investigation of decitabine in larger groups and for longer periods is warranted. Currently, "Decitabine for High-Risk Sickle Cell Disease" (NCT01375608) is an open-label, Phase 2 trial utilizing decitabine injections for up to 1 year in adults with SCD who have been refractory to or are unable to take hydroxyurea. The primary endpoint in this study, which is estimated to be completed in 2015, is the change in HbF level.

Vorinostat (Suberoylanilide Hydroxamic Acid, SAHA)

Vorinostat (SAHA) is a histone deacetylase inhibitor that binds directly to the catalytic site of the enzyme and blocks substrate access. SAHA is now being studied in clinical trials for the treatment of several forms of cancer. In a sickle cell mouse model (Hebbel et al. 2010), pulmonary vascular endothelial receptor VCAM-1 and tissue factor (TF) expression, both markers of endothelial activation, were significantly reduced following administration of SAHA. This inhibition of endothelial activation was seen in settings of acute and chronic administration of the compound. Additionally, SAHA induced expression of HbF and exhibited some functionality as an iron-chelating agent. Currently, a Phase 2 trial is recruiting adults with all genotypes of SCD and a history of clinically severe disease who have failed hydroxyurea therapy (NCT01000155). In this Phase 2 trial, SAHA is administered orally once a day, three times a week. The trial is designed to determine the efficacy of SAHA in inducing HbF levels over 2 years and to evaluate the safety of the treatment.

2,2-Dimethylbuterate (HQK-1001)

2,2-Dimethylbuterate (HQK-1001) is an orally-administered short-chain fatty acid butyrate derivative, which was shown to stimulate HbF production in vitro and in animal models. HQK-1001 was evaluated in a Phase 2 trial (NCT0160134) designed to evaluate its pharmacodynamics, efficacy, and safety in adults with HbSS or HbSβ^0thalassemia. The study was terminated early following a planned interim analysis that showed lack of effect in inducing HbF levels (Reid et al. 2014).

Lenalidomide and Pomalidomide

Lenalidomide and pomalidomide are immunomodulatory drugs that inhibit the production of the cytokine tumor necrosis factor (TNF)-α. In vitro, lenalidomide and pomalidomide slow erythrocyte maturation and increase the proliferation of immature erythrocytes. Additionally, these medications result in significant induction of HbF without evidence of cytotoxicity. When these medications were combined with hydroxyurea, they were found to have a synergistic effect on HbF production (Moutouh-de Parseval et al. 2008). In a mouse model, pomalidomide induced HbF levels with similar efficacy to hydroxyurea without myelosuppression; however, when pomalidomide was used in combination with hydroxyurea, no HbF was induced (Meiler et al. 2011). The results of a Phase 1 trial (NCT01522547) designed to determine the maximum tolerated dose and safety of pomalidomide in adults with SCA who had clinically significant disease are awaited and might provide important early evidence for continued investigation of this compound.

16.2.4 Modulators of HbO2 Affinity

The compound 5-hydroxymethyl-2-furfural (5HMF) is a naturally occurring aldehyde that has been shown to have anti-sickling properties. 5HMF is found in various food products including coffee, honey, dried fruits, juices, and wine, though concentrations are highly variable (Van Gorsel et al. 1992). When administered to sickle mice, the percentage of sickled cells decreased in a dose-dependent fashion. In addition, sickle mice treated with 5HMF had longer survival time under hypoxic conditions than sickle mice that were not exposed to the drug. The drug was unchanged and highly bioavailable after a single oral dose (Abdulmalik et al. 2005). The compound readily traverses the red cell membrane and binds to HbS. This binding allosterically shifts the oxygen dissociation curve to the left, thereby increasing the oxygen affinity of Hb and inhibiting sickling of Hb S. The drug also has the advantage of maintaining red cell ion and water homeostasis in vitro (Hannemann et al. 2014). A Phase 1 study of 5HMF (also known as AES-103) was completed and the drug was determined to be safe among adult patients with SCD (Kato et al. 2013). Investigators also report a dose-dependent reduction in pain, trend toward less hemolysis, and higher oxygen saturation and oxygen affinity. A Phase 2 study in adults is currently ongoing (NCT01987908).

A second compound, which also alters the oxygen affinity of the hemoglobin and thereby prevents sickling, GBT440 (formerly known as GTx011), has been shown to delay HbS polymerization and prevent sickling of isolated RBCs in vitro under hypoxic conditions (Dufu et al. 2014). Results of ongoing clinical trials in adults are expected soon.

16.3 Therapies with Downstream Targets

16.3.1 Anti-adhesives

Vaso-occlusion in SCD involves a complex cascade of events with interactions between adhesion molecules in erythrocytes, white blood cells, and platelets (Chiang and Frenette 2005). Selectins are a group of membrane adhesion molecules (E-selectin, P-selectin, and L-selectin) that mediate cellular adhesion between blood cells and the vascular endothelium and facilitate leukocyte rolling along the vessel wall. The potential involvement of selectins in vaso-occlusion has led to their evaluation as a novel therapeutic target in SCD.

GMI-1070 (E-selectin Inhibitor)

In mouse models, GMI-1070 (rivipansel) inhibited E-selectin-mediated adhesion and inhibited erythrocyte-leukocyte interactions, leading to improved microcirculatory blood flow (Chang et al. 2010). In a Phase 1 trial (NCT00911495), GMI-1070 was administered to 15 adult participants with HbSS. The study drug was well tolerated, and it significantly reduced biomarkers of endothelial and leukocyte activation, in addition to decreasing activation of the coagulation cascade (Wun et al. 2014). A Phase 2 trial (NCT01119833), utilizing GMI-1070, randomized adolescents and adult participants (12–60 years of age) with HbSS or Hbβ^0thalassemia who had been admitted to the hospital with an acute vaso-occlusive pain episode. This trial, which was designed to identify a reduction in the time to resolution of pain, has recently completed enrollment and results are forthcoming.

Poloxamer 188/MST 188

Poloxamer 188 is a nonionic block copolymer surfactant composed of hydrophobic polyoxypropylene and hydrophilic polyoxyethylene. It has been found to improve microvascular blood flow by lowering viscosity and adhesive frictional forces. The mechanism of action is not entirely known, but it is hypothesized that the hydrophobic portion of the molecule interacts with the hydrophobic areas of cells and leaves the hydrophilic chains free to interact with surrounding media, providing a barrier blocking adhesive interaction (Adams-Graves et al. 1997).

A randomized, double-blind, placebo-controlled, pilot trial enrolled 50 participants (>15 years of age) with any form of SCD admitted to the hospital for vaso-occlusive pain (NCT01737814) (Adams-Graves et al. 1997). Participants were randomized to receive either poloxamer 188 or placebo; those receiving poloxamer 188 may have had a reduction in duration of pain, narcotic utilization, and hospitalization time. A Phase 3 trial (NCT01737814), utilizing poloxamer 188 (MST-188), is currently enrolling participants (4–65 years of age) with any form of SCD who were admitted to the hospital for a vaso-occlusive pain episode. The study is designed to compare the duration of vaso-occlusive pain utilizing poloxamer 188 versus placebo. The estimated date of completion for this trial is winter 2015.

16.3.2 Anti-thrombotic and Anti-platelet Agents

At baseline, individuals with SCA exhibit elevated thrombin generation, microparticle formation, tissue factor expression, and platelet activation; in addition, individuals with SCD have depletion of natural anticoagulants and a reduced fibrinolytic activity (Ataga et al. 2008a; De Franceschi et al. 2011; Green and Scott 1986; Lee et al. 2006; Lim et al. 2013; Noubouossie et al. 2013; Tomer et al. 2001; van Beers et al. 2009; Westerman et al. 1999). These alterations are amplified during acute vaso-occlusive events, and although ameliorative therapies (hydroxyurea and chronic transfusion) decrease the hypercoagulation state, they are not able to completely correct it (Colella et al. 2012; Liesner et al. 1998; Nebor et al. 2013). Given that the hypercoagulable state worsens during acute complications and is only partially rectified with standard (hydroxyurea and transfusion) therapies, alternative therapeutic approaches that have anticoagulant, anti-platelet, and anti-adhesion effects are being investigated.

Heparinoids

Heparinoids [unfractionated heparin (UFH) and low-molecular-weight heparins (LMWH)] are highly sulfated mucopolysaccharides that bind to antithrombin via a high-affinity pentasaccharide sequence. Heparinoids exert their anticoagulant effect by increasing natural anticoagulant activity of antithrombin up to 1000-fold, and facilitate inactivation of thrombin (IIa) and factors (F) Xa, IXa, XIa, and XIIa (Björk and Lindahl 1982; Garcia et al. 2012; Hirsh and Raschke 2004; Rosenberg 1989; Rosenberg and Lam 1979; Verstraete 1990; Weitz 1997).

A single small cohort utilizing UFH has been reported in individuals with SCA (Chaplin et al. 1989). In this study, UFH (5000–7500 units subcutaneously twice daily) was administered for 12 months to four adults with HbSS who had severe, recurrent vaso-occlusive pain. No treatment related complications were identified. Cumulatively, patients had 73 % fewer days in the hospital and a 74 % reduction in the hours spent in the emergency room when compared to the year prior to initiating UFH. The use of LMWH molecules has also been evaluated. A prospective, randomized, double-blinded clinical trial utilized tinzaparin (LMWH) in individuals >12 years of age with HbSS admitted to the hospital for vaso-occlusive pain (Qari et al. 2007). In the 253 randomized participants, those who received tinzaparin had faster resolution of pain symptoms, correlating with shorter hospital stays and less overall days of pain reported.

Additional studies with different doses and forms of LMWH are necessary to confirm their benefit (van Zuuren and Fedorowicz 2013) and, currently, two trials of heparinoid medications are underway. The first is a feasibility study of UFH in adults with HbSS and ACS (NCT02098993). If feasibility of enrollment is documented, the corresponding larger trial would assess if UFH could decrease the duration of hospitalization or improve hypoxemia (caused by ACS) or pain. The second trial evaluating heparinoids is a prospective, randomized, double-blind placebo-controlled evaluation of dalteparin (a LMWH) in adults with HbSS or HbSβ^0thalassemia admitted for vaso-occlusive pain (NCT01419977). The primary outcome measure is reduction of hypercoagulable markers (D-dimer, thrombin antithrombin complex -TAT, prothrombin fragment 1.2, and thrombin generation assay), with secondary measures evaluating reduction in clinical pain scores.

Target-Specific Oral Anticoagulants (TSOACs)

Rivaroxaban (Xarelto©) and Apixaban (Eliquis©) are orally administered selective inhibitors of factor Xa that function independently of antithrombin.[1,2] In a Berkeley sickle cell mouse model, rivaroxaban normalized plasma levels of TAT without causing spontaneous bleeding (Sparkenbaugh et al. 2014).The drug is currently being evaluated in a single-center, double-blinded, randomized, cross-over trial designed to evaluate its effect on markers of inflammation, coagulation and endothelial activation in adults with HbSS (NCT02072668). In this trial, participants in steady-state are randomized to receive 4 weeks of either rivaroxaban or placebo; then, they undergo a 2-week washout period and are crossed-over to receive an additional 4 weeks of the alternative therapy. Additionally, a double-blinded, Phase 3 trial of Apixaban (NCT02179177) is being planned for adults with HbSS or HbSβ^0thalassemia with the primary endpoint being a reduction in pain.

Antiplatelet Agents

Currently, antiplatelet agents have not been proven to be safe or effective in ameliorating the complications of SCA; several trials are currently underway which may provide insight into this potential therapeutic class of medications.

Prasugrel (Effient©) and ticagrelor (Brilinta©) belong to the thienopyridine class of platelet inhibitors and reversibly inhibit the $P2Y_{12}$ ADP-receptor.[3,4] Recently, prasugrel was evaluated in a randomized, double-blinded, adaptive, Phase 2 study in

[1] 2014c. Eliquis (apixaban). *Package insert*, http://www.accessdata.fda.gov/drugsatfda_docs/label/2012/202155s000lbl.pdf.

[2] 2014d. Xarelto (rivaroxaban). *Package insert*, http://www.xareltohcp.com/sites/default/files/pdf/xarelto_0.pdf, Accessed 1 September 2014d.

[3] 2014a. Brilinta (ticagrelor). *Package insert*, http://www1.astrazeneca-us.com/pi/brilinta.pdf.

[4] 2014b. Effient (prasugrel). *Package insert*, http://pi.lilly.com/us/effient.pdf.

an adult population with any SCD genotype (NCT01167023) (Wun et al. 2013). Participants were randomized to receive 5 mg of prasugrel daily versus placebo for 30 days. Prasugrel decreased biomarkers of platelet activation, and there were trends in improvement in the intensity and frequency of pain episodes (Wun et al. 2013). Currently, an international, Phase 3, double-blinded, placebo-controlled trial of prasugrel in children is underway (NCT01794000). Eligible participants have HbSS or HbSβ^0thalassemia and clinically severe disease. Following randomization, participants are followed for 24 months with the primary endpoint being a reduction in vaso-occlusive events. Another antiplatelet agent, ticagrelor, is also being investigated in a pharmacokinetic and pharmacodynamic dose-ranging trial (NCT02214121) in children with HbSS or HbSβ^0thalassemia and clinically severe disease.

16.3.3 Anti-inflammatory Agents

Vaso-occlusion causes direct cellular damage from disrupted blood flow and resultant ischemia. Upon restoration of blood flow, the delivery of oxygen to the once ischemic tissue triggers a secondary, inflammatory reaction. The complex inflammatory cascade in ischemia-reperfusion injury involves activation of leukocytes and platelets and release of various cytokines, chemokines, and inflammatory molecules such as TNF-α, IL-1, IL-6, IL-8, monocyte chemoattractant protein 1 (MCP-1), platelet activating factor (PAF), leukotriene B4 and E4 and vascular endothelial growth factor (VEGF) (Hebbel 2014; Hibbert et al. 2005). Prevention of the activation of the inflammatory cascade has been a target of newer therapies for SCD. Historically, corticosteroids have been used to abate the inflammatory component of the disease; however, use of these agents has been associated with rebound vaso-occlusion and hospital readmission and has fallen out of favor (Bernini et al. 1998; Strouse et al. 2008). Other drugs being studied for their anti-inflammatory properties include agents that inhibit leukotrienes such as montelukast and zileuton, adenosine 2A receptor agonists, and HMG-CoA reductase inhibitors (statins).

Adenosine 2A Receptor Agonist ($A_{2A}R$)

Activated invariant natural killer T-cell NKT (iNKT) cells are elevated in individuals with SCD (Wallace et al. 2009) and have been implicated in ischemia-reperfusion injury through their ability to propagate the inflammatory cascade (Shimamura et al. 2005). The $A_{2A}R$ agent, regadenoson, functions by disturbing iNKT cell activation and reducing its activity. In a sickle mouse model, iNKT cells were present in greater numbers and were hyper-responsive to ischemia-reperfusion injury compared to wild type mice. Furthermore, disrupting activation of iNKT cells in these mice decreased pulmonary inflammation (Wallace et al. 2009). These preclinical data were the basis for a Phase 1 clinical trial of regadenoson in 27 adults with

HbSS and 14 healthy controls. The study demonstrated the safety of a low-dose IV infusion (1.44 mcg/kg/hr) during a painful vaso-occlusive crisis, as well as a reduction of iNKT cell activation compared to that of controls during steady-state (Field et al. 2013). No dose limiting toxicities were identified. A Phase 2 placebo-controlled study is underway (NCT01788631) to evaluate the impact of regadenoson on iNKT cells, as well as its impact on clinical parameters such as hospital length of stay, opioid use, and respiratory symptoms among patients with a painful vaso-occlusive crisis or ACS.

Utilizing the same principle of reducing iNKT cells activity, the humanized monoclonal antibody NKTT120, is also being tested in clinical trials. This drug was recently granted fast track designation by the FDA to facilitate development and expedite its review (Scheuplein et al. 2013). A Phase 1 study is being conducted in adults with SCD and is investigating safety and dosing (NCT01783691).

HMG-CoA Reductase Inhibitors (Statins)

HMG-CoA reductase inhibitors (statins) are used in the general population primarily for their lipid-lowering effects, and multiple clinical trials have demonstrated a reduction in mortality with their use (Palmer et al. 2014; Taylor et al. 2013). There is accumulating evidence that statins have pleiotropic effects as a result of enhancement of endothelial function and a reduction in inflammatory mediators (Marzilli 2010). A meta-analysis evaluating the impact of statin therapy on inflammatory factors in patients with rheumatologic disease found down-regulation of multiple inflammatory mediators (e.g., TNF-α, IL-1, and IL-6), and overall reduction in clinical symptomatology (Lv et al. 2015). Statins also reduce adhesion of monocytes to endothelial cells (Teupser et al. 2001), release of TNF-α and IL-1β from monocytes (Ferro et al. 2000), and expression of adhesion molecules (e.g., P-selectin, ICAM-1, and VCAM-1) (Stach et al. 2012; Yang et al. 2012). The activated coagulation system of patients with SCD might be responsive to the additional action of statins in reducing hypercoagulation. The mechanism involves decreasing both thrombin generation and platelet activation (Pastuszczak et al. 2010). Finally, statins improve NO synthase function, thereby reducing oxidant stress and mitigating the endothelial dysfunction that is a mainstay in SCD (Hebbel et al. 2009).

A Phase 1/2 study of statin use in 26 patients with SCD showed that NO levels increased and C-reactive protein and IL-6 decreased in a dose-dependent fashion (Hoppe et al. 2011). Sub-analyses demonstrated a potential additive effect of statins with hydroxyurea. Importantly, no serious adverse events occurred, and there were no apparent ill effects of lowering cholesterol in patients who are relatively hypocholesterolemic at baseline. This work has led to additional clinical investigations evaluating the impact of statins on endothelial dysfunction, vaso-occlusive pain, and albuminuria. Two trials are completed and awaiting results (NCT00508027 and NCT00072826) and two trials are currently enrolling (NCT01702246 and NCT01732718). Results of these trials will help establish the role of these agents in SCD.

Phosphodiesterase 9 (PDE9) Inhibitor

Phosphodiesterase 9 (PDE9) is another therapeutic target for SCD that has the advantage of being somewhat tissue specific, since its expression is high in hematopoietic cells. Inhibition of this enzyme prevents degradation of cGMP. Higher levels of NO and cGMP have been linked with decreased leukocyte-endothelial interaction, thus less inflammation (Almeida et al. 2008; Miguel et al. 2011). The compound BAY73-6691 is a PDE9 inhibitor that has shown some success in reducing the inflammatory state associated with SCD in mouse models (Almeida et al. 2012). When hydroxyurea was administered concomitantly with BAY73-6691 there was even greater inhibition of leukocyte adhesion, improvement in leukocyte rolling velocity, and greater plasma cGMP concentration, indicating a synergistic effect of the two agents.

16.3.4 Vaso-Dilators

Nitric Oxide (NO)

NO is a potent vaso-dilator that is critical to the maintenance of vascular tone and is a key modulator of ischemia-reperfusion injury. In SCD, there is both increased consumption and decreased production of NO (Morris 2014). Vaso-dilation is compromised as a result of NO deficiency and may contribute to the pathophysiologic mechanisms of vaso-occlusive events. Multiple clinical observations have been made of resolution of SCD-related complications after treatment with inhaled NO (iNO) (Chang et al. 2008; Montero-Huerta et al. 2006; Oppert et al. 2004). Therapeutic iNO was tested in 20 patients with SCD age 10–21 years who were experiencing painful vaso-occlusive crisis. Opioid consumption was reduced in the patients receiving iNO when compared to placebo and there was a reduction in pain scores in the iNO group (Weiner et al. 2003). In a larger clinical trial, 150 patients with painful vaso-occlusive crisis were randomized to iNO or placebo, but no difference was observed between the two study arms (Gladwin et al. 2011). Despite these results interest still exists in understanding the therapeutic role of iNO for ACS and in combination with other therapies such as transfusion and nitroglycerin.

Arginine

Arginine is an obligate substrate for NO and is converted through the enzyme NO synthase (NOS); thus, it indirectly affects vascular tone. Arginine deficiency is common in patients with SCD, who have relatively normal levels in childhood, followed by gradual decline associated with aging and acute decreases during SCD-related complications (Morris et al. 2000, 2005). Early studies of arginine therapy were unsuccessful, likely due to insufficient dosing and choice of suboptimal study endpoints (Morris 2014; Styles et al. 2007). Arginine therapy has been used for the treatment of SCD-related leg ulcers (McMahon et al. 2010), and anecdotally for priapism (Morris 2014). There are conflicting data on the use of arginine for pulmonary hypertension, though differences in the definition of pulmonary hypertension and the dosing of arginine may explain these findings (Little et al. 2009; Morris et al. 2003). A small placebo-controlled trial of arginine for painful vaso-occlusive crisis in children with SCD demonstrated a reduction in parenteral opioid use and lower pain scores upon hospital discharge without a difference in the hospital length of stay (Morris et al. 2013). Though arginine metabolism is clearly disrupted in patients with SCD, its therapeutic role still warrants further investigation. Multiple trials examining the role of arginine in various clinical SCD-related complications such as vaso-occlusive crisis, ACS, and leg ulcers (NCT01796678, NCT00029731, and NCT00004412) have been completed and results are pending.

Sildenafil

Another vaso-dilator of interest is sildenafil, a phosphodiesterase-5 inhibitor. Sildenafil has been shown to improve pulmonary hemodynamics and exercise capacity among adults in the general population with pulmonary hypertension (Galie et al. 2005). However, a multi-institutional randomized trial investigating this agent in SCD patients was terminated early due to an increase in hospitalizations for painful vaso-occlusive crisis in the sildenafil arm (Machado et al. 2011). As a result, momentum surrounding this drug has ceased and no active trials are in progress.

16.3.5 Anti-RBC Dehydration Agents

The sickling process is uniquely dependent on the intracellular concentration of HbS; the greater the HbS concentration, the shorter the lag time to polymer formation and the greater the propensity for sickling (Eaton and Hofrichter 1987; Ferrone et al. 1985). HbS concentration is directly dependent upon cellular hydration status with dehydrated RBCs having higher intracellular HbS concentrations. Three main pathways are involved in red cell dehydration: the calcium-activated potassium efflux channel (Gardos channel) (Vandorpe et al. 1998), the KCl co-transport channel (Brugnara et al. 1986), and the Na + pump (Joiner et al. 1986). Inhibition of any of these pathways could potentially prevent RBC dehydration and provide clinical benefit.

The combination of magnesium pidolate and hydroxyurea was investigated in a Phase 1 clinical trial in children with HbSS (Hankins et al. 2008b). A significant reduction of KCl co-transport activity occurred after introduction of oral magnesium pidolate, supporting previous reports of its membrane effects in SCD (De Franceschi et al. 1997, 2000). Subsequent clinical studies, however, have not been able to demonstrate the clinical benefit of using either magnesium sulfate or a Gardos channel blocker (Senicapoc) in reducing either vaso-occlusive events or duration of hospitalization (Ataga et al. 2008b; Goldman et al. 2013).

16.3.6 Anti-oxidants

L-glutamine, alpha-lipoic acid, and omega-3 fatty acid (docosahexanoic acid, DHA) have all been tested in SCD with mixed results. DHA was recently shown to improve red blood cell deformability in mice and reduce the rate of vaso-occlusive pain events in children, albeit with limited clinical benefit (Daak et al. 2013; Wandersee et al. 2015). It is not clear if anti-oxidants will have a significant role in preventing SCD-related complications, and their effects need to be confirmed in future larger clinical trials.

16.4 Conclusion

At present, only three treatments for SCD are considered standard of care: hydroxyurea therapy, chronic transfusion, and HLA-identical sibling donor HSCT. In the US, hydroxyurea is the only FDA-approved drug for SCD (as of December 2014, only for severely affected adults with HbSS). In Europe, the European Medicines Agency granted a favored marketing authorization and recommendation for the use of hydroxyurea in children and adults with SCA in 2007. However, with so many drugs in pre-clinical and clinical development today, one can only expect that we will most certainly have greater options of treatment in the next decade. Of all the clinical therapeutics currently under investigation, two classes of drugs seem poised to undergo a faster translation into clinical use: anti-adhesives (particularly anti-E selectin agents), and anti-inflammatory agents (particularly modulators of iNKT cells). New agents or modalities of treatment that are under investigation and are likely to alter the natural history of SCD are the HbO2 affinity modulators and gene therapy.

Gene therapy, especially the newest form of genetic engineering, gene editing, could have a powerful impact in ameliorating or curing the disease given its highly specific targeting ability. The combination of a newer agent with an established therapy (e.g., hydroxyurea) also appears to be an opportunity for rapid development since this approach could take advantage of drugs with different mechanisms of action and non-overlapping toxicity. An ideal drug regimen could combine upstream and downstream targets for maximum benefit. Moreover, as we investigate new therapies, especially drug combination therapy for SCD, careful choices of clinical and laboratory endpoints are necessary to provide the best opportunity to answer questions of efficacy.

Finally, widespread application of HSCT may become a reality with improvement in utilization of alternative graft sources, such as haplo-identical related donors and UCB from unrelated donors. The reduction in graft rejection and GVHD, coupled with decreased transplant-related mortality (using non-myeloablative and lower toxicity regimens), may provide the impetus for offering HSCT to many more severe, and, perhaps, less severe individuals living with SCD, including both adults and children.

In summary, after many years of sluggish "anti-sickling" drug development, it appears we have entered an era of true revolution in the development of new therapeutic opportunities for amelioration and potential cure of SCD. After more than 100 years since this condition was first described, it is finally time that we look forward to a day when we will have many choices to offer children and adults living with SCD.

Acknowledgments The authors are indebted to Dr. Winfred Wang, MD for editing of this work, Dr. Mitchell Weiss, MD, PhD for helpful discussions during the writing of this chapter, and Terri Davis, BS, for formatting and final editing.

References

Abdulmalik O, Safo MK, Chen Q et al (2005) 5-Hydroxymethyl-2-furfural modifies intracellular sickle haemoglobin and inhibits sickling of red blood cells. Br J Haematol 128(4):552–561

Adams-Graves P, Kedar A, Koshy M et al (1997) RheothRx (poloxamer 188) injection for the acute painful episode of sickle cell disease: a pilot study. Blood 90(5):2041–2046

Almeida CB, Traina F, Lanaro C, Canalli AA, Saad ST, Costa FF, Conran N (2008) High expression of the cGMP-specific phosphodiesterase, PDE9A, in sickle cell disease (SCD) and the effects of its inhibition in erythroid cells and SCD neutrophils. Br J Haematol 142(5):836–844

Almeida CB, Scheiermann C, Jang JE, Prophete C, Costa FF, Conran N, Frenette PS (2012) Hydroxyurea and a cGMP-amplifying agent have immediate benefits on acute vaso-occlusive events in sickle cell disease mice. Blood 120(14):2879–2888

Ataga KI, Moore CG, Hillery CA et al (2008a) Coagulation activation and inflammation in sickle cell disease-associated pulmonary hypertension. Haematologica 93(1):20–26

Ataga KI, Smith WR, De Castro LM et al (2008b) Efficacy and safety of the Gardos channel blocker, senicapoc (ICA-17043), in patients with sickle cell anemia. Blood 111(8):3991–3997

Aygun B, Mortier NA, Smeltzer MP et al (2013) Hydroxyurea treatment decreases glomerular hyperfiltration in children with sickle cell anemia. Am J Hematol 88(2):116–119

Bernaudin F, Socie G, Kuentz M et al (2007) Long-term results of related myeloablative stem-cell transplantation to cure sickle cell disease. Blood 110(7):2749–2756

Bernini JC, Rogers ZR, Sandler ES et al (1998) Beneficial effect of intravenous dexamethasone in children with mild to moderately severe acute chest syndrome complicating sickle cell disease. Blood 92(9):3082–3089

Berthaut I, Guignedoux G, Kirsch-Noir F et al (2008) Influence of sickle cell disease and treatment with hydroxyurea on sperm parameters and fertility of human males. Haematologica 93(7):988–993

Bhatia M, Jin Z, Baker C et al (2014) Reduced toxicity, myeloablative conditioning with BU, fludarabine, alemtuzumab and SCT from sibling donors in children with sickle cell disease. Bone Marrow Transplant 49(7):913–920

Björk I, Lindahl U (1982) Mechanism of the anticoagulant action of heparin. Mol Cell Biochem 48(3):161–182

Bolanos-Meade J, Fuchs EJ, Luznik L et al (2012) HLA-haploidentical bone marrow transplantation with posttransplant cyclophosphamide expands the donor pool for patients with sickle cell disease. Blood 120(22):4285–4291

Brachet C, Azzi N, Demulder A et al (2004) Hydroxyurea treatment for sickle cell disease: impact on haematopoietic stem cell transplantation's outcome. Bone Marrow Transplant 33(8):799–803

Brawley OW, Cornelius LJ, Edwards LR et al (2008) National Institutes of Health Consensus Development Conference statement: hydroxyurea treatment for sickle cell disease. Ann Intern Med 148(12):932–938

Brugnara C, Bunn HF, Tosteson DC (1986) Regulation of erythrocyte cation and water content in sickle cell anemia. Science 232(4748):388–390

Carr BI, Reilly JG, Smith SS, Winberg C, Riggs A (1984) The tumorigenicity of 5-azacytidine in the male Fischer rat. Carcinogenesis 5(12):1583–1590

Carroll D (2011) Genome engineering with zinc-finger nucleases. Genetics 188(4):773–782

Cavazzana-Calvo M, Payen E, Negre O et al (2010) Transfusion independence and HMGA2 activation after gene therapy of human beta-thalassaemia. Nature 467(7313):318–322

Chang WL, Corate LM, Sinclair JM, van der Heyde HC (2008) Continuous inhaled nitric oxide therapy in a case of sickle cell disease with multiorgan involvement. J Investig Med 56(8):1023–1027

Chang J, Patton JT, Sarkar A, Ernst B, Magnani JL, Frenette PS (2010) GMI-1070, a novel pan-selectin antagonist, reverses acute vascular occlusions in sickle cell mice. Blood 116(10): 1779–1786

Chaplin H, Monroe MC, Malecek AC, Morgan LK, Michael J, Murphy WA (1989) Preliminary trial of minidose heparin prophylaxis for painful sickle cell crises. East Afr Med J 66(9): 574–584

Charache S, Dover G, Smith K, Talbot CC Jr, Moyer M, Boyer S (1983) Treatment of sickle cell anemia with 5-azacytidine results in increased fetal hemoglobin production and is associated with nonrandom hypomethylation of DNA around the gamma-delta-beta-globin gene complex. Proc Natl Acad Sci U S A 80(15):4842–4846

Charache S, Terrin ML, Moore RD et al (1995) Effect of hydroxyurea on the frequency of painful crises in sickle cell anemia. Investigators of the Multicenter Study of Hydroxyurea in Sickle Cell Anemia. N Engl J Med 332(20):1317–1322

Chiang EY, Frenette PS (2005) Sickle cell vaso-occlusion. Hematol Oncol Clin North Am 19(5):771–784

Cokic VP, Smith RD, Beleslin-Cokic BB et al (2003) Hydroxyurea induces fetal hemoglobin by the nitric oxide-dependent activation of soluble guanylyl cyclase. J Clin Invest 111(2):231–239

Cokic VP, Andric SA, Stojilkovic SS, Noguchi CT, Schechter AN (2008) Hydroxyurea nitrosylates and activates soluble guanylyl cyclase in human erythroid cells. Blood 111(3):1117–1123

Colella MP, De Paula EV, Conran N et al (2012) Hydroxyurea is associated with reductions in hypercoagulability markers in sickle cell anemia. J Thromb Haemost 10(9):1967–1970

Creusot F, Acs G, Christman JK (1982) Inhibition of DNA methyltransferase and induction of Friend erythroleukemia cell differentiation by 5-azacytidine and 5-aza-2'-deoxycytidine. J Biol Chem 257(4):2041–2048

Daak AA, Ghebremeskel K, Hassan Z et al (2013) Effect of omega-3 (n-3) fatty acid supplementation in patients with sickle cell anemia: randomized, double-blind, placebo-controlled trial. Am J Clin Nutr 97(1):37–44

De Franceschi L, Bachir D, Galacteros F et al (1997) Oral magnesium supplements reduce erythrocyte dehydration in patients with sickle cell disease. J Clin Invest 100(7):1847–1852

De Franceschi L, Bachir D, Galacteros F et al (2000) Oral magnesium pidolate: effects of long-term administration in patients with sickle cell disease. Br J Haematol 108(2):284–289

De Franceschi L, Cappellini MD, Olivieri O (2011) Thrombosis and sickle cell disease. Semin Thromb Hemost 37(3):226–236

De Montalembert M, Bachir D, Hulin A et al (2006) Pharmacokinetics of hydroxyurea 1,000 mg coated breakable tablets and 500 mg capsules in pediatric and adult patients with sickle cell disease. Haematologica 91(12):1685–1688

DeBaun MR (2014) Hydroxyurea therapy contributes to infertility in adult men with sickle cell disease: a review. Expert Rev Hematol 7(6):767–773

DeSimone J, Heller P, Hall L, Zwiers D (1982) 5-Azacytidine stimulates fetal hemoglobin synthesis in anemic baboons. Proc Natl Acad Sci U S A 79(14):4428–4431

DeSimone J, Heller P, Schimenti JC, Duncan CH (1983) Fetal hemoglobin production in adult baboons by 5-azacytidine or by phenylhydrazine-induced hemolysis is associated with hypomethylation of globin gene DNA. Prog Clin Biol Res 134:489–500

DeSimone J, Koshy M, Dorn L (2002) Maintenance of elevated fetal hemoglobin levels by decitabine during dose interval treatment of sickle cell anemia. Blood 99(11):3905–3908

Dover GJ, Charache S, Boyer SH, Vogelsang G, Moyer M (1985) 5-Azacytidine increases HbF production and reduces anemia in sickle cell disease: dose–response analysis of subcutaneous and oral dosage regimens. Blood 66(3):527–532

Dover GJ, Humphries RK, Moore JG (1986) Hydroxyurea induction of hemoglobin F production in sickle cell disease: relationship between cytotoxicity and F cell production. Blood 67(3):735–738

Dufu K, Oksenberg D, Zhou C, Hutchaleelaha A, Archer RD (2014) GTx011, a potent allosteric modifier of hemoglobin oxygen affinity, prevents RBC sickling in whole blood and prolongs RBC half-life in vivo in a murine model of sickle cell disease. Blood 124(21):217, Abstract

Eaton WA, Hofrichter J (1987) Hemoglobin S gelation and sickle cell disease. Blood 70(5):1245–1266

Estepp JH, Smeltzer MP, Wang WC, Hoehn ME, Hankins JS, Aygun B (2013) Protection from sickle cell retinopathy is associated with elevated HbF levels and hydroxycarbamide use in children. Br J Haematol 161(3):402–405

Estepp JH, Smeltzer M, Kang G, Aygun B, Ware RE, Nottage KA (2014) Higher fetal hemoglobin following escalation of hydroxyurea to maximum tolerated dose provides clinical benefit to children with sickle cell anemia. Blood 124(21):85, Abstract

Ferro D, Parrotto S, Basili S, Alessandri C, Violi F (2000) Simvastatin inhibits the monocyte expression of proinflammatory cytokines in patients with hypercholesterolemia. J Am Coll Cardiol 36(2):427–431

Ferrone FA, Hofrichter J, Eaton WA (1985) Kinetics of sickle hemoglobin polymerization. II. A double nucleation mechanism. J Mol Biol 183(4):611–631

Ferster A, Tahriri P, Vermylen C et al (2001) Five years of experience with hydroxyurea in children and young adults with sickle cell disease. Blood 97(11):3628–3632

Field JJ, Lin G, Okam MM et al (2013) Sickle cell vaso-occlusion causes activation of iNKT cells that is decreased by the adenosine A2A receptor agonist regadenoson. Blood 121(17): 3329–3334

Fitzhugh CD, Wigfall DR, Ware RE (2005) Enalapril and hydroxyurea therapy for children with sickle nephropathy. Pediatr Blood Cancer 45(7):982–985

Galie N, Ghofrani HA, Torbicki A et al (2005) Sildenafil citrate therapy for pulmonary arterial hypertension. N Engl J Med 353(20):2148–2157

Garcia DA, Baglin TP, Weitz JI, Samama MM (2012) Parenteral anticoagulants: antithrombotic therapy and prevention of thrombosis, 9th ed: American College of Chest Physicians evidence-based clinical practice guidelines. Chest 141(2 suppl):e24S–e43S

Ghoshal K, Datta J, Majumder S et al (2005) 5-Aza-deoxycytidine induces selective degradation of DNA methyltransferase 1 by a proteasomal pathway that requires the KEN box, bromo-adjacent homology domain, and nuclear localization signal. Mol Cell Biol 25(11):4727–4741

Gladwin MT, Kato GJ, Weiner D et al (2011) Nitric oxide for inhalation in the acute treatment of sickle cell pain crisis: a randomized controlled trial. JAMA 305(9):893–902

Gluckman E (2013) Allogeneic transplantation strategies including haploidentical transplantation in sickle cell disease. Hematology Am Soc Hematol Educ Program 2013:370–376

Goldman RD, Mounstephen W, Kirby-Allen M, Friedman JN (2013) Intravenous magnesium sulfate for vaso-occlusive episodes in sickle cell disease. Pediatrics 132(6):e1634–e1641

Gragert L, Eapen M, Williams E et al (2014) HLA match likelihoods for hematopoietic stem-cell grafts in the U.S. registry. N Engl J Med 371(4):339–348

Green D, Scott JP (1986) Is sickle cell crisis a thrombotic event? Am J Hematol 23(4):317–321

Hankins JS, Ware RE, Rogers ZR et al (2005) Long-term hydroxyurea therapy for infants with sickle cell anemia: the HUSOFT extension study. Blood 106(7):2269–2275, available from: PM:16172253

Hankins JS, Helton KJ, McCarville MB, Li CS, Wang WC, Ware RE (2008a) Preservation of spleen and brain function in children with sickle cell anemia treated with hydroxyurea. Pediatr Blood Cancer 50(2):293–297

Hankins JS, Wynn LW, Brugnara C, Hillery CA, Li CS, Wang WC (2008b) Phase I study of magnesium pidolate in combination with hydroxycarbamide for children with sickle cell anaemia. Br J Haematol 140(1):80–85

Hannemann A, Cytlak UM, Rees DC, Tewari S, Gibson JS (2014) Effects of 5-hydroxymethyl-2-furfural on the volume and membrane permeability of red blood cells from patients with sickle cell disease. J Physiol 592(Pt 18):4039–4049

Hebbel RP (2014) Ischemia-reperfusion injury in sickle cell anemia: relationship to acute chest syndrome, endothelial dysfunction, arterial vasculopathy, and inflammatory pain. Hematol Oncol Clin North Am 28(2):181–198

Hebbel RP, Vercellotti G, Nath KA (2009) A systems biology consideration of the vasculopathy of sickle cell anemia: the need for multi-modality chemo-prophylaxsis. Cardiovasc Hematol Disord Drug Targets 9(4):271–292

Hebbel RP, Vercellotti GM, Pace BS et al (2010) The HDAC inhibitors trichostatin A and suberoylanilide hydroxamic acid exhibit multiple modalities of benefit for the vascular pathobiology of sickle transgenic mice. Blood 115(12):2483–2490

Heeney MM, Ware RE (2010) Hydroxyurea for children with sickle cell disease. Hematol Oncol Clin North Am 24(1):199–214

Hibbert JM, Hsu LL, Bhathena SJ et al (2005) Proinflammatory cytokines and the hypermetabolism of children with sickle cell disease. Exp Biol Med 230(1):68–74

Hillery CA, Du MC, Wang WC, Scott JP (2000) Hydroxyurea therapy decreases the in vitro adhesion of sickle erythrocytes to thrombospondin and laminin. Br J Haematol 109(2):322–327

Hirsh J, Raschke R (2004) Heparin and low-molecular-weight heparin. Chest 126(3 suppl): 188S–203S

Hoban MD, Cost GJ, Mendel MC et al (2015) Correction of the sickle-cell disease mutation in human hematopoietic stem/progenitor cells. Blood 125(17):2597–2604

Hoppe C, Kuypers F, Larkin S, Hagar W, Vichinsky E, Styles L (2011) A pilot study of the short-term use of simvastatin in sickle cell disease: effects on markers of vascular dysfunction. Br J Haematol 153(5):655–663

Horwitz ME, Chao NJ, Rizzieri DA et al (2014) Umbilical cord blood expansion with nicotinamide provides long-term multilineage engraftment. J Clin Invest 124(7):3121–3128

Hsieh MM, Fitzhugh CD, Weitzel RP et al (2014) Nonmyeloablative HLA-matched sibling allogeneic hematopoietic stem cell transplantation for severe sickle cell phenotype. JAMA 312(1):48–56

Jayabose S, Tugal O, Sandoval C et al (1996) Clinical and hematologic effects of hydroxyurea in children with sickle cell anemia. J Pediatr 129(4):559–565

Johnson FL, Look AT, Gockerman J, Ruggiero MR, Dalla-Pozza L, Billings FT 3rd (1984) Bone-marrow transplantation in a patient with sickle-cell anemia. N Engl J Med 311(12):780–783

Joiner CH, Platt OS, Lux SE (1986) Cation depletion by the sodium pump in red cells with pathologic cation leaks. Sickle cells and xerocytes. J Clin Invest 78(6):1487–1496

Kamani NR, Walters MC, Carter S et al (2012) Unrelated donor cord blood transplantation for children with severe sickle cell disease: results of one cohort from the phase II study from the

Blood and Marrow Transplant Clinical Trials Network (BMT CTN). Biol Blood Marrow Transplant 18(8):1265–1272

Kato G, Lawrence MP, Mendelsohn L et al (2013) Phase 1 clinical trial of the candidate anti-sickling agent Aes-103 in adults with sickle cell anemia. Blood 122(21):1009, Abstract

Kim H, Kim JS (2014) A guide to genome engineering with programmable nucleases. Nat Rev Genet 15(5):321–334

Kinney TR, Helms RW, O'Branski EE et al (1999) Safety of hydroxyurea in children with sickle cell anemia: results of the HUG-KIDS study, a phase I/II trial. Pediatric Hydroxyurea Group. Blood 94(5):1550–1554

Koshy M, Dorn L, Bressler L et al (2000) 2-Deoxy 5-azacytidine and fetal hemoglobin induction in sickle cell anemia. Blood 96(7):2379–2384

Krishnamurti L, Kharbanda S, Biernacki MA et al (2008) Stable long-term donor engraftment following reduced-intensity hematopoietic cell transplantation for sickle cell disease. Biol Blood Marrow Transplant 14(11):1270–1278

Lavelle D, Chin J, Vaitkus K et al (2007) Oral decitabine reactivates expression of the methylated gamma-globin gene in Papio anubis. Am J Hematol 82(11):981–985

Lee SP, Ataga KI, Orringer EP, Phillips DR, Parise LV (2006) Biologically active CD40 ligand is elevated in sickle cell anemia: potential role for platelet-mediated inflammation. Arterioscler Thromb Vasc Biol 26(7):1626–1631

Leikin SL, Gallagher D, Kinney TR, Sloane D, Klug P, Rida W (1989) Mortality in children and adolescents with sickle cell disease. Cooperative Study of Sickle Cell Disease. Pediatrics 84(3):500–508

Levasseur DN, Ryan TM, Pawlik KM, Townes TM (2003) Correction of a mouse model of sickle cell disease: lentiviral/antisickling beta-globin gene transduction of unmobilized, purified hematopoietic stem cells. Blood 102(13):4312–4319

Ley TJ, Anagnou NP, Noguchi CT, Schechter AN, DeSimone J, Heller P, Nienhuis AW (1983a) DNA methylation and globin gene expression in patients treated with 5-azacytidine. Prog Clin Biol Res 134:457–474

Ley TJ, DeSimone J, Noguchi CT et al (1983b) 5-Azacytidine increases gamma-globin synthesis and reduces the proportion of dense cells in patients with sickle cell anemia. Blood 62(2):370–380

Liesner R, Mackie I, Cookson J et al (1998) Prothrombotic changes in children with sickle cell disease: relationships to cerebrovascular disease and transfusion. Br J Haematol 103(4):1037–1044

Lim MY, Ataga KI, Key NS (2013) Hemostatic abnormalities in sickle cell disease. Curr Opin Hematol 20(5):472–477

Little JA, Hauser KP, Martyr SE et al (2009) Hematologic, biochemical, and cardiopulmonary effects of L-arginine supplementation or phosphodiesterase 5 inhibition in patients with sickle cell disease who are on hydroxyurea therapy. Eur J Haematol 82(4):315–321

Lobo CL, Pinto JFC, Nascimento EM, Moura PG, Cardoso GP, Hankins JS (2013) The effect of hydroxycarbamide therapy on survival of children with sickle cell disease. Br J Haematol 161(6):852–860

Locatelli F, Kabbara N, Ruggeri A et al (2013) Outcome of patients with hemoglobinopathies given either cord blood or bone marrow transplantation from an HLA-identical sibling. Blood 122(6):1072–1078

Lv S, Liu Y, Zou Z et al (2015) The impact of statins therapy on disease activity and inflammatory factor in patients with rheumatoid arthritis: a meta-analysis. Clin Exp Rheumatol 33(1):69–76

Machado RF, Barst RJ, Yovetich NA et al (2011) Hospitalization for pain in patients with sickle cell disease treated with sildenafil for elevated TRV and low exercise capacity. Blood 118(4):855–864

Marzilli M (2010) Pleiotropic effects of statins: evidence for benefits beyond LDL-cholesterol lowering. Am J Cardiovasc Drugs 10(Suppl 1):3–9

May C, Rivella S, Callegari J et al (2000) Therapeutic haemoglobin synthesis in beta-thalassaemic mice expressing lentivirus-encoded human beta-globin. Nature 406(6791):82–86

McGann PT, Howard TA, Flanagan JM, Lahti JM, Ware RE (2011) Chromosome damage and repair in children with sickle cell anaemia and long-term hydroxycarbamide exposure. Br J Haematol 154(1):134–140

McGann PT, Flanagan JM, Howard TA et al (2012) Genotoxicity associated with hydroxyurea exposure in infants with sickle cell anemia: results from the BABY-HUG phase III clinical trial. Pediatr Blood Cancer 59(2):254–257

McMahon L, Tamary H, Askin M et al (2010) A randomized phase II trial of Arginine Butyrate with standard local therapy in refractory sickle cell leg ulcers. Br J Haematol 151(5):516–524

Meiler SE, Wade M, Kutlar F et al (2011) Pomalidomide augments fetal hemoglobin production without the myelosuppressive effects of hydroxyurea in transgenic sickle cell mice. Blood 118(4):1109–1112

Miguel LI, Almeida CB, Traina F et al (2011) Inhibition of phosphodiesterase 9A reduces cytokine-stimulated in vitro adhesion of neutrophils from sickle cell anemia individuals. Inflamm Res 60(7):633–642

Montero-Huerta P, Hess DR, Head CA (2006) Inhaled nitric oxide for treatment of sickle cell stroke. Anesthesiology 105(3):619–621

Morris CR (2014) Alterations of the arginine metabolome in sickle cell disease: a growing rationale for arginine therapy. Hematol Oncol Clin North Am 28(2):301–321

Morris CR, Kuypers FA, Larkin S, Vichinsky EP, Styles LA (2000) Patterns of arginine and nitric oxide in patients with sickle cell disease with vaso-occlusive crisis and acute chest syndrome. J Pediatr Hematol Oncol 22(6):515–520

Morris CR, Morris SM Jr, Hagar W et al (2003) Arginine therapy: a new treatment for pulmonary hypertension in sickle cell disease? Am J Respir Crit Care Med 168(1):63–69

Morris CR, Kato GJ, Poljakovic M et al (2005) Dysregulated arginine metabolism, hemolysis-associated pulmonary hypertension, and mortality in sickle cell disease. JAMA 294(1):81–90

Morris CR, Kuypers FA, Lavrisha L et al (2013) A randomized, placebo-controlled trial of arginine therapy for the treatment of children with sickle cell disease hospitalized with vaso-occlusive pain episodes. Haematologica 98(9):1375–1382

Moutouh-de Parseval LA, Verhelle D, Glezer E et al (2008) Pomalidomide and lenalidomide regulate erythropoiesis and fetal hemoglobin production in human CD34+ cells. J Clin Invest 118(1):248–258

Nahavandi M, Tavakkoli F, Wyche MQ, Perlin E, Winter WP, Castro O (2002) Nitric oxide and cyclic GMP levels in sickle cell patients receiving hydroxyurea. Br J Haematol 119(3):855–857

Nathwani AC, Hanawa H, Vandergriff J, Kelly P, Vanin EF, Nienhuis AW (2000) Efficient gene transfer into human cord blood CD34+ cells and the CD34+CD38- subset using highly purified recombinant adeno-associated viral vector preparations that are free of helper virus and wild-type AAV. Gene Ther 7(3):183–195

Nathwani AC, Tuddenham EG, Rangarajan S et al (2011) Adenovirus-associated virus vector-mediated gene transfer in hemophilia B. N Engl J Med 365(25):2357–2365, available from: PM:22149959

Nathwani AC, Reiss UM, Tuddenham EG et al (2014) Long-term safety and efficacy of factor IX gene therapy in hemophilia B. N Engl J Med 371(21):1994–2004

Nebor D, Romana M, Santiago R et al (2013) Fetal hemoglobin and hydroxycarbamide moduate both plasma concentration and cellular origin of circulating microparticles in sickle cell anemia children. Haematologica 98(6):862–867

Nickel RS, Hendrickson JE, Haight AE (2014) The ethics of a proposed study of hematopoietic stem cell transplant for children with "less severe" sickle cell disease. Blood 124(6):861–866

Nienhuis AW, Persons DA (2012) Development of gene therapy for thalassemia. Cold Spring Harb Perspect Med 2(11), pii: a011833

Nottage KA, Ware RE, Winter B et al (2014) Predictors of splenic function preservation in children with sickle cell anemia treated with hydroxyurea. Eur J Haematol 93(5):377–383

Noubouossie DC, Le PQ, Rozen L et al (2013) Thrombin generation in children with sickle cell disease: relationship with age, hemolysis, transcranial Doppler velocity, and hydroxyurea treatment. Eur J Haematol 91(1):46–54

Oppert M, Jorres A, Barckow D, Eckardt KU, Frei U, Kaisers U (2004) Inhaled nitric oxide for ARDS due to sickle cell disease. Swiss Med Wkly 134(11–12):165–167

Orringer EP, Blythe DS, Johnson AE, Phillips G Jr, Dover GJ, Parker JC (1991) Effects of hydroxyurea on hemoglobin F and water content in the red blood cells of dogs and of patients with sickle cell anemia. Blood 78(1):212–216

Palmer SC, Navaneethan SD, Craig JC et al (2014) HMG CoA reductase inhibitors (statins) for people with chronic kidney disease not requiring dialysis. Cochrane Database Syst Rev 5, CD007784

Panepinto JA, Walters MC, Carreras J et al (2007) Matched-related donor transplantation for sickle cell disease: report from the Center for International Blood and Transplant Research. Br J Haematol 137(5):479–485

Pastuszczak M, Kotlarz A, Mostowik M, Zalewski J, Zmudka K, Undas A (2010) Prior simvastatin treatment is associated with reduced thrombin generation and platelet activation in patients with acute ST-segment elevation myocardial infarction. Thromb Res 125(5):382–386

Pawliuk R, Westerman KA, Fabry ME et al (2001) Correction of sickle cell disease in transgenic mouse models by gene therapy. Science 294(5550):2368–2371

Platt OS, Thorington BD, Brambilla DJ et al (1991) Pain in sickle cell disease. N Engl J Med 325(1):11–16

Platt OS, Brambilla DJ, Rosse WF et al (1994) Mortality in sickle cell disease – life expectancy and risk factors for early death. N Engl J Med 330(23):1639–1644

Qari MH, Aljaouni SK, Alardawi MS et al (2007) Reduction of painful vaso-occlusive crisis of sickle cell anaemia by tinzaparin in a double-blind randomized trial. Thromb Haemost 98(8):392–396

Reid ME, El Beshlawy A, Inati A et al (2014) A double-blind, placebo-controlled phase II study of the efficacy and safety of 2,2-dimethylbutyrate (HQK-1001), an oral fetal globin inducer, in sickle cell disease. Am J Hematol 89(7):709–713

Rivella S, May C, Chadburn A, Riviere I, Sadelain M (2003) A novel murine model of Cooley anemia and its rescue by lentiviral-mediated human beta-globin gene transfer. Blood 101(8):2932–2939

Romero Z, Urbinati F, Geiger S et al (2013) Beta-globin gene transfer to human bone marrow for sickle cell disease. J Clin Invest 123(8):3317–3330

Rosenberg RD (1989) Biochemistry of heparin antithrombin interactions, and the physiologic role of this natural anticoagulant mechanism. Am J Med 87(3 Suppl 2):S2–S9

Rosenberg RD, Lam L (1979) Correlation between structure and function of heparin. Proc Natl Acad Sci U S A 76(3):1218–1222

Sander JD, Joung JK (2014) CRISPR-Cas systems for editing, regulating and targeting genomes. Nat Biotechnol 32(4):347–355

Sankaran VG, Nathan DG (2010) Reversing the hemoglobin switch. N Engl J Med 363(23):2258–2260

Sankaran VG, Menne TF, Xu J et al (2008) Human fetal hemoglobin expression is regulated by the developmental stage-specific repressor BCL11A. Science 322(5909):1839–1842

Saunthararajah Y, Hillery CA, Lavelle D et al (2003) Effects of 5-aza-2'-deoxycytidine on fetal hemoglobin levels, red cell adhesion, and hematopoietic differentiation in patients with sickle cell disease. Blood 102(12):3865–3870

Saunthararajah Y, Molokie R, Saraf S et al (2008) Clinical effectiveness of decitabine in severe sickle cell disease. Br J Haematol 141(1):126–129

Scheuplein F, Thariath A, Macdonald S, Truneh A, Mashal R, Schaub R (2013) A humanized monoclonal antibody specific for invariant Natural Killer T (iNKT) cells for in vivo depletion. PLoS One 8(9), e76692

Serjeant GR (1995) Natural history and determinants of clinical severity of sickle cell disease. Curr Opin Hematol 2(2):103–108

Shimamura K, Kawamura H, Nagura T et al (2005) Association of NKT cells and granulocytes with liver injury after reperfusion of the portal vein. Cell Immunol 234(1):31–38

Singh SA, Koumbourlis AC, Aygun B (2008) Resolution of chronic hypoxemia in pediatric sickle cell patients after treatment with hydroxyurea. Pediatr Blood Cancer 50(6):1258–1260

Smith-Whitley K (2014) Reproductive issues in sickle cell disease. Blood 124(24):3538–3543

Sodani P, Isgro A, Gaziev J et al (2011) T cell-depleted hla-haploidentical stem cell transplantation in thalassemia young patients. Pediatr Rep 3(Suppl 2):e13

Sparkenbaugh EM, Chantrathammachart P, Mickelson J et al (2014) Differential contribution of FXa and thrombin to vascular inflammation in a mouse model of sickle cell disease. Blood 123(11):1747–1756

Stach K, Nguyen XD, Lang S et al (2012) Simvastatin and atorvastatin attenuate VCAM-1 and uPAR expression on human endothelial cells and platelet surface expression of CD40 ligand. Cardiol J 19(1):20–28

Steinberg MH, Hsu H, Nagel RL et al (1995) Gender and haplotype effects upon hematological manifestations of adult sickle cell anemia. Am J Hematol 48(3):175–181

Steinberg MH, Barton F, Castro O et al (2003) Effect of hydroxyurea on mortality and morbidity in adult sickle cell anemia. JAMA 289(13):1645–1651

Stevens MCG, Hayes RJ, Vaidya S, Serjeant GR (1981) Fetal hemoglobin and clinical severity of homozygous sickle cell disease in early childhood. J Pediatr 98(1):37–41

Strouse JJ, Takemoto CM, Keefer JR, Kato GJ, Casella JF (2008) Corticosteroids and increased risk of readmission after acute chest syndrome in children with sickle cell disease. Pediatr Blood Cancer 50(5):1006–1012

Styles L, Kuypers F, Kesler K (2007) Arginine therapy does not benefit children with sickle cell anemia; results of the comprehensive sickle cell center multi-center study. Convention of the National Sickle Cell Disease Program and the Sickle Cell Disease Association of America, Washington DC

Taylor F, Huffman MD, Macedo AF et al (2013) Statins for the primary prevention of cardiovascular disease. Cochrane Database Syst Rev 1, CD004816

Teupser D, Bruegel M, Stein O, Stein Y, Thiery J (2001) HMG-CoA reductase inhibitors reduce adhesion of human monocytes to endothelial cells. Biochem Biophys Res Commun 289(4):838–844

Tomer A, Harker LA, Kasey S, Eckman JR (2001) Thrombogenesis in sickle cell disease. J Lab Clin Med 137(6):398–407

Van Beers EJ, Schaap MC, Berckmans RJ et al (2009) Circulating erythrocyte-derived microparticles are associated with coagulation activation in sickle cell disease. Haematologica 94(11):1513–1519

Van Gorsel H, Li C, Kerbel EL, Smits M, Kader AA (1992) Compositional characterization of prune juice. J Agric Food Chem 40(5):784–789

van Zuuren EJ, Fedorowicz Z (2013) Low-molecular-weight heparins for managing vaso-occlusive crises in people with sickle cell disease. Cochrane Database Syst Rev 6, CD010223

Vandorpe DH, Shmukler BE, Jiang L et al (1998) cDNA cloning and functional characterization of the mouse Ca2+-gated K+ channel, mIK1. Roles in regulatory volume decrease and erythroid differentiation. J Biol Chem 273(34):21542–21553

Verstraete M (1990) Pharmacotherapeutic aspects of unfractionated and low molecular weight heparins. Drugs 40(4):498–530

Wallace KL, Marshall MA, Ramos SI et al (2009) NKT cells mediate pulmonary inflammation and dysfunction in murine sickle cell disease through production of IFN-gamma and CXCR3 chemokines. Blood 114(3):667–676

Wandersee NJ, Maciaszek JL, Giger KM et al (2015) Dietary supplementation with docosahexanoic acid (DHA) increases red blood cell membrane flexibility in mice with sickle cell disease. Blood Cells Mol Dis 54(2):183–188

Wang WC, Ware RE, Miller ST et al (2011) Hydroxycarbamide in very young children with sickle-cell anaemia: a multicentre, randomised, controlled trial (BABY HUG). Lancet 377(9778):1663–1672

Ware RE, Zimmerman SA, Sylvestre PB et al (2004) Prevention of secondary stroke and resolution of transfusional iron overload in children with sickle cell anemia using hydroxyurea and phlebotomy. J Pediatr 145(3):346–352

Ware RE, Despotovic JM, Mortier NA et al (2011) Pharmacokinetics, pharmacodynamics, and pharmacogenetics of hydroxyurea treatment for children with sickle cell anemia. Blood 118(18):4985–4991

Ware RE, Helms RW, SWiTCH Investigators (2012) Stroke with transfusions changing to hydroxyurea (SWiTCH). Blood 119(17):3925–3932

Weiner DL, Hibberd PL, Betit P, Cooper AB, Botelho CA, Brugnara C (2003) Preliminary assessment of inhaled nitric oxide for acute vaso-occlusive crisis in pediatric patients with sickle cell disease. JAMA 289(9):1136–1142

Weitz JI (1997) Low-molecular-weight heparins. N Engl J Med 337(10):688–699

Westerman MP, Green D, Gilman-Sachs A et al (1999) Antiphospholipid antibodies, proteins C and S, and coagulation changes in sickle cell disease. J Lab Clin Med 134(4):352–362

Wilber A, Tschulena U, Hargrove PW et al (2010) A zinc-finger transcriptional activator designed to interact with the gamma-globin gene promoters enhances fetal hemoglobin production in primary human adult erythroblasts. Blood 115(15):3033–3041

Wun T, Soulieres D, Frelinger A et al (2013) A double-blind, randomized, multicenter phase 2 study of prasugrel versus placebo in adult patients with sickle cell disease. J Hematol Oncol 6(1):17

Wun T, Styles L, DeCastro L et al (2014) Phase 1 study of the E-selectin inhibitor GMI 1070 in patients with sickle cell anemia. PLoS One 9(7), e101301

Xu J, Peng C, Sankaran VG et al (2011) Correction of sickle cell disease in adult mice by interference with fetal hemoglobin silencing. Science 334(6058):993–996

Yan JH, Ataga K, Kaul S et al (2005) The influence of renal function on hydroxyurea pharmacokinetics in adults with sickle cell disease. J Clin Pharmacol 45(4):434–445

Yang JC, Huang F, Wu CJ, Chen YC, Lu TH, Hsieh CH (2012) Simvastatin reduces VCAM-1 expression in human umbilical vein endothelial cells exposed to lipopolysaccharide. Inflamm Res 61(5):485–491

Yawn BP, Buchanan GR, Afenyi-Annan AN (2014) Management of sickle cell disease: summary of the 2014 evidence-based report by expert panel members. JAMA 312(10):1033–1048

Zhou D, Liu K, Sun CW, Pawlik KM, Townes TM (2010) KLF1 regulates BCL11A expression and gamma- to beta-globin gene switching. Nat Genet 42(9):742–744

Glossary

Acute chest syndrome (ACS) Pulmonary illness in sickle cell disease, characterized by fever and/or respiratory symptoms, typically defined by the radiographic finding of a new lung infiltrate.

Acute splenic sequestration Rapid trapping of cellular blood elements in the spleen, resulting in an acute drop in hemoglobin, often associated with thrombocytopenia and hypovolemia.

Alloimmunization Clinically significant development of new antibodies against erythrocyte antigens in the transfusion receiver; detected by direct antiglobulin testing (DAT) or through screening of irregular antibodies in the absence of clinical or laboratory signs of hemolysis.

Allosteric regulation Conformational changes of a protein, usually in an enzyme, which may modulate its affinity to the ligand at the active site.

Aplastic crisis Severe anemia with reticulocytopenia due to a temporary failure of the bone marrow to make red blood cells, typically caused by infection with parvovirus B19 in children with sickle cell disease.

Balanced polymorphism A stable polymorphism maintained by natural selection.

Band 3 clustering Abnormal clustering of the RBC anion exchanger Band 3 in sickle RBCs, due to binding to HbS hemichromes.

Cation loss/dehydration The loss of intracellular K+ and water through the Gardos channel and K/Cl cotransport system resulting in dehydration of sickle RBCs.

Cholelithiasis Gallstones.

Cytokines Low-molecular-weight (non-antibody) proteins that regulate the intensity and duration of immune responses and mediate communication between cells. Can be secreted by various cell types.

Dactylitis Painful swelling of the hands or feet due to vaso-occlusion that occurs in young children with SCD (also termed "hand-foot syndrome").

Damage-associated molecular patterns (DAMPs) Molecules that can initiate and amplify sterile inflammatory responses mediated via pattern recognition receptors (PRRs).

© Springer International Publishing Switzerland 2016

F.F. Costa, N. Conran (eds.), *Sickle Cell Anemia*,
DOI 10.1007/978-3-319-06713-1

Delay time The time between HbS deoxygenation and the onset of exponential polymerization.

Delayed hemolytic transfusion reactions Development of antibodies to antigen erythrocytes after transfusion, with the discernible clinical signs of hemolysis usually appearing from 24 h to 28 days after a transfusion and a positive direct antiglobulin test and positive elution test or newly identified erythrocyte alloantibodies in the serum of the receiver's serum, as well as an insufficient increase in post-transfusion hemoglobin.

Disease burden The overall impact of diseases and injuries at an individual level or at the societal level. May refer to the economic costs of a disease.

Downstream target In the context of sickle cell disease intervention therapy, target defined based on the temporal sequence of events according to the pathophysiology of the disease. A downstream target is one that occurs later in the process, such as the increased adhesivity of red blood cells.

Endothelins Peptides that induce vasoconstriction and, therefore, increase blood pressure.

Enhancer A short (50–1500 bp) sequence of DNA that can be bound to proteins to activate transcription of a gene or genes. Enhancers are often *cis*-acting and located far away from the gene. Enhancers can be upstream or downstream from the start site of the gene in the forward or backward direction.

Epistasis Interaction between alleles and their effect on a trait. If a quantitative trait results from adding up contributions from different loci, then it is said that there is no epistasis.

Erythrocytapheresis Extracorporeal blood separation method whereby whole blood is extracted from a donor or patient, the red blood cells are then separated, and the remaining blood is returned to the circulation.

F cell An erythrocyte containing sufficient HbF to be detectable by flow cytometry using anti-HbF antibodies. Usually, about 6 pg. of HbF per cell is required for an F cell to be detectable. For an F cell containing HbS as the predominant hemoglobin 10 pg. of HbF is needed to prevent deoxyHbS polymerization at physiologic oxygen saturations.

Flow mediated vasodilation The endothelium-dependent ability of blood vessels to dilate in response to an increase in shear stress.

Functional capillary density The number of perfused capillaries per volume of tissue.

Gene editing A form of genetic engineering in which DNA is inserted into, replaced within, or removed from the genome using nucleases.

Genetic modifier A gene that influences the expression or the effects of another gene.

Genome-wide association study (GWAS) Approach that compares genetic between people with a particular disease and unaffected individuals, often measuring SNPs that form haplotypes across the entire genome.

Genotype In the context of sickle cell disease, this refers primarily to the β-globin gene alleles inherited by the patient and responsible for the disease. With the identification of several other genes that modify the severity of the disease, the genotype may be extended to reflect these.

Haplo-identical hematopoietic stem cell transplantation A type of bone marrow transplant that utilizes a donor who is half-matched with the patient.

Haplotype DNA variations that are inherited together. The β^S-globin haplotype is a group of polymorphisms that are inherited together, along with the β^S mutation. Five major patterns have been described, some of which affect the phenotype significantly.

HbS-β thalassemia Compound heterozygous state wherein an HbS gene is co-inherited with a β (beta)-thalassemia gene, which causes the under expression of the β-globin gene. Can be divided into two subtypes; HbS-β^+ thalassemia and HbS-β^0 thalassemia, whereby HbS-β^+ thalassemia is generally clinically milder than HbS-β^0 thalassemia, as some Hb A is produced.

HbSC disease Inheritance of the HbS gene together with the HbC gene, also referred to as hemoglobinopathy SC.

HbSS Individuals homozygous for the HbS gene (β^S mutation), also known as sickle cell anemia.

Heme Molecule composed by iron linked to four groups of porphyrin released from hemoglobin during hemolysis. Extracellular heme exerts toxic effects via generation of reactive oxygen species and through the activation of innate immunity thereby triggering proinflammatory pathways.

Hemoglobinopathies Diseases caused by genetic variants that lead to one of the globin chains of the hemoglobin molecule inferring an abnormal structure on the hemoglobin protein or being abnormally produced (in excess or deficit).

Hemolytic anemia Anemia that results from the premature destruction of the red blood cell. This destruction can occur either outside the vasculature in the reticuloendothelial system where most normal erythrocytes are destroyed or within the vasculature. In sickle cell disease, up to a third of red cell destruction is intravascular.

Heterotropic regulation Modulation of the protein activity (usually enzymes) by different ligands outside the active site. The ligation with non-specific molecules can confer some conformational changes at the active site, changing its affinity for the native ligand.

Heterotypic cellular interaction Sickle RBCs can interact with endothelial cells and leukocytes through multiple receptors and adhesion molecules on their surface membrane. These heterotypic cell–cell interactions can induce inflammation and promote cell aggregation in the vaso-occlusive process.

Homotropic regulation Regulation of a protein's activity (usually enzymes) by its ligand at the active site. This ligation can also modulate other active sites of the protein by conformational changes.

Hydroxyurea Drug used in the treatment of sickle cell disease patients. Its main beneficial effect is the induction of fetal hemoglobin expression, with a subsequent reduction of the hemolytic rate and of vaso-occlusive crisis occurrence.

Hypercoagulable state (hypercoagulability) A state of increased activation of the coagulation process in which there is a higher risk of thromboembolic events.

Inflammatory mediator Varied cytokines and other molecules, such as histamine, bradykinin, prostaglandins, cell adhesion molecules and leukotrienes, that orchestrate the inflammatory response.

Integrin activation Integrins are transmembrane receptors that are expressed with low ligand-binding capacity. Intracellular signaling through cell surface receptors, for example, G-protein-coupled receptors (GPCRs), is required to induce conformational and avidity changes that greatly increase their affinity to ligands.

Intravascular hemolysis Process in which red blood cells suffer destruction in the circulation. In sickle cell disease this occurs due to polymerization of hemoglobin S, followed by sickling and rupture of red blood cells.

Intravital microscopy Intravital microscopy is a technique used to observe biological systems in live animals. Mouse cremaster muscle is a classical model tissue for studying leukocyte behavior during their recruitment and activation in the vasculature. Injection with low doses of fluorescent antibodies allows identification of differential leukocyte subset behavior during recruitment in vivo.

Irreversibly sickled RBCs (ISCs) Sickle RBCs with permanent shape change due to damage to membrane proteins and independent of hemoglobin polymerization.

Ischemia-reperfusion (IR) injury Tissue injury resulting from vascular occlusion (ischemia) or lack of oxygen, followed by the return of the blood (reperfusion) to the ischemic area.

Leukocyte adhesion cascade Recruitment of leukocytes requires adhesion and transmigration through the vessel walls. The classical model of leukocyte adhesion cascade includes selectin-mediated rolling, chemokine-triggered activation and integrin-dependent adhesion. These steps are followed by intraluminal crawling and paracellular and transcellular transmigration.

Linkage disequilibrium SNPs or genes that are inherited together more often than by chance alone.

Microvesicles Small particles derived from RBCs, platelets, monocytes, and endothelial cells that may greatly influence adhesive properties of RBCs and WBCs in SCD.

Neutrophil microdomain Neutrophils rapidly polarize to form leading and trailing edges during their recruitment. Polarization of neutrophils also induces rapid redistribution of surface receptors to form functional microdomains. These microdomains are important for the directional, chemokine-driven movement of neutrophils within blood vessels and across the endothelium.

Nitric oxide A signaling molecule with a short spatial and temporal half-life that is rapidly produced by endothelial cells to regulate a variety of vascular processes such as vasodilation, adhesion, inflammation, coagulation and vessel growth.

Phenotype The clinical characteristics that define the disease, and in a genetic disorder like sickle cell anemia, are directly or indirectly a result of the gene mutation.

Proliferative retinopathy Neovascularization of the retina, extending into the vitreous body.

Prostacyclins Metabolites of arachidonic acid, produced by the endothelium that inhibit platelet aggregation and regulate vessel diameter.

Prosthetic group An organic (such as a vitamin, sugar, or lipid) or inorganic (such as a metal ion) specific non-polypeptide unit required for the activity of an enzyme or other protein. In enzymes, they are often involved in the active site. Prosthetic groups are bound tightly to proteins and may even be attached through a covalent bond.

Reticulocyte Immature red blood cell found in the peripheral blood and used as a marker for bone marrow red blood cell production; elevated at baseline in sickle cell disease (reticulocytosis, elevated reticulocyte count; reticulocytopenia, decreased reticulocyte count).

Shear stress A longitudinal force exerted against endothelial cells by blood flowing along the vessel wall.

Sickle cell anemia Refers to the homozygous state, HbSS.

Sickle cell disease Caused by the inheritance of the HbS gene along with another abnormal Hb variant and encompasses the homozygous state, HbSS and other compound heterozygous states, e.g. HbSβ, HbSC, HbSD, $HbSO_{Arab}$ etc.

Silent infarcts Changes on magnetic resonance imaging (MRI) of the brain, consistent with infarction without any history of overt neurological symptoms or abnormal neurological examination.

Splenic sequestration Trapping of blood in the spleen that causes severe anemia in children with sickle cell disease.

Sterile inflammation Inflammatory response to non-microbial activators (DAMPs).

Thrombin generation The final result of the activation of coagulation, in particular activated factor X, culminating with the transformation of prothrombin into thrombin, a final mediator of the coagulation process.

Tissue factor A transmembrane protein found in several sub-endothelium cells of the vessel wall, being exposed in the flow after the occurrence of vascular lesions, and then triggering the activation of coagulation.

Upstream target In the context of sickle cell disease intervention therapy, target defined based on the temporal sequence of events according to the pathophysiology of the disease. An upstream target is one that occurs early in the process, such as the genetic lesion (single point mutation) resulting in the sickle mutation.

Vasoocclusion The obstruction of flow in blood vessels, usually in the microcirculation, initiated by the presence of sickle erythrocytes.

Vaso-occlusive crisis, also known as sickle pain crisis New onset of pain that lasts at least 4 h that can only be explained by vaso-occlusion and which may require analgesic therapy in a medical setting.